Stanley's Dream

The Medical Expedition to Easter Island

JACALYN DUFFIN

Carleton Library Series 247

McGill-Queen's University Press
Montreal & Kingston • London • Chicago

© McGill-Queen's University Press 2019

ISBN 978-0-7735-5710-9 (cloth)
ISBN 978-0-7735-5780-2 (ePDF)
ISBN 978-0-7735-5781-9 (ePUB)

Legal deposit third quarter 2019
Bibliothèque nationale du Québec

Printed in Canada on acid-free paper

This book has been published with the help of a grant from the Canadian
Federation for the Humanities and Social Sciences, through the Awards to
Scholarly Publications Program, using funds provided by the Social Sciences
and Humanities Research Council of Canada.

Funded by the   Financé par le   Canada Council   Conseil des arts
Government   gouvernement   for the Arts   du Canada
of Canada   du Canada

We acknowledge the support of the Canada Council for the Arts.
Nous remercions le Conseil des arts du Canada de son soutien.

Library and Archives Canada Cataloguing in Publication

Title: Stanley's dream : the Medical Expedition to Easter Island / Jacalyn Duffin.
Names: Duffin, Jacalyn, author.
Series: Carleton library series ; 247.
Description: Series statement: Carleton Library series ; 247 | Includes bibliographical
references and index.
Identifiers: Canadiana (print) 20190094478 | Canadiana (ebook) 20190094877
| ISBN 9780773557109 (hardcover) | ISBN 9780773557802 (ePDF) | ISBN
9780773557819 (ePUB)
Subjects: LCSH: Canadian Medical Expedition to Easter Island (1964–1965)
| LCSH: Skoryna, Stanley C. | LCSH: Medical expeditions—Easter Island—
History—20th century. | LCSH: Medicine—Research—Easter Island—
History—20th century. | LCSH: Medical care—Easter Island—History—
20th century. | LCSH: Easter Island—Environmental conditions—20th century.
Classification: LCC RA390.E27 D84 2019 | DDC 610.7209618—dc23

This book was typeset in 10.5/13 Sabon.

For

Tycho, Maxwell, Wolf, and Kensington Rose

Contents

13 Forgetting METEI and the IBP   353
14 METEI 2017   376

    Conclusion   413

    APPENDICES

A METEI Research   420
B Rapanui Health Data Gathered by METEI, 1964–65   426
C Rapanui Health and How It Changed, 1950s to 2017   434
D METEI Consultants, Ship's Officers, Cabins   438
E Maps of Rapu Nui   442

    Notes   445
    Bibliography   497
    Index   535

Tables and Figures

TABLES

TABLES IN APPENDICES

FIGURES

FIGURES IN APPENDICES

Acknowledgments

It is difficult to imagine how this book could have been written without the Internet, which located people and information on five continents. Once found and targeted, all the individuals named below contributed promptly with inspiring enthusiasm and generosity. Archivists at the University of British Columbia, Library and Archives Canada, and McGill University were patient and helpful as I mined their collections. Their colleagues elsewhere went out of their way to search for and provide documents: Lise Couillard and Annie Simard at the Archives de l'Institut national de la recherche scientifique (INRS); Pierre Payment at the INRS-Institute Armand-Frappier; Reynald Erard at the Archives of the World Health Organization in Geneva; Earl Spamer of the American Philosophical Society; Jeff Kerr at the Center for the History of Microbiology/American Society for Microbiology Archives; Debbie Taylor of the Alberta Trailer Company; Robert Hamilton of Woodbridge; Darren Yearsley at the Canadian Broadcasting Corporation Archives; and Barry B. Smith at the Nova Scotia Archives. In addition, librarians and archivists at Queen's University, particularly Deirdre Bryden, Bonnie Brooks, Jane Reeves, and the intrepid staff of interlibrary loan, gathered resources from around the world, cheerfully accepting half-formulated requests and viewing the tedious sleuthing as fun.

In looking for the material products of the Medical Expedition to Easter Island (METEI, pron. "mét-eye"), I benefited from the expertise of scholars and curators affiliated with many museums: Barbara Lawson of the Redpath Museum, Stéphanie Boucher of the Lyman Entomological Museum, and Heather McNabb of the McCord Museum, all in Montreal; Elise Rowsome, Sarah Smith, and Alan Elder of the Canadian Museum of History in Ottawa; Judy Chelnick, Adrienne Kaeppler, and David R. Hunt of the Smithsonian Institute in Washington, DC; Arleyn Simon, Christopher

Stojanowksi, and Gary Schwartz in the School of Human Evolution and Social Change at Arizona State University; Annamária Bárány of the Hungarian National Museum in Budapest; Silvano Landert of Culture Collection of Switzerland; Dr Guy Prod'hom and Professor Gilbert Greub of the Université de Lausanne; physicist Roy Bishop of Acadia University; retired curator Randall Brooks of the Canadian Museum of Science and Technology; Don McPhail, Eric Taylor, and the Beaty Biodiversity Museum at the University of British Columbia; and Dr Dirk Huyer.

Experts on Easter Island – its science and history, both remote and recent – responded with unfailing kindness to naive questions and put me in touch with people on Rapa Nui: Patricia Stambuk, Erika Hagelberg, George Gill, Sonia Flora Haoa Cardinali, Jo Anne Van Tilburg, Alice Hom, Jacinta Arthur, Rolf Foerster, Valentina Fajreldin, Betty Haoa, Jose Miguel Ramirez Aliega, Lilian López Labbé, James Joves, Hetereki Huke, and Pablo Howard Seward Delaporte. Ambassador Alejandro Marisio Cugat, Rodrigo Andres Meza Gotor, and the late Elena Bornand of the Chilean embassy in Ottawa understood the precious value of Georges Nógrády's collection of METEI records and worked to preserve, protect, and return them to Rapa Nui. Associated Medical Services provided a generous contribution for their digitization.

On Rapa Nui, energetic young scholars welcomed this project, inquisitive about their island from a time before they were born. They tracked down elders with memories and engaged fully with the notion of constructing a second Medical Expedition to Easter Island. It is an honour to recognize their contributions: Suvi Hereveri Tuki, Claudia Tuki, Marcos Astete Paoa, Vanessa Gomez, Camila Zurob Dreckmann, Lucía Tepihe, Lya Edmunds Hernández, Katherine Atán Retamales, Alejandra Edwards, Juan Pacomio, Madelena Hernández, Paula Valenzuela, Jimena Andrea Ramirez Gonzalez, Francisco Torres, Cristián Moreno Pakarati, Ana Maria Arredondo, Paola Rosetti, Leo Pakarati, and Jacinta Arthur (again! because she happened to be there). Those who shared their recollections of METEI include (but are not limited to) Alcalde (Mayor) Pedro Edmunds Paoa, Maria Teresa Ika Pakarati, Norma ("Tauranga") Hucke Atán, Bene Tuki Pate, Edmundo Edwards, Raúl Tuki, Ana Lola Tuki Chavez, Alberto Tuki, Manuel Tuki, Antonia Pate Niare, Maruka Tepano, Marcos Rapu, and Alfonso Rapu. Many others who heard me and my collaborators on the local radio or at our public talks sent ideas and questions.

Numerous colleagues and friends plunged into my quest with disarming charity and in a multitude of ways. They are James Boutilier, Anne Helene Kveim Lie, Dale C. Smith, Alan Richardson, Judy Segal, Susan Squier, Roy J. Shephard, Hugo Soudeyns, Jerome Cybulski, Ante Padjen, Fern

D. Charles, McGill University dean of medicine David Eidelman, Susan Lamb, Lucy Vorobej, Vivian McAlister, Kari Harrison, Gordon McOuat, and Bert Hansen. The late David Elder took on the labyrinthine process of obtaining endorsed letters of introduction through two national bureaucracies; I am saddened that he did not live to see the results.

The METEI alumni have sustained the intrusive probing into their youthful adventure with good grace, curiosity, and trust. Our many conversations, together with their diaries, letters, and photographs, constitute the most important sources for this research. They are Peter Beighton in Cape Town, Garry Brody in Los Angeles, Isabel Cutler in Naples (Florida) and Kennebunk (Maine), Ian Efford and Jack Mathias on Vancouver Island, Björn Ekblom in Stockholm, Harold Gibbs in Hampden (Maine), Einar Gjessing in Oslo, George Hrischenko in Mount Albert (Ontario), Robert Meier in Bloomington (Indiana), Cléopâtre and Denys Montandon in Geneva, James Nielsen in Clearwater (Florida), June and Gordon Pimm in Ottawa, Charles Fowler, David Murphy, and Charles Westropp, all in Halifax, and the late Armand Boudreault of Montreal, who was the first to read the entire manuscript but sadly died in October 2018. I was also privileged to interview former minister of defence the Honourable Paul Hellyer over tea and warm brownies at his Toronto residence. They have all become my friends.

Family members and acquaintances of the deceased METEI alumni have been equally forthcoming, long aware of the expedition, often protecting the objects and papers of the now absent travellers and wondering why METEI had been forgotten. They are John Cutler's widow, Isabel Cutler; Colin Gillingham's widow, Françoise Gillingham; Fred Joyce's children, Jim and Linda Joyce, and his son-in-law Ian Whitehouse; Eivind Myhre's son, historian Jan Eivind Myhre; Georges Nógrády's adopted niece and executrix, writer Judith Hermann, and his friends George and Dorothea Demmer; Helen Reid's children, anthropologist Judith Redfield and psychologist Douglas Chute; Maureen and Richard Roberts's daughter, criminologist Susan Roberts, their colleague (and mine!) geneticist Nancy E. Simpson, and Maureen's sister Dr Vanora Haldane; Al Taylor's widow, May Taylor, and his friend Dr John Baumbrough; Archie Wilkinson's widow, Sally Wilkinson, and her brother Tony Archer; Tom Galley's son Tom; Channing Gillis's widow, Mary Gillis, and his grandson Channing Guenther; Robert Manzer's son Bob and daughters Yvonne, Jackie, and Jennifer; Harry Crosman's sons George and Bill and grandson Chris; Bob Williams's son Rob and niece Heather Saunders; and finally Stanley Skoryna's extended family, including his widow, Jane Skoryna, son Christopher Skoryna, daughter-in-law Jean Skoryna, grandchildren Ana

Maria Warren, Michael Burnley, Halina Skoryna, and Mary Skoryna, nephew Woytech Skoryna, and friend and librarian Darlene Lake. They were sanguine about Stanley's foibles and exaltations. Important clarifications came from Al Tunis's son Andrew Tunis; Alexander Bearn's widow, Margaret Bearn; and Surendra Nath Sehgal's widow, Uma Sehgal, and their son, Ajai Sehgal.

Many METEI alumni and family members read this manuscript in draft, donating new information, spotting errors, and collaborating on the final result. The project was supported by a sabbatical leave from Queen's University in 2015–16 and by grants from Associated Medical Services through the Nova Scotia Health Research Foundation for digitizing the medical records and for the trip to Rapa Nui in January 2017.

A major incentive for digging deeper and "getting it done" came from the lively reactions of audiences at meetings of the Canadian Society for the History of Medicine and the American Association for the History of Medicine, from the microbiologists of the Université de Montréal, from historians and philosophers at the University of Leeds and the University of Leicester, from the Nursing Alumni of Kingston General Hospital, and from internists at St Michael's Hospital in Toronto. A talk at the University of King's College in Halifax in January 2019 drew two sailors from the Easter Island journey of HMCS *Cape Scott*, Reid Hall and Chez Walters, and numerous relatives of the METEI travellers, who added previously unknown stories late in my work. Kyla Madden and Philip Cercone at McGill-Queen's University Press believed in this research and its potential to become a book. Their colleagues Kathleen Fraser, Finn Purcell, Ryan Van Huijstee, and especially Robert Lewis oversaw its production with meticulous care and encouraging interest.

Ana Cecilia Rodríguez de Romo, my colleague, friend, and soulmate, took two weeks out of her busy life in Mexico City to participate in my Rapa Nui visit; without her companionship, sensitive comprehension, and indefatigable dedication, I would have missed a great deal. In myriad ways, not the least of which was their good-natured tolerance of my obsession, I was helped by my family: Joshua Lipton-Duffin, Jennifer Macleod, Jessica Duffin Wolfe, and Daniel Goldbloom. I have dedicated this book to their offspring, my grandchildren, hoping that they might read it some day. As always, Robert David Wolfe has shared this journey from its inception: the excitement, frustrations, discoveries, and disappointments. Steady, pragmatic, and imaginative, he solved myriad problems of technology, history, diplomacy, and prose. I am so grateful to him and to everyone else mentioned here. Thank you.

Abbreviations

ACFAS	Association Canadienne-Française pour l'Avancement des Sciences
APS	America Philosophical Society
ASM	American Society for Microbiology
ATCO	Alberta Trailer Company
BCG	Bacille Calmette-Guérin
BUN	blood urea nitrogen
CBC	Canadian Broadcasting Corporation
CCIBP	Canadian Committee for the International Biological Programme
CMA	Canadian Medical Association
CMAJ	*Canadian Medical Association Journal*
ECA	Empresa de Comercio Agrícola
HA	Human Adaptability
IBP	International Biological Programme
IBY	International Biological Year
ICSU	International Council of Scientific Unions
IGY	International Geophysical Year
INRS	Institut national de la recherche scientifique
IRPA	International Radiation Protection Association
IUBS	International Union of Biological Sciences
LAC	Library and Archives Canada
METEI	Medical Expedition to Easter Island
MRC	Medical Research Council of Canada
MUA	McGill University Archives
NFB	National Film Board
NRC	National Research Council of Canada
RCAF	Royal Canadian Air Force
RCN	Royal Canadian Navy
UBC	University of British Columbia
WHO	World Health Organization
WRCNS	Women's Royal Canadian Naval Service ("wrens")

STANLEY'S DREAM

Introduction

> This seems to me to be an imaginative scheme and one that will be
> helpful to Canada's international prestige, as well as contributing
> in a concrete way to the International Biological Year.
>
> Lester B. Pearson

Before dawn on 13 December 1964, a Canadian navy ship dropped
anchor off Easter Island (Rapa Nui). Passengers lined the rails, waiting
silently for something to happen. After a long month at sea, they were
breathless with anticipation, eager to set foot on this exotic island and
begin work. The sun rose, transforming the grey of a hulking volcano
into a bright green and bathing the sky in an orange glow. Then dozens
of long canoes appeared, filled with men and the occasional woman,
who rapidly closed the distance from shore to ship. Were they friendly or
angry? From the water, they began to wave carvings, wanting to trade.
A motor launch soon followed, and its uniformed officials boarded for
a formal welcome. This moment was the first contact between the members of the Medical Expedition to Easter Island and the Rapanui people,
who would tolerate, help, hinder, tease, love, and resent them for two
whole months. Islanders and travellers all remembered this remarkable
sojourn, but history soon forgot.

In 1964–65, Canada led an international, multidisciplinary scientific
expedition to Rapa Nui, the world's most isolated community. Already
an object of intense fascination for its massive *moai* (stone statues), dark
caves, evocative legends, and seclusion, it had been luring European
scholars for more than a century. Since 1888 it had belonged to Chile, the
mainland of which is more than 3,500 kilometres away; it was governed
by the military. The exploits of Norwegian adventurer Thor Heyerdahl
had made it a famous, seductive destination, described in his bestselling
books and Oscar-winning documentaries. But you couldn't visit easily.
Once a year, a supply ship brought goods, stayed a week, and returned to

the continent, conveying children headed to high school and the annual
crop of wool from a massive sheep farm. Since at least the mid-1950s,
Chilean authorities had been planning to open an airport suitable for
commercial flights – possibly by 1966.

The Medical Expedition to Easter Island (METEI, pron. "mét-eye")
was conceived and directed by surgeon and gastroenterologist Dr
Stanley Skoryna of McGill University in Montreal. His original plan had
two parts. First, before the airport was complete, the team would document the entire biosphere and examine the health of the population of
1,000 people. Second, the team would return some time after the airport
had opened to repeat the exercise, searching for the effects of increased
contact on how people and other living things had adapted (or not).
Skoryna's thirty-eight-member team and all their scientific equipment
travelled with the Canadian navy ship HMCS *Cape Scott* and her crew
of 230 sailors from Halifax through the Panama Canal. They were gone
four months, from mid-November 1964 to mid-March 1965. A final
report never appeared, and the follow-up visit did not take place.

This remarkable event happened in my lifetime, but I had never
heard of it until January 2014, when I had the privilege of visiting the
University of British Columbia (UBC) in Vancouver. The splendid lodg-
ings in Green College were a long way from downtown. During that
week, the weather was "typical BC" – chilly, cloudy, and rainy – and
I had loads of free time. At the UBC Archives, I idly typed in my usual
search terms – "medicine," "history," "disease" – and to my amazement
found three boxes of material labelled "Medical Expedition to Easter
Island, 1964–65 (METEI)."[1] They contained letters, reports, newsletters,
diaries, scientific journals, abstracts, conference proceedings, published
articles, lists of scientists, and clippings from newspapers and magazines.
The catalogue indicated that they were the papers of ecologist Professor
Ian E. Efford, who had deposited them in the 1970s. I assumed he must
be long gone.

I raced to my computer only to learn that next to nothing had been
written about METEI in the medical and historical literature. I found a
few articles in the 1960s medical journals, one authored by pediatrician Helen Evans Reid, who had been one of my professors in medical
school at the University of Toronto.[2] Reid's husband, Dr Laurie Chute,
was the dean, and our entire class had been out to visit their farm in
September 1970. I had no idea that she'd been to Easter Island and had
even written a book-length memoir about it.[3] Further digging produced
the excellent 1992 article by navy historian James Boutilier of Royal
Roads University; his paper focused on the navy aspects, logistics, and

itinerary, but it had once been buried in the *Rapa Nui Journal* – now fully open-access online.[4] In every spare moment that week in Vancouver, I pored over these documents, took photographs, and scrutinized the unfamiliar names of expeditionists from Canada, England, Scandinavia, Switzerland, and the United States, trying to trace what, if any, publications they had produced.

Library and Archives Canada in Ottawa and the McGill University Archives in Montreal turned up many more METEI records, including correspondence and reams of unpublished medical data. Deep excavation in the scientific databases, such as Web of Science, revealed numerous publications about Easter Island biology throughout the 1960s and 1970s authored by scientists who had not been on the expedition but who acknowledged access to its collections in the fine print.

The stupendous discovery of METEI waxed in promise when I realized that Efford had been only thirty years old at the time of the expedition. He could still be alive, but he seemed to have published nothing from his journey. Fortunately, his name is relatively unusual, and after repeated "Googling" over several months, I found him in British Columbia's Cowichan Valley; he was the author of a new book on rhododendrons, alive and well, and ready to talk. Efford was the first of the eighteen METEI alumni who contributed so generously to this book and who became my friends. It took more than three years to find them. Family members of the deceased were equally helpful. Their memories, diaries, photos, and confidences added life to the official reports, making the tale sparkle with intelligence, imagination, humour, irony, and regret. All are eager to see this book because they had been pondering the expedition's many mysteries for half a century.

The first big mystery was how Skoryna convinced the Canadian navy to give him a ship. The second was the absence of a final report. The third was the failure to return for the second survey. Many other mysteries followed. This amazing endeavour coincided with the launching of the International Biological Programme (IBP), which initially embraced METEI and then inexplicably dropped it. The expedition was immersed in the political tensions of the Cold War and growing interest in Latin America, and it witnessed the advent of democracy on Easter Island. METEI came at an exciting moment when Canada showed pride in its human and natural resources by launching new projects, enhancing its role on the international stage, contemplating other extraordinary expeditions, preparing for its Centennial in 1967, hosting that year's World's Fair, Expo 67, deciding on its own flag, and more controversially, reorganizing all its armed forces by unification.

METEI was one of the last missions that the Royal Canadian Navy would undertake as a separate entity.

Astounding though it was for Canada, METEI was just one more in a long series of medico-scientific expeditions and far from the first to visit Easter Island.[5] Insights from scholarly studies of past expeditions provided indispensable context for my project, especially when and where northerners had examined peoples of the tropical South.[6] In particular, Warwick Anderson's outstanding works on international investigations in Papua New Guinea, Fiji, Australia, and the Philippines emphasize the embedded racism and colonialism of their era.[7] Indeed, the majority of these historical works examine their subjects through the lens of colonialism. But colonialism was not quite the right frame for METEI. Rapa Nui was and still is a colony of Chile, and the Canadians operated with Chilean approval; however, even though invited, no Chileans participated. Canada itself was no longer a colony of Britain and never a colonizer of Rapa Nui, although it has been a colonizer of its own Indigenous peoples. METEI members watched, with tacit and often explicit approval, the islanders' bold steps to greater freedom. With respect to the International Biological Programme, Toby Appel, Frank Greenaway, and Simone Schleper explain the passion for collaboration across borders and the policy pitfalls that characterized science in the West following the Second World War and into the Cold War.[8] Abena Dove Osseo-Asare explores six case studies of how healing plants in Africa were leveraged into drug products; she details the complex relationships between Native peoples, scientists, and the pharmaceutical industry.[9] METEI's story also includes the discovery of a wonder drug from natural sources, well before the concept of "bioprospecting" had confronted legal and ethical boundaries.[10]

Skoryna and his collaborators were concerned with the possibility of new infections – the spectre of virulent organisms introduced to a vulnerable population. Observers had long described Rapanui outbreaks of an unknown *kokongo*, which arrived with visiting ships. But other infectious diseases were prevalent. His team included a microbiologist, a virologist, a parasitologist, and seven other physicians. In the mid-1960s smallpox had not yet been eradicated, Canada and Chile were still using Bacille Calmette-Guérin (BCG) vaccine against tuberculosis, and both countries were waging vaccine war on polio, soon extending it to measles. Leprosy had been introduced to the island about a century earlier; its ravages persisted, haunting the people not only due to its cruel mutilations but also because it became a pretext for depriving them of freedom to travel. Histories of these diseases, the policies intended to control them, and their treatment were also important to my study, as were considerations of the "new" travelling diseases that have emerged since METEI, namely AIDS, Ebola, SARS, West Nile, and Zika.

Although "medical" appeared in its name, METEI's objectives went well beyond medicine and health. It was to document the whole of the biosphere: humans, mammals, reptiles, fish, insects, birds, plants, microbes, and elements of soil and water. This agenda places it squarely in the early days of ecology. Historians of that discipline do not know of the expedition, but their works were essential for situating METEI at its birth.[11]

Similarly, genetics was just beginning its rise to prominence. The researchers who had resolved the structure of DNA had won the Nobel Prize in 1962. Although that nucleic acid could not yet be measured in a routine laboratory, proxy molecules had been identified, such as enzymes and hemoglobins. Genetics gave a materialist basis for ancient notions of heredity and population health. Its application to entire communities might elucidate their history and movements, as well as their proclivity for illness. METEI included a genetics survey for three reasons: first, to investigate the islanders' susceptibility to disease; second, to assess the extent of inbreeding, which constituted another form of vulnerability to disease; and third, to participate in the already well-established quest for the origins of the inhabitants of that remote speck of land. But the well-intentioned mid-twentieth-century studies relying on the new genetics slipped away from the promise of sorting out historical movements and entered the problematic terrain of scientific racism, making them a continuing source of debate for historians, philosophers, educators, and scientists.[12] Even with the most careful of modern techniques, Easter Island genetics is still not straightforward.[13] METEI was operating at the beginning of this new way of knowing.

Most historians of Rapa Nui know of METEI simply to mention it – because it coincided with political upheaval and the island's first free elections. Their writings elucidate the relationships between the colony and Chile.[14] It was surprising to find that they had often turned to the publications of Canadians Jim Boutilier, Helen Reid, and Douglas Porteous for details about the island's political past; METEI photographs and memories sometimes figured in their work. But these historians were baffled by METEI – where it came from, where it went, and why. They too were unfailingly supportive of my work. Without a final report, METEI had become one more riddle of the island that is famously defined by its secrets.

The structure of this book follows METEI in three parts. Part 1 examines its origins in the Cold War concerns of overpopulation, pollution, and conflict resolution that generated the International Biological Programme. Seeking to uncover the impact of greater outside contact, METEI was to contribute to the IBP's Human Adaptability section. Skoryna quickly leveraged his vision with an ambitious proposal, an international team, the permission of Chile, consent of the Canadian government, support of the World Health Organization, and extraordinary contributions from the Canadian navy. Part 2 explores METEI's island operations – scientific, personal, and even political – as it witnessed the rebellion and the first free elections. Its fraught group dynamics exemplify science as "bricolage," and the influence and difficulties of METEI women emerge from the privileged sources of their diaries and recollections. While awaiting METEI's completion, HMCS *Cape Scott* undertook a diplomatic mission to South America, inadvertently sailing into political turmoil, before returning to take METEI home. Part 3 turns to the published and unpublished findings in medical, biological, and social science, including more chauvinism, more "bricolage" in tracking the material products, and two surprise discoveries that brought improvement not only for the Rapanui but for global health too. It also investigates why METEI was dropped from Canada's IBP and, nevertheless, situates it within the overall output of that multi-nation venture. Finally, with my own journey to Easter Island, it embarks on an exploration of what METEI-2 might have found if the return visit had ever been attempted. If the present volume must declare a genre, it is the biography of a postcolonial scientific expedition and its offspring.

This book serves as a stand-in for Skoryna's never-written final report, placing the previously uncollected and unpublished findings in the public domain. At the end, with its modest step toward what should have become METEI-2, it begins a study that I hope others will complete. May it answer the questions of the islanders, team members, and scholars who have tried to understand METEI, and may it do justice to the indelible experiences of the travellers and the optimistic aspirations of the Rapanui people who welcomed them.

PART ONE

From Canada to Rapa Nui, 1962 to 20 December 1964

I

Dream Plan for a Troubled World

The Medical Expedition to Easter Island emerged from nearly two decades of international collaboration and competition, coupled with increasing concern about the environmental health and security of the globe. In this context, the ability to understand how human beings and other living organisms adapt to change seemed urgent. METEI's leader, Stanley Skoryna, and his friend Georges Nógrády were acutely aware of these concerns and possibilities; as immigrants from war-torn Europe, both physician scientists were in the process of adapting themselves to the bland safety of Canada. When they learned that the most remote community in the world was targeted for an airport, they realized its experience could be a laboratory of environmental adaptation.

POSTWAR INTERNATIONALISM AND ENVIRONMENTAL POLLUTION

At the end of the Second World War, high hopes for avoiding another cataclysm generated energetic plans for lasting peace and a better world. These efforts extended well beyond economic management tools, such as the International Monetary Fund, the General Agreement on Tariffs and Trade, and the World Bank, to increased collaboration across borders on matters of health, science, and culture. The United Nations, the World Health Organization (WHO), and other international organizations took aim at improving living standards and protecting the environment. The work targeted maternal and child health, nutrition, epidemiological notification, biological standardization, environmental sanitation, and control of specific infectious diseases, such as malaria, smallpox, tuberculosis, and venereal disease. Countries agreed that solutions to these problems required cross-border collaboration between scientists and healthcare providers.

Yet in this same period, suspicion arose between former allies in what became known as the Cold War, hampering international cooperation in peaceful, scientific projects and fostering destructive competition.[1] Testing of atomic weapons was a commonplace of the nuclear arms race as both experiment and deterrent. Until test ban treaties came into effect, it was practised widely by the United States, the United Kingdom, and Russia. Scientists soon realized that this form of aggression, unleashed twice on Japan in 1945 in a military setting, was waging an uncontrolled and devastating war against the entire planet. Following the dangerous 1946 atomic explosions at Bikini Atoll, for which the American navy had permanently "evacuated" the islanders, a 1954 test there spread a plume of fallout more than 160 kilometres. In 1953, after the "Dirty Harry" explosion in Nevada, radioactive rain fell on Chicago. By 1957 strontium-90 had contaminated cow's milk.[2] The public devoured terrifying novels and films about the environmental dangers of nuclear war and atomic tests. The 1954 film *Them* featured "mutant ants big enough to ruin any picnic."[3] Five years later, *On the Beach*, based on the 1957 book by Neville Shute, garnered Oscar nominations for having portrayed Ava Gardner and Gregory Peck awaiting imminent annihilation on the shores of Australia. In August 1958, in the middle of the Brussels World's Fair, the United States exploded a nuclear weapon in outer space.[4] By the end of that year, the first test ban was in effect. Remarkably, no tests were conducted until February 1960 when France flexed its colonial muscle and set off its first nuclear bomb, an ominous "test" in the Algerian desert, during that country's vicious civil war.[5]

National and international agencies were created to monitor and control the potential damage from fallout. The Health Physics Society, its name chosen over "Radiation Protection Society," was formed in 1956; the editorial board of its journal, *Health Physics*, boasted representation from seventeen nations. Soon it established "sections" in various countries, beginning – ironically – with France in 1961. That year the prominent Baby Tooth Survey out of St Louis appeared in *Science* to illustrate the effects of accumulated strontium in the teeth of children.[6] From these concerns, the founders of Physicians for Social Responsibility spoke out in the *New England Journal of Medicine* decrying the short- and long-term effects of thermonuclear war.[7] The International Radiation Protection Association appeared in 1965.[8]

Added to fear of radioactive contamination was a growing awareness that human activities were damaging all living things through pollution due to fertilizers, pesticides, petroleum emissions, and land-use practices. Biologist and conservationist Rachel Carson began her campaign against DDT following the American attempt to eradicate the gypsy moth in 1957. In her famous 1962 book *Silent Spring*, she published a long list of the harms wrought by that chemical, which had earlier won a Nobel Prize for its promoter. In that same year, social satirist Aldous Huxley published his last novel, *Island*, the story of an idyllic Pacific island whose healthy harmony is grievously threatened by the Western dystopian "gifts" of commerce, oil, and medicine.

Against this background of impending extermination arose a new and contradictory concern: overpopulation. With the ability to control certain diseases, improvements in water quality and supply, economic revival, the fragile peace, and increasing longevity owing to reductions in infant mortality, population numbers began to rise – and rise so quickly that they threatened to exhaust extant resources. Overpopulation posed yet another risk of war and, some contended, a threat to democracy and capitalism.[9] In other words, if human beings did not destroy the planet with weaponry and pollution, they would surely destroy it by consumption. Searching for better methods of birth control in developing nations increasingly became part of international aid programs, although in North America it met resistance from the Roman Catholic Church and some politicians who feared loss of votes. Biologists and physicians began to focus on adaptation, productivity, and energy use as they took stock of the importance of the environment to sustaining health.

The 1958–59 atomic test ban coincided with an unprecedented celebration of scientific collaboration: the International Geophysical Year (IGY). Proposed by the International Council of Scientific Unions (ICSU), the eighteen-month period from July 1957 to December 1958 witnessed a vast series of discoveries and open communication. Investigators studied the bottom of oceans, reporting on trenches and tectonic plates. They probed the heavens, shooting up rockets, identifying new moons, tracking meteors, and explaining the aurora borealis. Russia and the United States launched many satellites; Russia photographed the back of the moon. More than seventy countries analyzed Antarctica.[10] The *Annals of the IGY* filled forty-eight volumes published between 1959 and 1970. Contributing to all fifteen scientific disciplines, Canada's 190 IGY stations monitored weather, the ionosphere, atmospheric ozone, and glaciers, from Cape Race in Newfoundland to Sandspit in British Columbia and from Harrow in Ontario to Alert in the Northwest Territories.[11] All agreed that the IGY had been a huge success. Canadian geophysicist and expert in plate tectonics John Tuzo Wilson summarized the IGY as having led to a "vast increase in international cooperation in science" and the "transformation of earth science into planetary science." It was a useful "example of how international relations can be amiably and fruitfully conducted."[12] French biologist Henri Prat at the Université de Montréal and the Université de Marseille cited the IGY as a rare glimmer of hope in his essay on how the careless explosion of humanity could bring an end to the world, a destruction "aussi totalement stupide que stupidement totale."[13]

INTERNATIONAL BIOLOGICAL PROGRAMME

In March 1959, in the waning days of the IGY, the ICSU's president, Dr Rudolph Peters, was riding a train back to London from Cambridge with two colleagues. They fell to musing about how wonderful it would be if the same model could be applied to the new global problems of the environment, overpopulation, and strained resources: an International *Biological* Year. Peters chatted with scientists in the United Kingdom, Italy, and the Netherlands, particularly Giuseppe Montalenti, president of the International Union of Biological Sciences (IUBS).[14] Skeptics doubted that the biological sciences could lend themselves to such an ambitious notion. Specialists tended to imagine that, rather than addressing the amorphous global "problems," the initiative should promote their own disciplines: molecular biology and genetics, botany, medicine, conservation, and agricultural or marine productivity. Americans remained unconvinced of its value and suspicious of foreign influence. Everyone was concerned about who would pay for the added expense and complexity of cross-border collaboration. Would it result in decreased support for their ongoing programs at home?

But the idea of Big Biology would not go away, and it seemed to grow. The nature of biological research, with its focus on time and life cycles, would be cramped by a single year; the organizers soon began talking about an International Biological *Programme* (IBP) of several years duration, six, perhaps seven. In the end it was a decade, 1964 to 1974. C.H. Waddington, who succeeded Montalenti as president of the IUBS, found himself promoting the idea with mixed feelings in the summer of 1961.[15]

In August 1961 the prestigious British journal *Nature* reported on the IBP as if it were a foregone conclusion, planned "for some time."[16] *Nature* kept up this reporting with another item in late 1961, two more in each of 1962 and 1963, seven in 1964, and thirteen in 1965, ensuring that the IBP could not be ignored. For its part, the American journal *Science* printed the 1962 IBP report of G.L. Stebbins, who served as secretary of the IUBS from his academic home in Davis, California.[17] He outlined the basic goals of the program that had been hammered out at a meeting in Morges, Switzerland, in May 1962. The specialists had still wanted to organize the projects by their biological subdisciplines, but instead the IBP planners ordained projects to address those practical "problems" to which all disciplines could be applied. These problems were clarified as productivity in terrestrial, marine, and freshwater communities, productivity processes (i.e., physiology and energy transfer), conservation, use and management, and human adaptability. The IBP would examine those pressing new concerns about the environment, world population, and sustainability, and it would lay the groundwork for identifying solutions in the future.

At that 1962 meeting in Morges, E. Barton Worthington became the scientific director of the IBP, and anthropologist Joseph S. Weiner accepted the chair of its Human Adaptability (HA) section. Born in South Africa and trained in medicine, physiology, and zoology, Weiner had worked in England for Oxford University, the Medical Research Council, and the London School of Tropical Medicine and Hygiene.[18] He is considered a founding figure in physical anthropology and had participated in the 1953 exposure of the Piltdown skull hoax.

Earlier scientific projects in the era of European colonialism had made biological adaptation a subtext, if not a focus. For example, the Jardin Zoologique d'Acclimatation in Paris was founded to facilitate study of modifications to an organism "which render it able to live and to perpetuate its species under new conditions of existence."[19] Taming tropical nature and raising its degenerate "races" were deemed respectable goals, emphasized by the theory of evolution and predicated on convictions of European superiority and the idea that humans can be transformed.[20] Missions to tropical countries combined themes of "medical humanism, colonial development, and welfare policy," in which the power of "Christian caring" and human adaptation could best be proclaimed by "a leper cured of his disease."[21] Museums and parks, begun under colonial occupation, embraced narratives of biological improvement often with a nationalist agenda.[22]

Whether or not he knew of these precedents, Weiner decided to begin anew, in a spirit of *postcolonial* collaboration. To explore what might become the adaptability aspects of the IBP, he hosted a meeting in London in late 1962. He was excited by the potential to integrate the human sciences with the neophyte discipline of ecology. The meeting happened to coincide with the last great killer fog of 3–7 December, enforcing seclusion of the delegates and enhancing their own "productivity."[23] The

Table 1.1 International Biological Programme: Human adaptability themes

Worldwide

Human growth and development
Physique and body composition
Physical fitness
Climatic tolerance
Genetic constitution
Nutritional studies

Regional

High altitudes
Circumpolar and other cold climates
Tropical and desert climates
Islands and isolates
Migrant and hybrid populations
Urban and rural populations

Source: Collins and Weiner, *Human Adaptability*.

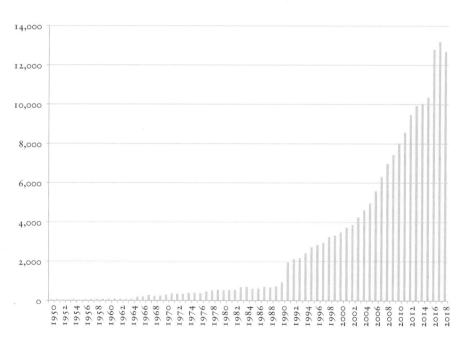

Figure 1.1 Number of articles with "ecology" as a topic word in scientific literature, 1950–2017. *Web of Science*, 8 January 2019.

smog probably also drove home a message about the role of environment in the future health of humanity. Six months later, Weiner held a symposium on human adaptability, from 29 June to 2 July 1964, at the Wenner-Gren Foundation in Burg Wartenstein, Austria, which resulted in a collection of essays.[24] Shortly after, on 23–25 July 1964, the First General Assembly of the IBP took place in Paris. Worthington continued as overall director, and Weiner officially became world convener of the HA section.[25] In response to the practical "problems" identified by the IBP planners, these meetings hammered out twelve themes that would define the IBP's HA section; some were worldwide and some regional based on climate and latitude (table 1.1).

The word "ecology," coined from the Greek word for "house" in 1873 by the German scientist Ernst Haeckel, now entered common parlance to express study of the relationship of living things to the environment.[26] The emerging discipline is reflected in the increasing number of scientific publications devoted to the topic, beginning as a trickle at the time of the IBP's creation in 1964 (figure 1.1).

STANLEY SKORYNA

Canadian government scientists had participated in many of the early stages of IBP planning (see chapter 13). But the program was being watched attentively at a much lower level by two doctors in Montreal, both immigrants from eastern Europe. The son of a physician, Stanley C. Skoryna was born in Warsaw, attended high school in Czechoslovakia, and studied medicine and surgery in Vienna. He had a bent for research anchored in the perception of humans as organisms within an environment. His focus became the gastrointestinal tract, which absorbs portions of the surrounding world in the form of food and drink, extracts essential nutrients and harmful elements, and expels the waste, only to repeat the cycle over and over again. Skin and lungs also mediate between the body and its surroundings, but the gut offered interesting possibilities for surgical intervention. Skoryna's mentor was Hans Finsterer, internationally known for his consummate skill in designing operations, especially for bleeding ulcers. Rather like Ambroise Paré long before, Finsterer was said to combine humility and religious faith. When he visited the United States in November 1949, he met President Harry S. Truman and praised God as he received the highest honour of the International College of Surgeons.[27] Still in Vienna, Skoryna completed a doctorate. Some of this research went into his 1946 article on the treatment of post-operative stomach cancer with the drug blastolysine. Derived from the cell walls of the bacterium *Lactobacillus bulgaricus* (commonly used for making yoghurt), blastolysine was thought to have effects against cancer and to boost the immune system.[28] His study represented a particularly early use of immunotherapy in cancer treatment.

In 1947 Skoryna came to Montreal on an Edward Archibald fellowship in experimental surgery. He embarked on more graduate work and in 1950 successfully completed a master's degree in science under the supervision of surgeon and physiologist Donald R. Webster. His thesis examined the cancer-causing effects of a fluorine derivative on the livers of rats. The research involved repeated operations to study the evolution of the experimental cancers. Not only did he address the causes and possible treatments of these tumours, but he also introduced a novel approach to cancer research that incorporated changes in lesions through time.

Soon Skoryna was directing McGill University's Gastrointestinal Research Laboratory, a position that he held for forty years. This research facility was housed in the newly built Donner Building, which later accommodated part of the Faculty of Dentistry until 2014. Skoryna also engaged in general surgery at St Mary's Hospital. It was with income from clinical practice that he supported himself, his Polish-born wife, Halina Irene Grygowicz, and their son, Christopher.

Skoryna usually worked in collaboration with others, often graduate students or resident trainees passing through the McGill program. There followed a series of publications, most involving experiments on rats or dogs, in which surgical skills were important but physiological and philosophical orientation was essential. On a fellowship with the National Research Council in 1951, he published an article in the *Journal of Experimental Medicine* that described an experiment to chemically induce cancer in 150 rats inbred from successive brother-sister matings and fed a strictly controlled diet supplied by the Purina feed company.[29] The positive reception of this paper led him to write to the journal's editor, Francis Peyton Rous, asking for 200 reprints and advice on how to obtain a grant from the Rockefeller Institute for a new project on extracting substances from autonomic nervous tissue. The elderly Rous had conducted extensive research on cancer-causing viruses, for which he would receive a Nobel Prize in 1966. He replied politely that he could not help because of his own "ignorance, sheer ignorance" of Skoryna's subject.[30] Rous wrote to Skoryna again, in 1960, expressing interest in the latter's 1958 article on a method of producing experimental penetrating gastric ulcers in rats and hormonal effects on healing.[31] That article proved to be Skoryna's most-cited publication. In thanking Rous for his thoughts, he confided that he planned to submit two more related studies to Rous and another philosophical article on cancer to *Nature*. None of these proposed articles ever appeared in those exact journals, although equivalents were published elsewhere. Of special note, Skoryna wrote about the bacterial flora in stomach acid of fasting humans in two articles that appeared in the *Canadian Medical Association Journal* (CMAJ) in 1966 and 1971. Two decades later, when Australians Barry Marshall and Robin Warren convinced a disbelieving scientific community of the role of bacteria in causing peptic ulcers, Skoryna would not have been surprised. If he had lived, he would have felt admiration, and possibly a twinge of jealousy, for their 2005 Nobel Prize.

Given Stanley's early views on the causes of cancer, his experimental interest in strontium was a logical next step. This radioactive element was a by-product of nuclear fission, with a long half-life of thirty years; like calcium, it localized to bone – a feature exploited in the Baby Tooth Survey. Following the wake-up call of Chicago's radioactive rain, the *New York Times* frequently commented on the great potential of strontium to do harm and the near impossibility of getting rid of it. In November 1955, Lewis Mumford warned against the folly of more nuclear tests and further contamination with the "deadly Strontium 90."[32] Others fretted about the disposal of nuclear waste from peaceful uses, although the promised power stations still had yet to be built. Would the toxic by-products be buried in deserts and mines, or carted round the ocean on barges, or projected into outer space?[33] In exploring the effects of this human-made pollutant on body systems, Skoryna was facing one of the greatest environmental fears of the Cold War. In 1957 he read a paper at the annual meeting of the Canadian Physiological Society about how he had created cancer in the bones of rats using radioactive strontium.[34]

That same year, Skoryna was awarded the medal in surgery of the Royal College of Physicians and Surgeons of Canada. This distinction extended the platform for his views on the complex nature of malignancies. His lengthy acceptance speech, delivered at the next annual meeting, was published in full by the CMAJ titled "Systemic Factors in Carcinogenesis."[35] A shorter version appeared in a letter to the editor of the *Lancet*.[36] In 1958 the CMAJ invited him to report on the Seventh International Cancer Conference in London, England; he deftly summarized the contributions of thirty-two Canadians, including himself, and wrote approvingly of keynote lectures delivered by future Nobel laureates Canadian-born Charles Huggins and Australian Sir Frank Macfarlane Burnet. He approved of the trend toward a "biological approach in cancer control" evinced by the conference.[37] Skoryna's engagement with strontium research predated 1961 reports in *Science* and the *New England Journal of Medicine* that consolidated medical concern; his work was on the cutting edge.

For Skoryna, to speak of "the cause" of any disease was naive and narrow: causes had to be both necessary and sufficient. A carcinogen could provoke cancer only if it was available in the surroundings and only if the organism was susceptible through genetics, physiology, or nutrition. He was interested in "stochastic processes," events that occur randomly through time, which, for large numbers, can be analyzed statistically. Perhaps because of his medal or because of the timeliness of his topic, he was able to publish more experiments with radioactive strontium on bone in the leading oncology journal, *Cancer*.[38] Next, he began work on a nine-article, multi-year series describing various methods to inhibit absorption of strontium from the gut – oft-cited work that promised antidotes for a poisoned future.[39] His research continued to appear in distinguished journals, including *Nature*, where he summarized his studies on strontium absorption.[40]

Skoryna's stature was growing, and he was invited to help organize and then edit the proceedings of a symposium on the pathophysiology of peptic ulcer disease. It would take place at the Second World Congress on Gastroenterology in Munich in 1962. With contributions by sixty-two authors from seventeen countries on five continents, his comprehensive volume on a perplexing and widespread disease was reviewed enthusiastically in the *Journal of the American Medical Association*.[41] Like his views on cancer, Stanley's closing paper laid out his vision of stochastic processes in the causes of peptic ulcers.[42] Because stomach cancer took the form of ulcers, the work consolidated his double fascination with malignancy and the gut.

Fluent in Polish, Czech, German, English, and French, Skoryna was intelligent and imaginative, a cultivated erudite who loved music and theatre and peppered his writings with references to historical precursors and philosophers, including Robert Koch, Bertrand Russell, and Albert Einstein. His favourite was William Beaumont, who, while stationed on Mackinac Island in 1822, took advantage of the hole accidentally blown in the stomach of French Canadian Alexis St Martin to conduct experiments on the physiology of digestion. Never shy and somewhat insensitive to social cues, Skoryna would approach famous leaders of medicine and government as equals, seeking favours, lobbying for science, and offering unsolicited advice. Many who worked closely with him called him "an operator."[43]

GEORGES NÓGRÁDY

A decade after Skoryna came to Canada, Georges L. Nógrády arrived from Hungary with his wife, Bernadette, both physicians. Georges had obtained his medical degree in 1945 in Kolozsvár (today Cluj-Napoca, Romania). During the war, he fell in love with a nurse, Ilona. Pregnant with their child, she died of sepsis contracted in her nursing work; the baby was lost too. Bernadette was born in the former Yugoslavia, and in the early 1950s, she had swum across the Danube to embark on medical studies in Hungary. As soon as she finished her doctorate in medicine in 1956, the Communist police moved to expel her during the Soviet invasion of Hungary. To protect her from arrest, Georges and Bernadette married quickly and fled as refugees. In Canada, Bernadette entered a residency in diagnostic radiology, becoming a much-loved teacher and researcher at the Université de Montréal. Although Georges held a medical degree, he did not see patients and stuck to his research, becoming a bacteriology expert at the same university. Remembered as a good teacher and adored by his students, he was known for his technical prowess, the man whose "stains always worked." Nógrády was an enthusiast and inveterate tinkerer who devoted meticulous attention to detail in all his restless pursuits, from the laboratory to scuba diving, photography, animal rescue, and the invention of eclectic devices. Unlike Skoryna, his scientific publications were few. The couple had no children. Friends recall that Nógrády's eyes would fill with tears at mention of Ilona or the war. At some point, Nógrády and Skoryna became friends.

The same age, with similar medical training in wartime eastern Europe and insatiable curiosity about the world, Stanley and Georges had many things in common. They both valued the freedom and opportunity of life in Canada, but they and their wives would also have encountered its less attractive, parochial qualities: prejudice, suspicion, discrimination, and, sometimes, outright mockery of immigrants who, notwithstanding their considerable linguistic abilities in both official languages (and many others), were neither Anglo-Saxon Protestant nor *québécois pure laine*. They seemed to rise above it and did not complain. They devoured the new books of travellers, scientists, and historians; Georges, especially, was a voracious reader. They followed the scientific and philosophical writings of Frank Macfarlane Burnet, whom Skoyrna heard speak in 1958 and who shared the 1960 Nobel Prize with Peter Medawar for the theory of immunological tolerance. Burnet's other famous biological contribution was clone theory.

In 1961, if not before, Skoryna and Nógrády began talking about the problems of the world: overpopulation, sustainability, pollution, radioactive fallout, and the ability of humans to adapt genetically and sociologically. They knew about the coming IBP and were inspired by the ecosystem programs and by the international collaboration that it recommended. They understood that the overall aim of the IBP would be to study specific ecosystems, aiming to predict consequences of natural or human-made disturbances and to improve capability for rational management of resources and control of environmental quality.[44] The HA section, in particular, stressed comparison of human populations in a wide variety of locations, assessing the interaction of both genetics and habitat, as well as the effects of changes in both.[45]

With Skoryna's views on the elemental causes of cancer and Nógrády's interest in bacteria, they dreamed up a plan to study an isolated population both before and after it was exposed to contact with the rest of the world. The community had to be small enough for a complete study, isolated enough that contact would provoke real change, and destined for an abrupt transformation. One place offered the perfect, natural experiment: Easter Island.

EASTER ISLAND: HISTORY AND HUMAN HEALTH TO THE 1960S

The most remote community in the world, according the United Nations isolation index, the volcanic island of Rapa Nui lies more than 3,500 kilometres from Chile, to which it belongs. It is a small triangle, measuring only 163.5 square kilometres. In 1960 its ravaged population hovered around 1,000. Served by a Chilean supply ship that came just once a year and stayed a week, it could be reached only by sea and that with difficulty because it lacked a deep-water harbour. But the extreme isolation was soon to end. Stanley Skoryna read that Easter Island was getting an international airport.

Thanks to recent books and films, Easter Island was also very famous. People longed to see its mysterious caves and the giant heads of its stone *moai*. Georges and Stanley wondered how these sheltered people would weather the barrage of tourists bringing new microbes, carcinogens, and useless but tasty nutrients. They imagined that the flora of the island, if not its entire biosphere, would shift toward adaptation or destruction. Here was the ideal HA project for the IBP. But they would have to move quickly.

Norwegian explorer and anthropologist Thor Heyerdahl had made Easter Island a household word with his astonishing South Pacific exploits in 1947 and 1955.[46] But the islanders had first met Europeans in the eighteenth century. Virtually every contact with so-called "civilization" was fraught with tragedy.[47] We know of several encounters thanks to the journals of the explorers. Dutch adventurer Jacob Roggeveen saw the island on 5 April 1722, Easter Sunday, naming it Paasch (Easter). His three ships lingered off shore until 11 April, and he estimated the native population at two or three thousand. On 10 April, a large landing party went to investigate, but to Roggeveen's apparent dismay, insubordinates shot "10 or 12" Rapanui dead and wounded others.[48] In 1770 two Spanish ships, under the command of Felipe Gonzalez, sailed from Peru and stayed for five days, making maps, erecting crosses on the highest point, and naming the island Isla de San Carlos after their king.[49] The Dutch and the Spanish had observed many tall, standing statues with topknots. Next came the ailing James Cook, who stayed from 12 to 18 March 1774; he sent explorers ashore, and they left a detailed description of the inhabitants. The people were docile and impoverished for "want of Materials and not of Genius." He found no water, the soil and sea were barren, and animals were scarce. "There is hardly an Island in this sea which affords less refreshments, and conveniences for Shiping than it does. Nature has hardly provided it with any thing fit for man to eat or drink, and as the Natives are but few and may be supposed to plant no more than sufficient for themselves, they cannot have much to spare to new comers." He estimated the population at 700, although he surmised that the women were in hiding. Cook's men shot an islander in the back for attempting to make off with a bag of supplies; they did not know if he died. Noticing discrepancies in his population estimate, the productivity of the land, the structure of canoes, and the many fallen statues, Cook doubted the accuracy of Roggeveen's account. But he also wondered if something dreadful had happened in the half-century between the Dutch visit and his own, for "this Isle is very different now to what it was then."[50]

In April 1786 the French naval officer Jean François de Galaup, Comte de Lapérouse, spent his intense stopover of only a few hours mapping and exploring. Aware of the pitiful state described by Cook, he brought gifts, animals, and seeds for plantation; however, he found the people healthier than expected and more numerous (approximately 2,000), and he was both annoyed and perplexed by the islanders' tendency to pilfer.[51] Lapérouse and other Europeans viewed the behaviour through a moral lens as gratuitous thievery; the idea that the concept of property might have been alien to these people without money or escape seems not to have arisen. He hoped they would view his abrupt departure as due punishment.

Sporadic contact continued into the nineteenth century with visits from Russian, British, and American vessels; some carried off islanders as slaves, or they kidnapped young girls for sex, later tossing them overboard to swim back to shore. At first welcoming and curious, the Rapanui grew suspicious; would-be visitors heard that they were hostile. In 1862 slave traders from Peru struck in several waves, removing 1,500 men and women, possibly half the population, and set them to work in guano pits off Peru. This action was widely publicized owing to the efforts of the French-born bishop of Tahiti, Florentin-Etienne Jaussen. The miserable captives were freed in 1863, but only a dozen had survived the brutality and sickness to return to Rapa Nui; however, they brought smallpox, provoking an epidemic that decimated the remainder. In 1864 came missionaries, who embarked on converting the island to Catholicism and setting up a school. One priest was grievously afflicted with tuberculosis, and by 1867 tuberculosis was rampant too.

The missionaries relied on transporters, one of whom was Jean-Baptiste Dutrou-Bornier, a French mariner, gambler, and arms dealer. He made the first land purchases in the island's history, eventually claiming almost all of its territory and setting himself up as governor with his stolen Rapanui wife as "queen." The sweeping grasslands, he thought, would make suitable grazing; as an agent for the company Maison Brander, he created a massive sheep ranch. To escape his irreligious cruelty, the missionaries evacuated nearly two hundred people to two other South Pacific islands: Tahiti and Mangareva (then called Gambier). Dutrou-Bornier was killed by an islander in 1876, and by the following year, the population had plummeted to 111.

In 1878 Alexander Salmon Jr came to Rapa Nui, bringing along twenty Tahitians and returning some of the Rapanui who had fled with the missionaries. Of Tahitian and European descent, he was the son of an English-Jewish merchant adventurer and brother of the Tahitian queen. Maison Brander, the Salmon family's company, held land and businesses in the southern hemisphere. A period of relative peace and increasing prosperity marked his decade as de facto ruler, although the visiting priests did not approve of him. Scholars cite this time as the moment when Tahitian influences blended into Rapanui culture, language, and tradition. Since the 1860s visitors had indulged in "*moai*-nappings," as Steven Roger Fischer dubbed them, and had stolen the coveted *rongorongo* tablets, which held (still) undeciphered script.[52] The plunder resides in the world's great museums, including the Louvre, the Smithsonian Institute, and the British Museum. In the 1880s Salmon guided the earliest archeological expeditions from England and Germany, and he assisted the surveying mission of the American USS *Mohican* in 1886. In this way, the theft extended to the trafficking of human remains. In 1895 the German anthropologist Wilhelm Volz reported his analysis of forty-nine Easter Island skulls, forty-six of which, he wrote, had been obtained through Maison Brander for a Berlin museum during the 1882 expedition of the ship SMS *Hyäne*.[53]

In early 1888 Salmon sold all his holdings in Rapa Nui to Chile, including the marginally profitable sheep farm. The island was annexed to that country by treaty, signed by Atamu Tekena and eleven chiefs of Rapa Nui and by Policarpo Toro, representing Chile.[54] From then on, it was managed by a consortium of entrepreneurs, which sent the annual supply ship. Leprosy came with the Chilean takeover, allegedly by their return of an afflicted Rapanui child. The vast sheep farm was leased to and managed by Williamson Balfour, a Scottish company based in Chile. Like prisoners in a concentration camp, the islanders were confined to the village of Hanga Roa, encircled by a wall, and not allowed to leave without permission. Several clergymen and physicians argued for better conditions, but sometimes well-meaning public health measures, such as the separation of people with leprosy by gender, exacerbated the imprisonment.[55] Finally, in 1953, Chile refused to renew the lease, and profits of the farm were nationalized; the island came under the control of the Chilean navy. The governor was an officer; however, as one historian put it, even though the rulers changed, the restrictions and neglect always stayed the same, "ambiguous with two or more foci of power ... usually of grossly unequal strength."[56] At each visit, the annual ship would drop supplies – flour, soap, sugar, clothing, shoes, toys, and medicine – and carry tons of wool back to Chile. It would also convey clergy and nuns on exchange missions and bright children (only boys) headed for high school education on the mainland. Some did not return.

The archeological expeditions raised interest in Rapa Nui's *prehistory*: the origin of its first human inhabitants, the carvings, the language, and the biology of the barren terrain, which, it soon emerged, had once been heavily forested. Theories of exploitation and catastrophic collapse were debated to account for a sorry past of conflict, rape, and cannibalism. The extent to which human exploitation generated the great changes has still not been resolved and is a focus of heated argument and ever more sophisticated scientific study in paleoecology.[57]

Sensitive investigators listened to the natives, among them archeologist Katherine Routledge of Oxford University. She spent thirteen months on Rapa Nui between late March 1914 and mid-August 1915. Her poignant, handsomely illustrated popular account was published in 1919 and dedicated to her mother, who had died during her absence.

Helped by islander Juan Tepano, Routledge studied ancient dwellings and *moai*, and she recorded the legends of the first king, Hotu Matu'a, who settled the island, and of the brutal rivalry between the Hanau Epe (Long Ears) and the usurping Hanau Momoko (Short Ears). The Long Ears stretched their earlobes with large ornaments, a practice noted by the early explorers that seemed to be reflected in the *moai*. A second edition of her book appeared the following year, but the planned "scientific" account was never completed. Without academic affiliations, Routledge was ostracized by scholars and sent to an asylum by her husband, Scoresby Routledge, who took control of her estate, although she was pursuing a divorce. Her extensive notes, maps, and photographs were lost until 1960; they now reside in London's Royal Geographical Society and formed the source for Jo Anne Van Tilburg's wonderful biography of 2003.[58]

Other investigators followed. In 1934–35 the Expédition franco-belge, led by Belgian archeologist Henri Lavachery, spent five months on Rapa Nui. Other participants included Swiss-born ethnologist Alfred Métraux and Chilean physician Israel Drapkin, who attended (and studied) the people afflicted with leprosy. Two decades after Routledge, they too relied on Juan Tepano as a useful guide, although scientists sometimes questioned the accuracy of his stories. They did not excavate, believing the soil to be too thin to avoid destabilizing the statues. Nevertheless, they spent their last weeks in December 1934 loading treasures into the hold of their ship. Lavachery documented the petroglyphs, and Métraux published a detailed ethnological study, although he is better known for his work on Haiti and on the Incas of Peru.[59]

Not long after their departure in 1935, Father Sebastian Englert, a Capuchin Franciscan, arrived to serve the islanders as priest, confessor, and champion. He remained for the rest of his life, beloved of his people. Educated and polyglot, Father Sebastian became a trusted authority on the monuments, history, and prehistory of the island. With Routledge and Métraux, he tried to connect oral traditions to material evidence in order to determine when humans first settled Rapa Nui and what their story had been prior to 1722. He created a small museum for bones and art objects, including carvings with sacred properties. This preoccupation prompted him, like them, to generate a list of rulers into the present; the thirty names that he collected, with an estimated fifteen years per reign, led him to conclude that Hotu Matu'a lived in the second half of the sixteenth century.[60] He also tried to distinguish between descendants of original Long Ears, the Short Ears, and those who had other Polynesian or Chilean blood. The Rapanui themselves advised him.

These lists were applied to tracing the geographic origins of the population through comparison of their facial features, blood, and eventually genetics with other groups around the South Pacific. As early as 1930, classical genetic markers, such as blood groups, were already under study for the Rapanui.[61] Father Sebastian was admired and respected by all the scientists who visited Rapa Nui. His lists were trusted for genetic studies, and he readily gave lectures. His approval of any visitor's research project always made the work much easier.

In 1947 Thor Heyerdahl and five fellow adventurers made a huge splash with their daring 8,000 kilometre Kon-Tiki odyssey from Peru to the Tuamoto Islands on a handmade raft. He was trying to prove the navigational skills of prehistoric people and to establish the intriguing possibility that at least some islands may have been settled east-to-west from South America rather than from Polynesia, as analysis of language and culture had suggested. His book became a bestseller, and the resultant documentary film won an Academy Award in 1951.

In 1955–56 Heyerdahl headed to Easter Island, this time travelling on a real boat as the leader of a distinguished archeological expedition. He took along his second wife, their toddler daughter, and his seventeen-year-old son by his first marriage, Thor Junior. The islanders called Heyerdahl "Kon-Tiki," and his son became "Kon-Tiki-Iti-Iti" (Small Kon-Tiki). The scientists began excavations at several different sites. Most statues had been toppled and lay on the ground, except for those sunk into the slopes of the quarry at the Rano Raraku volcano. Intent on proving his east-to-west theory of migration, Heyerdahl examined the islanders' personal caves, gathered their secret, sacred carvings, and sought evidence in the plants, architecture, and language to bolster myths about the island's prehistory. His team attempted to test genetic relationships through blood groups.[62] The team also engaged Rapanui men to help excavate around the *moai* and their *ahus* (platforms), and he challenged them to move and raise a statue to explore how it might have been done. They found an unusual "kneeling" statue that differed from the majority, and they attempted to relate their findings to the mysterious prehistory, correlating them with oral traditions.

The resultant 1958 popular book, *Aku-Aku: The Secret of Easter Island*, became another bestseller, although it came close to destroying Heyerdahl's reputation as a scientist. He described the Rapanui as "Polynesian, but of very mixed blood," superstitious, deceptive, and gullible. He exulted in tricking them into revealing their secret caves and giving away carvings; he shamed them when caught in stealing or lying; and he encouraged them to believe in his personal *aku-aku*, or great spiritual power.[63] An outing for schoolchildren to circle the island on his ship ended in disaster with three drowned: a teacher, a schoolboy, and the daughter of the mayor, Pedro Atán.[64] Heyerdahl told of his encounters with Chilean naval and air force officers who were already studying the island for a large-scale airport.[65] He also described *kokongo*, a febrile respiratory illness that afflicted islanders whenever a boat arrived. The same malady had plagued the Routledge expedition in 1914 and carried off thirty Rapanui in 1933.[66] The outbreak that Heyerdahl witnessed sickened the hapless mayor and killed his granddaughter.[67]

Shortly after Heyerdahl, in 1957–58, a German-Chilean expedition led by Thomas Barthel examined the ethnology and sociology of the island. This team challenged the Norwegian's origins theory and gathered many artifacts and skeletal remains that were a boon to scholars in Santiago; however, knowledge of this expedition was overshadowed by that of Heyerdahl, and memory of it was lost until Fischer re-examined the expedition in 2010.[68] French ethnologist Francis Mazière and his wife spent six months on Rapa Nui in early 1963; their exploits had yet to be published (see chapter 4).[69]

At times, the Rapanui had tried to resist the colonial oppression and unjust exploitation, retaining the names of several leaders of an early rebellion: Nicolas Pakarati Ure Potahi and the remarkable woman "prophetess" Angata.[70] In 1964 the Rapanui were still subjugated by the military government with puppet elections, kept uneducated, obliged to work, and denied permission to travel freely even around their own island.

STANLEY'S DREAM

How much of the long history of Easter Island's sad encounters with "civilization" was available to Skoryna and Nógrády is unknown, and many of today's origin theories about it had yet to be elaborated. But they did know about Thor Heyerdahl. Nógrády read *Aku-Aku* in late December 1962. He and Skoryna also read Routledge, and they likely saw the *National Geographic* photo essay in January 1962.[71] They reasoned that the forthcoming airport might simply fast-forward the transmission of germs that had happened so often in Rapa Nui's past, replicating the kind of tragedies that "first contact" had brought to the Indigenous peoples of the Americas. Sometime early in 1962, they dreamed up a study to analyze the human diseases and bacteria on Easter Island both before and after the airport. But they were in a hurry because they did not know when it would open; some sources suggested 1965. They missed the claims of Heyerdahl, Métraux, and others that the Rapanui were of "mixed blood."[72] They assumed that the extreme geographic isolation and recent population recovery would make them "genetically inbred," a special quality of vulnerability to disease that Skoryna had already tried to imitate in his laboratory with his 1951 study of rats. Aware of the interdisciplinary goals of the IBP, they consulted McGill anthropologist Richard F. Salisbury, who offered advice and outlined a sociological-anthropological research project in two letters in late 1962.[73] Puzzled by the repeated and long-reported outbreaks of *kokongo*, they also engaged the interest of Montreal virologist Armand Boudreault. A former student of Armand Frappier, Boudreault had written his doctoral dissertation under the direction of the French-born biologist Henri Prat, whose philosophical concerns about the population explosion and "the possibility of the end of the world" caused him to tilt toward eugenics.[74] Although he too was interested in the environment, Boudreault did not share these eugenic views.

What Skoryna and Nógrády did *not* know is that medical researchers in Chile had already embarked on similar studies of the "human ecology" of the Easter Island population with a team of scientists interested in blood, blood pressure, and genetics. Inspired by the rising vogue of population genetics, Raúl Etcheverry, Ricardo Cruz-Coke, and Ronald Nagel used the week-long visit of the military supply ship in the spring of 1963 to obtain data on approximately 17 per cent of the population. Eventually, they published twelve scholarly papers on their results between 1963 and 1967, many in English.[75] The Chilean team was also documenting the health effects of migration to the mainland.[76] All three researchers would go on to distinguished academic careers.

Omitting the social science aspects, Skoryna asked the World Health Organization to fund a project called Immuno-Epidemiological and Genetic Studies on the Population of Easter Island. His application emphasized the goals of the forthcoming IBP, the scientific expertise available in Montreal, and the possibility of international collaboration through his numerous European contacts, recently enlarged and strengthened by the 1962 gastroenterology meeting in Munich. In late 1963 the WHO gave Skoryna a one-year grant of US$5,000.[77] That same year, the WHO awarded a total of US$61,696 shared by fourteen individual researchers, including Skoryna, for an average of US$4,400. Skoryna's seemingly small WHO award was, therefore, above average.

Surely, Stanley and Georges were pleased. Were they surprised? Was it the full amount requested? We cannot know. All of Skoryna's own papers were destroyed in a flood after his death in 2003, and those once belonging to Nógrády languished in boxes before being shipped to a

Hungarian archive in Toronto, then moved to a private home in Ottawa, and finally, following his death in 2013, given to the Chilean embassy in Ottawa. Nógrády's correspondence and scientific manuscripts, like Skoryna's, are lost.

Stanley's dream was not yet a reality, but it had achieved international respectability – and with the prestigious WHO endorsement, he turned to a much more difficult task: convincing Canada to help.

2

Convincing Canada, Building a Team

With his grant from the World Health Organization (WHO), Stanley Skoryna set out to find other backers, arrange transportation, and assemble a team. To support his project, he had to work on many fronts at once, pursuing various sources of income, testing different angles, piling one small success on top of the last, and currying favour in unlikely places. He appealed to Canada's growing nationalism and sense of pride in its global profile.

COURTING CANADA'S NAVY AND POLITICIANS

Canada had engaged early with many of the projects of the WHO, partly because its first director general was Canadian military psychiatrist Brock Chisholm. In 1960 the National Research Council (NRC) created a special branch, called the Medical Research Council (MRC), its first head being Toronto's distinguished professor of internal medicine Dr Ray Farquharson. Skoryna hoped to find more funding there. He also had to seek permission from Chile and find a means of transportation. The annual supply ship would not help, as it stayed only one week – not long enough for the work plan – and neither Skoryna nor Georges Nógrády could devote an entire year to waiting for its return. Furthermore, they would need to take so much equipment that conveying those supplies to Valparaiso would be a major undertaking in itself. Even if they were permitted on the Chilean vessel, their supplies might not fit. They needed their own ship. Skoryna drew on his considerable imagination and ethnic connections. Finding collaborators willing to go to Easter Island was easy, but convincing Canada to support him would prove to be much more difficult than convincing the WHO.

From the beginning, Skoryna wondered if he could induce the Royal Canadian Navy to convey his expedition. Examination of the map revealed the "surprising fact" that, thanks to the Panama Canal, Easter Island was closer to Halifax than to Vancouver. He approached Surgeon Captain Richard H. Roberts, a senior navy doctor based in Halifax. English-born and trained, Roberts was serving as chief of medicine in the Canadian Forces Hospital in Halifax; his Scottish-born wife, Maureen, was also a physician, specializing in pediatrics and genetics and setting up a research laboratory at Dalhousie. They had met while interning in Liverpool and had served together in India during the war. Roberts met Skoryna at a conference of the William Beaumont Society of the US army – a gastroenterology organization of interest to them both. Roberts would have attended for the military aspects and because he had researched the incidence of peptic ulcer disease and obesity in navy personnel. Skoryna would have attended for the "gut" aspects of the conference, although I can't help wondering if he was deliberately stalking naval types in search of a ship.[1]

In his letter of 4 October 1963 to Roberts, Skoryna reminded the navy doctor of their earlier encounter, during which they had discussed plans for the Canadian Medical Expedition to Easter Island. He now informed Roberts of the WHO grant and asked if he would like to join the expedition, possibly with his pediatrician wife "since there is a large number of children on the island." Roberts replied quickly, "delighted" to hear from him and "delighted" to participate but needing to clarify whether or not he would be granted leave and insisting that his expenses be paid. Maureen was also interested, he wrote, especially if one of her mentors would join in, the distinguished McGill University geneticist Clarke Fraser.[2] Roberts observed that the Canadian navy usually plied the Pacific from Vancouver.

Now that he had hooked at least one naval officer, Skoryna replied to Roberts by return mail, moving deftly from personnel to transportation. "The question of transportation is difficult. I was thinking that if the navy can give us a hand, and since Halifax seems to be closer than Vancouver, it would be preferable to make our base Halifax rather than Vancouver." He now revealed that he had contacted some senior naval officers: "Admiral [Herbert S.] Rayner has mentioned that they might use either HMCS *Cape Scott* or HMCS *Cape Breton*. I suppose that these are stationed in the Atlantic."[3] Both built in 1944, they were aging escort maintenance vessels, or "mobile repair ships," loaded with workshops for electronics, machinery, and metal and wood working, with a top speed of only 11 knots. They each had a crew of more than 200 sailors and lots of room for cargo. But at this point, Skoryna had no approvals.

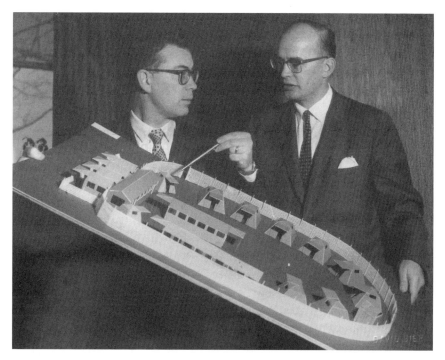

Figure 2.1 Virologist Armand Boudreault (*left*) and Stanley Skoryna with proposed model of METEI camp with tents. Boudreault Papers.

The Robertses supplied their photographs and biographies and suggested various other people, such as their friend Dr Margaret Corston, a "married lady doctor" with a 1942 medical degree, who had "done little medical work for some time" but would be "entirely competent to perform examinations and probably to help with the household chores."[4] The expectation that women physicians would naturally serve as housekeepers and cooks persisted throughout the entire adventure.

Rumours of the forthcoming journey spread across Canada. Soon a "memorandum" described the ambitious METEI project, its WHO funding, and its urgency. It would be a boon to international science and "the major Canadian contribution to the International Biological Year (IBY), set to begin in January 1965." "Any delays will jeopardize the objectives," as "the isolated status of Easter Island will be abolished by the proposed construction of an airfield on the island in 1965 for tourists and trans-Pacific travel." In this memo, Skoryna claimed organizational assistance from two Canadian government officials: Dr D.B.D. Layton of the International Division of the Department of Health and Welfare and

A.J. Pick of the Latin American Division of the Department of External Affairs. The claims were more hypothetical than firm. An accompanying statement on "Objectives and Organization" explained that the island did not have a good supply of fresh water and that McGill engineers were busy developing solar stills, a project that captured industry interest.[5] Facilities for housing the team and their laboratories were being researched by Hungarian-born Norbert Schoenauer of McGill's school of architecture; they anticipated using tents of lightweight plastic and aluminum for easy transport (figure 2.1). These memos went to would-be participants, targeted donors, and members of the government.[6]

Skoryna wanted support from the Canadian prime minister, Lester B. Pearson, whose Liberal Party had defeated that of Conservative John Diefenbaker in early 1963. Pearson had served in the previous Liberal government as minister of external affairs. In that capacity, his help in organizing the United Nations Emergency Force during the Suez Crisis had earned him the 1957 Nobel Peace Prize. Given the context of global anxieties over the environment and nuclear fallout, described in chapter 1, Pearson's 1963 victory implied a drastic change in Canada's foreign policy, making it seem closer to that of the United States. Five years earlier, rocky relations with the Americans had been aggravated with the death by suicide on 4 April 1957 of Herbert Norman, a distinguished Canadian sinologist and diplomat who, many believed, had cracked under relentless McCarthyism scrutiny. The Diefenbaker government had agreed to the construction of twenty-eight Bomarc missile silos on Canadian soil at North Bay, Ontario, and at La Macaza, Quebec. But Diefenbaker changed his mind about the missiles and declared that they should be armed with conventional weapons, not nuclear warheads. Because of this extraordinary new defence system, he cancelled the contract for the legendary Avro Arrow fighter plane on 20 February 1959, claiming it was no longer necessary. To the everlasting dismay of its planners, the results of ten years of Canadian work on the Arrow project were destroyed.[7]

Notwithstanding his Nobel Peace Prize, Pearson disagreed with Diefenbaker and supported the idea of allowing the United States to arm its two Bomarc missile sites with nuclear warheads. He argued that Canada needed to fulfil its international obligations through NATO and NORAD. Some saw this "Pearsonian" or "liberal internationalism" as an appropriate response to Canada's burgeoning nationalism: to become its own country, Canada needed to participate on a world stage. Others perceived his stance as a disastrous loss of autonomy, compounded by a decline in other traditional symbols of Canada's distinct status. In 1964 students staged demonstrations against the nuclear weapons, protesting war and American interference. Disputed analysis over Norman's death and the demise of the Avro Arrow entered the national psyche as founding myths that continue to stir hearts and minds more than half a century later. At the time, the situation was encapsulated in George Grant's famous 1965 book *Lament for a Nation.*[8] The world's second largest country was approaching its centennial in 1967, it was to host that year's World's Fair, Expo 67, and yet it did not have its own flag, nor did it control its own Constitution, and it was losing its fragile autonomy to the United States. The question of national identity dominated government, media, and culture for many years.[9]

Skoryna used these preoccupations to leverage moral support for his dream. One of his first acts was the creation of the Easter Island Expedition Society, which was granted letters patent in January 1964 with the help of McGill lawyers.[10] Its existence hinted that Skoryna and Nógrády had many supporters, although membership was small. The secretary-treasurer was Mrs Gerd Vold Hurum, who had served Thor Heyerdahl's expedition from a base in Lima and was now living in Montreal.[11] McGill's principal, surgeon H. Rocke Robertson, agreed to be president and, in that capacity, did Skoryna's bidding.

THE POLISH CONNECTION: DR STANLEY HAIDASZ

To reach the prime minister, Skoryna took an indirect approach. He targeted Dr Stanley Haidasz, Liberal member of Parliament for the Toronto riding of Parkdale. In early 1964 Haidasz was also serving as parliamentary secretary to the minister for health and welfare. Born in Canada to Polish immigrants, Haidasz was a Toronto-trained physician specialized in cardiology. He too was fond of medical history. Therefore, the two Stanleys had much in common; their frequent letters often closed with a few handwritten words in Polish.

On 13 January 1964, Haidasz described his first encounter with Skoryna to Prime Minister Pearson and Minister of Defence Paul Hellyer. "Last weekend I was conveying greetings" of the government to the Wilno Wing of the Royal Canadian Air Force (RCAF) "at their Tenth Anniversary in Montreal."[12] "During the festivities, I was approached by Professor Stanley C. Skoryna, consultant surgeon of the RCAF Auxiliary ... to seek your assistance in obtaining a Halifax-based, navy supply ship" that would convey his personnel and equipment "on a World Health Organization medical expedition to Easter Island." Haidasz outlined the relationship of the project to the IBY, the difficulty of using any other means of travel, and the "surprising fact" that Halifax was closer to Easter Island than Vancouver. Skoryna already enjoyed "consultative assistance" from the Department of Health and Welfare and the Department of External Affairs. He warned Pearson and Hellyer that they would soon be receiving an official request for a navy ship from the principal of McGill University.[13] Both letters were acknowledged quickly by staffers. Pearson's secretary, Mary Macdonald, took the liberty of forwarding it to the Latin American Division of External Affairs.

From this moment on, Haidasz was Skoryna's government champion for METEI and beyond. He blind-copied Skoryna on the letter to Pearson and Hellyer. The two men and their wives met again informally in Montreal before the end of January, and in thanking Skoryna for the warm reception, Haidasz confirmed his belief in the great scientific potential of the project.[14]

As predicted, by 3 February, Prime Minister Pearson had received "representations" from Robertson "on behalf of a medical scientific research expedition which will be going to Easter Island at the end of this year." The phrasing indicated that the plan was definite. Pearson punted to Hellyer and copied the minister of external affairs, the minister of industry, and Haidasz. He expressed his general approval of the idea: "This seems to me to be an imaginative scheme and one that will be helpful to Canada's international prestige, as well as contributing in a concrete way to the International Biological Year."[15]

On 18 February, Pearson shifted Haidasz out of the Department of Health and Welfare to become the parliamentary secretary to the secretary of state for external affairs, Paul Martin. The next day, Haidasz informed Skoryna of this potentially useful reassignment. He also forwarded information about Polish medical history and "the need of a bulletin devoted to history past and present and contributions to medical science."[16]

As the request for a navy ship and its accompanying memo, cited above, made their way around the various departments – Health and Welfare, Defence, External Affairs, Industry – they garnered cool commentary from bureaucrats reluctant to criticize a plan with WHO endorsement but equally reluctant to implicate their budgets. The Liberal Party had been elected on a platform that would support social programs; money for anything else was tight.

Career diplomat A.J. Pick, head of the Latin American Division of the Department of External Affairs, admitted that he was unable to judge the scientific merits of the project. A former ambassador to Peru and Bolivia from 1958 to 1962, Pick saw himself as a liaison between Chile's embassy in Ottawa and Canada's embassy in Santiago. He avoided direct involvement. "Dr. Skoryna rather overstates the assistance that I have been able to give him." Although the "imaginative scheme" would be "good for Canada's international prestige" and a "contribution to the International Biological Year (IBY)," the "Department of External Affairs would, of course, not be able to help in any material or financial way."[17] Hinting that the project itself might have flaws, he revealed that private sources had confirmed that Skoryna would find no support from the Department of Health and Welfare, although it had funded him for other projects in the past. He suggested that they approach either the Department of Industry through its minister, C.M. Drury, or the navy through Hellyer, something that Haidasz had already done.

Hellyer responded to all of Haidasz's letters, promising that the proposal was "under study" and that he was expecting a report from the navy on its feasibility. Skoryna and Haidasz kept up the pressure. On 6 March, now using special Easter Island Expedition Society letterhead with a distinctive green METEI logo, Skoryna invited himself to visit the House of Commons and meet with Haidasz.[18] The encounter took place four days later, and Haidasz even orchestrated a brief meeting with Hellyer, who again assured the pair that METEI was "under active consideration."[19]

Skoryna began inviting illustrious medical scientists and other dignitaries to become honorary consultants or patrons. In extending the same courtesy to Haidasz, he inquired about the advisability of similarly inviting the prime minister and the governor general. Haidasz immediately accepted for himself and telephoned his minister, Paul Martin, who assured him that inviting both the head of government and the head of state would be "perfectly proper."[20] The growing list of honorary consultants was intended to enhance credibility and entice donations (see appendix D, table D.1).[21]

THE MINISTER OF DEFENCE AND DR HELEN EVANS REID

First elected in 1949 at age twenty-six, Paul Hellyer had, to that point, been the youngest person ever to hold a seat in the House of Commons. Born on a farm in southern Ontario, he trained as an aeronautical engineer and pilot before serving with the RCAF in the Second World War. Defence had always been his special interest, and as minister under Pearson, he embarked on one of the most controversial projects in Canadian military history. Even as Haidasz, Skoryna, and the prime minister were asking about a navy ship for METEI, Hellyer was preparing a White Paper on unification of the armed forces. With his deputy,

Lucien Cardin, he tabled the document in the House of Commons on 24 March 1964. Strong opposition arose immediately from the army, the air force, and especially the navy. The rancour would eventually lead to the dismissal of Rear Admiral William Landymore and the forced resignation of several other senior officers.[22] Was the extraordinary request for a navy vessel to sail to Easter Island going to help or hinder his increasingly difficult relationship with the forces?

But Hellyer remembers that the greatest pressure over METEI came not from McGill nor from fellow members of Parliament, such as Haidasz, but from Toronto pediatrician Helen Evans Reid. She was married to Andrew Lawrence ("Laurie") Chute, physician-in-chief at Toronto's Hospital for Sick Children, head of pediatrics at the University of Toronto, and soon to be the dean of its medical school. Born in India, Chute was the youngest son of Baptist missionaries who had sent all four of their children back to Canada for high school so that they could continue their work abroad. Laurie and his older brother Ken were significantly younger than their other siblings. Hellyer believes that his mother probably heard an appeal through Baptist channels and readily offered the security of their family farm to the Chute boys. They were older than Paul; he recalls riding on Laurie's shoulders to visit the Canadian National Exhibition. But they became family, and when Laurie was attending medical school in Toronto and when he was serving in the Second World War, he would come "home" to the Hellyer farm, often bringing his good friend and medical school classmate Omond Solandt. Chute said that he felt closer to the Hellyers than to his own parents. In October 1939, Laurie married Reid, a medical graduate of the University of Alberta who was the daughter of a country practitioner. Their children – anthropologist Judith Omond Redfield and psychologist Douglas Lawrence Chute – still view Hellyer as "uncle Paul."

For the intrepid Reid, the minister of defence was her younger brother-in-law, and her husband's buddy Solandt was well connected with Ottawa intelligentsia, having been the first chair of the Defence Research Board until 1956. These relationships gave her special insight into the workings of government. Helen and her husband placed a high value on medical research and public service in aid of children around the world. As their former student, I know that they were dedicated teachers, honest, direct, and unafraid to broach delicate matters. They were the first couple that Hellyer had ever heard speak of "sexual intimacy" in public. Hellyer recalls that Helen had learned of METEI at a cocktail party, thought it a good idea, wanted to join, and told him to provide a navy ship. In fact, until he was recently shown the correspondence, he'd forgotten the near simultaneous lobbying of Haidasz, Skoryna, and Robertson. He remembered only Helen Reid.

Helen's cocktail-party "friend" was her neighbour William Harding Le Riche of South Africa, epidemiologist and department head at the University of Toronto. Originally slated to join METEI, he eventually dropped out owing to the press of work, but he remained an honorary consultant. Le Riche was interested in ecology and the spread of infectious disease via immigration. He had conducted a 1943 survey of child health in a South African township, exploring "epidemiology as medical ecology," which became the title of his 1971 book. Since at least 1956, he had made numerous television and radio appearances, and it is possible that Skoryna had identified him from his media profile. At the cocktail party, Reid expressed her envy of the opportunity to go to Easter Island. In reply, he suggested that she come along too and admitted that transportation was still a problem. "Maybe I can help," she said. Soon Le Riche invited Skoryna to Toronto to meet Reid and explain the needs. They dined at the Le Riche home. A large envelope in Reid's papers is labelled "How I got the Canadian Navy to Take the Exped. To Easter Island." It reveals that she approached Hellyer by letter on 9 January 1964, a few days before Haidasz, enclosing information about the journey and METEI materials from Skoryna.²³ She and Hellyer were unable to meet in person until 27 February when she came to Ottawa, although letters were exchanged in the interval. Helen's belief in the project, particularly its scientific merits, was convincing. Her previous experience in journalism, especially writing about medicine for the general public, led her to imagine an article about the project.

On 12 March, Cabinet approved Hellyer's recommendation authorizing the navy "to give transport for a scientific expedition to Easter Island for the purposes of medical research."²⁴ This approval came with no estimates for the necessary funds from the Department of Defence's budget, which had been voted by Parliament, something that would create problems for Hellyer the following year. By 7 April he had secured the navy's cooperation: the ship would be the maintenance vessel HMCS *Cape Scott*. Skoryna composed an exalted formal "statement" for internal consumption in which he lauded the Royal Canadian Navy for its collaboration with medical science, building on a tradition of similar endeavours aimed at "improvement of health standards for people throughout the world." With scientists "from six Canadian universities, Chile, Great Britain, Scandinavia, and the United States," he claimed, METEI would meet the goals of the Human Adaptability section of the International Biological *Programme* (no longer "Year"). Its claims to originality were considerable:

"a complete study of an isolated population has never before been carried out on so large a scale." He hoped that in addition to the "accumulation of significant medical data," the expedition would "provide valuable information for similar undertakings in Canada and elsewhere."[25]

CONVINCING CHILE

All agreed that the good news and the name of the ship had to be kept under wraps because the advancing expedition still did not have approval from Chile. A premature announcement would offend the host country. Furthermore, Canada's ambassador to Chile, G.B. Summers, had been raising objections.[26] How much Canada was aware of American involvement in the forthcoming elections in that country is not known: the CIA was busy pouring US$5 million into promoting the campaign of Eduardo Frei Montalva, the intellectual leader of the Christian Democratic Party, against the bid of the "communist" Salvador Allende.[27] Skoryna grew increasingly exasperated with official channels and decided, once again, to take matters into his own hands. He had dared to release names of three expedition members in late March, without explaining how the team would travel.[28] He decided to go after Chile's approval by a different route.

The Gastrointestinal Research Laboratory was a big consumer of Purina feeds for research animals. Skoryna knew the vivacious Polish Canadian who served as the company representative, Jane Polud (Paludkiewicz). She had been planning to go to Peru "to buy fish meal," but Skoryna began an active campaign to divert her to Chile. Once she consented to the new arrangement, he armed her with the names of necessary officials, including the ambassador, and tasked her with obtaining approval. Extroverted and exuberant, she had a wonderful time in Santiago and remembers several helpful people, including the minister of public health, Dr Francisco Rojas Villegas, and "at the hospital," Dr Raúl Etcheverry, who had a research interest in Easter Island. She convinced the authorities of the merits of METEI, assuring them that Chilean scientists would certainly be welcomed and that Chile would not be expected to cover any costs.

On 22 April, Haidasz received a letter from the Chilean ambassador in Ottawa, assuring him of his government's cooperation and granting tentative permission, provided more information was forthcoming. Did Haidasz feel a pang of glee when he conveyed the impending good news to A.J. Pick? The two Polish Stanleys had gone around the seasoned diplomat. With the name of the ship, a list of scientists, and commitment to include three Chilean collaborators, final Chilean approval

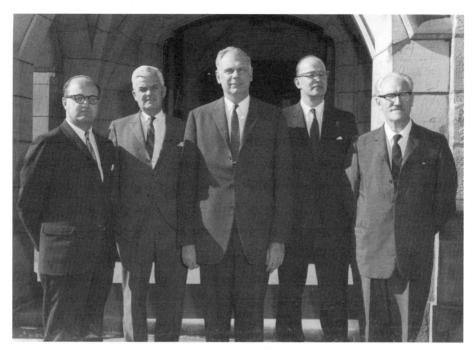

Figure 2.2 *From left*, Stanley Haidasz, John Easton, Paul Hellyer, Stanley Skoryna, and Chilean diplomat Juan Domeyko, Ottawa, 1964. Reid Papers, file 11.

came a month later.[29] A group photo, with Hellyer and a Chilean diplomat, celebrated the achievement (figure 2.2). Chile reminded METEI that conditions on the island were limited: food was monotonous and not plentiful, and there was no hotel, no electricity, and very little fresh water. By October 1964 the names of two Chilean scientists had been added to the METEI team to fulfil the stipulations: Gonzalo Donoso, a pediatrician and expert on nutrition, and Sergio Alvarado, an expert on radioactivity who would look for evidence of fallout.

FUNDRAISING

Skoryna also put an end to Pick's claim that METEI would receive nothing from the Medical Research Council. By approaching Dr Ray Farquharson directly, he had secured a grant of $10,000. Indeed, Skoryna had been lobbying the first director of the MRC since 1961, inviting him to visit the lab in the Donner Building at McGill, accosting him at meetings, complimenting him on his views, requesting reprints of his articles, and sending along his ideas for the education of medical scientists and a copy of an admired 1950 essay by Francis Boyer on the "research personality."[30] Were these gestures appreciated, or did they seem ingratiating?

The WHO and MRC grants were progress but still not enough. With them and navy support, the team moved into high gear, seeking funds from other Canadian sources, including both External Affairs and Health and Welfare. The undersecretary of state for External Affairs, Marcel Cadieux, took a long time to respond. With a background in law, Cadieux had served on United Nations commissions and would eventually become Canada's ambassador to the United States. On behalf of his minister, Paul Martin, Cadieux rejected all requests from Haidasz and Skoryna, denied that the upcoming ministerial tour of Latin America would entail a visit to Chile, and refused the position of honorary consultant for either Martin or Pearson because it might put them in the embarrassing position of financial responsibility. This response was in direct contradiction to what Martin had said in March about it being "perfectly proper" to ask. Haidasz then inquired about the governor general. Cadieux again declined, stating that "it would not be appropriate to ask the Governor General if the government is not prepared to give greater assistance than it has so far."[31] Weeks earlier, the influential Cadieux had prepared a detailed, skeptical memo to his minister, outlining the state of the METEI project and warning that the navy expense alone would be "upwards of $200,000."[32]

For his part, the minister of health and welfare, Dr Don Cameron, opined that the requested grant of $10,000 was far too much to spend outside Canada's borders. He also contended that, contrary to what Haidasz believed, Farquharson had not yet confirmed the plan to grant *any* MRC money to METEI and that, if he did, he had "in mind something between two and three thousand dollars," not $10,000. In closing, he pointed to a loophole that would allow for "training" of Canadians and apologized for sounding "so bureaucratic and obstructive."[33] Haidasz and Skoryna came back with a proposal to train young expedition scientists from Quebec in epidemiological methods. Still they were unsuccessful.

The Easter Island Expedition Society had raised almost no money, partly because the project had been kept secret until Chile granted approval. Haidasz encouraged Skoryna to appeal to private foundations – such as Atkinson, Molson, and Maclean (Canada Packers). In a "private and confidential" letter to his minister, Paul Martin, Haidasz lamented the sorry state of research in Canada, where scientists were denied modest funds for their work while money poured into development opportunities elsewhere.[34] Seemingly corralled by Cadieux, his own deputy, Martin suggested that they appeal to the External Aid Office; they did so, again without success – which is scarcely surprising since no actual "aid" was to be involved.[35]

ACCOMMODATIONS AND EQUIPMENT

Originally, the architects at McGill University, led by Norbert Schoenhauer, designed a self-contained encampment of tents that would enclose a private area with an opening at one end for reception, examination rooms, and laboratories (see figure 2.1). Soon, however, the advantage of portable dwellings in the form of collapsible trailers seemed a better prospect. Rain and wind were to be expected, and the delicate scientific equipment would suffer without more durable protection. The Alberta Trailer Company (ATCO), founded and owned by the Southern family since 1947, made – and still makes – collapsible trailers or cabins. A "shoebox model," measuring 3 by 6 metres and easily partitioned to create two cabins of 3 by 3 metres, could provide all the accommodation needed. It is not known if the architects or someone else suggested ATCO. Dr Garry Brody, who knew Skoryna and would join METEI, had known Ron Southern, the owner's son, at university in Alberta. Skoryna travelled to Calgary to examine the structures. He approved, and METEI ordered twenty-four trailers, valued at $2,300 each, for a total of $55,200. Schoenhauer and his students used the same basic layout, changing the tents to numbered cabins (figures 2.3 and 2.4).[36] The collapsed "shoeboxes" were shipped by rail – a big event for the company, which celebrated the global reach of its products. A group photo was taken in Halifax with members of the navy, the railway, and S. Don Southern, chairman of ATCO (figure 2.5).[37] The trailers were to be loaned and returned; however, Skoryna gradually realized that the landing and loading conditions were such that they could never be removed from the island. No one told ATCO.

Encouraging suppliers to donate equipment, Skoryna also began appealing to organizations to fund one trailer each. By the time METEI left Canada, only three trailers had been paid for. Nevertheless, the Ford Motor Company donated a four-wheel-drive truck, which would be left on the island. Picker X-ray donated machinery for taking radiographs, and thousands of films in different sizes were given by Dupont. The maker of the distillation unit, worth over $7,000, was willing to sell at a discount, although Skoryna hoped to bring that item home. A

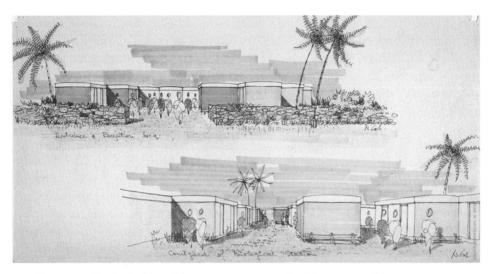

Figure 2.3 Revised plan of the METEI compound with ATCO trailers.
Norbert Schoenauer. McGill School of Architecture, http://cac.mcgill.ca/
schoenauer/index.htm.

nutritionist at McGill was engaged to calculate the correct amount of
food – largely nonperishables – that would keep METEI fed and happy.
Skoryna could not resist sizable donations of canned meat and pumpernickel bread, even if they were unpopular.

The files at McGill contain many letters to companies and organizations looking for financial support. A grant application went to the
United States Department of Health and Welfare asking for $30,000
and optimistically suggesting that METEI enjoyed the backing of
Canadian universities in the form of professors' salaries totalling more
than $64,000, with "applications pending" for $50,000 from the United
Nations Children's Fund and $10,000 each from the MRC, Canadian
Life Insurance Officers Association, and Canadian Department of Health
and Welfare.[38] Only the MRC grant came through.

With navy and Chilean approval, the naming of the ship's commanding
officer, and formal commitments to personnel, McGill removed the publication embargo, hoping to attract donors. On 23 July 1964 the *Montreal
Star* pulled out all the stops and filled almost the entire front page with
information about the expedition, *Cape Scott*, her captain, Skoryna, and
Easter Island (figure 2.6). The hype did little for the coffers, but it attracted
a flurry of attention from other newspapers, radio, and television. Not
until the actual departure would METEI enjoy greater media coverage.

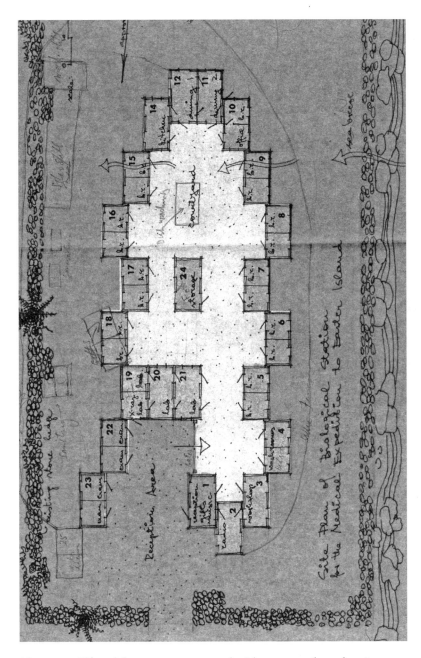

Figure 2.4 Plan of the METEI compound with ATCO trailers, showing sea-shore. The actual setup rotated the orientation to the sea by 180 degrees. The pencilled annotations show alterations made in practice and location of sanitary facilities and stills. Norbert Schoenauer. Reid Papers, file 5.

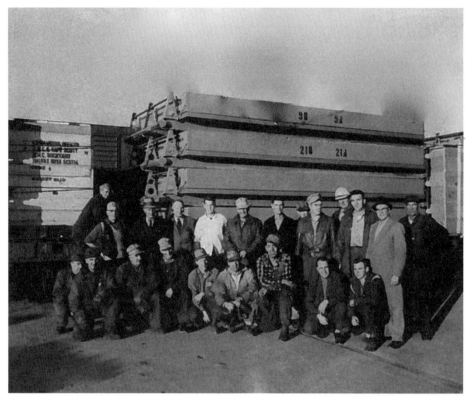

Figure 2.5 Some of the twenty-four palletized ATCO "shoebox" trailers shipped from Alberta by rail to Halifax for loading on HMCS *Cape Scott*. ATCO Archives, with thanks to Debbie Taylor.

BUILDING A TEAM

Even before the July announcement, word of the exotic journey generated a stampede of willing participants, and the project soon extended its original focus on human biology to sociology and anthropology. It would not stop at humans and their microbes but would include animals and plants too – all living things. Confirmation of HMCS *Cape Scott* meant that the numbers of researchers could expand. A broadened mandate would be more in keeping with the objective of the International Biological Programme (IBP) to study entire ecosystems. Because the IBP favoured international collaboration, Skoryna needed non-Canadians to join, as his April statement had implied. He hoped international prestige would encourage donors.

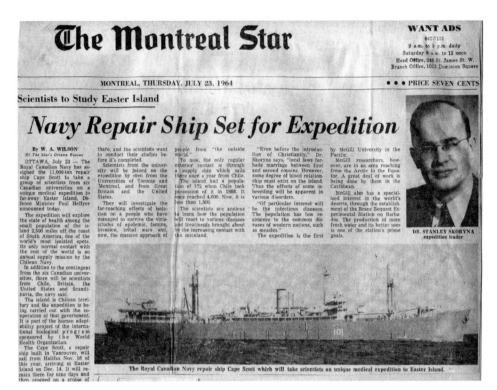

The Montreal Star

WANT ADS
842-7131
9 a.m. to 5 p.m. daily
Saturday 9 a.m. to 12 noon
Head Office, 245 St. James St. W.
Branch Office, 1013 Dominion Square

MONTREAL, THURSDAY, JULY 23, 1964   ● ● ● PRICE SEVEN CENTS

Scientists to Study Easter Island

Navy Repair Ship Set for Expedition

By W. A. WILSON
Of The Star's Ottawa Bureau

OTTAWA, July 23 — The Royal Canadian Navy has assigned the 11,000-ton repair ship Cape Scott to take a group of scientists from six Canadian universities on a unique medical expedition to far-away Easter Island, Defence Minister Paul Hellyer announced today.

The expedition will explore the state of health among the small population of the island 2,500 miles off the coast of South America, one of the world's most isolated spots. Its only normal contact with the rest of the world is an annual supply mission by the Chilean Navy.

In addition to the contingent from the six Canadian universities, there will be scientists from Chile, Britain, the United States and Scandinavia, the navy said.

The island is Chilean territory and the expedition is being carried out with the co-operation of that government. It is part of the human adaptability project of the international biological p r o g r a m sponsored by t h e World Health Organization.

The Cape Scott, a repair ship built in Vancouver, will sail from Halifax Nov. 16 of this year, arriving at Easter Island on Dec. 14. It will remain there for nine days and then proceed on a cruise of

there, and the scientists want to conduct their studies before it's completed.

Scientists from the university will be joined on the expedition by men from the Universities of Toronto and Montreal, and from Great Britain and the United States.

They will investigate the far-reaching effects of isolation on a people who have managed to survive the vicissitudes of epidemic, famine, invasion, tribal wars and, now, the massive approach of

people from "the outside world."

To now, the only regular exterior contact is through a supply ship which sails there once a year from Chile. The island had a population of 172 when Chile took possession of it in 1888. It once reached 4,000. Now, it is less than 1,500.

The scientists are anxious to learn how the population will react to various diseases and treatments brought about by the increasing contact with the mainland.

"Even before the introduction of Christianity," Dr. Skoryna says, "local laws forbade marriage between first and second cousins. However, some degree of blood relationship must exist on the island. Thus the effects of some inbreeding will be apparent in various disorders.

"Of particular interest will be the infectious diseases. The population has low resistence to the common diseases of western nations, such as measles."

The expedition is the first

by McGill University in the Pacific.

McGill researchers, however, are in an area reaching from the Arctic to the Equator. A great deal of work is being done by them in the Caribbean.

McGill also has a specialized interest in the world's deserts, through the establishment of the Brace Bequest Experimental Station on Barbados. The production of more fresh water and its better uses is one of the station's prime goals.

DR. STANLEY SKORYNA
expedition leader

The Royal Canadian Navy repair ship Cape Scott which will take scientists on unique medical expedition to Easter Island.

Figure 2.6 *Montreal Star* coverage of the announcement of the expedition, its director, and its ship, HMCS *Cape Scott*, following approvals from Chilean authorities, 23 July 1964. Wilkinson Papers.

Since March 1964, Skoryna's new secretary at the Donner Building, Mrs Isabel Griffiths, had been typing invitation letters on the special green and buff METEI letterhead. Like her predecessor, Mrs Ana Maria Eccles, she was Spanish-born and fluent in three languages. Both women were engaged by the mission early for their language and organizational skills. They had met when they first came to Canada and boarded with nuns; they soon shared an apartment. They both married young, and when Ana Maria left Montreal for Halifax with her husband, her job in Skoryna's lab slid to her beautiful, feisty friend Isabel.

Isabel recalls that McGill University was ambivalent about the program and its leader: on the one hand, it was avid for publicity and the exotic cachet; on the other hand, it worried about costs and obligations. Specifically, the university did not want Skoryna to use McGill letterhead so that it could avoid becoming financially implicated in what was proving to be an expensive proposition. That concern had prompted the creation of the Easter Island Expedition Society. She and Skoryna drew up forms for would-be participants to list their necessary equipment by volume and weight. The late March press release had already named Dr Richard Roberts, who would be "in charge of medical examinations," and Montreal engineer Robert O. Molson, who would look after mechanical and electrical matters and "applied science research projects," including radioactivity.[39]

Some team members came from Skoryna's contacts through McGill. Surgeon Garry S. Brody was a Canadian-born graduate of the University of Alberta. He had spent part of his residency at McGill conducting research with Skoryna. Having recently completed his specialty training in plastic surgery, he had moved into practice at Arlington, Virginia. By telephone, Skoryna invited him to be "assistant director." In advance of the journey, Brody went to the nearby Smithsonian Institute, offering to bring back anything useful; "Dr. [J. Lawrence] Angel" asked him to make plaster face masks of three islanders.[40] Although Brody's relationship with Skoryna had originated in Canada, his new American address enhanced the international profile.

Similarly, David Murphy had been an associate of Skoryna. After completing veterinary medicine in Guelph, Ontario, he turned to humans, earning his medical degree at McGill in 1960. As a student, Murphy thought of ways to earn extra money. Knowing that Skoryna needed help with his research on animals and planning on a career in surgery, Murphy had offered his veterinary skills to the Gastrointestinal Research Laboratory as soon as he started medical school. Murphy performed some experiments with Skoryna on dog pancreas. He knew Skoryna well as the "entrepreneurial" leader of the Donner lab who "really got it going." But he thought that Skoryna was a better gastroenterology researcher than a surgeon – notwithstanding his training, the Royal College medal, and his work at St Mary's Hospital. Similarly, secretary Isabel Griffiths (now Cutler) remembers that, although many people referred to Skoryna as a "surgeon," his forte was research.

In 1964 Murphy was almost finished his residency training in pediatric heart surgery at Boston Children's Hospital. He was married to physician Sonia Salisbury, and they were the parents of a little boy with another child on the way. Skoryna engaged him for METEI early on, principally for his veterinary skills, because the island had a vast number of domestic animals that would also need to be examined: sheep, horses, cows, chickens, pigs, and cats. Murphy could collect the blood samples, but he doubted his ability to handle the analytical aspects of the animal work. He suggested that they also include his friend from veterinary school Harold ("Hal") Gibbs, another father, with four children, the youngest only a year old. Born in Barbados but educated in Canada, Gibbs had completed his doctorate in parasitology at McGill's Macdonald College in 1958 with a thesis on hookworm in dogs and wolves. Since then, he had been happily working and teaching in the government's Animal Disease Research Laboratory near Ottawa. An entomologist at Macdonald College, D. Keith McE. Kevan, supplied Gibbs with an insect net, hoping he would collect specimens, although bugs were not Hal's "thing." Kevan was vexed not to have been invited to join METEI himself.

Wildlife was a different proposition. In March, Skoryna had approached zoologist and conservationist Ian McTaggart-Cowan, head of zoology at the University of British Columbia (UBC) in Vancouver. More importantly, from Skoryna's perspective, McTaggart-Cowan was a popular television personality, like Le Riche. His appearances raised awareness about the diversity of animal life and the need to protect the environment from pollution. His programs aired across Canada and in other countries too. His informal successor in this role is the famous geneticist David Suzuki, who was hired by UBC in 1963. McTaggart-Cowan agreed to join METEI in late March, sending along his biography and a photograph, but in July, he had to drop out, as he had become the dean of graduate studies. He recommended his young colleague, the Oxford-trained Ian Efford, who, at almost thirty years old and with a background in zoology and entomology, had been hired to develop the rising field of ecology. Married with two children, Efford recalls that he'd been in Vancouver only a few weeks when the invitation came "at the last minute." Time was so short that he had to receive all his injections for a tropical journey in one sitting with a warning that he might react. He asked to take along a student assistant. Skoryna replied that an assistant would be "acceptable provided it is a *male* student."[41] Senior undergraduate Jack Mathias could not believe his luck when he was chosen for the role. Planning to start his master's degree, he remembers that Suzuki advised him not to go. But the prospect of the romantic destination and the work with Efford was irresistible. He claims that it "opened [his] eyes to the world."

By April, Skoryna was sending around a tentative list of team members. The six Canadian universities referred to in his communications were McGill for Skoryna, Murphy, and Gibbs and the Université de Montréal for Nógrády and virologist Armand Boudreault, with researchers from the University of Manitoba, University of Toronto, Dalhousie University, and UBC. The home institutions were to continue the salaries of the professors, whereas costs of travel, meals, and accommodation would be borne by METEI. Student members would receive a stipend of $2,000 to defray expenses. However, the scientists also needed expensive equipment, which they looked to the expedition to provide.

Maureen Roberts was disappointed that her mentor Clarke Fraser would not be on the journey. In order to prepare for her fieldwork, she contacted Alexander G. Bearn, expert in genetics at the Rockefeller Institute, and she travelled to New York City to seek his advice on the collection of samples for genetic tests. In those days, DNA was well known as the vehicle of genetic information, James Watson and Francis Crick having garnered the 1962 Nobel Prize for resolving its structure; however, it could not yet be measured. Bearn recommended gathering serum for proteins that were markers of genetics – transferrins, haptoglobins, and group-specific antigens – for which he would be able to perform tests. Apologizing for the exorbitance, she sent Skoryna her travel expenses, and he quickly reimbursed them. Late in the planning and looking for more advice on collection and storage of red cells, she invited geneticist Nancy Simpson to Halifax. An expert on population genetics in Canada's North, Simpson was moving from the University of Toronto and considering Dalhousie before opting for Queen's University.[42]

Cardiologist T. Edward Cuddy of the University of Manitoba joined the project to conduct pulmonary function and cardiovascular research. He needed $4,000 for equipment, but that expense was not allowable through grants of the MRC, NRC, or Defence Research Board. Haidasz's office appealed to Tom Kent in the office of the prime minister. The request went to the secretary of the Cabinet, who replied two weeks later, saying that the matter had been discussed with the "relevant bodies" and denied, as it had come too late and was too expensive, $10,000 having already come from MRC coffers.[43] Cuddy dropped out.

Other names on Skoryna's preliminary list included hematologist Dr Ronald Denton and social anthropologist Richard F. Salisbury, both of McGill, the aforementioned epidemiologist William Harding Le Riche of Toronto, and physical anthropologist William S. Laughlin of the University of Wisconsin. In the end, none of these men would make the journey. As they abandoned METEI one by one, Skoryna grew frantic searching for others.

In replacing Toronto epidemiologist Le Riche, Skoryna turned first to J. Fraser Mustard. Interested in the project, Mustard could not leave home for so long, but he supplied materials for taking cholesterol measurements. He also recommended a young American-born hematologist working in his lab, Michael F.X. Glynn. Glynn prevaricated for a long time, and Skoryna appealed to Helen Reid several times to see if she could clarify his intentions about METEI and if he would need a technician. This correspondence went on for weeks and well into autumn.[44] In August, Hellyer noticed that Helen's name was not on the list of proposed travellers, although she had contributed so much; he offered to help.[45] She thanked Hellyer for his vigilance but looked after the omission herself by confronting Skoryna directly. He contended that she had failed to return forms sent to her two months earlier, although she seems not to have believed him. He sent new forms. By 27 August her name had been officially inscribed on the list of METEI members; Skoryna told the experienced pediatrician, "we plan to utilize you[r] well known talent for writing and human contact."[46]

Enraptured with the project, Reid plunged into a crash course in Spanish and helping with other preparations. She approached *Maclean's* magazine and Pierre Berton of the Canadian Broadcasting Corporation (CBC) to suggest METEI as a topic for an article or television program. She thought of items to take that the others had neglected and urged their donation from several companies: hundreds of garbage bags from the Polyethylene Bag Company, materials for diabetic testing, quantities of batteries from Union Carbide, and various gifts for the islanders, including soap, three thousand toothbrushes from Warner Lambert, Elizabeth Arden cosmetics, and toys. She even "sold" trailers to Mead Johnson and to Merck Sharp & Dohme for $2,300 each, and she arranged for Simpson Sears to donate four cooking stoves, which were shipped to Halifax dockyards. Reid gave Skoryna explicit instructions for sending letters of thanks and to whom. Beyond supplies, she offered suggestions about how data entry on computer cards could be accomplished by the "trapped" METEI members on the return journey, a notion that had been approved by Le Riche himself when she bumped into him on the city bus headed to her Spanish lesson. She also consulted Australian-born Roy Ellis, dean of dentistry at the University of Toronto, for pointers on how to examine the teeth of children. Instead of advising Reid, Ellis lectured her, insisting that METEI take a proper dentist and recommending that Skoryna look in the navy. "Who do you hear from oftener than from me?" Helen asked Stanley.[47] Conscious of her role in ensuring the transportation and unravelling the complexities, she told Hellyer, "I feel a personal sense of responsibility that the expedition should be a success. This feeling is very real to me even though it may seem presumptuous on my part."[48]

INTERNATIONAL OUTREACH

In his endeavour to find replacements for the numerous dropouts, Skoryna increased the international dimensions of his team. One of the new recruits was anatomical pathologist Eivind Myhre of Oslo, Norway. Although Myhre's special interest was in cancer, he eventually ended up replacing hematologists Denton and Glynn. Myhre had been at the Munich symposium on peptic ulcer disease in 1962; Skoryna had edited his paper on the effect of cortisone on ulcers for the resultant 1963 volume.[49] In addition to looking for cancer in the Easter Islanders, Myhre would study their blood groups. This kind of work had been done on earlier expeditions because blood groups and haptoglobins might reflect the genetics and geographic origins of the people. A genetic study would also be an additional tool to analyze claims for kinship in the present. However, previous attempts had examined only small samples of the population: 51 islanders by Heyerdahl's expedition[50] and 233 by Raúl Etcheverry and colleagues in 1963.[51] In all his statements, Skoryna emphasized the need for a total survey, a "sample" of "100 per cent," not only of humans but of all living beings.

Aside from the Robertses, who were Canadian citizens, the first British member of the METEI team was Dr Peter Beighton, who was doing his internal medicine residency when he spotted an announcement posted on the bulletin board of London's St Mary's Hospital. A McGill doctor was seeking medical personnel to join an international team of scientists bound for Easter Island; experience in tropical medicine would be an asset. This challenge appealed to Beighton, who had recently returned from military service as a United Nations medical officer in the Congo. With the necessary experience, a desire to see more of the world, and growing curiosity about research, he saw no reason to hesitate. His supervisor, Thomas Hunt, approved. Skoryna had directed Isabel to send the notice to Hunt, whom he had known by reputation and in person through their mutual research interests. For example, Hunt had founded the British Society of Gastroenterology, and he had presided over the entire 1962 World Congress of Gastroenterology, within which Skoryna's peptic ulcer symposium had taken place.[52] Isabel also remembers the visits to Montreal, referring to Hunt as a "classy gentlemen" who dropped by Skoryna's office. His name was on the list of honorary consultants.

The departure of the Canadian cardiologist Cuddy meant that experts in physiology were needed because the IBP vision of "adaptation" included physical fitness and training. Often athletes themselves, these researchers sought to understand the human ability to perform physical "work" by measuring muscle power, oxygen consumption, and the impact of training. Their machines included ergometers, stationary bicycles, and respirometers to measure the volume and composition of expired air. Because physical training can be a form of adaptation, such research had the potential to inform changes that might occur in response to new conditions of labour and environment. Consequently, exercise physiologists were early participants in the IBP in almost every country (see chapter 13).

In seeking an exercise physiologist, Skoryna was directed to Scandinavia. Cuddy had just returned to Winnipeg from a year in Stockholm working at the Karolinska Institute with leading exercise physiologists Irma and Per Olaf Åstrand and their graduate student Bengt Saltin, a physician. Cuddy may have suggested the Åstrands or Saltin. Or Eivind Myhre could have put Skoryna in touch with his Norwegian compatriot Karl Lange Andersen of Oslo, a distinguished physiologist. Andersen's work in exercise physiology looked at the effects of heat and cold on fitness and at temperature adaptation. He had contacts with several Canadian physiologists who were interested in the Arctic.

One September day, the phone rang in the Stockholm laboratory of the Åstrands, and graduate student Björn Ekblom answered. It was Andersen in Norway looking for Bengt Saltin, who had just completed his doctoral dissertation. He wanted to know if Saltin would like to go to Easter Island. Ekblom told him that Saltin was "out of the country." Andersen asked Ekblom, "without knowing [him] at all," if *he* could do the research and would like to go. Ekblom felt qualified, but he explained that he was "fairly broke." Not a problem, he was told; he would be reimbursed. The necessary equipment could be shipped ahead to Puerto Rico; and significantly, unlike the Canadians, it seems that the Scandinavians already owned it.

A Swedish champion athlete in cross-country running and orienteering, Ekblom was due to compete in Helsinki within a few days, but first he had to go west to Oslo to meet Andersen and then back east to Finland. That is how he joined METEI "by mistake." He borrowed the airfare from his father, an orthopedic surgeon. In the short time before his departure, he worked hard to perfect his technique in testing and repairing the machinery; he would have only a few spare parts and would have to maintain it himself.

More help would be needed to conduct the physiology experiments. Andersen had just been transferred to Bergen to become a department head. He could not easily leave the country. Like Thomas Hunt in

England, he posted on the bulletin board Skoryna's notice asking for an "experienced" student. Senior medical student Einar Gjessing spotted the notice. An avid reader of his countryman Heyerdahl, he could claim no expeditionary experience, but he proposed to compensate for this deficiency with considerable advance knowledge of Easter Island and deep motivation. He also hoped that the professor might be impressed by his interest in mathematics and physiology, together with his physical prowess, which included mountain climbing in the Alps and a Norwegian national championship in rowing. He dressed in his "finest clothes" and arrived for the interview more than a half-hour early. Andersen spent forty-five minutes talking to Gjessing, and when they opened the door, nineteen young hopefuls stood waiting outside. "I have found the man," said Andersen, and he sent all the others away. Thrilled to have been chosen, Gjessing also borrowed money from his parents. Ekblom did not yet know Gjessing but was confident that he would be an asset to the research "because he was a champion rower."

Andersen was responsible for one other METEI member, Danish American James ("Jim") McHenry Nielsen. Twenty-two-year-old Jim had finished his undergraduate degree and was headed for medicine, but his father and a family friend, who was a New York City orthopedic surgeon, thought that he would benefit from a "fellowship" year in research before medical school. Influential connections provided a spot with Andersen in Bergen. Nielsen knew that two famous athletes, Ekblom and Gjessing, had already been selected and that he was to assist them. Excited and eager to learn more about the destination, Nielsen telephoned Thor Heyerdahl Jr and went to meet him Oslo, where he was received in a home filled with artifacts and antiques. The others still wonder if Andersen selected young, distractible Nielsen simply to be rid of him. By Jim's own admission, research was never his goal.

REPLACING OTHER DROPOUTS

The Harvard-trained physical anthropologist William S. Laughlin was a logical member of the METEI team, although how Skoryna found him is not known. He had studied isolated populations on the Aleutian Islands and in Greenland. Like Andersen, his extensive work in the Arctic would have made his name familiar to Canadian anthropologists. Indeed, he served on the American Human Adaptability committee of the IBP and participated in the IBP collaboration between Canada and the United States concerning Arctic peoples.[53] But he too ran into commitments that prevented his leaving for several months in the middle of the academic year. He suggested that his graduate student Robert ("Bob") Meier be invited instead. The journey would constitute the fieldwork for Meier's doctoral dissertation. Meier remembers that it was a "spur of the moment" invitation. In advance of the departure, he went to Boston for training in odontology and learned how to make dental impressions, which are plaster casts of teeth. In New York City he met with Harry L. Shapiro at the American Museum of Natural History and contacted Alexander Bearn. Through Bearn, he contacted Maureen Roberts to learn about the plans for blood group testing because these results would be important for his physical anthropology studies.[54]

When William Harding Le Riche dropped off the list, Skoryna looked for others to represent Toronto, like Mustard, Glynn, and Reid. But he also needed an epidemiologist. Isabel remembers typing the letter that appealed to the US Department of Public Health. Two names were suggested, both American physician-epidemiologists from New York City. The first was John L. Cutler with degrees from Harvard University and Tufts University and a doctorate in public health; in June 1964, he was in Berkeley California conducting a survey of cardiovascular disease and stroke in the elderly.[55] The other was Morton Elliot Alpert, a graduate of Syracuse University; following his epidemiology residency in Albany, he was investigating a tuberculosis outbreak in a northeastern US medical school, soon to be published in the *New England Journal of Medicine*.[56] They both joined METEI.

The most spectacular dropout was McGill anthropologist Richard F. Salisbury, although it is not clear that anyone, other than Skoryna and probably Nógrády, ever learned of it. An expert in kinship and social structures, Salisbury had conducted fieldwork in New Guinea during the 1950s and was already a leading figure in the discipline.[57] Salisbury indicated that his collaboration with METEI in developing "economic" and "genealogical" surveys had gone back to late 1962, well before the WHO grant application; however, on 19 August 1964 he wrote a detailed letter to Skoryna confirming their conversation of the previous day, in which they had agreed that he must withdraw. He outlined his reasons for doing so in case they would be helpful, but his criticisms were scathing.

Salisbury was appalled at the haste, the poor preparation, the naive attitude to research methods, and the scholarly disrespect embedded in METEI plans. "To send an untrained worker would be completely wasteful." He could not justify the expense of time and money, "especially if professional workers later spend time in analyzing inaccurate data." He emphasized the importance of theoretical knowledge before gathering data. "Your suggestion that I might train such a worker by giving the equivalent of five years instruction in a two-month crash course I find to be impracticable." He went over the complex proclivities of Polynesian kinship patterns – with frequent pairings, adoptions, and divorce – and the imperative of speaking the local language. He decried the precautionary "arrangements to exclude the islanders from contact with the researchers" in the proposed living facilities.[58] Troubled by the withdrawal of hematologist Denton and not knowing about Myhre's willingness to cover for him, he foresaw the absence of serological and genetic studies as a serious impediment to the full analysis of sociological data. He dismissed as irrelevant the suggestion of Le Riche that the islanders' understanding of disease concepts should be explored. In closing, he offered to continue advising on statistical methods and promised to edit a "working dictionary"; he hoped that the expedition with more "limited objectives" would be "highly successful."

Skoryna was upset by this letter, arriving so late in his plans – although it was still less than a year since he had announced the voyage. Departure from Halifax had been fixed for 16 November 1964. Where would he find expertise to replace Salisbury, and would his negative opinion hamper the search and further damage Skoryna's reputation at McGill?

Soon after, sometime in September, surgical resident Denys Montandon wandered into Skoryna's office in the Donner Building, looking for research options. There he met the striking, articulate Isabel Griffiths. Newly arrived in July, Denys and his Greek-born wife, Cléopâtre, had come to Montreal from Switzerland for his postgraduate training in surgery. Isabel told him about the upcoming expedition. Denys set out to find Skoryna, curious about the plans. Skoryna was blunt. He had enough doctors already – too many. What he needed was a sociologist. Later that evening, Denys told Cléopâtre about the METEI plans; she sent him back to confront Skoryna. "My wife is a sociologist!" exclaimed Denys. "Of course, she cannot go without me." Denys was exaggerating. To fill her time in Canada, the polyglot Cléopâtre had already decided to enrol in a master's program in sociology at McGill. Indeed, she was *interested* in becoming a sociologist and later did so; however, in 1964 she was not yet qualified. Skoryna was desperate, his imagination infinitely vast. The energetic young couple seemed friendly and intelligent enough. Cléopâtre was hired and, with her, Denys. They had the added advantage of a home address in Geneva, which could only help ongoing relations with the WHO. Skoryna kept Salisbury on his list of honorary consultants and added Denys's father, Dr André Montandon.

WRITERS, PHOTOGRAPHERS, AND COMMUNICATORS

The Robertses appeared twice on television in Halifax, once with the captain of HMCS *Cape Scott*, to encourage donations. But it backfired; rather than raising money, the publicity raised the hopes of amateur photographers, archeologists, and even accomplished scientists who pestered them, wanting to "horn in on the loot," offering advice, asking how the work would be conducted, and wondering if METEI would accept outsiders' experiments.[59] Well before details were finalized, people eager to join the mission constructed elaborate arguments to justify their inclusion.

Along these lines, the young English writer and vivacious adventurer Carlotta Hacker had been making her way around the world, stopping to replenish her resources by working in Pakistan and Australia. Her original plan had included Easter Island, although she had no idea how she would get there. When word of METEI reached her, she mounted a no-holds-barred assault on Stanley Skoryna – a campaign worthy of his own techniques. Accustomed to the barrage of would-be travellers, he put her off. The determined redhead kept returning to Montreal to pursue him. Her relentless persistence wore him down, and he met her at the airport, expressing admiration for her perseverance and doubts about how she could help.[60] With a degree in history, she had no qualifications for science, but he finally labelled her role as "research assistant." Back in England, she met with Peter Beighton to discuss the upcoming journey.

George Hrischenko worked for CBC Radio. In his spare time, he was a skilled ham radio operator, as was his wife, Carol. The young father of five was also an avid consumer of world adventure stories, including the works of Heyerdahl. One day he was working on the popular current-events program of storied satirist Max Ferguson when he overheard an item about METEI, with the added information that the CBC was sending along director Bob Williams to make a film for national television. Hrischenko started a vigorous crusade for himself, demanding to know how METEI expected to communicate with organizers in Canada and homes in Europe and North America. He quickly discovered that little thought had been given to the problem. As anxiety mounted about this new complication, he assured the leaders that he was just the person to solve it. Knowing how ham radio operators patched their telephone calls through others, he was certain that a network of helpers would emerge eager to facilitate connections; a goal of every operator was to log time with many different places, the more remote the better. Eventually, he got the nod. The CBC would continue his salary as he worked on the audio for Williams's film and ran the METEI radio. For the winter, he moved his family from their farm to his in-laws' home in Windsor.

Publicity was an important objective for McGill as a means to recognize donors, encourage more contributions, and raise the university's profile. In autumn 1964 McGill's information officer, Albert A. Tunis, initiated correspondence with *Life* magazine. Before a contract could be signed, he and Skoryna went to New York City on 15 October 1964 to discuss mutual concerns and to meet the well-known photojournalist Carl Mydans. METEI organizers were thrilled when *Life* assigned Mydans to cover their story. A staff photographer and correspondent at the magazine for three decades, Mydans and his wife, Shelley, had covered the Second World War and the Korean War. Their riveting images defined the collective memory of those conflicts. *Life* insisted on stringent conditions: there could be no other non-Canadian photographers and no release of any photographs or news stories until it had published Mydans's article. This blackout was modified so that travellers could meet obligations that they had incurred in seeking backers at home; however, they would be allowed to publish only in Canada. *Life* would pay Mydans's salary and donate $5,000 to METEI.[61] It was a trade-off: delay might allow interest to wane, but METEI's anemic coffers stood to benefit from the infusion of *Life*'s prestige and wide circulation. *Life* assured Skoryna and Tunis that Mydans's story would appear quickly. They signed the contract and promised to make the other METEI members sign too. Only three days before departure, the CBC finally agreed to restrict distribution of the audio and visual material that Williams and Hrischenko would bring back.[62]

Two other media people joined METEI, both Canadian. Documentary filmmaker Hector ("Red") Lemieux would make a film for the National Film Board, and reporter David Bell Macfarlane, who had helped to generate the splashy coverage from July forward, would cover the expedition for the *Montreal Star* newspaper. Macfarlane got busy reporting news of upcoming events, naval plans, names of scientists, and fun facts about Rapa Nui. He would not be able to file stories after the mission left Panama, but he was creative in leaving behind information that could be added to short reports conveyed over ham radio through the McGill offices – that is, if the radio worked.

LABORATORY STAFF

Beyond the physical examinations, the medical aspects of the mission would rely on high-quality samples of blood, urine, nasal secretions, and fecal matter, requiring their immediate analysis and/or careful preservation for transport back to Canada. To that end, freezers were necessary and also a lyophilizer to turn liquid serum into powder. Denys Montandon was designated to run the lyophilizer, and he had to make a quick trip to New York City for instruction. Richard Roberts proposed the skilled laboratory technologist Fred Joyce, who had been with the navy's medical branch since the early 1950s. The married father of four lived in Dartmouth, across the harbour from Halifax, and was a skilled amateur photographer specializing in colour.[63] He would be in charge of the blood laboratory.

METEI also proposed to make X-ray examinations of the heads, chests, and teeth of all adults, as well as the hands and wrists of children to assess their "bone age." Chest films would afford an additional glimpse of the spine. The equipment could be left behind as a gift. Who would be in charge of these extremely technical tasks? Skoryna had engaged Montreal radiologist Robert G. Fraser as honorary consultant to METEI, but he could not absent himself from the Royal Victoria Hospital for so long. He designated his head technologist, G. Archibald ("Archie") Wilkinson, to go in his stead. Still single at fifty years of age, Archie was one of the older members of the METEI team. He would have to oversee the entire X-ray setup, including the taking and developing of films. Following a cursory examination by the nonspecialist doctors on the journey, the films would be taken back to Canada for interpretation. He plunged into the planning operations with gusto, and he placed his assistant, young Sally Archer, in charge of the hospital X-ray department during his absence. Archie's colleagues were excited for his adventure and gave him a big send-off, teasing him about his future with the exotic Polynesians. Like Hal Gibbs, Sally had been born in Barbados, and her father was an accomplished ham radio operator who had relocated to Yamachiche in Canada. Archie's many colleagues, friends, and parents began collecting newspaper reports and searching for information about Easter Island and Chile; they assembled a vast collection of clippings, sometimes in triplicate and quadruplicate copies. Sally's father was especially keen on following how METEI would maintain communications with Canada.

HMCS *CAPE SCOTT*, HER CAPTAIN, AND CREW

On 11 May 1964, the navy revealed that the captain of HMCS *Cape Scott* would be Commander C. Anthony Law. Born in London, England, and raised in Quebec and Ontario, Law was an award-winning artist who had studied with Frank Varley and Percyval Tudor-Hart. He presented his first one-man show in 1937. He was also a sailor who had once constructed his own boat. When the war broke out in 1939, Law enlisted first with the army and then with the navy. He was assigned to motor torpedo boats, serving in coastal waters, and he took part in action against the German battleship *Scharnhorst* and sorties in the English Channel just before the Normandy invasion. He was awarded the Distinguished Service Cross. Law was named war artist, and after the conflict, he served on the Arctic patrol ship HMCS *Labrador* and as commanding officer of the destroyer HMCS *Sioux*. His appointment to command *Cape Scott* on its Easter Island journey was meant to be a quiet, end-of-career reward that would provide ample time and unusual subjects for painting.[64]

During May and June 1964, the navy began planning for the expedition – both for METEI and for provisioning the ship and crew for the voyage. The ship's officers, engineer Robert Molson, and Skoryna met to discuss logistics on 11 and 12 June on board *Cape Scott*. Departure in mid-November would allow the team to be on Easter Island just before the arrival of the annual supply ship, which notoriously brought with it an epidemic of *kokongo*. METEI would want blood samples both before and after its arrival.[65] They relied on a twenty-two-page list of cargo prepared at McGill in twenty-four categories detailing all the food and equipment, from which they determined locations for storage.[66] Using the ship's estimated speed of 10.5 knots and its fuel consumption of 9.4 barrels per hour, they calculated the dates of landfall at the various ports and the volume of fuel needed for the entire voyage – a total of 16,000 barrels, or 6,000 barrels above the ship's annual allotment. Extra provisions, equipment, and fuel could be taken on at Puerto Rico's San Juan (spelled "San Wan" in the first documents of the Royal Canadian Navy), at Balboa, and at the ship's goodwill stops in South America. The designated staging area was Building D-17 at HMC Dockyard Halifax, where the ship would be altered and provisioned. Hatches were to be enlarged and consideration given to expanding the forward ballast tanks in order to increase the ship's range by 1,000 barrels.[67]

McGill engineer Robert Molson, who had been working on designs for the distillation units, suffered a serious skiing accident in the late winter of 1963–64 and had to withdraw from the expedition, although he remained interested in all its endeavours. Bitterly disappointed, he joked with Roberts that the proposed cargo contained no evidence "of supplies for plaster casts (ha, ha, ha)."[68] He corresponded with experts in Barbados about distillation units, and he hoped that the navy would see fit to include the helicopter that he'd spied sitting on the deck of

Cape Scott in an official photo that had been circulated. He and Skoryna decided that they also needed a radio operator, a cook and helper, two or three technicians, and ten crew members, and they hoped the navy would supply them. He drafted requests for Roberts to sign because "your name will pack more of a wallop to the Navy than ours."[69]

With the expanded scientific goals and the tight relationship with the navy, Skoryna decided to replace the injured Molson with a director of the "physical plant," a former military officer with leadership experience. Retired Air Vice Marshal John A. Easton was a "security expert" who had held a number of senior positions with the Royal Canadian Air Force following the war. In 1957 Easton had witnessed a nuclear test from a distance of 153 kilometres; it nearly blinded him, although he was wearing sunglasses.[70] His involvement with the fated Avro Arrow resulted in his leading a Canadian team sent to California to study alternate systems in 1958. It also meant that he was interviewed by many of the numerous authors who explored that famous story; the Avro Arrow's plans had to be destroyed, he believed, because it was "too damn good."[71] Easton would run interference between Skoryna, the scientists, and the navy to ensure that all operations ran smoothly. Few of the scientist travellers remember him, suggesting either that he had little to do or that he did his work well.

But Roberts and Law were getting worried. There were far too many loose ends. Since early 1964 Roberts had been thinking of important matters that Skoryna had never addressed in his communications with would-be travellers. What about passports? What about malpractice insurance while METEI worked in a different country? What about surgical equipment, inoculations, and documentation? Exactly how many people were travelling, and how many would be female? What about support staff? On 25 August he sent another lengthy letter to Skoryna citing the ambiguities that he and Tony Law needed him to clarify and insisting that Skoryna and his "tame Air Vice Marshal (whose name I have forgotten)" come to Halifax for another face-to-face meeting. Skoryna needed to write to all members about vaccinations. Noting that Panamanian authorities were "very strict," he wrote, "*Please* insist on certificates as doctors are notoriously careless about their personal immunization status and by no means always truthful."[72]

Roberts and Law discovered that Surgeon Rear Admiral Blair MacLean was "not too favorably inclined" to METEI since "we are taking away part of his important repair facilities for four months."[73] Consequently, Roberts recommended working around him through Minister of Defence Paul Hellyer or waiting for MacLean's retirement and replacement by the more amenable Surgeon Commodore Walter Elliot. Confusion over whether the personnel requests should come from navy men Roberts and Law or from Skoryna as the leader meant that some fell through the cracks. Just five weeks before departure, Skoryna announced in a cryptic single line, "We have got a cook!"[74] For Roberts, the lack of clarity on logistical details was a source of mounting anxiety that heralded much greater conflict to come.

In addition to the seamen who would support the ship and move her cargo, the armed forces contributed team members to METEI. Major Alexander Taylor was a dentist serving with the Royal Canadian Dental Corps based with the navy in Halifax; his role would be to examine the teeth of the islanders and take plaster impressions. Roy Ellis, dean of the University of Toronto's dental school, later claimed to have recruited Taylor for METEI, although he left out the key role of Dr Helen Reid. As an inveterate researcher with a special interest in children, Ellis provided Taylor with materials for making the impressions of teeth.[75] Taylor's addition to the team came as welcome news to Bob Meier, who had been worried that he would not be able to do the dental procedures properly.

Like the laboratory technologist Fred Joyce, other METEI members came from the navy. Petty Officer Tom Galley was assigned to take photographs.[76] Two members of the Women's Royal Canadian Naval Service (WRCNS, or "wrens") were also part of the mission, both single and both having served in Canada's navy during the Second World War. It would be the first time in the navy's history that women had been included on any naval voyage longer than a single day's duration, a fact frequently touted in the press.[77] Lieutenant Rita Katherine Dwyer held a degree from the University of Toronto and, with fluency in Spanish, had worked in Cuba and with Canadian embassies in Argentina, Portugal, and Turkey before returning to the navy in 1959. Lieutenant Mary Olive King had a background in science, served in the statistical office of Atomic Energy Canada, and was a much-appreciated volunteer at the Spitz astronomical observatory in Halifax. She owned a Questar 3.5, considered the "Rolls Royce" telescope of its day, which she packed along for the METEI journey and later donated to the Royal Astronomical Society Centre Library in Halifax.[78] Some contend that Dwyer got the nod because of her language skills and that King was sent along as female companion and chaperone. The navy's decision to allow women influenced Skoryna's willingness to take Hacker and probably also Reid and Cléopâtre Montandon.[79]

Chief Petty Officer Harry Crosman and Able Seaman Robert A. Fulton were also assigned to the team that would remain on the island; they were to look after mechanical and electrical equipment. Several naval officers, some nearing retirement, were posted to *Cape Scott*, most at the rank of lieutenant commander. They plunged into their METEI duties with gusto, loading and managing cargo as well as planning for the camp's setup, water, and sanitation. HMCS *Cape Scott* also had her own doctor, Surgeon Lieutenant Gilbert Joseph Bérubé, admired for his operatic singing voice (see appendix D, table D.2).

The youngest naval officer was tall, handsome Lieutenant Charles L. Westropp, whose memories of METEI remain vivid. Born in London, England, but raised in La Paz, Bolivia, because of his father's foreign-office posting, he went to sea at age fifteen, crossing the equator several times as he travelled the globe with the merchant marine. He joined the Canadian navy at age twenty-one in 1958. By 1964 he was "getting on well" and moving up the naval ladder, but one day he was summoned by his career officer, who "told" him that he'd been posted as navigator to the aging, slow *Cape Scott* with "old and spent" officers. "You must be out of your flaming mind, sir," said the affronted rising officer.

"Shut up and listen," came the reply.

For Westropp and his aging mates, Easter Island was a "great opportunity," "like a holiday with pay," and they were eager to participate. The logistical nightmare of unloading an entire village – complete with a laboratory, clinic, radio station, truck, and all the housing, food, fuel, and supplies for a thirty-eight-person team – onto a remote island with no harbour was a delicious challenge, one that would allow the threatened navy to shine. Westropp would navigate the journey of 9,012 kilometres by sextant.

In one short year, Skoryna had convinced the Canadian government to donate a naval ship and crew, garnered approvals from Chile, identified qualified (and less than qualified) scientists and support staff, and assembled the equipment and facilities needed for research and living on the remote island. He had not yet, however, secured sufficient funding. But the planned airport was looming, and he needed to get going. He prepared his dream for liftoff.

Table 2.1 Members of METEI who travelled to Rapa Nui

Member	Specialty	Origin
Alpert, Dr Morton Elliot	Epidemiology	Albany, NY
Beighton, Dr Peter	Medical examination	London, UK
Boudreault, Armand	Virology	Montreal, QC
Brody, Dr Garry S.	Medical examination	Arlington, VA
Crosman, CPO[a] Harry	Mechanics, electricity, RCN	Halifax, NS
Cutler, Dr John L.	Epidemiology	Berkeley, CA
Donoso, Dr Gonzalo	Nutrition	Santiago, Chile
Dwyer, Lt Rita Katherine	Interpretation, RCN	Ottawa, ON
Easton, AVM[b] John A.	Physical plant	Montreal, QC
Eccles, Ana Maria	Interpretation	Halifax, NS
Efford, Ian Ecott	Ecology, biology	Vancouver, BC
Ekblom, Björn Thoreson[c]	Work physiology	Stockholm, Sweden
Fulton, Robert A.	Mechanics, electricity, RCN	Dartmouth, NS
Gibbs, Dr Harold C.	Human, animal parasitology	Hudson, QC
Gillingham, Thomas Colin	Kitchen, catering	Ottawa, ON
Gjessing, Einar Tandberg[c]	Work physiology	Bergen, Norway
Griffiths, Isabel	Interpretation	Montreal, QC
Hacker, Carlotta	Research Assistance	Farnham, UK
Hrischenko, George	CBC, radio communication	Windsor, ON
Joyce, CPO[a] Fred	Laboratory technologist, RCN	Dartmouth, NS
King, Lt Mary Olive	Research assistance, RCN	Armdale, NS
Lemieux, Hector ("Red")	NFB filmmaker	Dollard des Ormeaux, QC
Macfarlane, David Bell	*Montreal Star* journalist	Montreal, QC
Mathias, Jack[c]	Ecology	Vancouver, BC
Meier, Robert John[c]	Anthropology	Madison, WI
Montandon, Dr Denys M.	Medical examinations and laboratory	Montreal; Geneva, Switzerland
Montandon, Cléopâtre[c]	Sociology	Montreal; Geneva, Switzerland
Murphy, Dr David A.	Animal and human medicine	Boston, MA

Mydans, Carl	Photographer for *Life* magazine	New York City, NY
Myhre, Dr Eivind	Pathology	Olso, Norway
Nielsen, James McH.[c]	Work physiology	Hackensack, NJ
Nógrády, Georges L.	Microbiology	Montreal, QC
Reid, Dr Helen Evans	Medical examinations	Toronto, ON
Roberts, Dr Maureen	Medical examinations	Halifax, NS
Roberts, Dr Richard H.	Medical examinations	Halifax, NS
Skoryna, Dr Stanley C.	Director	Montreal, QC
Taylor, Dr Alexander G.	Ondontology, RCN	Shearwater, NS
Wilkinson, G. Archibald	Radiography	Montreal, QC
Williams, Robert	CBC filmmaker	Halifax, NS

[a] Chief Petty Officer; [b] Air Vice Marshal; [c] medical or graduate student

3

The Journey Out

Before the age of space travel, many "expeditions" for scientific and exploratory purposes conveyed people, equipment, dwellings, laboratories – entire "villages" – by sea. The Royal Canadian Navy embraced the Medical Expedition to Easter Island with enthusiasm, possibly because it would showcase the navy's distinctive abilities in the face of Minister of Defence Paul Hellyer's imminent merger of the armed forces. The navy personnel examined the logs of Easter Island explorers and recent descriptions of the island, which emphasized the total absence of a harbour and electricity, the paucity of fresh water and trees for construction, and the marginal existence of the islanders, whose meagre provisions must not be further stressed by the presence of the Canadian sailors and METEI travellers. The planners also noted the past history of *kokongo* epidemics provoked by visiting ships, recognizing that their arrival might bring similar "first contact" illness.[1] In conveying large numbers of people and all their provisions to a shore that had no port, the navy drew on its expertise from the Normandy landings twenty years earlier. Perhaps the officers also studied the meticulous plans for polar expeditions that had transported necessities for the survival and work of the scientist-explorers.

Several teams had visited Easter Island in recent years: an American group led by archeologist William Mulloy raised the seven statues at Ahu Akivi in 1960; Francis Mazière, from France, stayed several months in 1963 or early 1964; and from the 1950s to the early 1960s, Chilean teams had attempted health surveys on genetics and disease, including on the prevalence of leprosy.[2] The 1963 Chilean surveyors enjoyed funding from the Rockefeller Institute and travelled on the annual supply ship to obtain blood samples; they published several articles, including one in *Nature* in January 1964.[3] METEI did not know of these recent precedents until after it reached Rapa Nui. The revelation would provoke dismay as well as annoyance with Stanley Skoryna for his rushed, uninformed planning.

METEI ASSEMBLES IN HALIFAX

Departure was fixed for 16 November 1964. For several weeks, navy officials had been busy calculating distances and estimating times and quantities of fuel. HMCS *Cape Scott* lay in her berth at Halifax, ready to receive the estimated 100 tons of cargo, itemized on the twenty-four-category manifest prepared at McGill University.[4] In the navy's stilted lingo, the logistical plan "was somewhat nullified due to the non-delivery of materials from the originating companies." Less than a month prior to departure, "approximately 90% of the cargo had not generated."[5]

The material began arriving with only a week to spare. Under the leadership of Lieutenant Robert Manzer, the seamen scrambled to stow it all safely and carefully, trying to keep track of its location on board. They had to split up into several teams, later trying to combine their lists of items in each hold. Nevertheless, some boxes could not be found until they were off-loaded weeks later. "Many peculiar storage problems arose such as the Super Frozen Culture Media, which had to be maintained at minus 70 degrees C (–90 F)."[6] The flattened ATCO "shoebox" trailers were stored on the deck, both fore and aft.

Commander Tony Law and his artist wife, Jane Shaw, enjoyed a tremendous farewell party hosted by their Boulderwood neighbours, who had composed musical parodies to celebrate the forthcoming journey. Law packed all their creations for recycling in the onboard entertainments: "Disenchanted Island" (to "Some Enchanted Evening"), "Easter Island Lament" (to "Lovely Bunch of Coconuts"), and "Tony and the Statue" (to "The Lion and Albert").

Several travellers gathered in Montreal. Bob Meier and Jim Nielsen joined Montrealers David Murphy, Hal Gibbs, Armand Boudreault, Archie Wilkinson, Denys and Cléopâtre Montandon, Georges Nógrády, and Stanley Skoryna. METEI cook Colin Gillingham came from Ottawa. The media were invited to snap their photos as they boarded the train for Halifax on 14 November (figure 3.1). They met in the "bar car" for a celebratory drink while the train chugged east through the Gaspésie and into Nova Scotia. Gibbs remembers Boudreault pointing out the Acadian part of the Maritimes, a traditional home to francophones. Helen Reid described her impression of Boudreault as "a distinguished virologist ... aggressively Canadian."[7] Cléopâtre recalls the virologist fretting over his

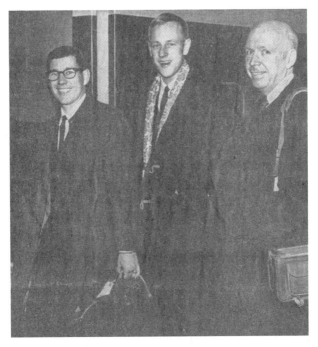

Figure 3.1 *From left*, Robert Meier, Jim Nielsen,
and Archie Wilkinson bound for Easter Island.
Montreal Star, 16 November 1964, section 3, 31,
Wilkinson Papers.

cells and freezers, which had to be kept deeply frozen or his collections
would be ruined; he was using dry ice on the train. Based on these casual
conversations, Meier told his diary, "it would seem that a great deal
of organization and integration of the research program is needed; too
much overlap and confusion are inevitable."

Carlotta Hacker bumped into Helen Reid on another train coming
from Toronto to Halifax. A rigorous interrogation by the pediatrician
with "alarmingly acute intelligence" made Carlotta feel fraudulent and
outclassed, although she soon realized that Reid was a great tease.[8] Helen
flew from Halifax to Boston to say goodbye to her daughter, Judith, an
anthropology doctoral student at Harvard University. Carlotta checked
into a hotel for her last night on *terra firma*. The following morning,
Maureen and Richard Roberts took her home for a hot lunch libated
with large glasses of gin. Then they went to the airport to collect "a
Norwegian physiologist and an English doctor" before boarding *Cape*

Scott together with the Montreal travellers who arrived directly from their train.[9] Archie Wilkinson was left alone at the railway station guarding the luggage until a navy truck came to collect it. Shipboard cocktails, followed by a lively press conference, put travellers in good spirits as they searched for their cabins and new cabin-mates, some of whom were complete strangers. Bob Meier found that he had a cabin to himself, but his carefully packed luggage had been "misplaced."

DEPARTURE AND STORM AT SEA

On Monday, 16 November, a pipe over the ship's broadcast system roused the company at 6:30 a.m. Carlotta went exploring and found Isabel Griffiths – the "most beautiful woman" she had ever seen.[10] No one else was around. Together they set out in search of food and found a splendid buffet waiting in the ward room; meals were to be self-serve, as no table was large enough for all the officers and the METEI members. The morning papers in Halifax and Montreal were once again full of METEI and *Cape Scott*; the press conference had been a success. Back in Montreal, Al Tunis hoped it would translate into more donations.

Everyone crept out on deck. It was cold, with light snow falling. The families of sailors had gathered on the pier with naval dignitaries for the final farewell. Student musicians from the teacher's college delivered a fanfare, and a naval marching band played "Auld Lang Syne" and a rousing version of "Heart of Oak," which is the official march of both the British and Canadian navies. Lines were let go, and the ship slowly drifted away (figure 3.2). METEI passengers were surprised when, in answer to the crowd on shore, a *Cape Scott* piper appeared on the upper deck above their heads, kilted in Nova Scotia tartan, to play "Tangle o' the Isles," "Will Ye No Come Back Again?" and "Speed Bonny Boat."[11] Cléopâtre wrote in her diary that "little by little the silhouette of the port drifted into the horizon, uniting itself with the land, until it too soon disappeared."[12]

The first day out was calm, and passengers enjoyed meeting each other and learning about their scientific projects. Denys and Cléopâtre were grilled by David Macfarlane for the *Montreal Star*, and they found themselves at the captain's table for dinner with Bob Meier and Skoryna. She wore her best dress, something that, Carlotta decided, "looked as if it had come straight from Dior."[13] Law regaled them with his adventures in the Arctic. Skoryna wanted to know the name of the Swiss president because he would send greetings to the leaders of all the nations of METEI members. Meier was impressed with the "tasty and substantial" food and relieved when his luggage was located in the machine shop.[14]

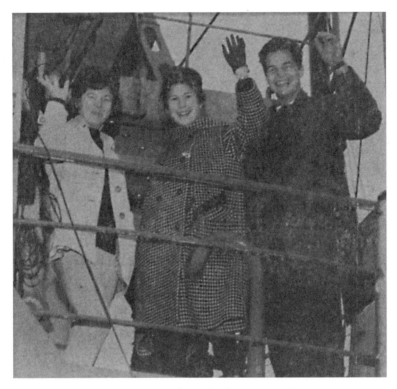

Figure 3.2 Carlotta Hacker (*left*) with Cléopâtre and Denys
Montandon waving goodbye on board HMCS *Cape Scott*. Is that coat
Dior? Halifax *Mail Star*, 16 November 1964, LAC, Law Scrapbook,
vol. 3, by permission of the Halifax *Chronicle Herald*.

But a sudden low pressure system swept down from north west of
Newfoundland, and *Cape Scott* found herself in the midst of a raging
North Atlantic gale. In the words of the captain, it "seemed to cover the
ocean" with "huge angry mountains and hurricane force winds."[15] A massive jolt roused Denys and Cléopâtre and sent all the drawers and loose
objects in their cabin flying. The electricity failed. Meier reported that
everyone felt "a little woozy"; he and Jim Nielsen ate breakfast alone.

The winds continued at 60 knots for two days. Cléopâtre described
the rolls with swells, some twelve metres high, that tilted the ship 15
degrees off the vertical in either direction. Reid too wrote of the lengthy,
apprehensive waiting: "When you have nothing to do but lie and feel the
ship struggling and straining, you become aware of all her sounds and
motions ... a shudder passes along her length and she rolls crazily ... she

hangs between sky and sea and then the long protesting shudder as if the task were repugnant. She braces herself for the next roll and tortured wallow and starts the cycle of protest again."[16]

During the storm, Skoryna convened the first formal meeting of METEI members, but a big wave washed in, disrupting the decorum. "Quite a sight," Meier wrote. Hacker described the "wall of water two feet high" that crashed across the room and splashed down to the galley, provoking "shrieks of laughter" from below.[17] The "chaos" of that meeting seemed prophetic of greater trouble ahead; some METEI members swore off ocean travel forever.[18]

The METEI cargo stored on deck made the ship unstable. On top of the ATCO trailers forward of the bridge, the navy had placed "a huge box" containing another trailer destined for the Royal Canadian Air Force VS880 Squadron in Bermuda. At 17 metres across, it was "so wide that it extended the full breadth of the ship and so high that it obscured the view from the bridge for anyone under six feet tall."[19] Rather than fight the storm, the captain decided to steer a cautious course to the southeast. As many travellers later remembered, they were going to Easter Island but were pointed at Africa. "That's rubbish," maintains navigator Charles Westropp a half-century later; the adjustment was a wise manoeuvre to weather the storm. Law wrote to Jane that "the only safe course" was to "run before the wind," heading "towards Africa." His cabin was "a mess," the gift rubber plant, meant to keep him company, destroyed. "We buried it at sea."[20]

The next day was "draggy," Meier wrote; the speed at 10:00 p.m. was only 2 knots, and they had made "4.8 miles in four hours." "Wow! Easter Island here we come."[21] Cléopâtre also noted the "somnolence."[22] Law fondly remembered *Cape Scott* as the only ship that, with its engines going full speed, could be overtaken by a seagull.[23] The promised Spanish lesson was cancelled because no one was likely to attend. Finally, on 19 November, the weather was fair, no cargo had been damaged, and the only casualty was thirty hours from the schedule. Skoryna attributed this fortunate outcome to the impressive skill of the captain.[24]

LIFE ABOARD AND BERMUDA

With the calm, Law held his first art class for twelve students; he recommended certain oil paints for purchase at the next port. The sailors would make palettes for the budding artists in the ship's carpentry shop. Expeditionists could also study their mimeographed Rapanui dictionary of 1,500 words, and, finally, the Spanish lessons began in earnest.

Isabel Griffiths and Ana Maria Eccles organized the twice-daily language sessions around simple greetings and basic communication that would help interactions with the islanders. Skoryna deemed the lessons important, although not compulsory. Peter Beighton was a devotee and learned quickly, one of the best pupils. Law tried to follow the teaching too but confessed to Jane that he was having as much difficulty with this new language as he did with French, which he was trying to use with the Montandons and Boudreault. Isabel taught songs to improve the accents of her students, sympathizing with them because of her own troubles pronouncing English. With her unerring ear, Hacker overheard Isabel consulting an American: "When you say 'esheep,' doing you mean something that says 'ba-a-a,' or do you mean this boat we are in?"

"I never say 'esheep,' baby," the man replied.[25]

Cape Scott came alongside the Canadian naval station at Bermuda at 6:00 p.m. on 20 November. This stop had not been part of the original plan but was added to serve the navy's wish to transport the large trailer. Law was delighted to be rid of it; now all his officers could see from the bridge.

METEI members sent their first letters home. Skoryna wrote to Tunis to thank him for his "wonderful help," expressing the hope that the "bad weather" and "poor beginning means a good end." He also inquired about the extent of the "blackout" imposed by the *Life* magazine contract. He advised Tunis to inform Red Lemieux, who was still in Canada, about these rules and reported that Macfarlane, Reid, Rita Dwyer, and Fred Joyce, who were writing for Canadian news sources, had "signed" the contract and would abide by it too. Many others were asking about the embargo on news, and Skoryna did not relish imposing restrictions on photographs or interviews at various ports of call, nor did he want the publishers of *Life* to "feel that we are doing anything behind their back."[26]

At Bermuda, the local naval liaison officer, Lieutenant Commander Douglas J. Fisher, invited METEI members and senior officers to his home in Hamilton for a glittering cocktail party. They were regaled with sailor stories and by Skoryna, who described his immigrant beginnings in Montreal with self-deprecating wit. Enchanted by the lush island, the younger members regrouped at the Hotel Princesse, found the bar Gazebo, and wandered the moonlit streets in the perfumed air, returning to *Cape Scott* at 2:00 a.m.

The ship sailed again at first light, but METEI members barely noticed. Everyone was feeling a little worse for wear. Meier wrote that it was a "bad morning and meeting!"[27] The hangover was so powerful, Cléopâtre observed, that even the naval officers abstained from alcohol at their noon meal.[28] METEI scientists were reminded of the importance of understanding each other's work to avoid duplication and inefficiencies. A kind of uneasiness lurked under these discussions, as if they realized that the planning had been too hasty and too rough around the edges; much more should have been done before they left Halifax. Carlotta admitted to one of the Americans that she did not know what she would be doing; he laughed and replied that neither did he.[29] Soon it was decided that the daily meetings should take place in smaller groups devoted to similar tasks. Cléopâtre made friends with the American epidemiologists John Cutler and Elliot Alpert and offered to help with their census; they, in turn, would help with her survey.[30] Those expecting to examine patients revised the paper forms that Richard Roberts had developed, which had multiple choices with boxes for check marks that would allow easy transfer to punch cards.[31]

Law reported to his superiors about the entertainments. "To keep my ship's company and the Expedition members amused in their off-duty moments, a variety of activities have been organized; these include movies, bingo, volleyball on the flight deck, swimming in two canvas pools that have been built on the forecastle and the flight deck, and 'cook outs.' Probably the most popular are the 'cook-outs'; two 45-gallon drums serve as barbecues for the evening meal. When the food is finished, members of the ship's company and the scientists stage an impromptu talent show."[32] Cléopâtre thought it was "very interesting to see the ways these men found to amuse themselves as they passed long days between the sky and the sea."[33] She did not like the first movie, an English comedy, although Bob Meier enjoyed *Stitch of Time* (1963) and *Rhino* (1964), "shot in Zululand [with] good photos of fauna."[34] The talent shows featured Skoryna and a Ukrainian sailor on their accordions, David Murphy and Jim Nielsen with their banjos, and Cléopâtre and Denys singing and playing guitar, and later filmmaker Lemieux served as master of ceremonies (figure 3.3).[35]

Sundays were to be days of rest throughout the entire mission, marked with a short religious service. Carlotta was pressed into playing a portable organ, although she claimed to know only one hymn.[36] Skoryna, Dwyer, and Lieutenant Commander Channing D. Gillis read the Bible lessons, and John A. Easton led the naval hymn (figure 3.4). Commander Law was moved by the occasion: "This must be the first time that Protestants and Catholics, both men and women, have joined together in prayer aboard one of Her Majesty's Canadian ships."[37] Cléopâtre and Denys were amazed by these quaint, eclectic devotions – "prayers for sailors, the Queen of England, and the Virgin Mary, accompanied by a few canticles" – rituals that had long faded from their European home.[38]

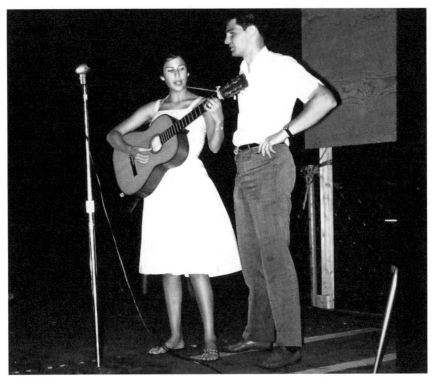

Figure 3.3 Cléopâtre and Denys Montandon at shipboard talent show.
Photo Georges Nógrády.

The temperature rose as *Cape Scott* entered the Caribbean, stifling during the day and uncomfortable at night, leading some to sleep on deck. Volleyball and sunbathing on the lounge chairs on the flight deck were popular fair-weather activities for the women and a few men (figure 3.5).

A bikini caused a stir. Cléopâtre now denies that she wore a bikini while aboard, but all the men remember otherwise, and her journal proves her wrong: she wore it at least once but "did not really feel at ease." Cléopâtre was in the early weeks of pregnancy. She and Denys learned the news just before departure; however, if everything went as planned, they should be back in Canada well before the baby was due. They did not announce her condition. A medical member of METEI, who wishes to remain anonymous, cannot now remember exactly when the pregnancy became public knowledge, but he recalls the episode vividly. Cléopâtre was "well-endowed in the front," he said, and with her scant attire, the heat, the sun, the torpor of the engines, and "the waft of pheromones," the dozens of

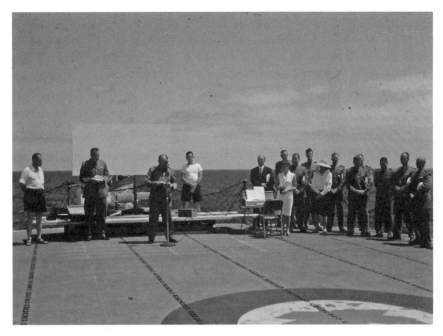

Figure 3.4 "Church service" on board HMCS *Cape Scott*, 6 December 1964. Harold Gibbs (*left*) and Commander Tony Law (*at microphone*) with Stanley Skoryna and Carlotta Hacker (*at organ*). Photo Georges Nógrády.

red-blooded seamen were spellbound; "the ship almost came to a halt." He recalls that the captain asked her not to wear the bikini, although her discomfiture suggests that he had no need. Young Jack Mathias confided in his diary, "God! What a bikini! She drives all the METEI guys and all the sailors out of their minds."[39] In Hacker's memory, Cléopâtre's bikini "practically caused a mutiny." The captain did not restrict attire, but he confined sunbathing to the bridge, at the opposite end of the ship from the pool. There is no doubt: Cléopâtre wore that bikini.

The novelty of women passengers added both levity and curiosity to the journey. Law observed to Jane that the "girls" were "good sports" and had survived the storm better than the men, although "Mrs. Roberts" was laid up for days.[40] Hacker remembered the surprising patience of the officers and crew, as the women would get lost, or deliberately use incorrect labels for the ship's anatomy, or "accidentally" contravene navy protocol.[41] On Sunday, 29 November, "all eight girls really dug in" to prepare an on-deck "cook out" of hamburgers and hot dogs for the entire crew of 230 men; Law reported to his wife that "the sailors really

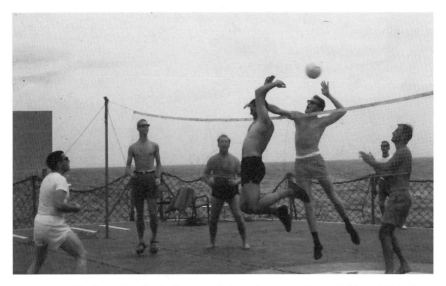

Figure 3.5 Shipboard volleyball. From *left*, unknown, Björn Ekblom, Eivind Myhre, Elliot Alpert, Red Lemieux, unknown, and Peter Beighton. Photo Georges Nógrády.

enjoyed that," telling her, once again, that "the girls were all very good sports – or I should say the ladies."[42]

At sea while enjoying the substantial navy cuisine, METEI members realized that their own designated "chef," a twenty-four-year-old, seasick lad from Inverness, Scotland, had no cooking experience at all. No one remembers how or why young Colin Gillingham was hired; his address was a large house in Ottawa's Lower Town, and he had come to Canada with the air force, having worked as a steward and correctional officer. Helen Reid believed that he had served in a diplomatic household.[43] She and Maureen Roberts adopted the young man, instructing him in basic culinary skills; he became proficient at making bread. Every traveller was aware that the female participation was a precedent. For the most part, it was a matter of pride.

The company realized that METEI did not have its own flag. The lab tech Fred Joyce described what happened for the Canadian papers. Commander Law sketched the METEI logo on some green cloth scavenged from unused pennants, and "the ladies of the company invaded the sail-maker's quarters and put sewing machines to work," stitching the green logo to a white background and trimming loose ends "with manicure scissors" (figure 3.6).[44] This unique and respectable ensign was flying high on 24 November as *Cape Scott* reached Puerto Rico, docking at the American naval base in San Juan – which the navy's logistics plans continued to refer to as "San Wan."[45] The new banner was a popular backdrop for photographs.

PUERTO RICO AND THE TEAM GROWS

At San Juan, new expeditionists joined the group, among them Evind Myhre, Björn Ekblom, David Murphy, and Carl Mydans. On shore, Law, Skoryna, and Easton dined with Mydans and his wife, Shelley. They had been the first husband-and-wife photojournalist team on staff for the Time Life company. In 1941 they had been captured by Japanese soldiers and interned as prisoners of war, first in Manila and then in Shanghai. They were not released until a prisoner exchange in 1943. Mydans's photographs of the destruction caused by a 1948 earthquake in Japan are legendary. METEI members were given to understand that Mydans was, in the words of both the captain and the navigator, "the world's greatest living photographer"; they were to treat him with awe and deference. Mydans lost no time interviewing his fellow travellers, extracting bits of information that they would rather not reveal. In particular, in the case of the Montandons, he probed their future plans. Cléopâtre admitted that she was not "yet" a sociologist.[46] Subjected to the same, Garry Brody found him to be "very serious about his work but aloof" and doubted the sincerity of his compliments.[47]

Skoryna dashed off another letter to Tunis, claiming that the *Life* photographer "[C]arl is happy." But Stanley kept worrying about media coverage and its relationship to the debt. The Ottawa papers had described the journey, and he was relieved that, unlike the captain, they did not use "Mrs." when referring to Maureen Roberts. There were "only two married couples ... all scientists." He asked Tunis to "write to the *Ottawa Journal* and/or *Ottawa Citizen* to suggest that Lt. Dwyer will prepare special reports for them if they wish (with my help). This will appeal to the secretarial staff in Ottawa, which forms about 60% of the population."[48] Did this scrupulousness over female sensibilities and professionalism stem from a tiny streak of feminism or from his growing financial despair?

Again, METEI members left the ship to go exploring, although rules of the American base did not make it easy. Law was disappointed in San Juan as a place of shore leave for his crew – too far from town, too few police, "and a great deal of knifings, etc."[49] There were receptions, dinners, strolls in the old town, visits to the beach, a trip to the Yunque

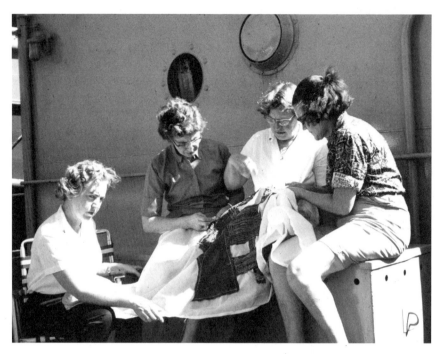

Figure 3.6 Four "ladies" sewing the METEI flag from scraps. *From left*, Lieutenant Rita Dwyer, Dr Maureen Roberts, Lieutenant Mary King, and Dr Helen Reid. Photo Fred Joyce.

rainforest by taxi, and a lot of shopping at the PX store. Several members invested in camera equipment. Some fell ill after eating paella in a traditional restaurant. Reid became so dehydrated that she needed intravenous therapy; the ship's doctor sat up with her all night.[50] Cléopâtre and Denys were curious about the relations between Puerto Ricans and Americans; did the islanders not want independence?[51] Wilkinson wrote his parents a fourth letter since sailing on 16 November, reporting on his adventures, his photography, and his sunburn, closing always with, "take good care of yourselves." He warned that, soon, the only contact would be radio. Impressed with the interesting new places and solemn about his responsibilities, Archie was homesick.

At San Juan, *Cape Scott* racked up another delay of four hours because some equipment, which had been too late for loading in Halifax, had failed to catch up. When the team found out that it was still in Baltimore, Brody made arrangements to have it air-lifted to Balboa, the last stop. He recalls that one missing item was the washing machine, which arrived without its lid and a bill of $1,500 for transport – a bill that was never paid. Now *Cape Scott* was thirty-six hours behind schedule, but "a following wind and favorable current" enabled her to make up time, and she had reached the Canal Zone back on schedule by 1 December. Wrapping up his monthly report for November, Commander Law wrote, "Cape Scott has spent 13 days at sea, 17 days in harbor, and covered 2494.5 miles."[52]

George Hrischenko kept to himself, preferring the company of the crew. The sailors had their own mess, and when he learned that all the food came from the same galley, he decided to eat with them – "my people," he said. During the stops, he worried about future radio communications. Things were working fine on the ship, although he had to stop transmitting whenever the captain needed the ship's radio. But he knew that Rapa Nui had no trees, and he was not sure if his signals would be heard. He made a point of gathering long bamboo poles to serve as potential antennae. He also bonded with the navy's radio operator and those he met on shore, seeking tips for how to stay in contact with home. Westropp remembers tension over the radio; Hrischenko remembers the captain's impatience when he wanted to take to the air.

PANAMA AND THE TEAM IS COMPLETE

Crossing the Panama Canal promised excitement for the METEI members. All the filmmakers and photographers, professional and amateur alike, assembled at the railings to document each step. At 5:30 a.m. on 1 December, *Cape Scott* was taken over by an American pilot and his special crew, who were to guide her for the six-hour journey covering 77 kilometres. Locks rose up from the Atlantic to a central artificial lake, and then there were more locks down to Balboa and the Bridge of the Two Americas at the Pacific. The fee was 90 cents a ton, "an expensive transit for you the taxpayer," Tony Law wrote to Jane.[53] Still aware of her own role in implicating the navy, Helen told her family how great a draw it would be on "your good taxpayer money. Guilty me!"[54]

George Hrischenko was delighted to observe the reaction of the crew of an American destroyer headed in the opposite direction and berthed in a lock beside *Cape Scott*. METEI's "shapely secretaries ... in their bikinis" – a "new invention" at the time, George noted – were sunbathing on the helicopter deck at the fantail of the ship; these "nearly naked women (and guys) guzzled booze and beer." Word spread quickly on the destroyer, and so many American sailors crowded the rail to observe this scene of wonder that George thought their ship would capsize. He couldn't resist. As they slowly descended and *Cape Scott* slowly rose, obscuring their view, the nondrinker ham radio operator raised his Moosehead beer and yelled, "What navy did you guys join?"[55]

At Balboa, five more members came aboard. Ecologists Ian Efford and Jack Mathias from British Columbia had spent the previous week studying small *Emerita* sand crabs in Costa Rica. Dr Garry Brody and National Film Board director Red Lemieux also arrived. "God protect us from all these photographers!" Cléopâtre wrote.[56] Dr Gonzalo Donoso, the Chilean pediatrician-nutritionist came aboard too; however, the two other Chilean scientists, including Sergio Alvarado, never materialized, and no explanation was given. At first, Donoso exuded a "superior attitude," which Cléopâtre pardoned "because it is always disagreeable to find strangers viewing the people of one's country as underdeveloped."[57] Helen Reid had the same impression: "He is sensitive to the attitude of some of the members that we are going to visit a remote and backward people. He says they will know more about us than we know about them ... He is on the defensive and my feelings are with him ... To be patronizing is to insult with feelings of superiority."[58] Rooming with Donoso, Brody decided that he was a "typical anti-American socialist, leaning but prob[ably] not a violent Communist."[59]

Distracted with preparing their equipment, the ecologists seemed "little interested in the rest of us," Cléopâtre wrote;[60] however, they joined the Spanish lessons. Bob Meier celebrated his birthday, suffering from diarrhea and sorely missing his pregnant wife, Carol, and their baby daughter, Heidi.

Back in Montreal, David Murphy's wife, Dr Sonia Salisbury, was soon to give birth to their second child. Devastated at his departure, she could not stop crying. Anticipation of the baby's arrival was building, and Hrischenko had been alerted that the news would come soon. Engineers at the Canadian Broadcasting Corporation's International Service rigged up a "phone patch" by placing electronic equipment on the roof of the Montreal building; it would provide reliable daily contact for METEI and people at McGill. In late November, Hrischenko made advance contact with Montreal through a ham radio operator, but the connection was weak. The uncomprehending Montrealer was so excited to have raised METEI that he told the newspapers a cockeyed story: Murphy was at home in Canada while his wife, great with child, was one of the researchers on the distant boat.[61] On 2 December an eight-pound girl was born, and the newspaper corrected its error with a glorious photograph of mother and children, all doing well and talking to Dave through the radio (figure 3.7).[62] *Cape Scott* celebrated this news.[63]

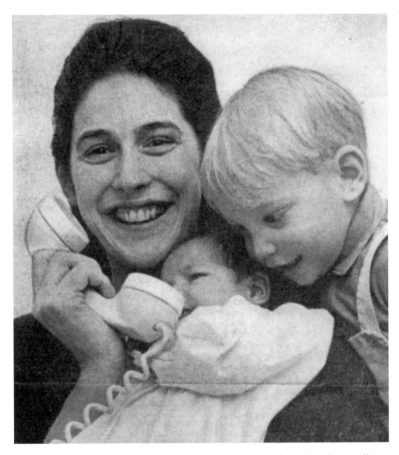

Figure 3.7 Dr Sonia Salisbury with her son and infant daughter talking to her husband, Dr David Murphy, via ham radio and telephone. *Montreal Star*, 28 December 1964, 4, Wilkinson Papers.

COMMUNICATING FROM THE SOUTH PACIFIC AND TROUBLES BEGIN

The ham radio connections afforded no privacy. Many people could be listening, including friends, neighbours, and utter strangers. George Hrischenko was used to it and kept in touch with his family several times a day, giving advice about homework, finances, house maintenance, and car repairs. But Commander Law found it "difficult to carry on a normal conversation on the radio" and was at a loss for words. Meier got around the inhibition by making little lists of things to discuss when he was able

Table 3.1 HMCS *Cape Scott* itinerary, Halifax to Rapa Nui, 1964

Date	Details
15 November	27 METEI members join the ship; press; conference and cocktails
16 November	10:00 a.m. depart Halifax
20 November	6:00 p.m. arrive Bermuda
21 November	6:00 a.m. depart Bermuda
24 November	3:00 p.m. arrive San Juan; more Canadians, Europeans, and Americans join
27 November	1:30 p.m. depart San Juan
1 December	5:30 a.m. boarded by American pilots to traverse the Panama Canal
2 December	2:00 p.m. depart Balboa; 5 more members join
5 December	Crossing the equator
13 December	7:00 a.m. arrival at Cook Bay, Rapa Nui

to connect. Carol's baby was not due until after his return, but he worried about her, sent maternity clothes from San Juan, and asked after the results of her doctor visits. He was sad when little Heidi made no sound.

Armand Boudreault wrote to his boss, Armand Frappier, thanking him for the "opportunity to live a unique experience" and hoping that this "new stage in the history of the lab would be a source of satisfaction in spite of all the preoccupations it had caused." He reassured Frappier that the freezers were working and described the storm, which had reduced the company to "crouching in corners, surviving on sandwiches." But with the ensuing calm, he fell under the spell of the exotic life at sea, with "a poet, a painter and several musicians in our midst," a choir of sailors, an orchestra, and games of chess and bridge. He too was learning Spanish, and the scientists took turns giving lectures about their planned research. "A Swedish pathologist and two Swiss from Geneva spent an entire evening with me on the bridge discussing Jean Paul Sartre and Teilhard de Chardin." Nights spent "contemplating the sea in clear moonlight, under a sky twinkling with stars could stir up sentiments that would turn a man into a poet in spite of himself." Nevertheless, like Archie Wilkinson and Garry Brody, he missed home and family: the romantic feelings were "not enough to erase a certain sense of solitude," and "my mind turns often to those I left behind."[64]

In fact, Boudreault was worried about his special freezers. He had been going down to the hold of the ship every two or three days to check the temperature. One day he was upset to find that a freezer had been moved and connected to the wrong power supply, 110 volts instead of 220 volts; the temperature had dropped, putting his precious cells in danger. Nevertheless, he got on with his work. One of his tasks would be to uncover the cause of *kokongo*, which arose with visiting ships. After clearing the Panama Canal, Boudreault and Fred Joyce took blood, throat, and nose swabs from fifty sailors in the little sick bay on board and from anyone who had cold symptoms.[65] Only too aware that *Cape Scott* might bring *kokongo* or some other infectious disease, he wanted to look for viral culprits in the sailors and be able to compare the findings with those of the sick in the event of an outbreak.

CROSSING THE EQUATOR

On the night of 4 December, "Davy Jones," the "herald of Neptune Rex," as Cléopâtre called him, boarded the ship to conduct the navy shenanigans for admission to the "Ancient Order of the Deep." Tradition required an inspection of the ship to see if it was "clean" prior to the "crossing the line ceremony" the next day. *Cape Scott* was old and ugly and crawling with cockroaches; it could never be more than nominally clean. The rite began on 5 December when "Neptune" (bearded, husky Chief Petty Officer Neil P. Chambers), his "Queen" (a sailor in drag with saucepan breasts), and their entourage strode over the decks and set up court. They started with the captain himself, who may have had the worse treatment. Cléopâtre described it in detail (figures 3.8, 3.9, and 3.10).

Cape Scott was deemed "filthy." Consequently, Law was awarded the Order of the Fish and then paraded before the "doctor," who wore a cap and a mask and was "judge over all impurities of body and soul." Cléopâtre wrote, "Found to be dirty, badly shaved, and poorly groomed, [Law] was forced to drink his 'potion' (rum), then dragged to the pool, daubed with 'soap' (plaster) from a marine paint brush (a broom), and, with barely a chance to catch his breath, he was grabbed by a 'barber' wielding a foot-long razor, and tipped backwards into the water where four big blokes, each labeled 'BEAR,' enjoyed plunging him a dozen times or more, during which he spewed salt water like a hydrant whenever he resurfaced."[66] Shivering with cold, the captain

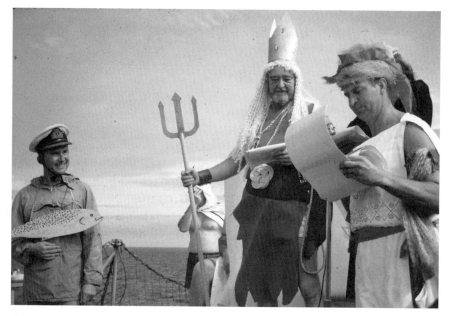

Figure 3.8 Neptune giving Commander Tony Law the Order of the Fish, 5 December 1964. Photo Fred Joyce.

was allowed to watch as every "tadpole" of his ship's company was subjected to the same treatment, marking the transition to "shellback." No one was eager to participate, and Neptune's henchmen snatched the recalcitrant travellers. Next came Gillis, then Skoryna, all the sailors, and all of METEI, including its women. Only a few, including Westropp and Lieutenant Robert Manzer, were exempt, having already sailed across the equator several times. Cléopâtre faced immersion in her best dress. More navy "firsts" were noted when *Cape Scott* extended this hoary rite to "wrens" and civilians, both male and female – more than 150 people in all.[67] A costume party followed (figure 3.11).

On 6 December everyone could atone for their pranks at "church." Jack Mathias thought he looked "real goofy" in a tie with a brush cut as everyone gathered following "church" for the METEI group photo (figure 3.12).[68]

PREPARATIONS, REALIZATIONS, AND TREPIDATIONS

Rapa Nui was still a long way off. Additional planning took place. The naval officers and crew arranged details for off-loading cargo and setting up the METEI *campamento* (figure 3.13).[69] The rough sea foiled attempts

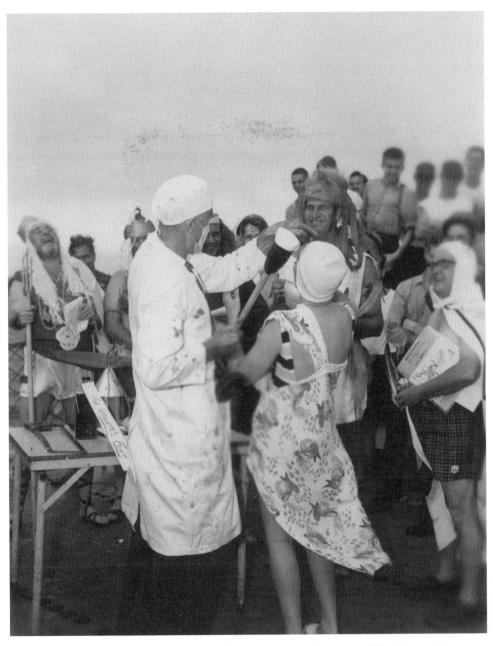

Figure 3.9 Crossing the equator ceremony, 5 December 1964. The "doctor" administers "medicine" to Rita Dwyer while Neptune laughs and Denys Montandon (*fur hat*) and John Easton (*glasses*) look on. LAC, Law Scrapbook, vol. 3.

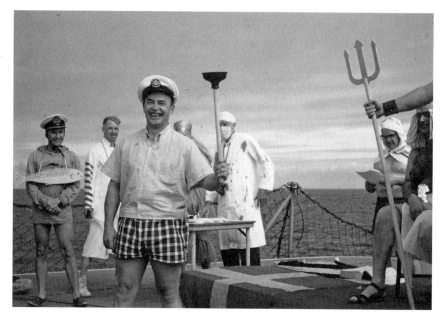

Figure 3.10 Commander Tony Law with the Order of the Fish and Stanley Skoryna awarded a plunger at the crossing the equator ceremony, 5 December 1964. Photo Fred Joyce.

at shifting cargo in readiness.[70] *Cape Scott* would drop anchor about a mile off shore and materials would be conveyed back and forth. They had brought a 26-ton mechanized landing craft (LCM3) borrowed from the Department of Transport, similar to those used in the Normandy invasion. *Cape Scott* also carried two personnel landing craft vehicles (LCVPs), or Higgins boats, suitable for carrying people and smaller objects.[71] A Zodiac and divers were at the ready for an underwater survey of the landing site if needed. They were equipped with blasting equipment if the landing proved too shallow for their work.

Officers and sailors established a detailed list of items to be off-loaded first. A small winch – 5-ton capacity – resided on a quay at the landing place, called Hanga Piko. The red, four-wheel-drive Ford truck, always referred to as the "Jeep," would go early to drag the large ATCO pallets to the campsite, whose location could not be known precisely until after they arrived. Despite the careful planning in the autumn, the naval officers realized that they needed to manufacture many fittings and components. They also partially prefabricated the solar distillation unit and other equipment while on board the ship. Law and his officers

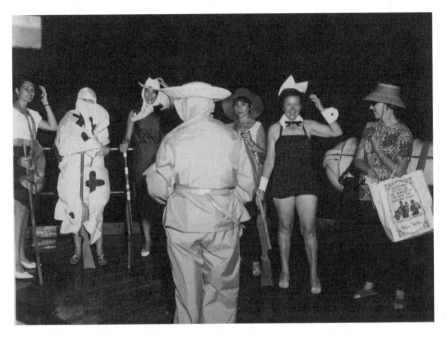

Figure 3.11 METEI "ladies" in costume at the crossing the equator ceremony, 5 December 1964. *From left*, Isabel Griffiths, Carlotta Hacker (*possibly*), Cléopâtre Montandon, Mary King (*facing away*), Ana Maria Eccles, Helen Reid, and Rita Dwyer. Yes, that is Dr Reid as a Playboy bunny. LAC, Law Scrapbook, vol. 3.

estimated that the setup would take at least six days, and the scientists were assigned various tasks to help. During that time, women would have to remain on board *Cape Scott* a mile offshore.

Clarity began to emerge for the scientists. The budding, young sociologist Cléopâtre observed two types of reaction to the long days and the serious, tedious meetings. One group was relaxed, enjoying the "holiday," seemingly confident that the work would go well; these included the Scandinavians and the young ecologists from British Columbia. She wondered if their insouciance was a national character trait or a product of their youth or of the type of work they would do. A second group grew increasingly tense, among whom she numbered Skoryna, Nógrády, Boudreault, the Robertses, and other older members of the team "with grey hair," who had left behind important positions and had a lot riding on the research results. In addition, "the whole band of journalists, filmmakers, and photographers ... loitered uselessly around the ship

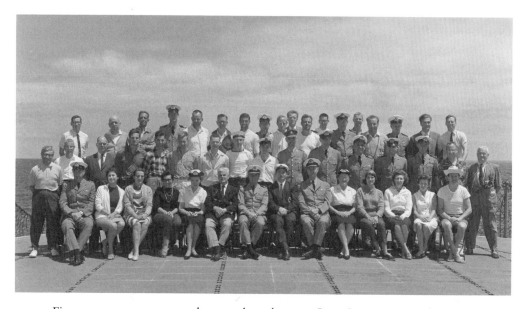

Figure 3.12 METEI group photo on board HMCS *Cape Scott*, 6 December 1964. *Front row from left*, Lieutenant Commander Channing D. Gillis, Cléopâtre Montandon, Helen Reid, Ana Maria Eccles, Lieutenant Rita Dwyer, John Easton, Commander Tony Law, Stanley Skoryna, Richard Roberts, Lieutenant Mary King, Isabel Griffiths (later Cutler), Maureen Roberts, Carlotta Hacker, and Gonzalo Donoso. *Middle row from left*, Carl Mydans, Fred Joyce, Robert Williams, Denys Montandon, George Hrischenko, Ian Efford, Colin Gillingham, Robert Fulton, Harry Crosman, Al Taylor, one unknown officer, Lieutenant Robert Manzer, two unknown officers, Garry S. Brody, and David Macfarlane. *Back row from left*, Robert Meier, Archibald Wilkinson, John Cutler, Charles Westropp, Harold Gibbs, Armand Boudreault, Elliot Alpert, unknown officer, Jim Nielsen, Red Lemieux, Peter Beighton, Jack Mathias, unknown officer, Björn Ekblom, Eivind Myhre, unknown officer, Georges Nógrády, and David Murphy. *Missing*: Einar Gjessing and Charles Fowler (who was on the return journey only). National Defence Photograph Tom Galley. LAC, Roberts Papers, vol. 1, file 23; also in Reid, *World Away*, opposite 22.

contributing nothing."[72] She acknowledged the difficulty of building a coherent team from forty independent souls. Helen Reid also noted the rising tension: "There is a perversity to the whole ship ... ever since we left Puerto Rico ... a gentle but increasing tension."[73] Reid attributed it to the unaccustomed confinement, the diversity of views, and the constant

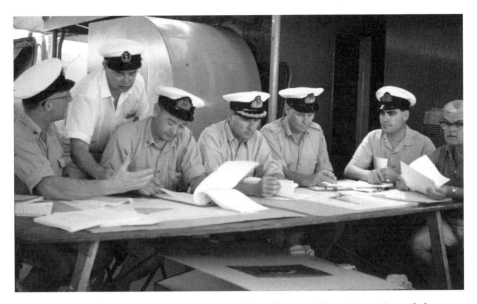

Figure 3.13 METEI planning meeting on board HMCS *Cape Scott*. *From left,* unknown, Stanley Skoryna, Lieutenant Commander Channing Gillis, Commander Tony Law, unknown, Lieutenant Commander Alfred Shaw, and Air Vice Marshal John Easton. Photo Fred Joyce.

presence of the media, even during scientific meetings, when Lemieux would "point his huge microphone at speakers like a ray gun."[74] With "over two hundred people on board, ... over two thousand opinions" were expressed. "Expedition members were clearly divided. The 'split' had come early and remained, with only a few changes, throughout the entire expedition."[75] Archie Wilkinson confessed his sense of betrayal to Helen Reid: many things that he had been led to expect weren't true; the prospect of "research" seemed hollow before it began.[76]

At each stop, the arrival of newcomers had enlivened discussions and provoked controversy. Over a San Juan supper of paella, Cléopâtre had been surprised to hear Ekblom criticize the choice of Easter Island for the study; it was the first time she'd heard anyone utter a critical comment, but she admitted that "more than one member surely shared the same reflections."[77] After Balboa, Reid wrote that "bright," "argumentative" Ian Efford "spread dissension." Over dinner at the captain's table, he startled listeners by announcing "that the navy was finished"; *Cape Scott* was a "sitting duck," and only submarines would survive. Efford then told the Spanish-born members "just what ailed Spain." The others "looked down in embarrassment." Even Efford's young assistant, Jack Mathias, thought his boss was "not very tactful." Commissioned Officer James R. Barlow "excuse[d] him because he is young" and his considerable success "has gone to his head."[78] A half-century later, Efford himself offered this explanation: "I was a pain ... not because 'it had gone to my head,' but rather involvement with graduate training at Oxford for four years consisted of critical analysis and argument about anything that was discussed! I took this training to heart!"

A system of edifying lectures was created for the evenings. Team members would explain their fields of interest, describe their protocols, or pass on interesting bits of information gleaned from reading about Easter Island. Nógrády spoke about the geological and natural history of the volcanic island, illustrated with diagrams and images. He had prepared with love and enthusiasm, ripping apart four or five crates in the hold to locate his slides; however, the result was too long and erudite for the crew and too erroneous for the ecologists.[79] Mary King compared *rongorongo* script to that of the Indus Valley; unfortunately, we do not know her sources. Gonzalo Donoso gave a lively presentation about Chile that was so entertaining and informative that it left his audience eager to visit his country.[80] When it was Carl Mydans's turn to talk about photography, he could not conceal his vexation over the many amateurs who turned up with their own cameras hoping to glean a few useful pointers.[81]

Cléopâtre completed the questionnaire that she would use to conduct her sociological survey.[82] But when she took it to Isabel to have the questions translated into Spanish, she was unpleasantly surprised to discover that Isabel had translated something similar for Helen Reid. Cléopâtre was angry and hurt. "The blood went to my head." How could Helen not know that sociology was *her* role? The pediatrician was supposedly in charge of *medical* examinations of children; what was she trying to prove going beyond her mandate when her Spanish skills were barely serviceable? Isabel tried to calm her, explaining that the physical well-being of the island children depended on their families and their way of life. She suggested that Cléopâtre talk to Helen. But Cléopâtre would have none of it; Helen should come to her. She admitted that the incident showed how rumours got started and stories were embellished. Oblivious to Montandon's vexation, Reid had made no secret of her own survey, discussing it with anyone who would listen, including the student Jack Mathias. At the same time, using her clinical eye, the pediatrician, a mother herself, surmised that the young woman was pregnant and disapproved of the deception.[83]

Carlotta was designated as a "research assistant" to Nógrády and Joyce. Georges began giving her lessons in bacteriology and recipes for "cooking" sterile culture media. He illustrated his teaching with diagrams portraying the secret ways of microbes and the life cycles of parasites. He would ask a question and then answer it: "How do we prepare the media? Ah! We prepare it like this."[84] She enjoyed his verve and his meandering, didactic style, which incorporated tales of his near-death experiences in wartime.[85] His cabin was bursting with a wild variety of objects: cameras, maps, books, compasses, a life jacket that he had designed himself, provisions for three days, and many hats. The Montandons also visited Georges in his cabin and came away with the same impression: "a special personality ... well prepared with everything one could imagine."[86]

Easton sidled up to Carlotta one day and asked, "Have you ever done any book-keeping?" She soon found herself trying to balance columns of figures; the worries of the unpaid bills began to haunt her. Skoryna handed over a receipt for thirty-two mouth organs that he had acquired as gifts in the last port of call.[87]

With his contacts back at McGill, Skoryna devised a scheme to support the mission by selling special METEI seals and postcards for one dollar apiece. These items were ordered in vast quantities. Canadian stamp collectors who wanted them cancelled by the Chilean post could place their orders through McGill and include a few cents more for postage. METEI had been organized to investigate the health status of the islanders, but it had no pretentions to actually *improving* their health. Indeed, they had no idea if the Rapanui needed medical care or not. At best, the study might *protect* them from future unknown onslaughts. Nevertheless, these seals took on the allure of well-known, successful campaigns for specific charities, furnishing small tokens in exchange for tiny contributions that donors could place on envelopes to display their philanthropic zeal. For example, Christmas seals had first appeared in Denmark to raise funds for tuberculosis; however, by 1907 and 1908 they were widely used across the United States and Canada. Similarly, Easter seals were created in 1934 to serve the American National Society for Crippled Children. Both programs were flourishing in the early 1960s and had broadened their mandates to support research and care for other lung diseases and all forms of disability.[88] Frustrated with the lack of support from government and charitable foundations for his ATCO bill, Skoryna was hoping to tap into the success of these stamps in order to stir a groundswell of public enthusiasm. He allowed news reports to dissemble their purpose: McGill's special seal would "promote health on the island."[89]

Travelling with *Cape Scott*, David Macfarlane managed to file a couple of stories about the stamps with the *Montreal Star* before leaving Balboa. They were printed while the ship was still at sea in the Pacific Ocean. One such article featured a large photo of Stanley Skoryna, Archie Wilkinson, and Hal Gibbs watching Lieutenant Mary King address Christmas cards.[90] Readers were encouraged to place their orders for stamps. Macfarlane cited Skoryna: "We have brought these trailers a long distance, and it would seem illogical that we should take them back to Canada when we visualize the important uses for them on the island – uses that will help the islanders and also promote international knowledge of disease through follow-up studies."[91] The message to the government and ATCO was clear, although no one seemed to notice. Another report, aimed specifically at stamp collectors, pointed out that Chile was opening a post office on Rapa Nui just for the occasion; if they acted quickly, collectors could possess its first franking.[92] It was a leap and not a very successful one: the amount eventually retrieved from well-intentioned, philatelic Canadians was $2,000, not quite enough for one trailer.

Security was another concern for Skoryna. Ever since the first European visits, the islanders had been described as light-fingered and especially fond of taking hats. Thor Heyerdahl too had emphasized their habit of stealing. He was shocked that the famous priest Father Sebastian Englert had seemed more distressed by thieving than by the tragic accidental drownings; the priest explained, "We all have to die, but we don't have to steal."[93] Less ethnocentric observers contended that, in a society without money, bartering was a form of trade and everything on the island was collectively owned.[94]

This concern over theft, along with the Polynesian openness to matters of sexuality, the loose kinship traditions, and the distant history of cannibalism, appeared among the topics explored during the meetings, with input from Donoso.[95] These issues meant that Skoryna fretted over safety, especially for the women of his team. He was glad the navy insisted that the ladies remain on board the ship until the camp was complete with a secure fence constructed around it. He made a rule that women should not go about the island alone. Cléopâtre was furious at the restriction but did not speak up, hoping that he would change his mind after their arrival.[96] According to Westropp, Myhre enjoyed teasing gullible females, especially "wren" Rita, about what they should expect from men on the island; she was frightened.

Skoryna had also surmised that the islanders respected people who wore hats. Where he derived this impression is unknown – possibly from the early European tales of hat theft or from the archeological information that many *moai* had once worn red stone topknots. Whatever the origin of the idea, he was rarely photographed without headgear and recommended that METEI members always wear their hats too. Hacker thought that his choice of a yachting cap for attire on the naval vessel demonstrated a certain amount of nerve.[97] Mathias was astonished when sixty cowboy hats labelled "L.B.J." were distributed to the team as gifts of "the government," although he did not specify which one; Efford replaced the label with his own initials, I.E.E.[98] Brody, who transported them, thought that they were "well received."[99] Few photos depict anyone, other than Skoryna, wearing these hats; they may have joined the goods for trading.

In the final days of the voyage, the planning issues demanded much pondering, although they were largely imponderable. Would the islanders be friendly? How many people could be examined in one day? Would the equipment need guarding at all times? How should the many gifts be distributed? They carried 900 dresses, 500 shirts, bolts of fabric, soap, cosmetics, perfume, toys, fish hooks, carving tools, mouth organs, toothbrushes, and cigars. Skoryna did not want METEI to give out cigarettes for fear of setting a bad example, and he believed that cigars were healthier. Some members gave up smoking; others stocked up on supplies. Father Sebastian had asked METEI not to bring alcohol to the island, but many members exempted themselves from his request. The cargo manifest indicates a "musical instrument," which David Murphy remembers as a pump organ brought for the island church at the insistence of Mary King, possibly the one Carlotta had played for Sunday services on the ship.[100] On the matter of gifts, George Hrischenko later observed, "we were all stupid": the islanders owned cameras and radios; what they needed were film and batteries, but of course METEI had none to spare. Several members described a meeting around 10 December that agonized over how the trove of gifts should be revealed – all at once or gradually? Community gifts were to be directly distributed: playground equipment, sewing machines, and carving tools. But an hour-long argument ensued over the "philosophy of gift-giving" and the meaning of the word "bribery": the gifts would be expressions of gratitude for cooperation; they were not "bribes."[101] A silent majority suspected otherwise.

Just days from arrival, a shouting match ensued between John Easton and Richard Roberts over plans for the water supply.[102] Brody saw "the only hint of non-co-operation" in Roberts, who was "very stubborn" and had "unrealistic ideas."[103] Reid's anxiety over the value of the mission increased. She wrote in her diary of the "tension and shortness of temper here and there ... [and] jockeying for position in the trading market, which seemed to me revolting ... It's difficult to sit back and watch the display of boorishness, which seems a part of the expedition – among certain members. I forecast there will be no adaptability here – that aggressiveness will be the criterion."[104] Meanwhile, Macfarlane maintained his upbeat reporting, announcing the imminent "E-Day" and explaining that "the expedition is a dream child" conceived by the "energy, drive, and imagination" of Stanley Skoryna.[105]

Finally, on the evening of 12 December, Commander Law reduced the speed to half, slowing *Cape Scott* to make her appointed rendezvous on time. She dropped anchor. As confirmed by Chilean radio from Rapa Nui, the governor, doctor, and manager of the airport (with no flights) were expected to greet her at 7:00 a.m. At dawn, the smooth, treeless hulk of the island emerged silently from the grey gloom; soon, however, the sun rose behind a volcano and the scene was flooded with orange light. Within minutes, six long, narrow canoes, bearing fifty men and two women, headed out from shore to surround the ship. Others joined in, and at one point, Bob Meier counted more than a hundred islanders in boats.[106] Myriad white specks dotted the shore; the ecologist opined that they might be sheep, but Peter Beighton knew they were people.[107] Rapa Nui had been watching all night with giant bonfires blazing so that the Canadian ship would not pass it by.[108]

After a month of travel, METEI had finally reached its destination. Most team members had revelled in novel sights and adventures along the way and were full of admiration for the navy crew. But this was not a holiday. Uncomfortable friction swirled among them. And as they reached their destination, they were afflicted with a growing awareness that preparations had been inadequate for the task ahead.

4

Raising Camp Hilton

FIRST CONTACT

"Iorana!" yelled Jim Nielsen over the side of the ship. "Iorana! Hallo dere," came the reply. With his fair hair and blue eyes, the Danish American was immediately identified by the islanders as Thor Heyerdahl's son, who had been on Rapa Nui ten years earlier. Known ever after as "Kon-Tiki-Iti-Iti" (Small Kon-Tiki), Nielsen enjoyed the title and the special privilege that came with it – although, as a recent undergraduate, he considered himself the least member of the team.[1]

From sacks lying in the canoes came wooden carvings, including the cachectic, crouching figure of the Cava Cava Man and the Birdman with his male body and long, curved beak. These were the statues that Heyerdahl had criticized for being unoriginal, although they were expertly carved.[2] The islanders made it clear that they wanted cigarettes. METEI members were not allowed to oblige them, but the sailors felt no such inhibition. Well before departure, the navy had identified tobacco as "Rapa Nui's unofficial currency."[3] The islanders also accepted soap, shirts, and cheap perfume, which rained down on their canoes while ropes carried up the carvings to the happy shoppers. Bob Meier reported that the brisk trading went on until 10:00 p.m., although some islanders took time off to fish (figure 4.1). The young anthropologist observed their physical characteristics and was struck by the remarkable variability in appearance.[4] What genetic homogeneity was this?

Meanwhile, the official welcoming party arrived as planned: Governor Jorge Portilla, who was a Chilean naval officer; the medical doctor Guido Andrade, also of the navy; and Sergio Piñero of the Chilean air force (figure 4.2).[5] They stayed only a short time. As bartering continued at the ship, Commander Tony Law, Stanley Skoryna, Gonzalo Donoso, Peter

Beighton, George Hrischenko, and Denys Montandon followed the governor in a landing craft vehicle to make official visits. With them went the journalists, of course – Carl Mydans, David Macfarlane, Bob Williams, and Red Lemieux – and another small party charged with selecting the site for the METEI camp: John Easton, Lieutenant Commander Robert Billard, and Isabel Griffiths. Navigator Charles Westropp and the beach master, Lieutenant Commander Ernest ("Pony") Moore, went to survey the coastline and to mark the narrow channel into the government wharf at Hanga Piko (figure 4.3). They stationed a sailor with a walkie-talkie on shore. The Zodiac and divers were readied to assess the safety of the approach to the little jetty. But Westropp determined that the harbour was deep enough for their landing craft at all tides; the diving inspection and blasting were not needed. By noon, Easton's crew had settled on a site for the METEI camp, situated between the sea and Hanga Roa, the only village; it had ready access to salt water for the distillation units and proximity to the island homes, but it was some distance from the landing site.

The jetty was covered with people, mostly curious women and children who had not been able to go out in the canoes. Spanish-speaking Denys Montandon conversed at length with Mario Arévalo, an engineer from the little airstrip, which, the Chilean said, was "the only one in the world that never received planes."[6] He learned that the islanders wanted to leave, their preferred destination Tahiti, not Chile. This desire was thought to reflect political aspirations for a federation of Pacific islands connected to France; therefore, it was unpopular with Santiago. According to the Chilean hosts, the islanders were a "bizarre mix of many races since most of the ships that passed by had left a few souvenirs and, in some cases, entire families."[7] This diversity had been known to other Easter Island expeditions, including Heyerdahl's. So much for Skoryna's notion of inbreeding. Arévalo professed sympathy for the Rapanui but emphasized their differences in mentality and culture. Notwithstanding the genetic mix, he said, "we are Latins; they are Polynesian." This conversation took place in the engineer's home while a "young woman" sliced pineapples for the visitors to enjoy.[8]

The Chileans had a few military vehicles on the island (between two and six, with reports varying). Skoryna, Donoso, and Denys, perhaps others, were invited to eat at the home of Gustavo Montero, who ran the sheep farm. His wife had prepared a delicious meal of soup, chicken with maize, tea, and fruit. Denys grasped something that he consigned to his journal: "these Chileans received me as if they were at home, in their own country, but on the other hand, they did not feel native. I realized that Easter Island belongs to Chile, but Easter Island is not Chile."[9]

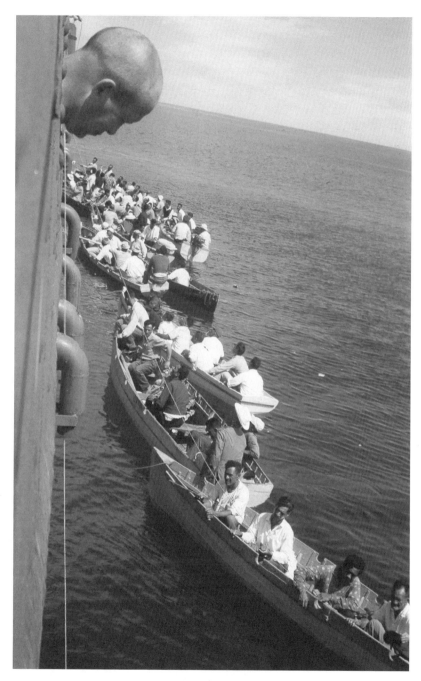

Figure 4.1 Trading over the side of HMCS Cape Scott, first morning, 13 December 1964. Photo David Murphy.

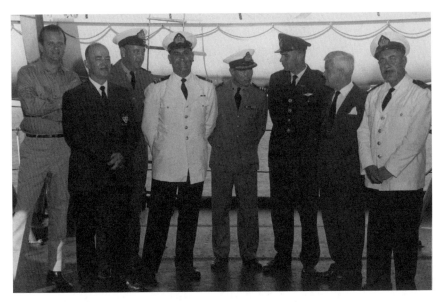

Figure 4.2 Welcoming party, first morning, 13 December 1964, 7:30 a.m.
From left, Dr Gonzalo Donoso, Dr Stanley Skoryna, Lieutenant Commander
Channing Gillis, Governor Jorge Portilla, Commander Tony Law, unknown
(possibly Sergio Piñero), Air Vice Marshal John Easton, and Dr Guido
Andrade. LAC, Law Scrapbook, vol. 3.

DAY ONE

During the first day, while leaders visited and inspected, the sailors began
the off-loading operation using the mechanized landing craft and following the plans that had been so carefully arranged during the journey.
First, at 2:00 p.m., went the four-wheel-drive vehicle, with farm wagons,
a generator, and tools for Beach Master Pony Moore. On every trip of the
landing craft, extra space was filled with a few of the 45-gallon barrels of
diesel fuel. The sea was relatively calm, but even the normal swell made
the off-loading dangerous. In "frustrated rage" at being forced to remain
on board, Carlotta and Helen spent the day hanging over the rail, watching the crew, and staring at the island through binoculars. They marvelled
at the dexterity and precision of the sailors. Carlotta observed how "the
trailer swung from a crane over the landing barge, lower and lower ... and
then a wave took the barge and crashed it up into the hovering trailer.
Trying to fit the heavy trailer into the continually moving [barge] was as
difficult as threading a needle during a fit of coughing. And considerably

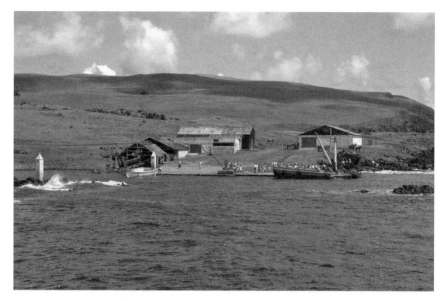

Figure 4.3 Hanga Piko jetty with landing craft and small crowd. The barren Rano Kao volcano is behind. Photo Ian Efford.

more dangerous."[10] Helen wrote, "A miscalculation and the load could plunge right through or be shattered by the upward impact ... a breathless danger riding in every swell ... Indeed, one seaman just saved his life by diving overboard from the craft as it crashed against the ship's side."[11] Jack Mathias watched in horror "as men went flying" and "two of the large cables controlling the swing of the loading boom pulled over the fender and roof of the METEI truck and bashed the fender all in" (figure 4.4).[12] The experienced navy mechanic Harry Crosman was horrified by what he viewed as careless damage to the beautiful new truck.

Laden with cargo, the landing craft was driven skillfully by Leading Seaman Thomas Picco to the Hanga Piko landing; however, the approach was treacherous – a narrow, tortuous channel surrounded by jagged lava rocks. Law wrote, "at times the pier was awash with the breaking surf and the huge swell."[13] The landing craft negotiated the channel with care, and the small winch onshore was used to unload its contents (figure 4.5).

On that first day, the landing craft and its crew also conveyed six ATCO trailers – one erected at the pier and one at the campsite for the security guards, each with two beds, two sleeping bags, and tinned food. The landing craft also carried plumbing equipment, pumps for salt water, the solar still, the mechanical still, and more diesel fuel barrels as fill.

Denys made a brief trip back to the ship to visit his "petite femme," who was "biting her nails" in vexation at having been left behind. He discovered that he was "on call" and had to return to the trailer erected at the jetty to watch over the landed materials. He was supposed to contact *Cape Scott* via walkie-talkie every fifteen minutes all night long. However, Portilla and the captain of the air base came to collect him, assuring him that nothing would be stolen. Over a fine whiskey, "the most expensive liquor in Chile," the governor explained his complex life as a farmer, judge, and military chief. The island had a jail that could hold one person. The governor's young Chilean wife had found life on Rapa Nui difficult at first, but she had adapted to the island's calm. Its people were "primitive," she said, but was unable to explain why. Then Denys was taken back to his post by jeep. His radio wasn't working, but he didn't even try to fix it and slept well.[14] Meanwhile, Armand Boudreault and one other had been sent to guard the equipment at the chosen campsite. Warned of theft, Armand grew anxious when a band of people approached, but they wanted only to talk, playing music and singing into the night. He was charmed by their friendliness.

Peter Beighton also went ashore on that first day. With one other young man, he explored the island, looking for *moai* and climbing the barren hills to get a sense of the land. That night, the pair did not return to the ship and slept rough. Skoryna was angry over their inconsiderate adventure, which had alarmed him and the other leaders. Back at *Cape Scott*, Peter said that the landscape, with its barren hills and stone fences, reminded him of Scotland.[15]

DAYS TWO TO FOUR

The morning of the second day was clear and calm, and the landing crafts were busy going back and forth. Easton's chosen site for the *campamento* was a lengthy 2 kilometres from the landing jetty. The scientists were pleased with the choice: it met anthropologist Richard Salisbury's concern that the expedition should not isolate itself from the people. But Denys could tell that the location was a "source of friction" between Skoryna and the naval officers. At the campsite itself, the divers conducted a survey of the rocky beach and deemed it unsuitable for landing anything but the smallest boats. Therefore, every ATCO trailer, at 2.5 tons, would have to be dragged the entire distance from the Hanga Piko jetty. This decision would complicate and delay the setup. But the governor solved the problem for METEI when he "volunteered his agricultural tractors and native labour" (figure 4.6).[16] Bright turquoise with orange roofs, the trailers made a colourful statement.

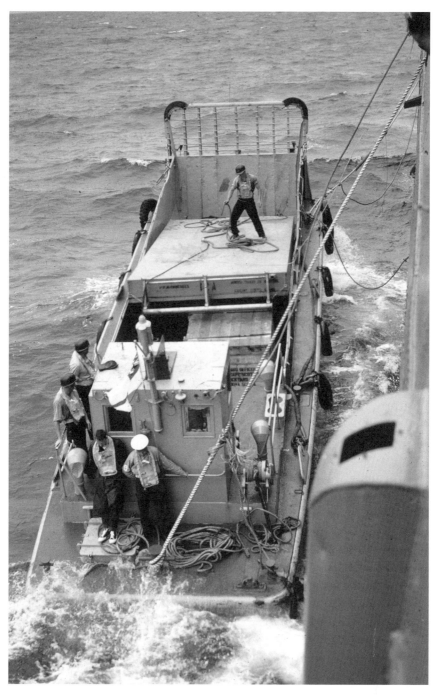

Figure 4.4 Loading an ATCO palletized "shoebox" trailer onto the landing craft. Photo Fred Joyce.

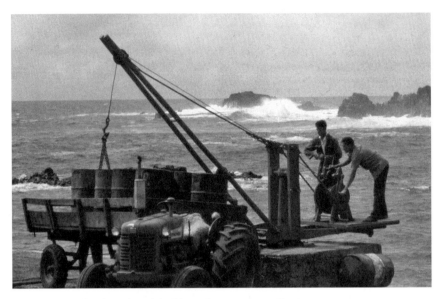

Figure 4.5 Unloading diesel fuel barrels at Hanga Piko jetty.
Photo Peter Beighton.

To shorten the turnaround time for each landing-craft trip, a crew
was stationed on the beach from dawn until 10:00 p.m. Remarkably
little damage ensued after the front fender of the truck had been dented:
a barrel of formalin plunged to the ocean floor, and a large slab of plywood slithered into the harbour but was quickly retrieved by a spon-
taneous cluster of sailors, Rapanui, and METEI scientists, including Al
Taylor, Bob Meier, and Jim Nielsen. The navy arranged for feeding the
crews – an estimated total of 300 mouths, including the island workers
– in round-the-clock shifts at three different sites: Hanga Piko, the *campamento*, and the ship.[17] To help out, Helen Reid took up mess duty for
the crew remaining on the ship.[18] Most male members of METEI made
their first contact with the island on this second day. Meier admired the
beautiful village with its simple houses nestled in gardens and the open
friendliness of the people and their children.[19]

Also on the second day, the navy men concentrated on the water supply. The suction basin was 137 metres from the storage tanks with a lift
of 6 metres. To supply 500 gallons each day, the mechanical distillation
unit would need 5,000 gallons of salt water. The solar unit was to supply
another 200 gallons, but it never worked well, possibly because it was
missing parts. By noon the wind had picked up, "increasing the swell

and causing the ship to roll heavily." Meier made it back to *Cape Scott* in rain over rough seas and felt "some excitement boarding ship from rope ladder."[20] Law suspended all activity at 3:45 p.m. and ordered the landing craft and teams to remain at Hanga Piko overnight.

Women were still confined to the ship, but the Montandons noted with envy and annoyance that – despite being female – Isabel had gone ashore to translate and Maureen Roberts had taken lunch at the governor's home. The aggrieved women remonstrated with the captain over the "intolerable" delay after so many weeks at sea.[21] Law said the work building the camp was hot and heavy, and he confessed that his biggest concern was the descent down the rope ladder from the ship into the landing craft: a person could be crushed between the two boats careening unpredictably on the waves. He had responsibilities to their husbands and parents. They plied him with Drambuie, and he lifted the restriction.[22] Cléopâtre Montandon made a brief trip to shore on 14 December while the others stayed behind.

On 16 December – day four – all the women finally made it to shore (figure 4.7). They were relieved to be on *terra firma* for the first time in two weeks and excited to see the island for themselves. Like their fellow travellers, they were astonished to find friendly people and lively, tiny children riding horses bareback, sometimes three and four together (figure 4.8). Ian Efford adjudged it a form of babysitting: small children were placed on horseback with an older sibling; too small to get off, they stayed in place, and the horse could always find its way home. But Helen detected a kind of "hunger in their faces, food hunger, work hunger, and the long hunger of loneliness and boredom." She was enraptured with the tropical beauty: "The island wraps you instantly in its downy silence. Time disappears and there is only the reality of the sea, the chirping of tiny birds, the peace is like a soft cloud that flows up on the earth. Surely the theists must feel the all-pervasive presence of their individual Gods. Hotu Matu'a is here." But at the jetty and the campsite, the "ordered confusion of a tremendous moving operation" reigned supreme.[23]

Already nine trailers stood on-site, another nine were awaiting placement, the stills were working sluggishly, and lavatories were being dug, supervised by Hal Gibbs, who also helped Fred Joyce and Eivind Myhre to construct the laboratory (figures 4.9 and 4.10). A fuel dump for the 180 drums was set up at the rear of the compound. A ready-supply system fed the three 25-kilowatt diesel generators that the navy electrical team was connecting to the wiring built into each trailer by the manufacturer, performing necessary repairs as they went. The camp was a hive of

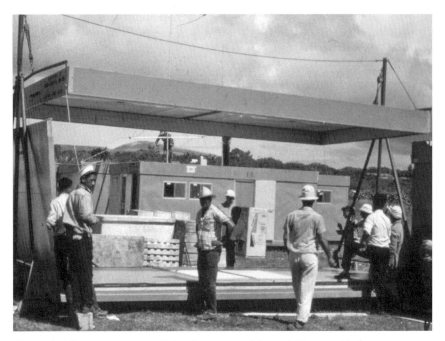

Figure 4.6 Raising an ATCO "shoebox" portable with Rapanui helpers.
Photo Peter Beighton.

activity, and the Rapanui were working hard too. Surgeon Garry Brody
was needed to "sew up one sailor," and with David Murphy giving the
anesthetic, he treated "another who had dislocated his elbow."[24]

Carlotta "had never known people who were so eager to work." But
she admitted that the Rapanui had been well prepared. They understood that METEI was there *for them*, not for their famous statues, caves,
or prehistory – the focus of most previous expeditions.[25] On his first
day ashore, Bob Meier also recognized the "good workers." Law was
impressed too: "Everything I have heard about Polynesian islanders is
balls. They are very kind and charming people and have been most helpful ... in setting up the campsite and getting the cargo ashore."[26] Brody
wrote, "It seems the most striking thing here is the misinformation we
had about the island. The natives are hard-working. Very friendly and
pleasant. There is no real consanguinity."[27]

Skoryna was pleased with the architecturally designed setup – a loose
rectangle, open only at one end – the west – where the laboratories,
examining rooms, reception area, and radio station were located (figure 4.11). The living, eating, and washing quarters were at the far end,

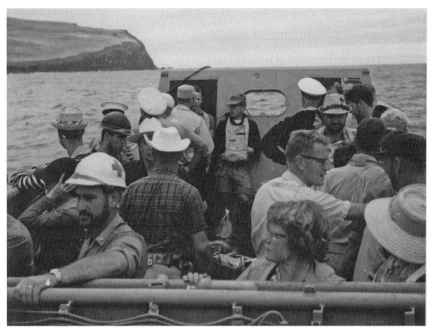

Figure 4.7 METEI team members in personnel landing craft. Front right, Mary King and Rita Dwyer (*hat*). Behind, Red Lemieux, Harold Gibbs, Cléopâtre and Denys Montandon, and Al Taylor. *Back centre*, Robert Meier. *Left*, Björn Ekblom (*facing island*). LAC, Law Scrapbook, vol. 3, envelope CS 1152.

closed to "penetration" by the islanders. But Carlotta observed that the friendly, uninhibited Rapanui had already "penetrated." They were everywhere, gathering on the hillside to watch, leaping unbidden to lend a hand, and looking through windows. When she went to her cabin for a nap, she found three island girls scrubbing the floor.[28]

The work went faster as the islanders learned the procedures. Law reported that by the fourth day, "the production rate doubled," and "all the trailers and large cargo had been discharged." On this day, Meier helped to build a stone breakwater to protect the water pumps. Boudreault's freezers containing tissue cultures were unplugged, brought up from the ship's hold, and left on deck in the blistering heat for many hours before being transported to the *campamento*. He was distraught, although several METEI alumni remember his relative sangfroid in the face of calamity.[29] He recalled that if he seemed "cool," it was due to his earlier experience on the voyage; this unloading incident was the second time he had reason to worry about his precious Hela cells and K cells.

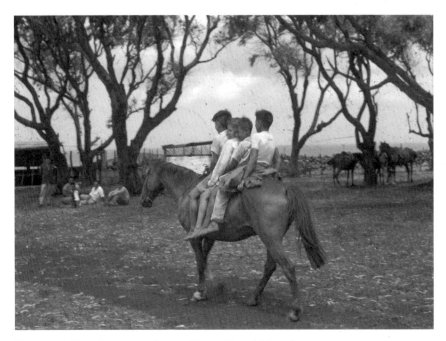

Figure 4.8 Four boys on a horse. Photo David Murphy.

Were they alive or dead? Boudreault would not know if his work had any meaning until he returned to Canada months later.

Also on day four, Denys visited the little "hospital," where the nurses made it a point of honour to describe their work, and three nuns took him to see Father Sebastian Englert. Legendary for his three decades of service on the island, Heyerdahl had called him the real "king" of Easter Island. The missionary Franciscan received the Swiss doctor in his "austere little room behind the church." It held "a desk with a packet of letters, a few shelves with all the literature about the island, some yellowing folders, an old clock, a couple *soutanes* hanging from a nail, a crucifix, and a portrait of the pope over the bed, from under which peeked his hiking boots. Voilà, the entire décor!"[30]

Denys asked about the airport. The priest put his head in his hands, saying he'd rather not reveal his opinion. Instead, he read a passage in a letter from the bishop of Tahiti that predicted its damaging influence on the population: prostitution, corruption, and so on. They discussed the desire to emigrate, the use of traditional foods and medicines, the recent improvement in health, the near-disappearance of leprosy, and belief in spirits. The sheep farm, the priest thought, was beneficial. Father Sebastian

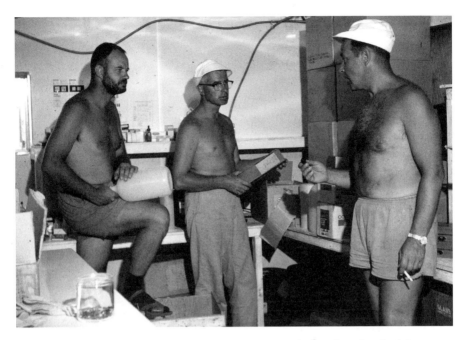

Figure 4.9 *From left*, Harold Gibbs, Fred Joyce, and Eivind Myhre building their lab. Photo Fred Joyce.

also displayed a remarkable command of Ancient Greek, which he had learned in Germany.[31] It was evident to the Montandons and to Carlotta Hacker, although possibly not to the METEI leadership, that it was Father Sebastian who had prepared the way for METEI. He told the islanders that they "had been chosen of all the people of the world" for this important research. His flock was "very flattered" and "also a little apprehensive."[32]

Later in the afternoon of 16 December, an assembly took place at the school (figure 4.12). The nuns gathered the children outside in the courtyard, and Helen Reid delivered a little speech in Spanish to describe the purpose of the expedition.[33] Photographs show that Rita Dwyer, Georges Nógrády, Fred Joyce, Carlotta Hacker, and a few *Cape Scott* sailors accompanied her. The children then performed the traditional *sau sau* dance in grass skirts and feathers, followed by an impressive rendition of the twist. How much the youngsters grasped from Reid's words is unknown, but their mothers, holding infant siblings, crowded into the compound too, listening carefully. They seemed to like the lady doctor and the other female newcomers. Cléopâtre witnessed this encounter too. She was fascinated by the children's songs, dances,

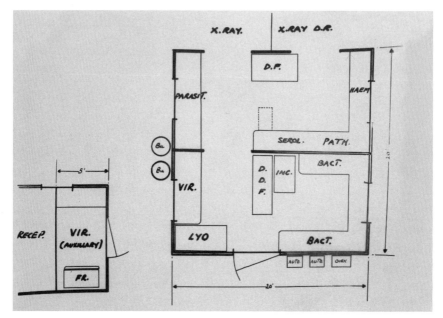

Figure 4.10 Diagram of METEI labs with sections for virology, bacteriology, serology, parasitology, hematology, pathology, freezers, and lyophilizer. The X-ray unit is next door. LAC, Roberts Papers, vol. 1, file 23.

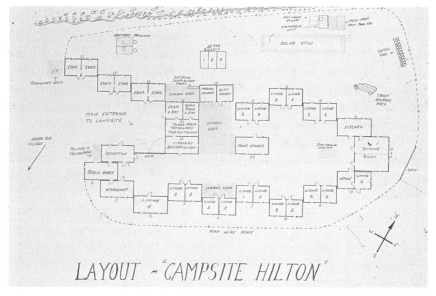

Figure 4.11 Final layout of Camp Hilton with cabin numbers. Sanitary (*top left*), generators (*top centre*), water distillation and showers (*top right*), and fuel depot (*extreme right*). Wilkinson Papers.

and affection and surprised that they adopted her "as a mother" with their disarming warmth and trust.[34]

The colourful school artwork reminded pediatrician Reid of Canadian children; they were the same all around the world. She commissioned some pictures to take home (figure 4.13). She also recorded her meeting with the teachers in great detail. With one notable exception, all were nuns from the order of Hermanas Misioneras Catequistas, which also ran the small leprosarium. Sister Maria Petronila was the principal and taught grade 5. The others were Sister Maria Francesca (grade 1), Sister Maria Emiliana (grade 2), Sister Maria Esperanza (grade 4), and Sister Maria Luisa (grade 6). The sisters told Helen about the subjects taught, the meagre diet of the children, and several cases of domestic abuse. The one nonclerical exception was Alfonso Rapu, a twenty-two-year-old Rapanui man, "very handsome and intelligent," who had returned in November 1963 from his education in Chile to serve as the grade 3 teacher.[35]

FIRST GLIMMER OF POLITICAL TROUBLE

From the earliest encounters ashore, most METEI members, like Denys, sensed that something was not quite right. On the first day, they learned that the regular naval supply ship, *Presidente Pinto*, "had failed to appear for its scheduled annual visit." It was at least one month overdue, although Tony Law understood it was three.[36] The islanders were short of essential foodstuffs, including flour, oil, yeast, sugar, tea, and supplies such as antibiotics, soap, shoes, batteries, film, and cigarettes. This short-term failing compounded the long-term grievances. For example, the islanders had ordered and paid for special roofs to catch rainwater; however, five years later, they had not appeared. Carlotta kept hearing the expression "Chileno malo," although she had not met any Chileans that she could deem "bad"; some she "quite liked."[37]

The chronic neglect provoked resentment and grumbling, but the tensions ran far deeper and extended into politics. The islanders had an elected council, but women could not vote, and all candidates had to be approved by the governor. In addition, every man had to spend one day each week working for the government, without pay, on roads, walls, cutting grass and planting trees, or making various improvements. Worse, they could not leave without permission; even circulation around the island was difficult.[38] According to Law's letter to his wife, Jane Shaw, Easter Island essentially ran on a "feudal system," but an unnamed "French couple" had come to settle there and had begun to spread "communism or democracy," which will always breed well under

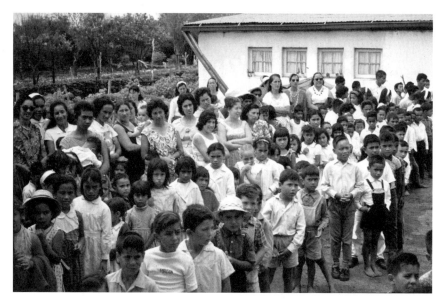

Figure 4.12 Rapanui schoolchildren, in lines by class, their mothers and infant siblings behind, listening to Dr Helen Reid describe METEI, 16 December 1964. Photo Fred Joyce.

such conditions. Law understood that the schoolteacher Alfonso Rapu "fell under the spell" of this French couple.[39] Others contend that Rapu's education, his fostering with a liberal family on the continent, and his native intellect helped him to think well for himself. He agreed.

Forty years later, Rapu told Patricia Stambuk that he had never spoken with the French couple, although he knew about them. His so-called "radicalization" began well before. In 1962, on a visit home from his school in Santiago, he travelled on the annual supply ship, where he met the wife and three daughters of Salvador Allende. After three failed attempts beginning in 1952, the leftist politician would be elected president of Chile in 1970. While the Allende visitors stayed on Easter Island, they became great friends with Rapu, who escorted them to the main sites. He saw the lamentable conditions with new eyes – their eyes – although they did not speak of it directly. They all travelled back to mainland Chile together on the supply ship, and he became a frequent guest in their home, although he never met the politician father, Salvador.[40] Also, in 1962 Rapu had a brutal and close encounter with the arbitrary "justice" of the military rulers. His brother, Carlos, was molested by a dentist named Julio Flores, but when the boy complained to the

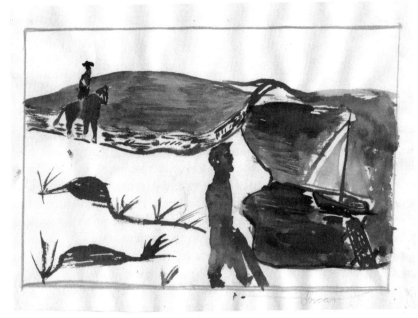

Figure 4.13 Two of the thirty-six pieces of artwork by Rapanui schoolchildren that Helen Reid brought home to Canada. *Above*: Life on the island with *moai*, horseman, and boat, by Oscar. *Below*: Is it a bulldozer? by Bernabé Teao. Reid Papers, file 3.

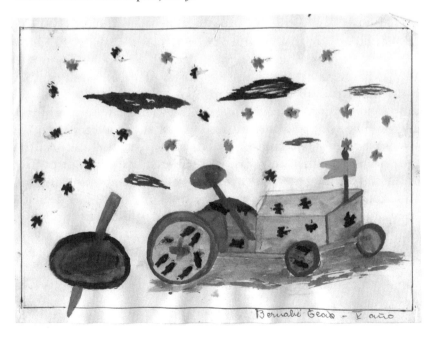

governor of the time, John ("José") Martin – a friend of the dentist – the lad was scolded, stripped, beaten, and thrown in the little stone jail, an experience that marked him for the rest of his life. Three decades later, he told his painful tale to the historical truth commission.[41]

The Chilean election of a new president, Eduardo Frei Montalva, in October 1964 and the prospect of international attention with the December arrival of METEI inspired Rapu and his friend Germán Hotu to draft a two-page letter to Frei enumerating their complaints, many of which concerned Portilla's administration. They also made recommendations. On 8 December, shortly before METEI's arrival, the islanders had staged an election and chosen Rapu as their *alcalde* (mayor). Portilla contended that the island already had a mayor in Lazaro Hotu, and he deemed this election illegal. He appealed to Chile for help, knowing that his actions would be watched closely once METEI arrived.

Five days later, *Cape Scott* sailed smack into the middle of this rising rebellion. On that day, Rapu was not immediately in evidence, nor was there any turmoil, other than the sense that "something was not right." The first mention of Rapu is the school encounter in Helen Reid's diary of 16 December. But all METEI members soon became aware of the problems. The island doctor, Guido Andrade of the Chilean navy, had been part of the official welcoming party, and he offered a cocktail party for METEI members at his home on the evening of day four, 16 December. He too had supported these democratic aspirations. The islanders opened up to the travellers, describing their frustrations and aspirations with the naval administration. The women startled Helen Reid and Carlotta Hacker with their frank expression of views: the governor's punishments were inappropriately severe; he should be shot.[42] Sister Maria Francisca explained to Helen that the previous governor was "a big, strong, powerful man" who gave out heavy sentences: "for example, theft of a wrist watch" could result in "one year in jail with chains."[43] At least one woman's head had been shaved by the governor (or her father) for a "crime" that was never made clear. Both Helen and Carlotta kept track of the many incompatible reasons given for the "cutting of Maria's hair": she wanted to start a brothel; she sang "naughty" songs; she stole something, and her father wanted to kill her, but the governor intervened, cutting her hair instead; the governor was in love with her and resented her rejection; she was too attractive and lured many strangers to Rapa Nui, risking leprosy (governor) or marriage with Chileans (father).[44]

Others have identified the devious "French couple" of Law's account as ethnologist Françis Mazière and his Tahitian wife, Tila, who spent several months on Rapa Nui between 2 February 1963 and the summer of

1963 or 1964, if his later publications are to be believed.[45] The Chileans gave METEI members to understand that their visit had ended only "eight weeks" earlier in October 1964;[46] however, no "French couple" can be identified from that period. In contrast, Law told Jane that Mazière had come "a few years ago."[47] Rapu, who never met them, returned in late 1963; therefore, the French influence is in doubt. In his 1965 book, Mazière excoriated Chile's military rule: the country that had produced Pablo Neruda, he wrote, should understand that improving the wretched conditions on Easter Island was a matter of honour.[48] Not only did he criticize the Chilean administrators, but he also ridiculed all previous scientific expeditions, including that of Heyerdahl. He claimed that he had listened to the islanders with deeper sympathy and used their legends to uncover mysteries that had defied or duped all his predecessors. His book would sell more than 1 million copies in France and enjoy several translations. But in 1964 it had yet to be published, and it would not appear in English until 1968. Mazière predicted that the book would "earn us violent abuse from certain mandarins of science, prudent skepticism from others."[49] Indeed, serious writers about the island largely ignore this book, its merit cribbed from Englert's work of 1948; otherwise, they contend, it is "weak on scholarship but strong on emotion."[50]

No evidence suggests that METEI members knew of Mazière or the democracy movement until after their arrival. Nor does anything back the notion that Mazière was operating on the island for French national interests. Reid described the couple without naming them and situated their departure only eight weeks before METEI's arrival: "the Tahitian wife went about the island in a topless sarong."[51] Law too cited their influence, suggesting that his source was Governor Portilla, who was about to demand a favour of Canada.[52]

FEEDING THE ONE THOUSAND

On day four, the Chilean naval authorities asked *Cape Scott* to supply the deprived islanders with food from her stores and, upon her departure, to convey various Chileans, island schoolchildren, three nuns, a borrowed bulldozer, and the harvest of 72 tons of wool back to the mainland. The proceeds of the wool – about CDN$50,000 yearly – belonged to Chile and were applied to the greater annual costs of running the island – about CDN$151,100.[53] With a ship headed for the mainland, Governor Portilla also decided to expel Dr Andrade to face a disciplinary tribunal for his support of the democracy movement. Dr Gonzalo Donoso would be leaving too, abandoning the METEI nutrition project before it began.

Some wondered if Donoso had participated in the political activities over the few days of his island sojourn; indeed, corresponding to the earlier assessment of his cabin-mate, Brody, Donoso frankly told Reid that he was a communist.[54] From speaking with the priest or the governor, Law thought that Portilla had "banished" both Chilean doctors by the end of METEI's first week.[55] How much METEI members understood of this political situation at that moment is unknown. Nor is it clear that the Rapanui knew that their popular Andrade was under a cloud.

But Skoryna soon grasped that his expedition was in big trouble – a double bind. He could not risk offending the governor; however, if the islanders believed that Chilean authorities approved of METEI, they would not cooperate. The Rapanui seemed to like the Canadians, but a woman told her "amiga" Carlotta that refusing to participate in the examinations was imperative – a way of "striking back."[56] Gone with the notion of genetic homogeneity would be METEI's goal of a 100 per cent sample. As the political tension mounted, Skoryna labelled it "a domestic matter" of no concern to Canada, and he forbade METEI members to mention the political strife in radio conversations with their families. But he knew that he had to communicate with Rapu and that *Cape Scott* had to donate its extra food.

For the distribution of supplies, Law sought permission from his Canadian navy superiors; they consented. Then he agonized over how to proceed. He turned to Father Sebastian, who informed him that the Rapanui did not trust the Chileans and advised the captain to organize it himself. Law handed the task to his supply officer, Lieutenant Commander Alfred Shaw, who set the date for "feeding the multitude" as Saturday, 19 December – day seven.[57] This plan gave Shaw two days to pack the supplies and arrange the handout procedure. It also allowed the navy to complete raising the *campamento*.

By day five – 17 December – all the METEI cargo had been landed, but electricians were still tinkering with the trailers' wiring and the laboratories. Adjacent to the camp, they erected a playground with swing sets and slides for the children. Simultaneously, *Cape Scott* was slowly being loaded with wool from the small Rapanui boats, but the transfer sped up when Law allowed use of the Canadian landing craft. Bob Meier was on guard duty that night while the islanders held one of their *sau sau* parties, which left him tired the following day. On the afternoon of 18 December, the camp was complete, and the METEI members moved from the ship into their new quarters, now dubbed the "Rapa Nui Hilton" (figures 4.14, 4.15, and 4.16). The Canadian navy, like God, had created a new world in just six days.

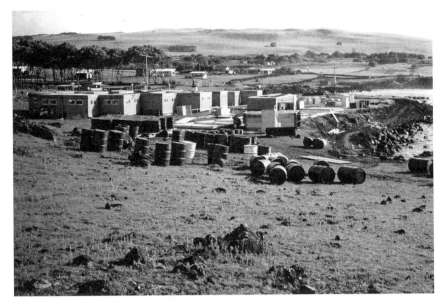

Figure 4.14 METEI's Camp Hilton almost complete, without fence, from the hill to the northeast. The *moai* of Plaza Hotu Matu'a is in the middle distance to the right of the radio antenna. Photo Fred Joyce.

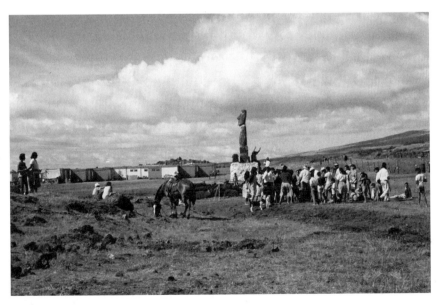

Figure 4.15 METEI's Camp Hilton from the southwest with the *moai* of Plaza Hotu Matu'a. Photo David Murphy.

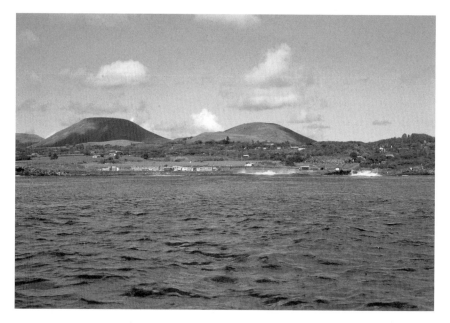

Figure 4.16 METEI's Camp Hilton and Hanga Roa from the sea looking south-southeast. The camp lies along the shore, with the white church higher and to the right. The Puna Pau volcano is in the distance (*centre*). Photo Ian Efford.

Denys and Cléopâtre tried to make their trailer homey: two beds, a folding table, two collapsing lawn chairs, and a little lamp made from an empty bottle of Grand Marnier.[58] Reid was shocked by the *campamento* "kitchen" and its lack of utensils and supplies. "Badly planned, poorly organized, inadequately staffed, it became a thrice daily test of manners and cooperation, and not everyone passed the test. It was five weeks before there was running water in the kitchen or a proper sink and hot water for washing up." She worried about how the cook, Colin Gillingham, would cope. He "had to feed about forty people each meal" without "a single bowl ... no platters or serving dishes, no mixing spoons, no vegetable peeler, cheese grater, rolling pin; no pie plates or large enough roasting pans, no beaters, no shelves for supplies or dishes, no drawers for boxes of cutlery." The only jugs for powdered milk and juice had been borrowed from the departing *Cape Scott*. Why had METEI transported 50 pounds of chili powder but no rice and 300 pounds of pancake powder but no griddle?[59] Maureen Roberts also found the kitchen arrangements challenging. She pitched in, "glad to

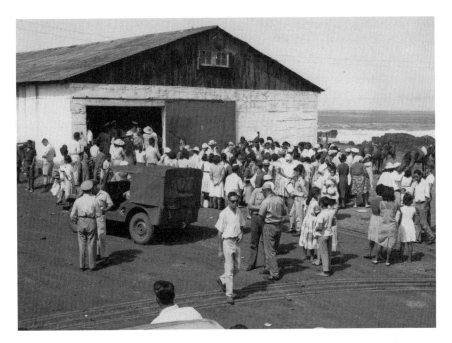

Figure 4.17 Feeding the one thousand. Crew of HMCS *Cape Scott* distribute extra supplies at Hanga Piko, 19 December 1964. LAC, Law Scrapbook, vol. 3, envelope CS 1179.

help," as cooking was "an interest"; but the rations, determined by a Montreal dietician thinking of office workers, were "only about half adequate for our younger members who were working like stevedores and carpenters." They depended on "carbohydrates to make up the calories, and this was not appreciated as every loaf of bread had to be made by hand and this put a terrific strain on the cook, and the masses of pumpernickel alternative was not at all popular."[60]

METEI took its first meal in the *campamento* dining room, a pleasant affair, despite the culinary challenges – "sympathique," Cléopâtre wrote.[61] Skoryna chaired a meeting to discuss the next steps. The conversation was dominated by concerns over organization of the research and security measures: what was to be done about the many islanders who entered the compound at will and at all hours? They could be found staring through windows or standing with their horses in front of the trailer doors. A fence was part of the plan; once it was erected, Skoryna predicted that it would solve the matter, although some wondered about the hostile symbolism. Access would be limited to the open end with examining rooms and laboratories. Denied entry to the inner courtyard, islanders clustered at the gate, singing, dancing, and watching.

On the morning of Saturday, 19 December, the day designated for distributing food packages, "all 300 families" of islanders assembled at Hanga Piko (figure 4.17). Using the census provided by the governor, which John Cutler and Elliot Alpert were updating for the study, Shaw had devised a sliding scale of quantities determined by family size; none of the offerings were large. Onlookers included Portilla, Father Sebastian and his assistant, Father Ricardo Rainer, "official" mayor Lazaro Hotu and his council, and various members of METEI. The people were "terribly happy" with these gifts, Law told Jane: "they threw their arms around me and gave me the Polynesian hug, and placed beads around my neck made out of sea shells. They all went home with their families on horseback as happy as can be." Later, singers and dancers, mostly teenagers, came out to *Cape Scott* and performed for the ship's company with their "wonderful harmony."[62]

DR ANDRADE'S LECTURE ON RAPANUI HEALTH

That same afternoon, Dr Andrade gave a lecture to METEI members about the diseases he had seen in his two years on the island and the operations he had performed (figure 4.18). Helen Reid, Bob Meier, and David Murphy, possibly others, took detailed notes, expecting that they would be useful to the METEI study. Andrade had attended 107 deliveries, most in hospital with two at home.[63] Having spent a residency year at the Mayo Clinic and another in Detroit, he was fond of surgery and had performed an astonishing number of operations: 191 surgical cases, including 76 cholecystectomies. He claimed to have lost only one patient despite the rudimentary facilities in the hospital. Medical members of METEI were skeptical that this prolific surgical work had been necessary. Did Rapa Nui have a higher incidence of gall bladder disease than elsewhere? Advance word of Andrade's surgical proclivities had already caused Helen to skip his cocktail party: "He has done 200 major operations in the two years he has been here, 75% of them gallbladder removals. A remarkable figure in a population of 900!!"[64] In his lecture, which she did attend, Andrade delivered a complete breakdown of births, deaths, and the causes of disease in his more than 700 consultations over the two years; many people suffered from more than one condition (table 4.1). Helen changed her mind: he spoke with "dignity and much erudition," and she respected the people's affection for him. She later annotated the passage: "at this time I didn't know of his political activities."[65]

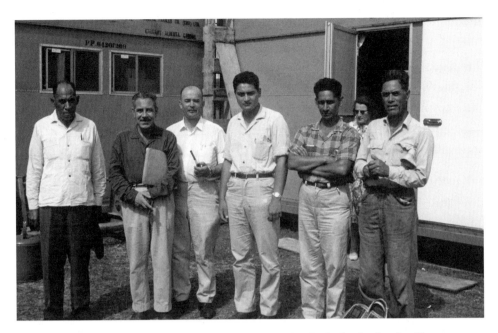

Figure 4.18 *From left,* Mayor Lazaro Hotu, Dr Guido Andrade, Stanley Skoryna, future mayor Alfonso Rapu, Germán Hotu, Helen Reid, and unknown. Possibly occasion of Andrade's lecture, 19 December 1964. Photo David Murphy.

Andrade discussed what he called the psychology of the islanders, revealing the derogatory view of the colonial masters. "Very sensitive" and imaginative, they could distinguish good from bad. But, he continued, they are "terrific liars." As for social conditions, 46 per cent did not have their own beds. Acute alcoholic intoxication was a problem whenever a well-stocked ship arrived. Delinquency was rising because there was no employment. Prostitution did not exist, he claimed, as free sex was well accepted in their society. He confirmed the impression that the islanders were not inbred; consanguinity was frowned upon. A girl who worked in the hospital was "related to everyone" and could marry no one on the island, a unique predicament oft-repeated in diaries and media. The meat consumed was 99 per cent lamb, available all year. They ate fish during the winter months of June, July, and August and occasionally milk and eggs. Helen had already discovered that the children were given milk and bread at school once or twice a day; the nuns opined that, for some, it was their only meal. She and David Murphy both annotated their extensive notes with "insufficient data on nutrition."[66]

Table 4.1 Dr Andrade's report of health on Rapa Nui, 1963–64

A. Deaths in hospital: 7 (6 children, 1 adult)

Bronchopneumonia with asthma: baby four months old
2 intoxications (accidental poisonings): 3 years old, Dieldrin (an insecticide); and age illegible, "Gamma tox" [hydroxybutyric acid?]
Congenital heart disease: newborn
Dehydration: child
Asphyxia neonatorium: newborn
Biliary peritonitis with subphrenic abscess (following gall bladder operation)

B. Important diseases

Tuberculosis	23 new cases: 3 genital, 1 peritoneal; BCG program for newborns
Leprosy (based on a 1962 WHO visit by Brazilian leprologist)	18 ambulatory cases, 6 in sanatorium, 4,763 smears, only 7 suspected active cases
Asthma	42 cases of severe bronchial asthma
Tetanus	1 case
Eosinophilia (sign of parasites)	61 of 183 adults tested, 50 children
Anemia	15 adults, 16 children
Smallpox	No evidence of smallpox
Typhoid	No typhoid vaccine
Polio	No polio vaccine

C. Medical consultations, 1963–64:
Diagnoses and numbers of consultations (total 992)

Abscess	19
Amenorrhea, primary	1
Bronchitis (smoking related, aggravated by northwest wind)	190
Colds	326
Congenital malformation (amaurosis)	3
Cough	339

Dermatological problems	18
Endocrine disturbances	2
Enteritis	160
Erysipelas	5
Furunculosis	41
Headaches	392
Idiocy	2
Influenza	620
Moniliasis	80
Muscular pain	79
Mycosis (no athlete's foot)	32
Nasal/sinusitis	75
Neuroses/hysteria	35
Oligophrenia (mental retardation)	3
Otitis	3
Parasitosis	109
Parotiditis (mumps)	3
Pelvic inflammatory disease (no gonorrhea)	27
Pharyngitis	89
Pneumonitis viral	7
Pyelonephritis	9
Stomach pain	45
Tonsillitis	162
Varicose ulcers	2

Source: Based on Murphy Diary, nd; Reid Diary, 17 December 1964, and nd, 101v–102.

Andrade – or a predecessor – also had a proclivity for performing skin biopsies for leprosy through a crescent-shaped incision under the left eye. So many people were "marked" in this manner that Carlotta and Helen wondered if the scar was, in fact, a tribal custom that the Rapanui were shy to explain. When asked, the islanders provided the dubious response that it came from falling off horses; but then, one day, a boy came in with a wound under his left eye after he fell from a horse.[67]

Some METEI members told me that Andrade was a "terrible doctor" who had been sent to the island to pay off gambling debts.[68] Helen heard

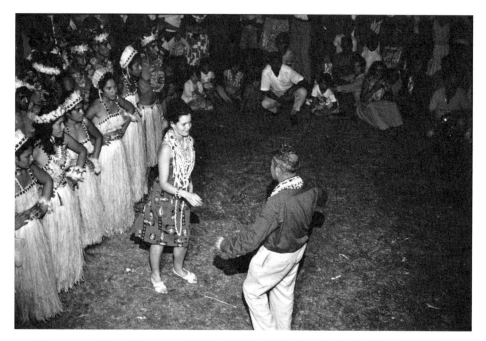

Figure 4.19 Farewell *sau sau* for Dr Guido Andrade, who is dancing with his wife, 19 December 1964. Photo Fred Joyce.

that he was "an alcoholic." One afternoon, Efford and Gibbs found the doctor blind drunk and lying "among the fig trees in the centre of the island"; they "loaded him onto [the] truck and took him home and put him to bed."[69] Nevertheless, the people loved him, and his intoxication may have been in response to his impending expulsion. A farewell dinner of chicken, lobster, salad, and fruit was held in his honour, with more singing and dancing. Helen was puzzled by his wife's "detached and remote" expression as they danced together and walked off hand in hand (figure 4.19).[70] If the doctor was a prisoner, his arrest was understated. Accustomed to the comings and goings of various officials, the islanders accepted his departure with sadness but without probing deeply into the reasons why.

As for Dr Donoso, some sources suggest that he was not banished but had decided to leave of his own accord. He may have imagined that without Andrade, the authorities might force him to remain when the Canadians left – an indefinite sentence that he wanted to avoid. Reid wrote that he "suddenly remembered" a commitment in Trinidad.[71] The Montandons understood that he had a contract to begin work for the

United Nations on 1 February, and no one expected a Chilean supply ship before that date.⁷² Indeed, the delayed supply ship was now said to be "cancelled." With *Cape Scott* about to depart, Donoso's prospect of rescue became even more remote. He could not keep a rendezvous for 1 February if he did not take advantage of a sailing in December. His decision to leave meant that no Chilean was participating in METEI, something that Chile had demanded prior to granting permission.

EARLY EXPLORATIONS AND THE BULLDOZER CONTROVERSY

The next day was Sunday – the day of rest. Many METEI members and Tony Law went to Father Sebastian's little church. "All the Polynesians with two hundred or more voices sang the entire time during the service. Their voices and harmony [were] wonderful," he told Jane. "I enjoyed that service and will never hear another like it again." The Canadian naval surgeon Gilbert Bérubé sang a solo in his "wonderful operatic voice." The captain took lunch with the mayor, Father Ricardo, and Father Sebastian, "a wonderful old man of eighty-one." Again, the grateful islanders gave Law many presents, including carvings and fruit.⁷³

Bob Meier tried to explore the island on a rented horse, heading northeast to its only beach at Anakena. But the animal was so tired that he gave up half-way, somewhere in the hills, and had to pull his mount most of the way back. The sun went down, and he discovered the daunting, profound darkness that made nocturnal movement almost impossible. For his part, Jim Nielsen wandered the island like a celebrity, trading on his "Kon-Tiki-Iti-Iti" persona and oblivious to its repercussions; islanders would offer him a good horse every day, and he never had to pay. Long after the journey, he learned that his popularity irritated Skoryna, who tried to get rid of him by sending him off with *Cape Scott* until Peter Beighton and others intervened on his behalf.⁷⁴

That night, while a farewell party feted the ship's officers, Rapu and his followers sabotaged the borrowed bulldozer. According to both Garry Brody and Helen Reid, this act was the spark that ignited the strife that would follow (see chapter 6). The bulldozer had been on the island because of the parlous condition of the old Mataveri "airport," a grass strip that had received rare exploratory flights since at least 1951. In 1964 no plane had landed in one or two years. The planned airport improvement was not for tourism, nor was it for the islanders. The upgrades were needed for joint American and Chilean interests to serve a "top-secret satellite tracking station."⁷⁵ Ostensibly built to monitor weather, the station was a Cold

War tool designed to track Russian ships and South American communications. When the airport plans were confirmed, the American ambassador to Chile decided to inspect its future location. In 1962 or early 1963, his party set out with two planes, both DC-6BS, one bearing the diplomats and the other carrying supplies. Upon landing, the first plane sank into the soft earth of Mataveri and stuck. Watching the situation from on high, the pilot of the second plane decided not to land and returned to Chile. A Chilean navy vessel rescued the stranded Americans and brought along a bulldozer, borrowed from the city of Valparaiso, to liberate their plane; however, the earth-encased aircraft had already been "liberated" by sixty islanders wielding shovels under the direction of Governor Martin. *Cape Scott* presented a "golden opportunity" because she was the first visiting ship large enough to take the bulldozer home.[76]

But the islanders wanted the bulldozer to stay. They were using it to improve their roads. Carlotta Hacker claimed that ownership of the bulldozer spawned rumours. Some said that it did not really belong to Chile; the Americans had intended it as a gift.[77] When they heard that *Cape Scott* would take it away, Rapu and his mates disabled it by removing some parts, possibly the carburetor, although a recent account from Rapa Nui suggests it was the main axle.[78] "Valparaiso has lots of bulldozers," they argued, "and this one was needed on the island." Their act of insubordination enraged Portilla, who ordered Rapu's arrest and demanded return of the missing part within twenty-four hours. Rapu went into hiding, and the part was not returned.

There are many versions of the rest of this story, and the exact sequence of events is not clear. Eventually – either before (Hacker) or after (Reid) the departure of *Cape Scott* – Skoryna finally met with Rapu and/or two or three of his "illegal" councillors. He also negotiated with the governor. METEI could proceed if it met several conditions: women and children were to be examined only by female doctors; no blood, other than a finger prick, was to be taken from children under age seven; and only 25 millilitres of blood were to be taken from everyone else, although it became 40 millilitres. No gynecological examinations were to be performed unless medically indicated. James Boutilier and Reid indicate that the governor and his advisory council laid down these rules as early as the night of Andrade's lecture.[79] Rapu's group wanted no examinations until after the repeat election scheduled for mid-January. Skoryna's correspondence suggests that he was meeting with both sides, possibly without revealing his double negotiations.[80] Whatever the origin of the stipulations, Skoryna agreed to all, except Rapu's wish for a delay.

This agreement was a form of damage control, quickly communicated to the METEI team. The two women doctors were going to have to do most of the work. They also realized that, without Andrade or Donoso, METEI would be the sole medical (and surgical) support for the entire island until Chile sent another doctor. This caregiving task had never been part of the original plan; however, METEI physicians accepted it, adding a call schedule and hospital duties to the responsibilities, and they began making daily rounds with designated interpreters in the little infirmary.[81] Military nurses would alert them when emergencies arose.

GOODBYE HMCS *CAPE SCOTT*

The camp was complete, and the navy was now ready to leave. Skoryna took the opportunity to scrawl a report to Al Tunis back in Montreal, a missive full of hope: "I have spent the last few days negotiating with the Governor and the Eldermen [Rapu et al.] ... As you may well imagine these two factions do not agree ... However, thanks to our approach and (again) the assistance of the Navy by giving gifts to the Islanders – the plan is to examine 100% of the population and I hope it will be possible." He also praised all the METEI members who helped "physically" with the raising of the camp. It was his "hope" that the "excellent" "spirit of cooperation" would persist. Then he explained how much money would be needed for Chilean stamps for the postcard scheme – at least $1,000. The stamps would have to be purchased in Chile before the return of *Cape Scott*. Skoryna enclosed a report by Mary King for Toronto's *Globe and Mail* and another by Rita Dwyer for the *Ottawa Citizen*, and he asked Tunis to forward them, clarifying that he had no prior arrangement with either paper. He wrote, "If [the newspapers] would be willing to contribute to the Expedition ... [all] the better. In any case, it is good for the Expedition to have reports." Finally, he stated what had been suspected all along: the landing was difficult "due to the Pacific swell & it will be almost impossible to take those trailers off the Island. Commander Law has promised to talk to the Can. Ambassador in Santiago to convince the Can. Foreign Office to purchase the remaining trailers. All I can say, I hope it works. If not, I think we will have to finance the remaining trailers until we find the money."[82] Meanwhile, Mrs Gerd Hurum was closing the books of the Easter Island Expedition Society for 1964; she estimated the debt at $20,000.[83]

Reid also wrote one last letter to family at home. In earlier messages, she had enthused about the great adventure, the interesting people, her fondness for the navy, and her love of *Cape Scott*. Now she admitted to

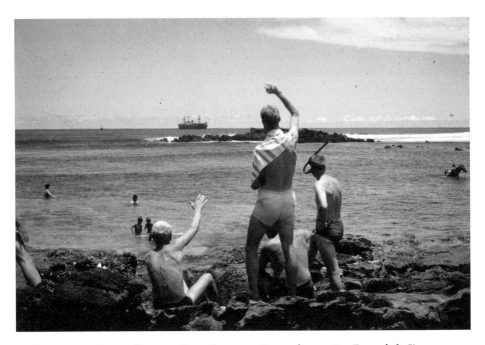

Figure 4.20 Farewell HMCS *Cape Scott*, 21 December 1964. *From left*, Jim Nielsen, Björn Ekblom, unknown, and Ian Efford, with a child on horseback in the sea (*right*). Photo Fred Joyce.

apprehension about the mission: "Poor Colin, the cook, finds the going hard, so we try to help ... We have a lot of deadwood in camp and I feel trapped. If we make a mess I will feel personally responsible to the navy. I have to work, and they slack all the more."[84]

Monday morning, 21 December, Meier and the other men were sent to raise the chain-link fence; "damn hot work," he wrote. It provoked more controversy. Some contended that the fence was superfluous and would aggravate relations by an implied lack of trust; others thought it was necessary for security and privacy. At noon, as METEI members worked and watched, *Cape Scott* weighed anchor and "slowly sunk into the horizon. [I will] see her again I trust," wrote Meier, but he had doubts: "she had trouble with evaporators" (figure 4.20).[85] Her human cargo included forty-two Chileans, of whom twenty-six were schoolchildren, three nuns, the island's dentist, and the agronomist, as well as Dr Donoso and Dr Andrade with his family. Two stowaways, found hiding in the wool, were returned to shore. David Macfarlane claimed it was four. With their restricted freedom, Rapanui often hid as stowaways on departing ships. One was found upon METEI's definitive departure in February 1965, and no fewer than twelve were hiding on a Chilean vessel in April 1965.[86]

At sea between Easter Island and South America, Tony Law typed another letter to Jane. He described the challenging and dangerous work that the navy had accomplished and his immense satisfaction with the crew: "I am very proud of my officers and men. They all did an extremely fine job of getting the material ashore, and building the Hilton Camp Site, as well as installing the Solar Still and the Mechanical Still, which are both providing fresh water ... The power generators were installed quickly and are providing all kinds of power to meet the needs of the scientists. I have successfully completed my part of the agreement; now it is up to the Medical Expedition to get down to their medical work."[87]

Law knew that the navy gift of provisions to the islanders would encourage their cooperation. He told Jane of the two "banished" doctors. Andrade was obviously seen as a prisoner by the navy men and some METEI members; Westropp and Gibbs both remember that he was metaphorically led away "in chains." The captain described his low opinion of "the mad Doctor Skoryna." "He is extremely difficult as he lives on cloud nine and his feet ... never touch earth. I think poor little Air Vice Marshal Easton has his hands full with such an abstract, way out 'Nut' ... Many of the members do not have much use for him. The Doctor is extremely clever but way out." Law also harboured reservations about Skoryna's premise for the research on "these *primitive people* – who can do the twist much better than [we] and have outboard motors on their boats. They also have many horses to a family, land, and cows and sheep. They are much better off than we crazy whitemen ... Their children cannot get candy and pop etc. They are a very healthy group."[88]

With many others, Law might have been surprised to learn that Skoryna and Nógrády agreed with him. His attitude reveals a misunderstanding of the objectives of the expedition for which he had done so much. METEI's concern had always been to characterize the current – as it turned out, good – state of health in order to uncover what might happen once the airport opened and the world's microbes and bad habits flooded in. The error about "inbreeding" aside, never had they pretended that Rapa Nui was backward or unhealthy, nor had they presumed that the two-month sojourn could improve things. They wanted merely to document and do no harm. Law's views of METEI were coloured by the media, by the missionary zeal that lurked around the project – for example, in the stamp campaign – and by his loathing of Skoryna.

Personal animosity and scientific confusion notwithstanding, Law shared Skoryna's hopes for the expedition: "I wish them luck with their project." He told Jane how the governor had failed to catch Rapu for deportation before *Cape Scott* set sail: "I am glad [Rapu] did not come with me as the Islanders might have made it very difficult for the Medical Expedition to carry out [its] research and studies."[89] With three nuns in the cabin next door, he predicted that he would be a "reformed character by the time I reach Halifax." Little did he know that one of those nuns, Sister Esperanza, was carrying the letter of complaint from Germán Hotu and Alfonso Rapu to President Frei. It is not clear that Law ever knew how it found its way into the Chilean papers (see chapter 8).

Despite the many unforeseen complications – political, logistical, meteorological, and personal – the creation of Camp Hilton was complete within the anticipated six days. Even if METEI accomplished no science at all, the safe transport of an entirely self-sufficient research station, with living quarters, laboratories, clinic, kitchen, toilets, water, and power, over a distance of more than 9,000 kilometres was a monumental achievement all by itself – unique for Canada, possibly unique for the entire world.

Stanley's dream was still not a reality, but now it entered the tangible realm of possibility.

PART TWO

Rapa Nui to Canada, 21 December 1964 to 17 March 1965

5

The Study Begins

After the departure of HMCS *Cape Scott*, the medical members and the physiologists of the Medical Expedition to Easter Island had to wait for the completion of the clinics, laboratories, X-ray unit, and ergometer before they could examine people. In the meantime, the ecologists and veterinarians got busy with their research (see chapter 7). Christmas would come on Friday, bringing more interruptions, and it would soon be followed by another Sunday break. They were getting restless. Some attended a ceremony to mark the last day of school on 23 December, during which certificates were given and prizes offered to the children. Helen Reid noticed that Alfonso Rapu was absent, but three nuns carried on regardless.[1] Laid out on a table were little gifts: crayons, toys, clothing, and other small objects. The lad with the best marks went first. Armand Boudreault was deeply affected by the boy's choice: a bar of soap.

In the "reception area," METEI set up a Christmas tree, transported from Nova Scotia in the ship's refrigerator and brought to the camp by Garry Brody with the dented METEI truck (figure 5.1). With a star on top, it was decorated with red balls, silver bells, and "icicles" made from tinfoil that had been used to cook fish; its needles were crispy and turning brown.[2] The tree proved a popular attraction for children and amateur photographers; some islanders contend that it was the first one they had ever seen. Skoryna used a colour photograph of himself with children and the little tree as his personal Christmas card in 1965 (figure 5.2).[3]

The clinical facilities, with six examining rooms, occupied three trailers, in typical ATCO turquoise, arranged in a staggered line extending west out from the main compound. Nearby, at right angles, three white trailers were joined on their long sides to form the labs and the X-ray unit. Not only would Rapanui be thoroughly inspected, measured, and imaged, but they would also donate samples of their fluids, excreta, skin, and hair, and

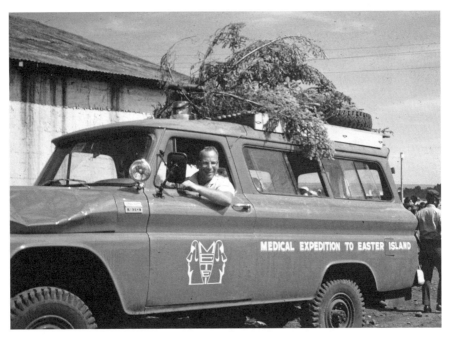

Figure 5.1 Garry Brody in the dented Jeep Mea Mea driving the Christmas tree from Hanga Piko to Camp Hilton. Photo Fred Joyce.

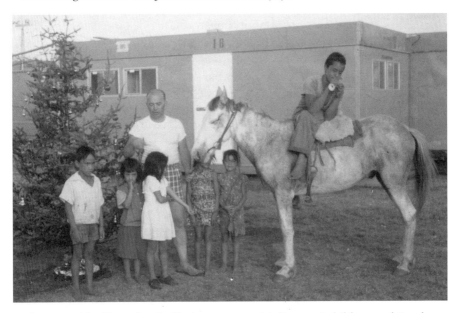

Figure 5.2 The Nova Scotia Christmas tree with Rapanui children and Stanley Skoryna, who used this photo as his 1965 Christmas card. Reid Papers, file 15

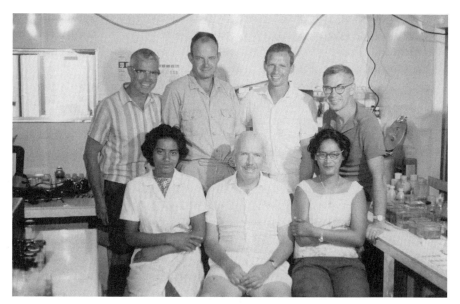

Figure 5.3 METEI lab team. *Back row from left*, Fred Joyce, Harold Gibbs, David Murphy, and Armand Boudreault. *Front row from left*, Norma (later "Tauranga") Hucke Atán, Archie Wilkinson, and Margarita Tepano Kaituoe ("Uka"). Photo David Murphy.

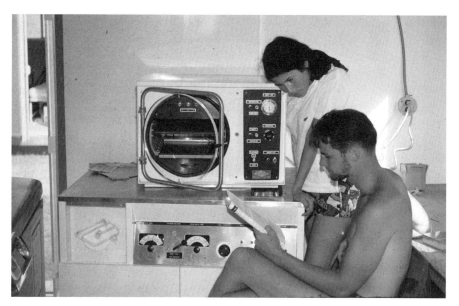

Figure 5.4 Cléopâtre and Denys Montandon with his lyophilizer. Photo Fred Joyce.

swabs were taken from their noses, throats, and anuses. Some specimens were scrutinized on the spot in the evenings; others were stored for return to Canada. In addition, to create reasonably reliable conditions for diabetic screening, the team used a simplified glucose tolerance test: everyone over age seven was to down a sugary drink of 100 grams of glucose; one hour later, a urine sample was requested (for glucose, protein, and pH) and a blood sample drawn (for glucose, among many other things). From the blood, serum fractions would be collected, divided, and placed in tubes for immunology and chemistry tests, including cholesterol levels, as requested by Fraser Mustard. Elliot Alpert and Fred Joyce were placed in charge of the sugar and cholesterol collection and analysis.[4]

Archie Wilkinson set up his X-ray machine in a space of 3 by 3 metres in one of the white trailers. It was not ideal; he had to reposition the machine several times for each person's size and body part. They would undergo X-rays of chest, head, and teeth – and if they were children, hands and wrists too. The other half of his small space served as his dark room, for Archie had to develop, as well as shoot, all the images taken on Rapa Nui. To do so he needed abundant water, and water proved a problem.[5] The space was hot, humid, cramped, and dark, and the work was heavy. Dressed mostly in a T-shirt and shorts, he managed to examine almost thirty people every day, taking and developing a daily average of 105 films. Archie liked the happy children and would tousle their hair. They knew him as the man who would ask them to "take a deep breath and hold it," which he could pronounce in flawless Rapanui: "Haka naro te hangu!" They called him by that name. It stuck, and ever after, his extended family back home called him "Haki."[6]

The laboratories were the domain of several people: navy technologist Fred Joyce, virologist Armand Boudreault, bacteriologist Georges Nógrády, physician Maureen Roberts, parasitologist Hal Gibbs, and pathologist (masquerading as hematologist) Eivind Myhre (figure 5.3). Joyce, Gibbs, Myhre, and Boudreault did a lot of the building, putting up shelves and creating benches. Unfortunately, the people would have to march through the lab to have their blood taken. Worried about contamination and privacy, Boudreault chose a little corner for his virology work as far from the traffic as possible. Also, using a piece of plywood, he walled off a space of less than 2 by 2 metres in the reception trailer, where he hooked up his freezer. In so doing, he made the astonishing discovery that in all their carefully assembled provisions, METEI had brought no nails.

The laboratory had facilities for taking blood in syringes and by finger prick, cupboards for reagents, thousands of test tubes, glass slides, workbenches, microscopes, freezers, fridges, a lyophilizer for turning

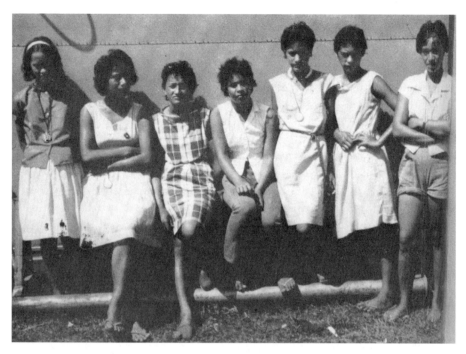

Figure 5.5 The Rapanui girls who helped METEI. *From left*, Elena Huke Atán (14), Norma (later "Tauranga") Hucke Tepihe [Atán] (17), Ana Teao Atamu (13), Maria Bernardita Huke Atán (15), Maria Raquel Paoa Huki (13), Ana Rosa Laharoa Hei (13), and Teresa Tepihe Hotus (17). Names from METEI records may not be correct. Reid, *World Away*, opposite 55; original in Reid Papers, file 17.

liquid serum samples into powder, and many dishes for holding special agar media for growing bacterial cultures. Brody sometimes helped take blood, and Denys Montandon was in charge of the lyophilizer, newly trained in its mysteries from his trip to New York (figure 5.4).

Margarita Tepano Kaituoe, the thirty-five-year-old laboratory technician from the local infirmary, came to assist. Several teenage girls also contributed to washing equipment and cleaning the facilities (figure 5.5). Nógrády and Reid recorded their names, some erroneously, as Norma Hucke Tepihe [Atán] (17), Elena Huke Atán (14), Maria Bernardita Huke Atán (15), Ana Rosa Laharoa Hei (13), Maria Raquel Paoa Huki (13), Ana Teao Atamu (13), and Teresa Tepihe Hotus (17).[7] Georgina Sonia Riroroko Tuki also appears in the laboratory in photos taken by Fred Joyce and Armand Boudreault. Sixteen-year-old Jorge Ika Pakarati joined the team a little later. Carlotta Hacker never quite understood his purpose, as all she ever saw him do was pass bottles to Nógrády. "Just what does Jorge do?" she asked Georges one day. "Oh, he is very useful," came the reply. "He hands me bottles when I ask for them."[8] The laboratory precinct absorbed the most electricity of the camp, even more than the kitchen.

The people who helped METEI were not paid in cash, which would have been useless to them. They were paid in donations of food from the METEI stores and often in goods, such as dresses, fabric, soap, or cosmetics. At the end of the sojourn, Skoryna gave each of the clinic girls a fob watch, which they wore round their necks like medals.[9] The grown men were given McGill University badges.

EXPLORING THE ISLAND

In the slow days before the holiday and the onset of the physical examinations, Helen Reid and many others went exploring on horseback. She expected to have little free time later. Having read about the island's history and prehistory, METEI members studied maps and were eager to see the statues, volcanoes, caves, and remains of ancient dwellings.

Triangular Rapa Nui is surrounded by sea, but it has only one big beach at Anakena in the northeast. Thor Heyerdahl had camped there in 1955, and that is where he had goaded Rapanui men into raising a *moai* that still loomed (and continues to loom) over the shore. A smaller beach, called Ovahi, lay just to the east of it. Several burned-out volcanoes pocked the island. As Bob Meier had discovered, Anakena was a long way from Hanga Roa, almost 18 kilometres, a hike of three and a half hours. The two volcanic destinations favoured by METEI (and tourists today) were Rano Raraku, where hundreds of *moai* had been carved, many left to accumulate half-buried on the slopes, and Rano Kao, closer to Hanga Roa village and Camp Hilton. Both volcanoes encircled reedy crater lakes. Villagers used Rano Kao as a source of water when rain supplies were low. On its lip were Birdman carvings and the remains of an old village, Orongo, where oval rings of stone defined the foundations of dwellings that had once been covered with branches and leaves. From Orongo, in 1868, the English ship HMS *Topaze* had taken the great *moai* called Hoa Hakananai'a ("lost or stolen friend"), which still resides in the British Museum despite vigorous calls for its repatriation. Looking west from Orongo, the three tiny bird islets – Moto Nui, Motu Kao Kao, and needle-like Motu Iti – were clearly visible as jagged specks in the blue sea. Only the bravest METEI members would visit those islands.

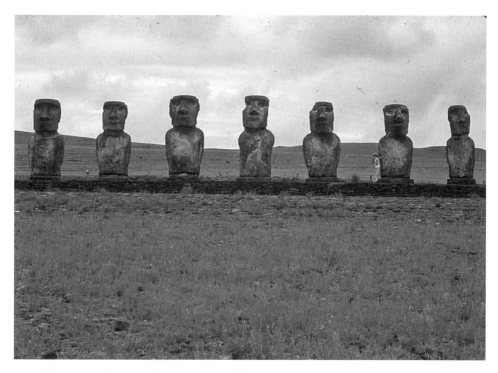

Figure 5.6 Carlotta Hacker at Ahu Akivi, reconstructed in 1960.
Photo Archibald Wilkinson.

As for the *moai*, most lay on the ground, toppled by warfare, weather, and tidal waves – except for those on the slopes at Rano Raraku. But in 1960 the American archeologist William T. Mulloy and his Chilean colleague Gonzalo Figueroa García-Huidobro had raised seven statues on a platform at Ahu Akivi, located inland on the barren plain to the northeast of the village (figure 5.6). At the time of METEI, it was the only reconstructed site. The travellers were impressed with the solemn figures but had already absorbed the notion that it faced in the "wrong" direction. Not too far from Hanga Roa was the small Puna Pau volcano, with its rock quarry, which had been the source of the red, cylindrical topknots. None of the *moai* wore topknots in 1964. These reddish stones had migrated widely, and Bob Meier spotted a few making up the foundation of a barn.[10]

Two other destinations attracted the scientists: first, the sheep farm at Vaitea in the centre of the island, which boasted 38,000 sheep; and second, Mataveri, southwest of Hanga Roa, lying between it and Rano Kao, site of the governor's home, his farm, and the airstrip. The more adventurous searched for the many caves that Heyerdahl had made famous; some featured wall paintings and carvings; others could be entered only by climbing down daunting cliff faces at dizzying heights over sharp lava rocks in the restless sea. Alone, Helen went to as many of these places as she could on her rented horse, Marko, who "cost" a bottle of perfume and a bar of soap each day.[11]

CHRISTMAS ON EASTER ISLAND

On Christmas Eve, Father Sebastian Englert celebrated Midnight Mass for the islanders and METEI travellers. He wore new white and gold robes, sent from Franciscans in Canada. Even those not given to attending religious services went along to witness the musical celebration, marvelling at the familiar carols rendered in Rapanui and at the clear, sweet voices with one odd, raucous sound – "like a eunuch," wrote Cléopâtre Montandon. Jim Nielsen and Archie Wilkinson made recordings. Reid offered prayers for the unfortunate people she'd seen: a disabled boy crawling on all fours; a lonely old woman tending graves in the cemetery. She also prayed for the expedition itself; her spirits were low, and she was weary of her own anger and perversity.[12]

Denys Montandon was on call with Stanley Skoryna at the hospital. Immediately after Mass, they made the rounds, checking on its three patients: two men and a woman suffering, respectively, from asthma, diarrhea, and a ventral hernia sequela of a cholecystectomy performed by Dr Guido Andrade.[13] With a handful of expedition members, Carlotta was invited to the home of her friend Georgina for a *sau sau* of dancing that went on till morning. Georgina became an endless source of information about island gossip and politics.[14]

On Christmas Day, a *curando* feast took place at an islander's home. Fascinated to discover that the "oven" was a hole in the ground 2 metres wide and 1 metre deep, Cléopâtre drew a diagram (figure 5.7) The islanders began with hot rocks and coals, laying wood on top, followed by leaves; when the pit reached the right temperature, they put in whole fish and chunks of meat, covered with more leaves and cobs of corn. Never had they eaten more perfect tuna and beef.[15] Carlotta and Helen also went to a *curando*, possibly the same one, although they ate pork, at the home of Carlos Teao Ika ("Big Carlo") (figure 5.8).[16] Back at Camp Hilton, Maureen Roberts spent Christmas morning preparing a traditional, festive meal, complete with plum pudding. The already well-fed METEI members devoured that repast too. Helen and sailor Harry Crosman fabricated a centrepiece of wire and red geraniums in the shape of a Christmas tree.[17]

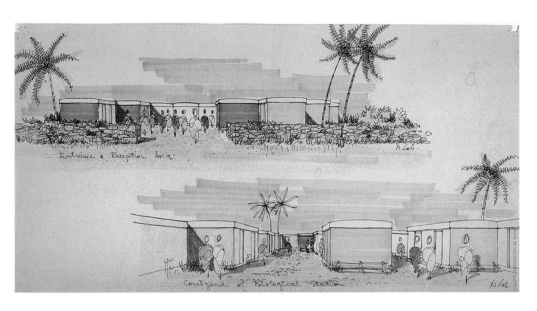

Figure 2.3 Revised plan of the METEI compound with ATCO trailers. Norbert Schoenauer. McGill School of Architecture, http://cac.mcgill.ca/schoenauer/index.htm.

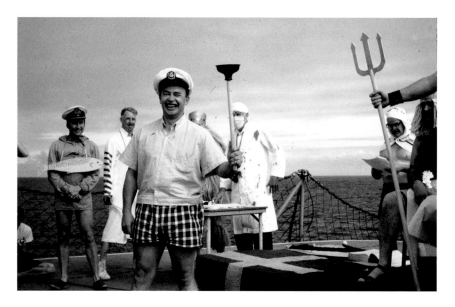

Figure 3.10 Commander Tony Law with the Order of the Fish and Stanley
Skoryna awarded a plunger at the crossing the equator ceremony,
5 December 1964. Photo Fred Joyce.

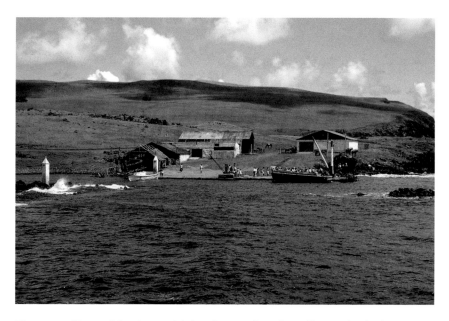

Figure 4.3 Hanga Piko jetty with landing craft and small crowd. The barren
Rano Kao volcano is behind. Photo Ian Efford.

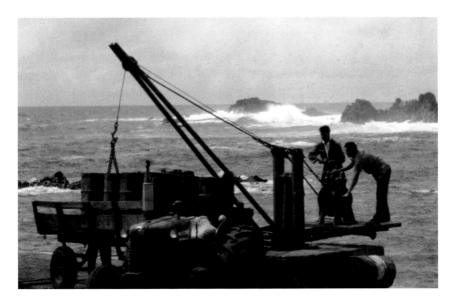

Figure 4.5 Unloading diesel fuel barrels at Hanga Piko jetty.
Photo Peter Beighton.

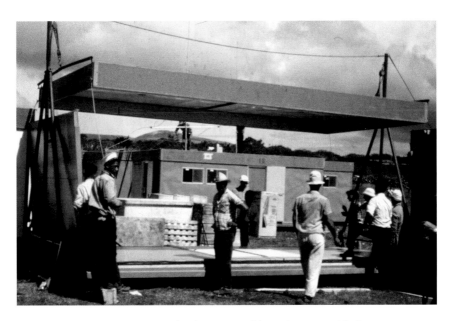

Figure 4.6 Raising an ATCO "shoebox" portable with Rapanui helpers.
Photo Peter Beighton.

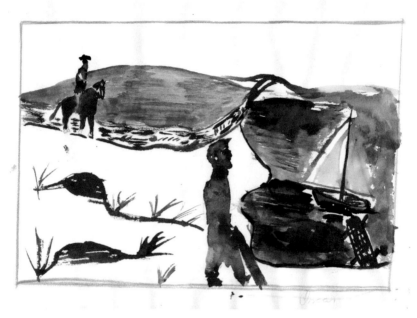

Figure 4.13 Two of the thirty-six pieces of artwork by Rapanui schoolchildren that Helen Reid brought home to Canada. *Above*: Life on the island with *moai*, horseman, and boat, by Oscar. *Below*: Is it a bulldozer? by Bernabé Teao. Reid Papers, file 3.

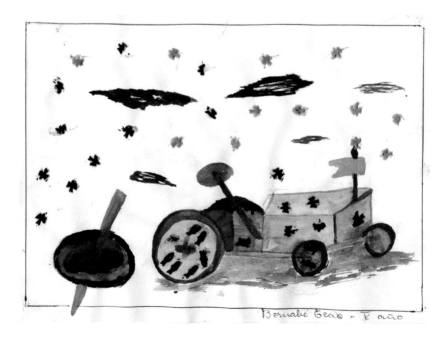

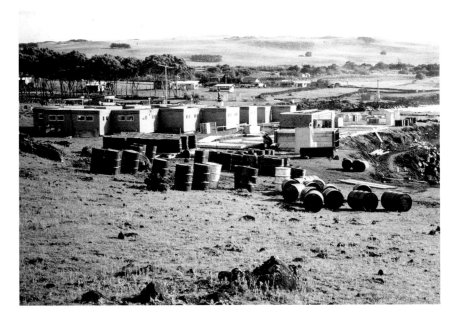

Figure 4.14 METEI's Camp Hilton almost complete, without fence, from the hill to the northeast. The *moai* of Plaza Hotu Matu'a is in the middle distance to the right of the radio antenna. Photo Fred Joyce.

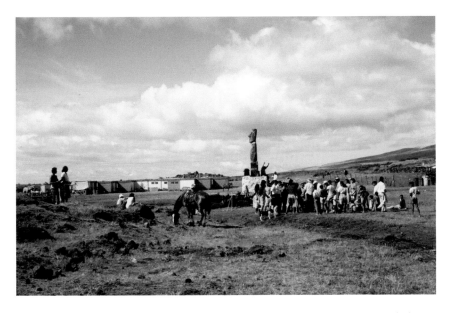

Figure 4.15 METEI's Camp Hilton from the southwest with the *moai* of Plaza Hotu Matu'a. Photo David Murphy.

Figure 4.16 METEI's Camp Hilton and Hanga Roa from the sea looking south-southeast. The camp lies along the shore, with the white church higher and to the right. The Puna Pau volcano is in the distance (centre). Photo Ian Efford.

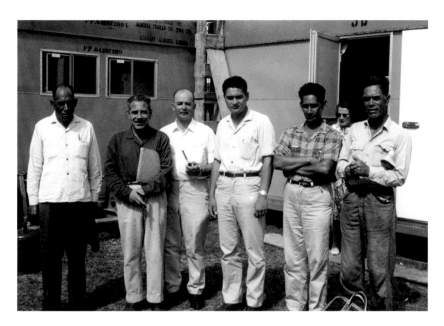

Figure 4.18 *From left*, Mayor Lazaro Hotu, Dr Guido Andrade, Stanley Skoryna, future mayor Alfonso Rapu, Germán Hotu, and unknown. Possibly occasion of Andrade's lecture, 19 December 1964. Photo David Murphy.

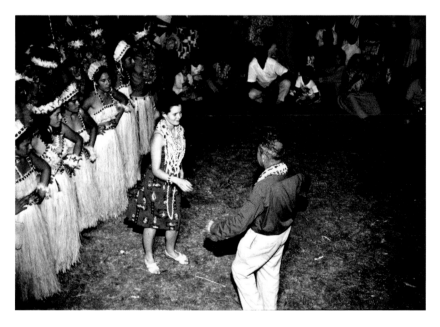

Figure 4.19 Farewell *sau sau* for Dr Guido Andrade, who is dancing with his wife, 19 December 1964. Photo Fred Joyce.

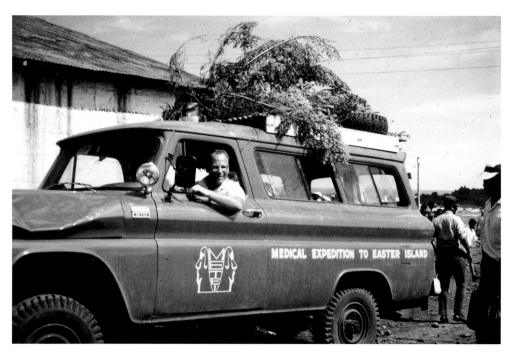

Figure 5.1 Garry Brody in the dented Jeep Mea Mea driving the Christmas tree from Hanga Piko to Camp Hilton. Photo Fred Joyce.

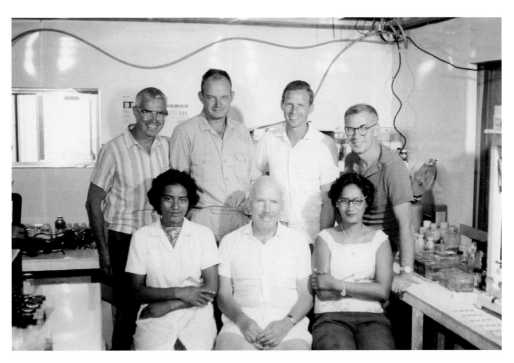

Figure 5.3 METEI lab team. *Back row from left*, Fred Joyce, Harold Gibbs, David Murphy, and Armand Boudreault. *Front row from left*, Norma (later "Tauranga") Hucke Atán, Archie Wilkinson, and Margarita Tepano Kaituoe ("Uka"). Photo David Murphy.

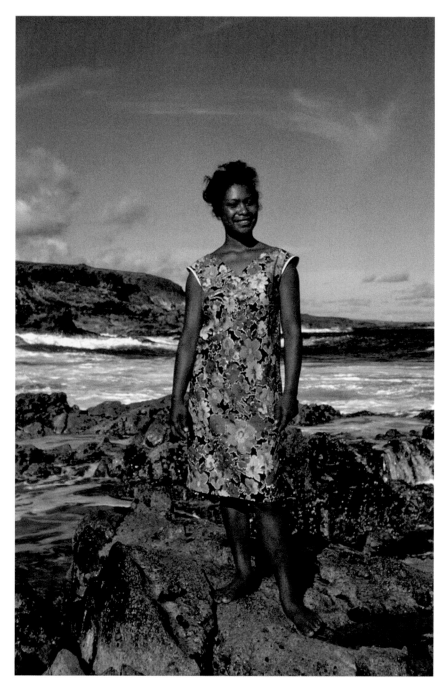

Figure 5.21 Maria Teresa Ika Pakarati, age eighteen. Photo Peter Beighton.

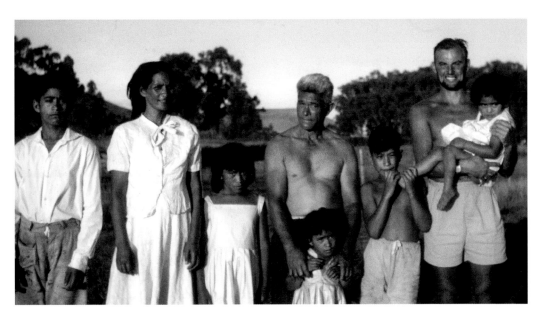

Figure 5.22 Some of the Ika Pakarati family. *From left*, Jorge (16), mother Luisa Pakarati Atamu, Ana Maria Carmela (10), father Enrique, Maria Jovita (5), and Carlos (11), with Dr Peter Beighton holding Antonia (3). Photo Peter Beighton.

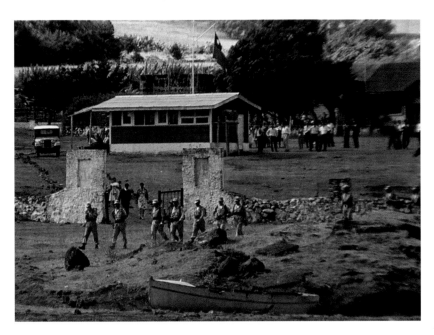

Figure 6.3 Troops from Chilean ship *Yelcho* at the Jefetura building near Camp Hilton. Photo Archibald Wilkinson.

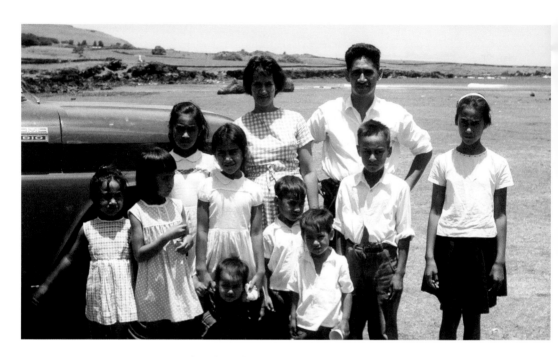

Figure 6.8 Hotu Hey family with Jeep Mea Mea: mother Maria Amalia Hey Paoa and father Germán Hotu Chavez with children Teresita (12), Maria Fatima (11), Victoria (9), Matias Aquiles (8), Maria Rubelinda (7), Melania Carolina (5), Urbano Matias (4), Pedro (3), and Sonia Margarita (18 mos). Germán was elected as a councillor with Alfonso Rapu. The family was examined a week after the election on 19 January 1965. A lying *moai* is visible behind the mother. Photo David Murphy.

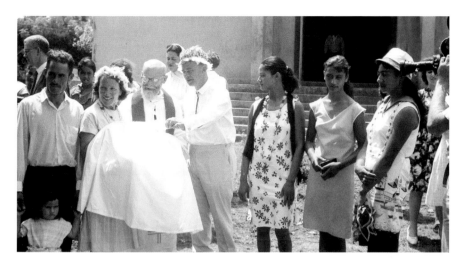

Figure 6.14 Outside the church following the baptism of Halina Irene Pont Pate ("Mi Poki"), 31 January 1965. The baby is held by Dr Helen Reid. *Also from left*, baby's father Aurelio Pont Hill and sister Ana Margarita, Father Sebastian Englert, Dr Stanley Skoryna, mother Maria del Rosario Pate Niare, and aunt Antonia Pate Niare. Photo David Murphy.

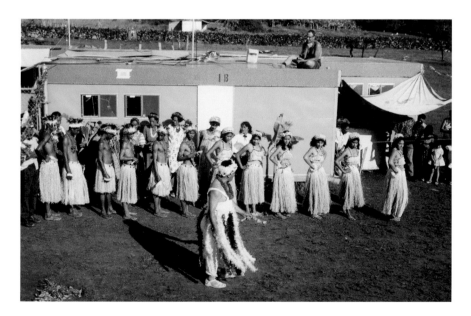

Figure 6.15 Papa Kiko – Luis Pate (later Luis Avaka) – leading dancers in reception area of *campamento*. Garry Brody is on the roof of the trailer. Photo David Murphy.

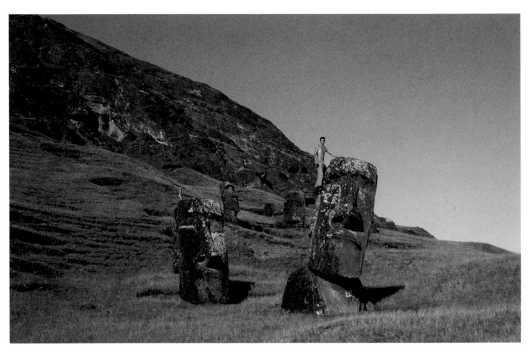

Figure 7.1 Jack Mathias atop *moai* at Rano Raraku. Photo Ian Efford.

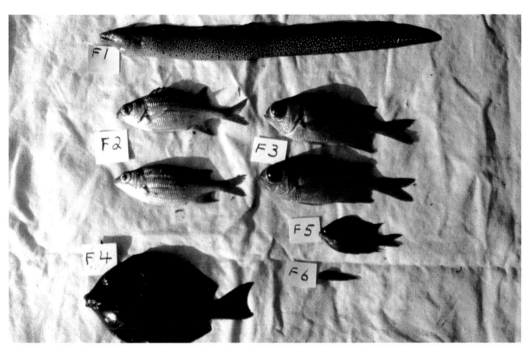

Figure 7.4 Rapanui fish. Photo Ian Efford.

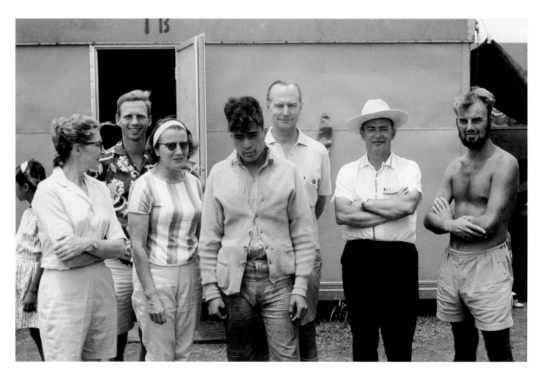

Figure 7.21 "The last patient," Nelson Teao Hey, with the doctors, 5 February 1965. *Also from left*, Maureen Roberts, David Murphy, Helen Reid, Richard Roberts, Stanley Skoryna, and Peter Beighton. Photo David Murphy.

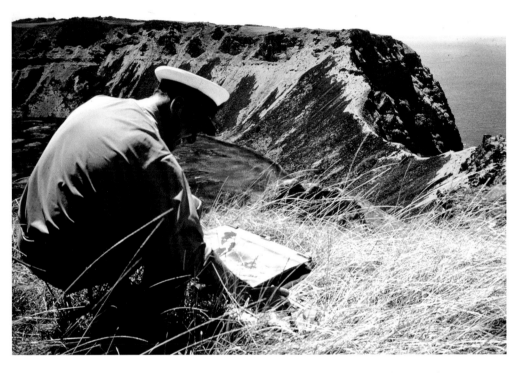

Figure 8.2 Commander Tony Law taking a moment to paint at the rim of Rano Kao crater, February 1965. Photo Fred Joyce.

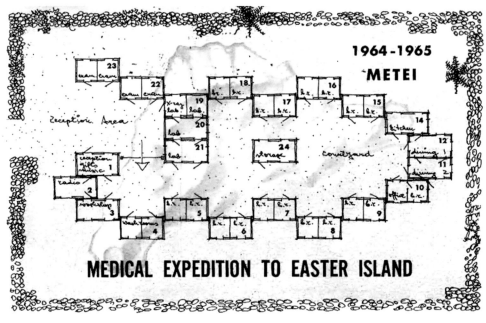

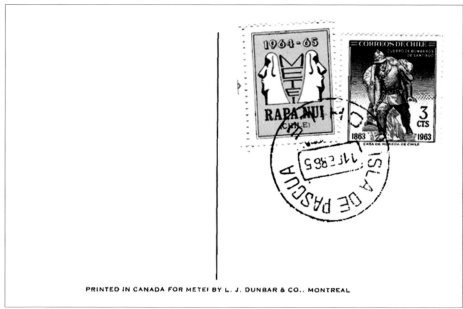

Figure 8.7 Both sides of an unused METEI postcard stamped and franked at the Easter Island post office. It featured a map of Rapa Nui superimposed with an architectural plan of the camp. The small break between trailers 18 and 19 is missing, and trailer 24 was not in the centre but on the upper left as the third clinic trailer. Note the METEI seal. Wilkinson Papers.

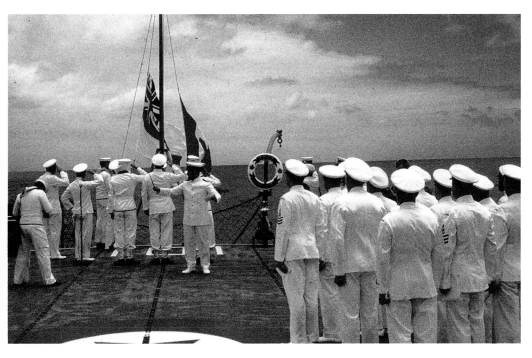

Figure 8.9 Singing "O Canada" as the White Ensign is lowered and the new flag is raised on board HMCS *Cape Scott*, 15 February 1965.
Photo Archibald Wilkinson.

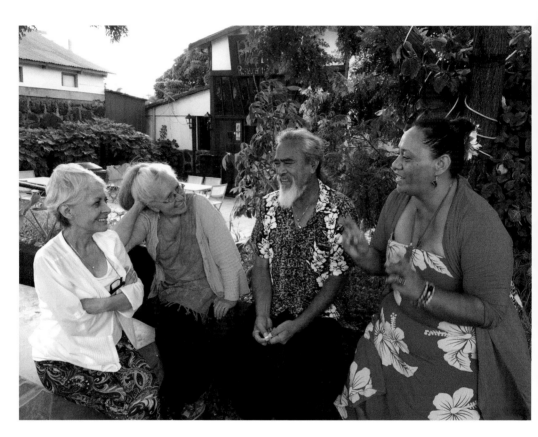

Figure 14.5 *From left*, Ana Cecilia Rodriguez de Romo, author Jacalyn Duffin, Marcos Rapu Tuki, and Suvi Hereveri Tuki at Hanga Roa, 20 January 2017. Photo Robert David Wolfe.

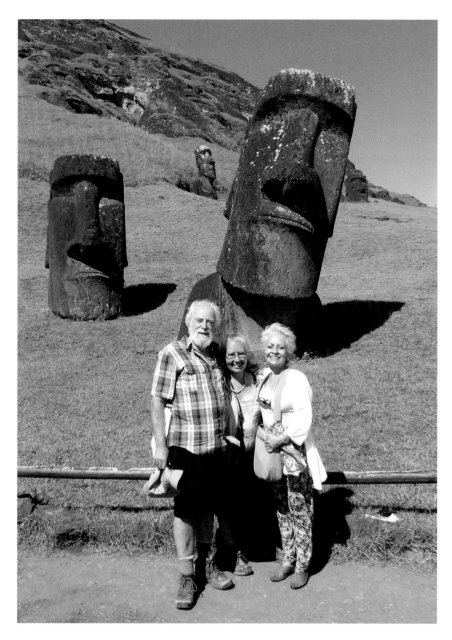

Figure 14.6 *From left*, Robert David Wolfe, author Jacalyn Duffin, and Ana Cecilia Rodriguez de Romo at Rano Raraku. No climbing allowed. Compare with figure 7.1, where Jack Mathias is atop the *moai*.
Photo Robert David Wolfe.

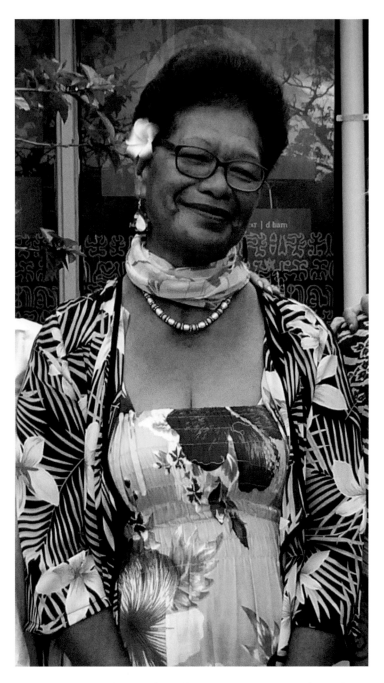

Figure 14.7 Maria Teresa Ika Pakarati, January 2017. She is also in figure 5.21. Photo Robert David Wolfe.

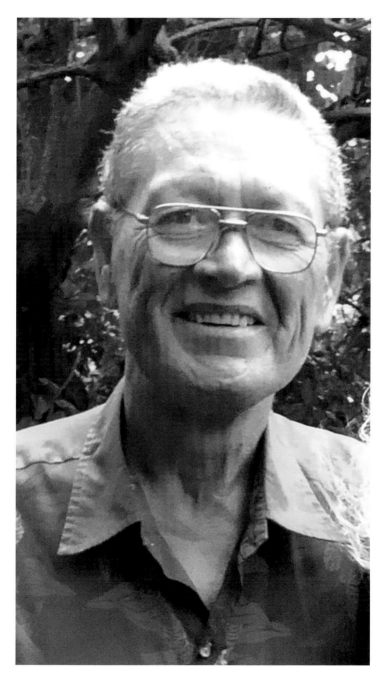

Figure 14.8 Alfonso Rapu, January 2017. He is also in figure 4.18, the figures of chapter 6, and figures 8.4 and 8.12.
Photo Robert David Wolfe.

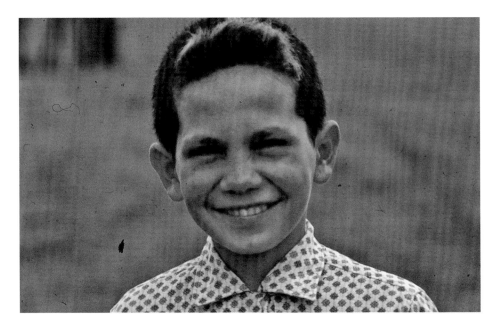

Figure 14.9 *Above*: Pedro Edmunds Paoa in 1965. Photo Archibald Wilkinson. *Below*: Pedro Edmunds Paoa, long-time mayor of Rapa Nui, in 2017. Photo Robert David Wolfe.

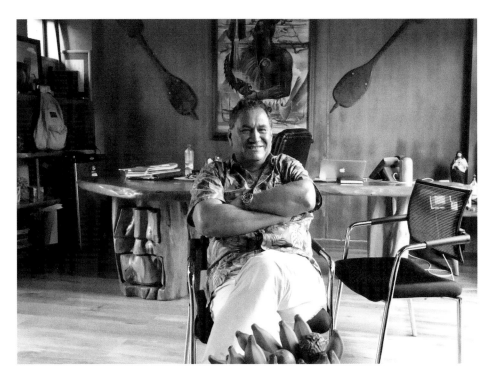

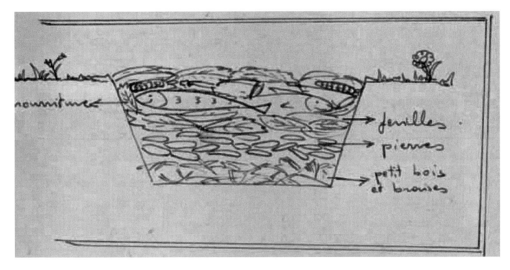

Figure 5.7 Diagram of a *curando*. Sketch in Montandon Diary.

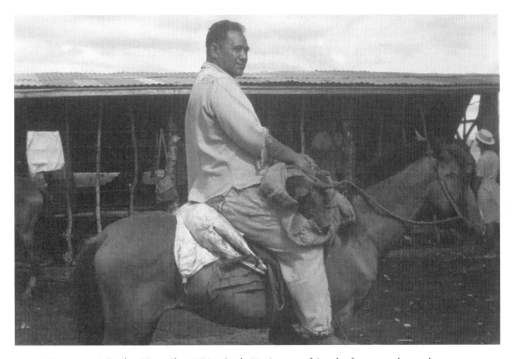

Figure 5.8 Carlos Teao Ika ("Big Carlo"). A great friend of METEI, he and spouse Livia Chavez were examined along with six of their children on 28 December 1964. Photo David Murphy.

Most METEI members spent Christmas afternoon exploring. The expedition leaders, John Easton, Reid, and the Montandons, set out in the truck to visit Ahu Akivi and Anakena Beach, splendid in the setting sun. Helen then went looking for more caves on her own, while Carlotta hoped to nap in their shared cabin. But young girls invaded and insisted on teaching her the *sau sau*; by dinner time, twenty-five Rapanui were crammed into the small trailer asking for Coca-Cola.[18]

Some members were visibly unhappy to be so far from home. Hal Gibbs unwrapped the present he'd carried since November and found a framed photograph of his four children. Bob Meier enjoyed a meal of fresh beef and watermelon, a gift from his new friend, Juan Tuki, who had agreed to do carvings for him. The young anthropologist wrote in his diary, "very lonely without my Carol and Heidi." He watched a "couple movies," projected on the white wall of George Hrischenko's radio shack. During the entire sojourn, islanders would gather in this open area outside the compound to see films; they were mesmerized by scenes of Canadian winter, especially those of skaters gliding and falling on the stiff water. The health film that showed weight reduction with a vibrating belt made them laugh in disbelief.

FINISHING TOUCHES

Over the next few days, Carlotta practised her skills at mixing media for bacterial cultures. Fred Joyce assured her that it "was only cooking and a bit of common sense." By the week's end, she was making "relatively germ-free agar."[19] She also organized the numerous volunteers, hoping to maximize their willingness and minimize their incidental confusion. The young girls loved her and imitated her hairstyle and dress; her "drastic haircut," administered by "a Scandinavian doctor" (likely Eivind Myhre), started a fashion trend, and twenty young girls cut their hair.[20] Older women liked Carlotta too. Around 28 December, Maria Atán decided to give Carlotta "a cow," which turned out to be a bull (or a steer; reports differ), intended to be the main course of a feast. But first it would have to be killed and butchered (figure 5.9).[21] The team looked to the vets, Hal Gibbs and David Murphy, who made themselves scarce: slaughter was not their job.

While on *Cape Scott*, possibly earlier, Richard Roberts had created an elaborate, multipaged form for recording the examination of each person in a manner suitable for transfer to computer punch cards. The doctors and their assistants were to note measurements, abnormal findings, and significant normals. Each examination could take an hour or

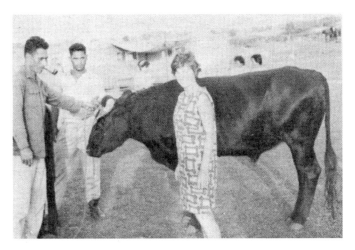

Figure 5.9 Carlotta Hacker with her gift "cow." Photo originally published in Hacker, "Aku Aku and Medicine Men."

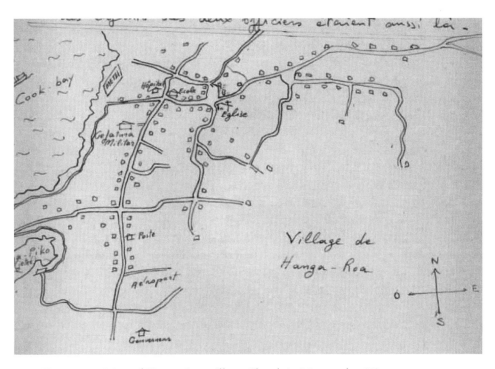

Figure 5.10 Map of Hanga Roa village. Sketch in Montandon Diary. Compare with sampling map in figure E.1, which includes family numbers.

more. The X-rays and laboratory data would be reported using the same identification numbers, and later the information could be integrated on the computer cards.

METEI had been provided with a relatively recent census by Governor Jorge Portilla. Soon after arrival, the epidemiologists, John Cutler and Elliot Alpert, assisted by Cléopâtre, Rita Dwyer, and Gonzalo Donoso, began exploring and mapping the village to update the census with births, deaths, and departures to the continent (figure 5.10). They assigned a three-digit number to every house, which they painted above the door; it became the number of the family who dwelt within, from 001 to 222. Each person who lived in the family group also had a number, which was tacked on to the end of the family number: 01 for the head of household, usually a man; 02 for the spouse, usually a woman; 03 for the first born; 04 for the next; and so on. Therefore, every Rapanui individual had a unique five-digit number, ranging from 00101 to 22002 (figure 5.11). One family (088) had eighteen members and two (003 and 083) had fourteen. The youngest children in a family were often adopted, or they were grandchildren of the head of household, but their parentage could not be established with certainty. Two stragglers were added at the end of the study as the sole members of "families" 230 and 231, a two-year-old boy and a sixty-two-year-old woman.

At least 140 non-Rapanui lived on the island, fifty of whom received salaries for work on the farms, at the airport, in the hospital, or in various offices. METEI ignored them until near the end of its stay (see chapter 7). Only the German-born Father Sebastian and Chilean Sergio Piñero turned up in their official records, simply because Archie took X-rays prompted by specific health concerns: the former's chest infection; the latter's injured elbow.

Following their survey of the island, Cutler and Alpert discovered that forty-two families were on the continent – "en conti," as the Rapanui said. These families were also numbered, but how many members each contained is unknown. This preparation work created a list of 967 individuals to be examined in the thirty-three to thirty-nine days that remained (six working days each week). That meant the doctors and their assistants should examine thirty people every day, a comfortable average of five or six people per day for each METEI doctor. But 575 of these people were under age sixteen, and 195 of those over that age were women. Therefore, according to the new agreement, the two women doctors would be expected to examine 770 people, more than 75 per cent of the population, which would convert to an uncomfortable average of about twelve every day for each of Helen and Maureen. The age restriction on "children" had

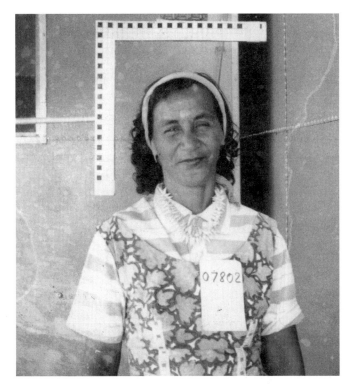

Figure 5.11 Josefina Pate Pacomio being measured with her METEI ticket and number. She and her husband, Juan Nahoe, welcomed METEI, becoming friends with Helen Reid and many others. Her family members, including eight of her ten children and one daughter-in-law, were examined on 6 January 1965. Photo probably by Lieutenant Mary King. Reid Papers, file 22.

to be modified to allow boys over age seven to be seen by male examiners. That left 603 people for Helen and Maureen to examine – two-thirds of the population – for an average of nine a day each. In addition, the dentist and the anthropologist were to examine all people over age eighteen (344 individuals). Working separately, the physiology team, Björn Ekblom and Einar Gjessing, aimed for a sample of one-third of people over age nine (approximately 180).

As for the labs, the plan was to X-ray the chests of everyone over age two (869 individuals), the hands and wrists of those under age nineteen, and the skulls of those over age seventeen. Blood was to be drawn from everyone over age seven, but finger pricks for blood grouping were to be

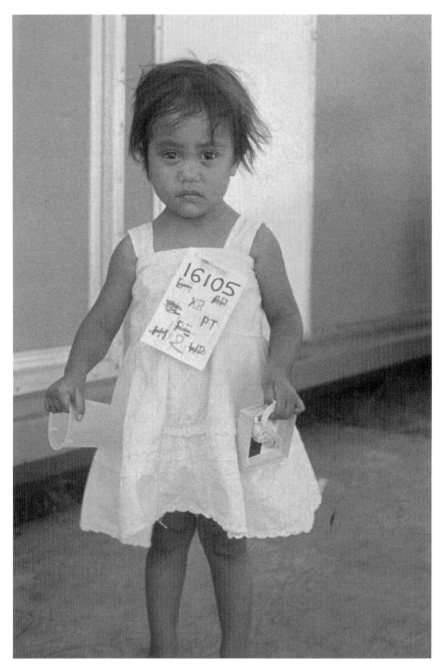

Figure 5.12 Rosa Verónica Hito Pate, age two and a half, wearing her METEI ticket and number. She was examined on 22 January with her mother and two siblings. Photo Peter Beighton.

permitted even in toddlers. Some older children and the small or squeamish could not always provide the 25–40 millilitres required, and some tests had to be eliminated. Each person was asked to provide urine and stool samples and was given cups to take home for collecting them.

The nonmedical team members sorted the traffic flow through the clinic and labs. Carlotta and Isabel devised a system of paper "tickets" or badges to be pinned on each person, bearing the identification number and list of stations through which they must pass. Each step would be crossed off on the ticket to ensure that nothing was overlooked. Peter Beighton still remembers this solution as an excellent device, which he later borrowed for other studies (figure 5.12). Despite the efficiency and anonymity, Bob Meier found the numbered tickets disturbing for their historical analogies.

During this period of waiting, METEI members forged links of genuine friendship with the Rapanui, which inadvertently contributed to the work of their mission. They also tried to comprehend the baffling political situation. Alfonso Rapu had been gone for almost a week, and they heard varying accounts of his whereabouts and the gravity of his actions, coloured by the varying sympathies of their sources. Meier, Hacker, Reid, Tony Law, and the Montandons described two distinct factions: on the one hand, Chilean naval authorities; on the other, islanders who wanted more democracy and respect. Some Rapanui were in contact with Rapu, moving him from cave to cave at sites scattered over the island.[22] Skoryna insisted that these problems were not part of METEI and that members should not take sides.

Everyone admired Father Sebastian, who championed the needs of his flock in view of harsh Chilean rule (figure 5.13). But the priest could not relinquish his main agenda of spreading Christian morality. He was especially disturbed by theft and female "lasciviousness." That Alfonso Rapu did not go to church, and allegedly discouraged others from doing so, became another vexation. Consequently, the priest's stance on the brewing rebellion was ambivalent. Those expeditionists (often older) who spoke with the Chilean authorities doubted the rebel tales of unfair or brutal treatment; those (often younger) who were growing close to the youthful Rapanui were more sympathetic. Restrictions imposed on islanders' movement and travel were incomprehensible to METEI members, and the fact that women could not vote was yet another injustice. People friendly with Jack Mathias prevailed on him to ask Skoryna about borrowing the rifle that the ecologists used for gathering birds. He did talk to Skoryna and was not disappointed when the request was denied, but it was awkward. Would violence be justified? Was it inevitable?

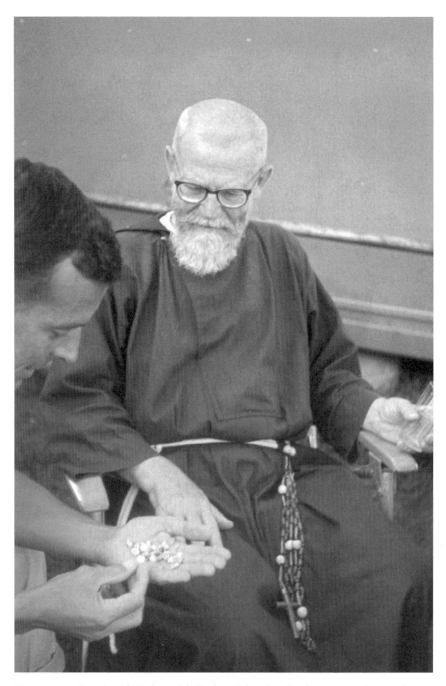
Figure 5.13 Dentist Al Taylor with Father Sebastian Englert examining teeth found at gravesites. Photo Peter Beighton.

THE FIRST PHYSICAL EXAMINATIONS

At 8:00 a.m. on Monday, 28 December, the day appointed for the start of the physical examinations, Skoryna stood waiting at the reception area wearing "a ten-gallon hat." He and his medical colleagues were ready to receive, but no one appeared. At this point, both Carlotta and Helen reported, two emissaries from Alfonso Rapu appeared, insisting once again that no exams take place until after the new elections. A bit later, a group of women came to say that they too needed to wait for Rapu's orders. Frantic that the whole mission would fall apart after his lengthy preparations, Skoryna sprang into the truck – now called "Jeep Mea Mea" (Red Jeep) – and drove into Hanga Roa. Somehow, he persuaded a family to return with him.[23] The team leapt into action.

That day, twenty-one people (fourteen under age eighteen) were put through the METEI clinics, including all nine members of the family of Carlos Teao Ika and Livia Chavez, and seven of the eight members of the family of Juan Atán Pakomio and Verónica Hotu; Verónica herself was examined the following day. Archie took X-rays of all but a baby and a three-year-old. The other four subjects examined that day – two men and a woman in their twenties and thirties and a teenage boy – may have been workers at the camp. It wasn't yet the hoped-for thirty examinations, but it was a start. For his part, Meier "ran through only seven" adults in the morning "confusion."[24] Reid found that the first day unmasked inefficiencies, and the team held a meeting to sort out how to improve the flow. Archie's anxieties "manifested in an outburst," of which he was later ashamed.[25] Meetings took place in the dining trailer or out of doors in the inner courtyard (figures 5.14 and 5.15).

Incentives were important to encourage participation. Lieutenant Mary King (dubbed "Mellyking") got the idea to offer a Polaroid group photo to every family who came for examination; it became part of the ritual. A chance to ride in Jeep Mea Mea was also a draw. John Easton insisted on personally testing every potential driver. With Easton's blessing, plastic surgeon Garry Brody became the designated chauffeur and transported willing families to the camp on the appointed day. Carlotta admired Skoryna's ability to turn the family examination into a status symbol; people who refused to make a METEI appointment were just not "*with it.*"[26] To emphasize their participation as a significant scientific contribution and to display his own commitment, Skoryna loitered at the reception area, greeting the islanders as they arrived for registration by Ana Maria Eccles, Rita Dwyer, and Isabel Griffiths. He often

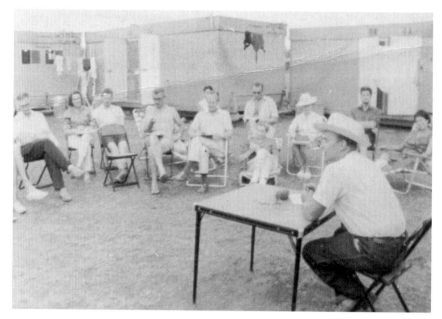

Figure 5.14 The only photo found of a METEI meeting held in the Camp Hilton courtyard. Stanley Skoryna is at the table. *From left*, Georges Nógrády, Helen Reid, Red Lemieux, Armand Boudreault, Isabel Griffiths (*hidden*), Richard Roberts, Maureen Roberts, Eivind Myhre (*behind Maureen*), Rita Dwyer, and Denys and Cléopâtre Montandon. Photo probably by Lieutenant Mary King. Reid Papers, file 22.

appeared in the family group photos. Everybody knew "Koreena," or "Eskoryna," and recognized him as the leader.

The next day with the traffic flow revisions in place, METEI surpassed its target with thirty-one examinations; all but three tiny children were X-rayed too. Meier examined twelve. That same day, Commander Law and his *Cape Scott* sailed into Valparaiso and even deeper political waters (see chapter 8).

THE RESEARCHERS DESCRIBE THEIR WORK

While David Macfarlane and Carl Mydans took masses of photos, both Bob Williams and Red Lemieux filmed documentaries – Williams with the audio help of Hrischenko for the Canadian Broadcasting Corporation (CBC) and Lemieux for the National Film Board (NFB). Their work brings the story alive. Both films feature the journey and the

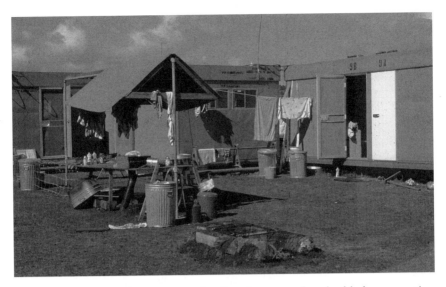

Figure 5.15 Camp Hilton courtyard, a laundry space that doubled as a meeting area. Trailer 9B (*door open*) was shared by Helen Reid and Carlotta Hacker. The dining trailer is behind (*left*). Photo Archibald Wilkinson.

raising of the camp, but Williams, in particular, focused on the scientific research. For a major part of Williams's film, Dr Richard Roberts acts as the master of ceremonies, standing stiffly in the reception area of the *campamento*, an Alcan company label prominently displayed over his shoulder, as he introduces each project leader in turn. Then the camera turns to the researchers; one by one, they explain details of their work, in their own words, sometimes as a "voiceover," while another team member is seen going through the motions described.[27]

In introducing the medical examinations for Williams's camera, Roberts explains the importance of updating the census through baptismal and gubernatorial records. Following registration as the families came to the camp, measurements were taken of height, weight, pulse, and blood pressure. He emphasizes the importance of having the same observer make measurements to avoid variations in the figures. Garry Brody is seen taking the blood pressure of a little girl and then of a man; Brody also scrutinizes their hands, as it was his particular clinical interest. Isabel then guides the subject to King, who takes an individual Polaroid photograph, which is affixed to each record "for identification purposes." Next, they move on to "Spanish-speaking" Denys Montandon for a "basic medical history," which was sometimes difficult to elicit from mothers with up to eleven children. Then subjects are sent to Archie Wilkinson for X-rays, which requires what Roberts calls "a major undertaking ... an enormous amount of work, [and] a great deal of finicky adjustment." The skull films of "a selected group of adults" were "required by Dr [*sic*] Meier," who did not yet have his doctorate. The hand X-rays were "for Dr. Helen Reid's study of child development." Wilkinson stands back from the machine as he shoots each image in the small space, but he does not appear to have a lead shield or apron to protect his own body from scatter.

Roberts then explains that, because no radiologist has come on the journey, the X-ray films will be read by Archie's boss, Dr Robert Fraser, back in Montreal; however, a group of clinicians met three evenings a week to go over the X-rays taken in the previous two days, doing their nonexpert best to assess the presence of disease in order to treat it expeditiously. In this manner, they would uncover five new cases of suspected tuberculosis, although Roberts does not say that on camera.

"Then we come to the clinical examination proper," Roberts says, "a careful examination of the whole person, done in a completely orthodox way." While Peter Beighton examines a man, Roberts details the elements of his assessment: build, skin ("always on the lookout for leprosy"), hair, extremities, eyes, ears, gut "from the mouth right down," chest, heart, neurological system, and an electrocardiogram on anyone over fifty years of age. "We had to agree at the beginning that all the women and all the older girls are examined by female doctors. The people are rather shy." Roberts admits that this rule, coupled with examination of children, means that the two women doctors have "perhaps the bulk of the work to do." Perhaps?

Williams's camera next turns to Helen Reid, who is sitting in the examination room with one of her young helpers (figures 5.16 and 5.17). She describes the complete physical once again, while images show Maureen Roberts examining an unhappy little girl. Head circumference was part of the inspection of children. Reid states, "I am particularly interested in the development of the children, and from having seen so many here on the island, I have some distinct impressions. To me, the children all seem small ... but they are very active, healthy, energetic." Over scenes of cheerful children busy playing on the swing sets brought on *Cape Scott*, she reports little evidence of deficiency diseases or the "pudgy," "overfed" children we sometimes see in Canada (figure 5.18). "There's another impression that I have ... the women on the island age ... very early." The pediatrician's evidence on aging came from overall appearance, lax skin, and "eye changes" that appeared ten to fifteen years earlier than in North America. Many

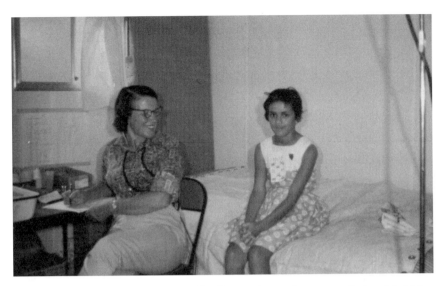

Figure 5.16 Sonia Flora Haoa Cardinali, age eleven, in METEI clinic with Helen Reid. For the special occasion, her mother made the dress from a tablecloth. Sonia is now an archeologist, researcher, and leader in the preservation of the island's heritage. Photo Peter Beighton.

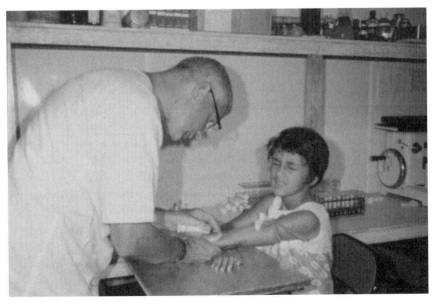

Figure 5.17 Sonia Flora Haoa Cardinali, age eleven, in METEI lab with Fred Joyce, 27 January 1965. Photo Peter Beighton.

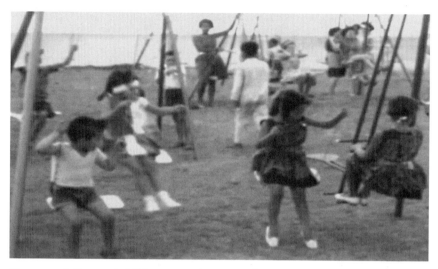

Figure 5.18 Rapanui children on swings outside METEI *campamento* with the sea behind. Film still from CBC, Williams, and Hrischenko, *Canadian Expedition to Easter Island*, part 1, at 18 mins, 30 secs, with thanks to Janice Belanger.

scenes show examiners recording the results on Roberts's multipage form with carbon paper for duplicates.

The lab is next. Eivind Myhre explains that, as a pathologist, his scientific interest is in cancer. But he has found little sign of it, even after examination of a few vaginal smears and some sputum samples, the latter prompted by the high rate of smoking. He thinks its absence may be due in part to the young age of the population. He is then shown pricking the finger of a little boy who sits on his mother's lap; Myhre mixes the drop of blood with reagents on an Eldon card to determine the boy's ABO and Rh blood groups. "We should have brought a hematologist on this expedition," he says, "but unfortunately we haven't ... So I was told to be in charge of the blood sampling." While Fred Joyce fills a syringe with blood from a woman's vein, Myhre describes the many destinations of the sample in the form of cells or serum to be examined, frozen, dried, and stored – for Boudreault, Nógrády, and the World Health Organization. Joyce drops portions of the serum samples in tiny test tubes labelled for "[Maureen] Roberts" and "[Alexander] Bearn."

Roberts then introduces Armand Boudreault, who stares intently at the camera, possibly reading from a cue card, to declare that he is carrying out a "survey of the viral flora of the island." He explains in careful English the sources of his samples from body orifices and blood, noting that some are inoculated into living cells, incubated, and then frozen at –95° Celsius for shipping back to Montreal. Georges Nógrády follows. He speaks with a Hungarian accent and in broken English, facing the camera while his eyes, behind black-rimmed glasses, wander around the room. Because the human population "lives close together with animals," the study has expanded to look for diseases shared between them. His samples come from people, animals, soil on the surface and in caves, water in the sea and wells, and cows' milk. Hair is inspected for pathogenic fungi; nasal swabs are inoculated on media looking for leprosy and pathogenic staphylococci; throat swabs are plated for streptococci; intestinal microorganisms are sought in rectal samples. As Nógrády speaks, his helpers, Carlotta Hacker, Margarita Tepano, and Jorge Ika Pakarati, work inside the lab, and Alpert collects soil and water outside. To date, Nógrády says, they have gathered "more than 2,000 cultures," and it is now "our duty to keep them alive" for transport and distribution to "different expert laboratories."

Physical anthropologist Bob Meier appears next, describing the observations he makes on adult subjects, usually on the same day as their medical examination. He uses a variety of rulers and calipers to measure limbs, digits, and facial features; and he takes prints of palms and fingers. Each study takes about thirty minutes, he says. Meier was also interested in the blood samples, as his investigation would serve as a baseline to describe the islanders and as a possible indicator of their distant geographic origins. By the end, he had detailed measurements on more than 300 people over eighteen years of age. In addition, Father Sebastian allowed him to measure thirteen skulls in his museum, items that had been found at burial sites near *ahus* (platforms). Over the previous century, many other bony remains – skulls and complete skeletons – had been carted off to laboratories in Europe and America. The priest's small collection was to protect the samples from pilfering, but he was also very interested what they could reveal about the origins of human life on Rapa Nui.

Meier shared his research space with navy dentist Al Taylor, who follows in Williams's CBC film, explaining his survey of 239 adult subjects. Slightly apprehensive, Isabel Veriveri, a twenty-six-year-old mother of three, allows Taylor to take plaster impressions of her teeth while he speaks off camera. He states that the people are generally healthy but have poor dentition, stemming from lack of dental care and poor hygiene. He handed out toothbrushes for the families. In their shared premises one day, Meier helped the dentist to "fix a girl's jaw."[28] Taylor also examined teeth that Carlotta, Einar, and Lemieux had collected in the Cave of the White Virgins for Father Sebastian's museum.[29]

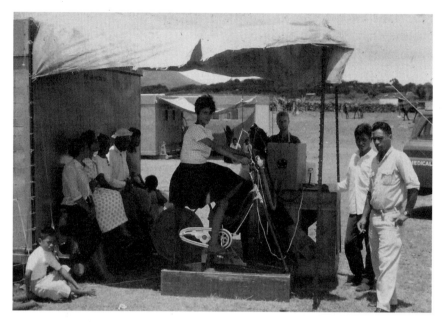

Figure 5.19 Work physiology setup with Björn Ekblom (*back centre*) and Jeep
Mea Mea (*right*). Photo Georges Nógrády.

Williams's camera then turns to Björn Ekblom, who explains the work
physiology project. In the background, forty-one-year-old Humberto
Lazaro Pont Hill pedals away on the bicycle ergometer as Einar Gjessing
takes notes. Ekblom then explains the collection and analysis of
Humberto's expired air to determine how much oxygen was absorbed
and how much carbon dioxide released. A further study on eight selected
workers (five men and three women) will assess energy expenditure and
fitness during a working day. They are fitted with transistors for pulse
and monitored by telemetry, and they wear large sacks for gathering
expired air eight to ten hours throughout the day. The three women were
housewives with many children to care for; the men were farmworkers
or unemployed.[30] Reid put it this way: "With the ergometer and chemistry they studied just how hard the Pascuense *could* work. The next question was how hard *did* they work."[31] The champion runner Ekblom tells
Williams's camera that his fitness survey shows that "these people don't
work as much as we do, at least in Europe, in my hometown in Sweden."
    Many islanders had never seen a bicycle, and they were baffled by the
stationary device that, despite their best efforts, did not move and accomplished no work (figure 5.19). Ekblom and Gjessing offered bars of soap for

cooperation; if the people applied themselves well, two bars – and on rare occasions, for outstanding performances, three. Priding herself on her physical prowess, fifty-three-year-old Helen Reid wanted to try out the ergometer and goaded the Scandinavians into letting her have a go. It looked easy – "a pleasant morning spin." When she "staggered off the machine at the end," a mere sixteen minutes later, she was "in a state of near collapse." "You vere vunderful! No?" said Einar. "Better than the average North American voman. No? And as good as the average Scandinavian voman."[32]

Ekblom tried to keep up with his running while on Easter Island – but the food was terrible and insufficient. He felt hungry all the time and lost weight. In addition, while taking pictures of the waves on lava rocks, he fell in the sea and tore his Achilles tendon – a grave injury for anyone, especially a competitive runner. Although the facilities were primitive, plastic surgeon Garry Brody stitched the tear, which healed well and quickly with no infection.

At the end of Williams's segment on the medical examinations, Mary King photographs a nine-person family group standing with Skoryna in his ten-gallon hat. She hands the product to the people as a "straight gift," says Roberts, which is "very much appreciated, particularly when it is in colour."

The film made no mention of the logistics of obtaining urine and stool samples. Around 12 January, Reid noticed that no one had been checking on the urine tests, and she saw the sample cups being used as drinking glasses in island homes.[33] She then launched an active campaign to encourage people to produce specimens, but the resulting total of 303 samples from 301 people (91 female, 208 male, and 2 unknown) came from just one-third of the population and reflected the inadequate toileting arrangements at Camp Hilton. Boys and men could dispense with the task easily, but girls and women could not; they took the specimen cups home, often forgetting to bring them back. Nevertheless, twenty-five male heads of households did not provide a specimen, whereas their wives and children did. Hal Gibbs encountered similar difficulties with the fecal samples: of the cups and paddles distributed, only 207 came back; some were dessicated and others contained urine and stool mixed together.[34]

On the return voyage, METEI members updated the census to incorporate the date of each person's examination. From it, we can generate a chart to illustrate the relentless pace of the work (figure 5.20). With an average of 27 examinations daily (range 1 to 45), most islanders were seen in the allotted time – a total of 958 people. No examinations were conducted on Sundays. Even the cook had that day off, and teams of METEI members took turns preparing meals for the whole company. The work did not slow during the personal, political, and military upheaval that ensued.

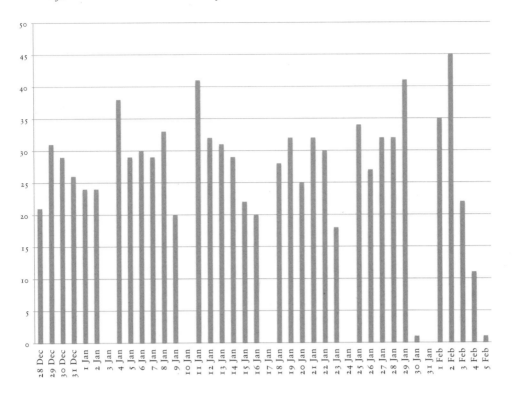

Figure 5.20 Number of daily physical examinations by METEI on Rapa Nui from 28 December 1964 to 5 February 1965. Note no examinations on Sundays. "METEI Census on the Population of Easter Island," UBC Archives, Efford Papers, METEI box 1.

SOCIAL LIFE

New Year's Day came and went with little fanfare. METEI members partied with Lowenbrau beer in the Camp Hilton courtyard until 3:00 a.m. Skoryna announced that he would give ten cases of beer to Father Sebastian and save the rest "for a blowout at the end of research."[35] Reid enjoyed a wonderful meal of lobster salad with her new friends Josefina Pate Pacomio (see figure 5.11), Juan Nahoe, and their nine children; Cléopâtre and Denys were guests of Esteban Pakarati.[36]

On Sundays when Colin Gillingham was given a break from the relentless cooking, the travellers had the adventure of fending for themselves alone or with island friends. For his turn, Garry Brody remembers that he and a couple of Rapanui "trekked out to Anakena after dark ...

with a diesel-soaked torch" to bring back "a load of crabs – delicious!"[37] After dinner in a Rapanui home, a little crowd of people, unbidden, would typically accompany the guests back to Camp Hilton, singing as they walked.

By now the travellers had well-established patterns of socializing with the islanders, and the youngest members were falling in love with the beautiful, willing vahines. "The women threw themselves at you," one METEI traveller recalled, adding that he was lucky that his wife had allowed him to go. The island had a strict embargo on kinship marriage – the origin of which was obscure, but it had been observed and documented by Alfred Métraux, endorsed by the Catholic priests, and justified by outsiders in the genetic risks of consanguinity.[38] METEI members were intrigued that Rapanui youth could choose partners from only a handful of families, and these limitations attracted media reports.[39] Anthropologist Bob Meier delved into unravelling its manifestations.[40]

On Rapa Nui, no stigma was attached to illegitimacy: when the census was nearing completion, 166 "illegitimate" children had been identified.[41] These babies were loved just as much as the others and fully integrated into their families. Many had unknown fathers, long gone with passing ships, but often people extolled the nationality of their absent progenitors as a matter of pride: Norwegian, French, German, Dutch, English. The nationality of a distant ancestor could be a reason for special "kinship" with the newcomers.[42] Carlotta's single friend Georgina had four children by different fathers; she was proud of them all.[43] From the first contact, as Meier observed from the rail of *Cape Scott*, the genetic homogeneity anticipated by METEI was revealed as complete fiction – yet one more sign of bad planning.

Ecologist Ian Efford, a husband and father, found the open attitude of the "aggressively outbred" islanders a refreshing contrast to the repressed sexuality and stigmatizing of illegitimacy that he had known in England. Many others said it "opened their eyes" to the stringent social taboos of home; the enlightened, easy ways of these supposed "primitives" contrasted with the hypocrisy of so-called civilization. Helen recorded the phrase "Nice girl for you?" – trotted out frequently by eager mothers, aunties, grandmothers, and married sisters whenever newcomers arrived.[44] One of the teenage girls who helped in the clinic fell in love with the young cook, Gillingham. Several travellers still remember how she pursued him, singing songs, getting underfoot, and trying to help and impress. "He barely survived," one told me. At only thirteen years old, Ana Rosa Laharoa lived alone with her younger brother; their mother was in Chile, and an aunt was directing her wooing strategy.[45]

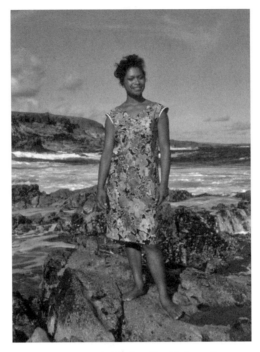

Figure 5.21 Maria Teresa Ika Pakarati, age
eighteen. Photo Peter Beighton.

In their diaries, both Cléopâtre and Helen wrote of the romantic
exploits of the single men – Peter, Elliot, Jim, Jack, and Einar – some
in their early twenties and in love for the first time.[46] By Christmas,
many had found steady partners. "But of course, we all had girlfriends,"
said Peter Beighton fifty years later. Two of the travellers gave me the
names and photographs of their lovers. "Conquistador Beighton," with
his dashing beard and athletic frame, was considered by everyone to be
the most immersed and best adapted of all; he could even speak some
Rapanui. METEI members referred to his beautiful girlfriend, Maria
Teresa Ika Pakarati, as "The Mrs." (figure 5.21).[47] She was intelligent,
learned English more quickly than anyone Skoryna had ever met, and
was eager to help, although Beighton thought she should avoid the camp.
He was captivated by her entire family, who lived simply and shoeless
as shepherds: father Enrique, his second wife, Eloísa Pakarati Atamu,
and at least seven children, including son Jorge, who worked in the lab,
eleven-year-old Carlos, who could ride horseback like the wind, and a
three-year-old sister, Antonia, disabled with flaccid paralysis and unable

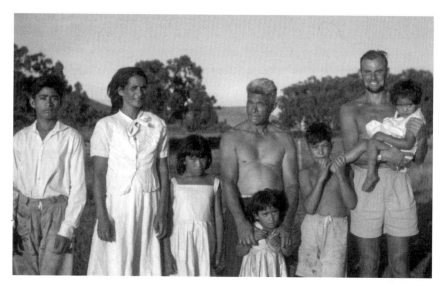

Figure 5.22 Some of the Ika Pakarati family. *From left*, Jorge (16), mother Luisa Pakarati Atamu, Ana Maria Carmela (10), father Enrique, Maria Jovita (5), and Carlos (11), with Dr Peter Beighton holding Antonia (3). Photo taken by Maria Teresa for Peter Beighton.

to walk (figure 5.22). Georges Nógrády was also a great friend of this family, and they accompanied him on his travels.[48]

Reid tried to puzzle through the origins of these liberal mores that had become combined with the more conservative restrictions on consanguineous marriage, both of which seemed to predate the advent of Catholicism.[49] What depressed her was not the free sexual expression – she seems to have admired it – but the many ways that the sailors and METEI members readily exploited it. Even married men whom she liked took advantage of teenage girls and bragged about their exploits in seduction and avoiding venereal disease. "This island will change me ... I will not be the same person when I come home," she told her husband. The irony was not lost on her: this process, she mused, was something akin to "adaptation."[50]

Adaptation – the focus of the METEI journey – forms a thread throughout Reid's diary. She analyzed it in the mutual reactions between the Rapanui and the travellers, and she blamed failures to adapt on a lack of communication, direction, and understanding. "Some individuals blend with the landscape and disappear. Others have learned a great deal of the language – some are able to carry on their private explores and plans. The area where adaptation is most difficult is in the compound itself."[51]

Armand Boudreault noticed adaptation to heat; the Rapanui sweated hardly at all, whereas he was drenched after only a few minutes work. He also detected an adaptation effect that METEI was having on the Rapanui: greater contact fed a certain "snobbisme." Working in the camp, hosting expedition members for a meal, and having prized gifts became status symbols, added to others already established, such as the surgical scar from an Andrade operation. In church, he was impressed to see how the islanders adapted the METEI gifts (bribes) for participation to their living conditions: the women added sleeves to the sundresses; they wore high-heeled shoes on strings around their necks until they reached the church door, where they put them on their feet. These people were human, and so were the travellers.

PERSONAL CONFLICT

Richard Roberts disagreed with Skoryna over many aspects of the study. Some have labelled their conflict as a "personality clash." METEI's astute translator, Isabel, now disagrees and believes the tension emerged from their differing management styles, military versus academic. Roberts was a naval officer and, according to Helen Reid, a "perfectionist," "firm," and "uncompromising." Skoryna was "more compromising, more pliable," and, I might add, conflict averse.[52] Carlotta Hacker described his proclivity to listen, agree that a suggestion was a good idea, and then ignore it, carrying on with his original plan. If one remonstrated that no change had been made, he'd shrug and say that it *might* be a good idea, who knows? Then he'd smile.[53] Roberts thought that Maureen and Helen were overworked. Rather than a rush job on Skoryna's infernal 100 per cent, he believed that the study could yield equally valuable results if it were confined to a thoroughly examined sample of a few hundred people. Roberts did not perform electrocardiograms on "all people over age fifty," as he claimed in Williams's film, but on 80 per cent of the adults over fifty (51 of 64 people) and 12 per cent of those between the ages forty and fifty (8 of 68 people). His electrocardiograph machine was not working properly, and he didn't bother to fix it. He and Maureen refused to conduct examinations beyond 4:00 or 5:00 p.m. each day.[54] Roberts also worried about Archie Wilkinson and Fred Joyce, who were obliged to toil well into the night in order to complete the handling of images and samples gathered during the day.[55]

Cléopâtre, however, found that the much older Armand "never missed an opportunity to grumble" and that the even older Archie did not bother to "explore the island and know the islanders."[56] She probably did not understand how much their work kept them in the lab or how familiar

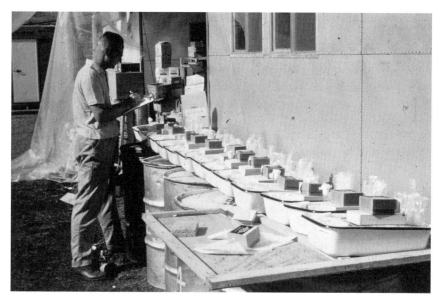

Figure 5.23 Richard Roberts with sample trays laid out for the day.
Photo Fred Joyce.

Archie had become with the island children. Some METEI members sided with Roberts. Others were loyal to Stanley, who had brought them to Rapa Nui and whose imagination stimulated their research.

The published memoirs, discussed in chapter 9, are discreet about these differences, but they admit that there was trouble. Reid described how Skoryna's "single-minded vision" provoked "eruptions that were sometimes acrimonious and a strain on personal loyalty." She also indicated how Roberts's formal manner and habit of "clamping his jaw" could shut down discussion. You could call him "Dr. Roberts, or Richard, never 'Dick.'" She saw the trouble as a "perfect personality clash" and blamed its exacerbation on the hovering media men (figure 5.23).[57]

Carlotta described a miserable luncheon on a scorching hot day about two weeks after the examinations had begun. Everything ran awry. She'd made up a batch of media and set it outside to cool, but a sudden downpour ruined it and she had to start over. The lunch menu promised yet more tinned meat and pumpernickel. Roberts voiced his opinion that the "ridiculous" pace was too much. Skoryna answered "in such a devious manner that no one believed him." He popped a piece of pumpernickel in his mouth and "smiled innocently." Coupled with his iron will, Carlotta wrote, he had "very tough" skin, "even the spikiest barbs just bounced off

... leaving him smiling, agreeable and bearing no malice. But often leaving the barb thrower in a fury of frustration." She wondered if a menu of lobster thermidor might have averted that particular meltdown.[58]

Almost thirty years later in his own brief memoir, Skoryna minimized these difficulties and justified his actions in the exact manner that Carlotta had described and as if he had had a world of experience in expeditionary research: "The dual personality of all people became evident in the small community of 38 members ... personality problems are typical under such circumstances. For instance, those who chose their cabin-mates on the ship wanted to 'divorce' them a few days after landing. Those who wanted to examine only 50% of the population started to work harder when they realized that our goal, a 100% sample, would be met regardless. I had to make these people believe that they were 'right' in their judgment even when they were wrong, to prevent rebellion."[59] He was ever confident in his dream.

A full half-century after METEI, the younger travellers now recall the strife vividly and are blunt, although they too are loath to name names and their opinions are divided. "I had never before seen a grown man act like a four year old," said one traveller of Roberts's petulant outbursts. In contrast, another thought that Roberts would have made the better leader for being more precise, firm, and organized. Yet another thought that Roberts, being a naval officer, *wanted* to be leader and that therein lay the problem. One is adamant that Roberts wanted the expedition to fail in order to hurt Skoryna's plans. Most agreed with Carlotta that relations were strained and that nerves were frayed by the endless canned meat on pumpernickel, the relentless heat, and the hovering cameras. A METEI member recalled that Carl Mydans had recognized the unruly behaviour as natural, akin to what he'd seen in in the close confinement of a prisoner of war camp. Another remembers a crisis when supplies of liquor ran short, causing "a little frisson among the Americans." The diaries are similarly candid about the strife.

Camp Hilton degenerated into cliques: young versus old, scientists versus clinicians, military versus academics, parents versus singles, optimists versus pessimists, media wallahs versus researchers, drinkers versus teetotalers, churchgoers versus atheists, Scandinavians and Spanish and French speakers versus parochial anglophones, and Americans versus everyone else. The rubrics seemed endless; cliques, so refined, sometimes contained only one person.

Even the media set, which so annoyed the researchers and the navy, was fractured from within by intense rivalry. "You did not want to be accused of stealing someone else's ideas," George Hrischenko explained. Tiptoeing around the small expedition on the small island were four men in three teams bursting with cameras, notebooks, recording equipment, and giant egos.

The "Group" was the word used by both Helen Reid and Carlotta Hacker to refer to an obstructive band of dissenters who stuck together, ready to party, criticize, and complain.[60] This characterization was later contested by expedition alumni. Some explained that their disaffection stemmed from METEI's poor planning; the bright minds sank into whining and misbehaviour when they had far too little to do. Helen wrote to her husband that members of the Group "spend all their time drinking. They came for a cruise, they don't work, and jobs they are asked to do are beneath them."[61] In her diary, she tracked three broad factions on a chart containing names and annotated with arrows that showed who, in her estimation, left the Group and who joined from among a majority cadre of hard workers and a middle cohort of the more or less oblivious, which included secretaries, the "wrens," Taylor, Beighton, and Nógrády. Later arrows relocated Mary King from the "oblivious" to the hard workers, and other arrows moved Efford from the workers to the Group and Lemieux from the Group to the workers.[62] The same day that she constructed her chart, Helen – an avid reader, possibly a fan of George Orwell, also inscribed a list of animals in her diary: "these I can't abide: wolves, skunks, snakes (in the grass), cats ... foxes, female dogs, mules, ... rats, pigs, chicken[s], weasels, and grouse."[63]

Epidemiologist John Cutler, married with children back in California, was a noisy, exuberant member of the Group. One night he sat on Carlotta's trailer step, marvelling over the magic of the island, his unexpected freedom, and the improbability of the whole adventure. "Just think," he said to her, "it will never be like this again. Me sitting here in the sun while you pound your washing on that board and wring it dry on the handle of your garbage can. Boy, this is the life!"[64]

Helen herself misbehaved and recorded it in her diary. One evening over supper, Skoryna asked Denys Montandon if he could deliver a baby because an island woman was soon due. "I hear *you* are going to have a baby, Denys," Helen remarked "casually" in front of the astonished company. Denys was "covered with confusion and said 'Yes, but not soon.'" Cléopâtre added that she was "only four months along the way." Helen concluded this entry, "Quel expédition!"[65] She was probably not the only one to have guessed their secret, but it seems that this moment was the first time that the pregnancy became public knowledge – something else that Cléopâtre could hold against Dr Reid. For her part, Helen thought that the Montandons' deception of Stanley and METEI was irresponsible and "immoral" – one of her favourite concepts. Morality, for Helen Reid, was a philosophical notion that bears consideration, although I am not confident that I understand what she meant. She carried on an extended conversation about it with one of the naval officers (see chapter 8). It was not about drinking, or sex, or stealing, or lying but had more to do with service, duty, coherence, and decency.[66] She remembered that one reason, among many, for hematologist Michael F.X. Glynn's decision not to join METEI was his wife's pregnancy. By making an announcement that was not hers to make, she revealed to all what she and others had known for weeks. She may also have lost friends.

In early January 1965, Reid told her husband that "the expedition is a poor, poor thing ... scientifically it is so poor, in so many ways [that] it is pathetic ... There is no nutritionist." She listed the unexpected findings that should have been expected: "the people are not isolated – there have been two ships since *Cape Scott* left and we expect another within the week; ... the islanders are of all races and colours; ... they have many comforts, 7 jeeps now, electricity." She also described the tense personal animosity:

> Morale is at rock bottom. People scream at each other ... The epi-
> demiologists having taken a census, object to washing their dishes.
> There is dishonesty. Stores of gifts are rifled for trade goods. There
> were to be no cigarettes except for personal use; one non-smoker
> brought 15 cartons. They are trading rum with the natives and now
> they are taking butter for trading and they never stop bitching at
> Harry [Crosman] and Bob [Fulton], the saints the navy left behind
> who have a 24-hour job keeping even drinking water available – the
> food they rant at, etc, etc. Lest you think it is a total loss there are
> about 15 people of integrity and honour. I am embarrassed for the
> others. Confinement with them for three months is hell. As far as
> I am concerned the whole thing is a nightmare to be endured. The
> only happiness I have is my roommate [Carlotta] and the work I
> am doing. Guilt enters into it, that I should have let the navy in for
> this terrible ... experience. My problem is to keep perspective so that
> what I write for *Maclean's* will not undercut Paul [Hellyer].[67]

She continued this epistolic lament on the following day, having been cheered by a good radio connection with her family that morning: "I am still depressed and bitter, but I know I will survive it." Then she described the work and the friction with other doctors: "Public health types of examinations are very dull, don't you think? There are a large number of diffusely enlarged thyroids in females. A crazy surgeon we have aboard wants to stick a needle in them all for biopsy ... What will it prove? Teeth are terrible ... there are no old people ... and signs of aging are present about 20 years ahead of us, people of thirty [years] have opacities of the lens [cataracts]."[68] She hoped to send the lamenting letter with one of the departing Chilean ships.

In the course of the examinations, Reid also told her husband that she'd found a family of five children all with low diastolic blood pressure, two of whom also had distinctive systolic murmers. She wondered if they had patent ductus arteriosis (PDA) and described their murmurs and X-rays. "Of course, our ECG [electrocardiogram] had to break down, but Dr. Richard Roberts, who is an adult heart man, says my *guess* of PDA is wrong."[69] Reid's attempt to diagnose – not "guess" – the abnormal findings meant that she had needed to "stick her neck out. The other clinicians won't hazard a guess."[70] Dismissing her interpretation of the enlarged thyroids and the heart murmurs – even to the point of labelling her findings as uninteresting – was yet another way that she felt her male colleagues put her down as an older woman trying to keep her hand in the clinical game. Unbeknownst to Roberts and Reid, a 1963 survey of 183 Easter Islanders had found thyroid enlargement (goiter) in seven adults simply by looking, not touching.[71] With METEI doing palpation (feeling) of the neck and given that goiter is more frequent in women, this information would have vindicated Reid's judgment.

In my interviews, three people – two METEI alumni and one offspring – asked if I had ever read William Golding's 1954 novel *Lord of the Flies*, "for that's what we had become." Carlotta said as much when she concluded her passage on the luncheon argument: "it looked as if we were going to degenerate into one of those depressing novels where civilized adults become savages."[72] Helen told her family that METEI was exactly like *Lord of the Flies* and instructed her husband to pick up a copy in the book department at Eaton's.[73]

METEI began its inspections of the bodies and abilities of the Rapanui and found friends, enemies, and lovers. But the lack of planning and interpersonal conflicts cast a pall over the expedition that the Sunday excursions and evening socializing could not relieve. Stanley's dream had taken shape, and for many it was a nightmare.

6

Revolution, Politics, and Disease

By the end of the first week, Stanley Skoryna worried that too many things were conspiring to derail his plans. Dissent within Camp Hilton was challenging the enthusiasm and cooperation upon which the study relied. Outside the *campamento*, political tensions were coming to a head between the Chileans and the Rapanui population, within which several divisions could be found. Members of the Medical Expedition to Easter Island had begun to make friends and were taking sides, and each faction suspected all the others of lying. Skoryna needed the approval and trust of everyone or his elaborate mission would fall apart. He did not know that a small revolution was about to occur – one that, historians agree, would forever change the political destiny of the island.[1]

THE MARINES ARE COMING

On 29 December 1964, officers at the airport informed METEI that the military ship *Yelcho* was on its way from the mainland, bringing marines and Dr Guido Andrade. Several islanders claimed that the Chilean soldiers were going to kill Alfonso Rapu. John Easton conveyed the governor's view to the team: Rapu had been ordered arrested "on civil charges [for stealing] bulldozer parts"; the governor agreed to "overlook" the teacher's earlier protests "if Rapu would cooperate. Rapu wouldn't. He want[ed] to be king of the island." The Chileans alleged that Rapu had been plotting for a union with Tahiti under France.[2] METEI travellers doubted this version and sympathized with the islanders. Skoryna insisted on their silence about the political situation during their radio calls home. He walked a fine line between Governor Jorge Portilla's administration and the goodwill of the Rapanui, and he reasoned that strict neutrality in the face of what he kept insisting was a "domestic problem" would be the only way that they could continue. Some, like Helen Reid and Maureen Roberts, obeyed assiduously: in her detailed but anodyne description of life on the island, Maureen described *Yelcho*, which she did not refer to by name, as a "small Chilean vessel" that had come "for some government business," offering her a chance to mail a letter.[3] Others, however, ignored Skoryna's order.

On 31 December both the *New York Times* and Toronto's *Globe and Mail* published short reports from two sources – United Press International and the Associated Press – announcing that Chile was sending a troopship to quell a rebellion on Easter Island.[4] During her New Year's Day radio call, Helen Reid was astonished when her anxious family asked if she was safe. They told her that marines were coming to put down a "revolution" and helpfully suggested that "P.H." (Minister of Defence Paul Hellyer) might get in touch with her for inside information.[5] Their alarm was especially jarring since the New Year's Eve festivities on Rapa Nui had proceeded in merry harmony.

Someone was leaking, Helen thought, despite Skoryna's caution. She suspected it was Carl Mydans of *Life* or Bob Williams of the Canadian Broadcasting Corporation. We "gave our word ... the fact that Stanley allows them to get stuff out ... bugs me no end."[6] Who else could draw the attention of America's most important newspaper? However, Mydans could not have known of Santiago's decision to send the marines unless he had contacts in Chile. This possibility becomes probable because, some contend, Mydans had his own radio. Furthermore, *Life* was rumoured to have paid $15,000 for the privilege of Mydans travelling with METEI; in fact, it was only $5,000.[7] Nevertheless, Mydans may have felt that the price exacted by METEI organizers exempted him from Skoryna's authority. Plus it was a great story. Who could resist?

But a leak does not have to be the explanation. Unknown to METEI, *Yelcho*'s preparations were no secret in Santiago and Valparaiso, certainly after HMCS *Cape Scott* reached the Chilean mainland on 29 December and possibly well before. Governor Portilla may have asked for help at the first sign of trouble with Rapu's upstart election back on 8 December or possibly on 20 December when the islanders sabotaged the bulldozer. Also, once *Cape Scott* reached Valparaiso, Rapu's letter received wide coverage, garnering commentary from a former Rapanui *alcalde* (mayor) in Santiago who was said to have conveyed the "principal aspirations" to the Ministry of the Interior and the secretary of state.[8] Even the bulldozer was mentioned in the newspapers with sympathy for the islanders.[9] Therefore, the Canadian ambassador to Chile, G.B. Summers, would have known of the military plans for Easter Island and informed Ottawa; American diplomats would have done the same. (For more on this episode from Commander Tony Law's perspective, see chapter 8).

Back in Montreal, Al Tunis began fielding anxious phone calls and letters. John Cutler's father in New York City demanded news of his son and what McGill University was doing to protect his safety.[10] Radio contact with the willing "hammies" was stepped up. On 2 January, Mydans talked to Tunis "to give him an 'official' report," wrote Helen sarcastically. That day, Toronto's *Globe and Mail* published a soothing statement that the situation was "quiet" on Easter Island and that work was proceeding normally; the source was radio operator George Hrischenko via a contact in Halifax.[11] But by now everyone in Canada and on Easter Island knew that a Chilean ship was on its way with "forty [actually thirty-seven] marines" to put down the secession movement.

FRENCH INTERFERENCE?

Suddenly, on 2 January 1965, the French frigate *Amiral Charner* appeared offshore. Hacker wrote cynically about its "extremely significant" timing: "the warship ... happened to be passing, ... heard there was a revolution going on and decided to call in to see if it could help."[12] "Quelle coïncidence!" wrote Reid.[13] Chileans were concerned that Rapanui aspirations for more democracy would lead them toward Tahiti and French control. In fact, several days earlier, the French navy had been denied permission to go ashore at Easter Island, a decision reported in the *Washington Post* on 29 December. Privately, officials blamed the recent demonstrations "for independence from Chile on agitation from crewmen of another French ship, which visited Easter Island nearly a year ago."[14] (Was this another reference to Francis Mazière?) Americans hoping to build a satellite station also wanted Chile, rather than France or any other country, to keep control. Respecting the order, *Amiral Charner* posed no threat, although people on Easter Island were uncertain. In the end, it left the same day after only a few hours. France was not about to claim Rapa Nui for itself. And Alfonso Rapu remained in hiding. Meanwhile, the examinations, the photographs, the X-rays, and the blood tests went on as before.

Nothing of this anxiety or the orders forbidding a landing had been conveyed to METEI, although many, like Carlotta Hacker, suspected the French ship's motives. A little party of its officers came to shore and asked for a guided visit of the island. Happy to meet fellow francophones in the midst of the South Pacific, Armand Boudreault became the designated tour guide. At the end of the day, along with Cléopâtre and Denys Montandon,

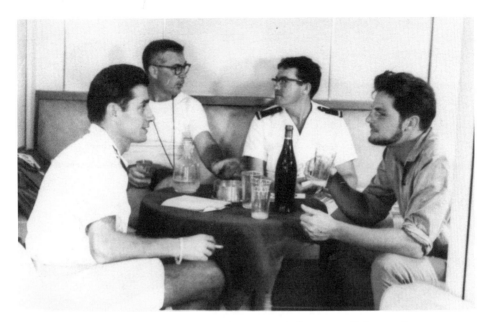

Figure 6.1 On board the French frigate *Amiral Charner* with Armand Boudreault (*2nd from left*) and Denys Montandon (*right*). Montandon Diary.

he was taken out to the frigate for "un bon souper"; they had a marvellous time chatting *en français* with the captain and the ship's doctor. "C'était si bon ce petit Pernod!" wrote Cléopâtre with nostalgia; the Proustian *madeleine* had become *pastis*. She later pasted a snapshot of the gathering in her scrapbook (figure 6.1). The French doctor gave them a 20-litre cask of red wine (figure 6.2). Thrilled, they brought it back to Camp Hilton to store for the upcoming *sau sau* in honour of the family of Juan Atán, at which Carlotta's "cow" would be consumed.

The following day, 3 January, was a Sunday, and the Montandons went out exploring, while less fortunate members of METEI participated in the inexpert slaughter and ghastly butchering of the hapless bovine. Veterinarians David Murphy and Hal Gibbs deliberately stayed away. While Denys and Cléopâtre were touring, the wine was stolen. She described the crisis: "Unfortunately, the members of the American group of *intelligentissimi* decided to help themselves and put the wine in the dining room for general consumption"; they had already diminished it considerably. "By an Olympian effort," Denys reclaimed the wine for storage, but "this action agitated our friends; tongues and spirits grew heated, and a diplomatic incident ensued." Skoryna intervened as

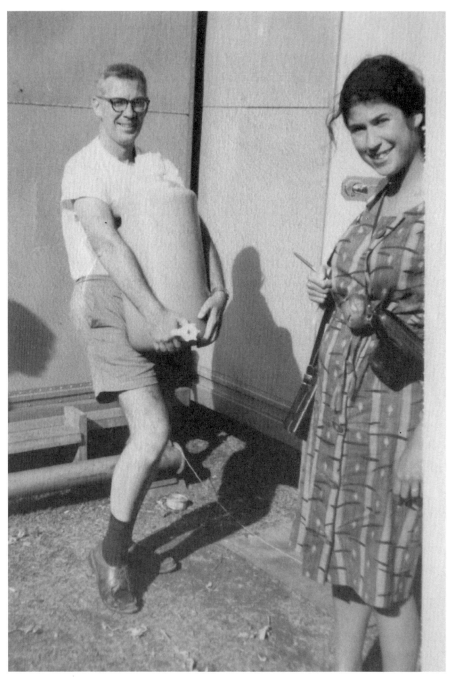

Figure 6.2 Armand Boudreault and Cléopâtre Montandon with their cask of red wine. Photo Armand Boudreault.

mediator, and the Montandons backed down, "not because we needed the friendship of those who would never be our friends – real friends always remain – nor to demonstrate our 'superiority.' It was simply to do no harm to the famous expedition 'team spirit' that had never really been established."[15] Boudreault did not mind the theft as much as he objected to the disrespect of the precious wine: he was shocked to discover that Skoryna had helped himself to a large glass of red to accompany a dish of canned pork and beans.

That night, Meier, at least, enjoyed a "very good meal with red wine. The Atáns were here in force." In the aftermath of the tiff, Carlotta noticed members of the Group deliberately (and childishly) bumping into Cléopâtre as they reached for the butter.[16] *Quel expédition!* At this distance, it is poignant to note that the Montandons disliked the antics of the Group and reporters as much as did Helen Reid, Carlotta Hacker, and Mary King; yet Reid had considered the young couple charter members. Language, culture, age difference, and the stress of isolation eroded nerves and dulled perception.

The tiff within the camp paled in contrast to the political tensions that mounted while everyone waited for the marines. On the evening of 3 January, Helen Reid was walking with a Rapanui woman when the governor sped by in his unarmed jeep. Her companion "looked at the stone wall and said, 'It is just right – a gun over the wall would kill the governor. Some go with a gun here (she put her hand to the left armpit) and some here (she put her hand to an imaginary holster). There will be blood.'" Helen "asked if the people would fight with guns. She replied 'Yes.' No more."[17]

THE TROOPS TAKE CONTROL

Finally, on 5 January, the much-anticipated *Yelcho* arrived with its marines and two jeeps. It had covered the great distance in just five days. Prepared to put down an armed rebellion, the soldiers set up camp in camouflage tents near Hanga Piko. METEI members worried that their arrival might escalate the tension. But a battery of Rapanui women formed the reception committee, overwhelming the invaders with flowers, song, and the welcoming words "Nice girl for you?" Rapu's mother watched, neither singing nor giving flowers (figure 6.3).[18]

The commander was Guillermo Rojas Aird. He brought along John Martin, the former governor of Easter Island, whom, Reid claimed, had been well liked.[19] Later testimony challenged that view: Martin and his wife could speak Rapanui and had mingled with the people, but his

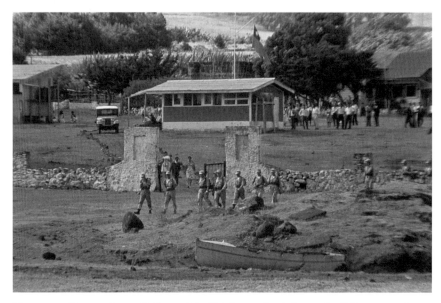

Figure 6.3 Troops from Chilean ship *Yelcho* at the Jefetura building near Camp Hilton. Photo Archibald Wilkinson.

unbending cruelty is still remembered.[20] It was said that Dr Andrade was somewhere on board, being held prisoner.[21] Helen wondered why the beloved doctor would have been brought back to the island. Was he to be "tried at the site" as a "terrifying example" to "make it seem impartial" and frighten the people? She detected posturing: "the acts are played, and the puppets make the ordered dance."[22] No one from METEI set eyes on Andrade during the ten-day sojourn of *Yelcho*, and they did not yet know the outcome of his court-martial, which had already taken place. He was found guilty of sedition, sent to prison for a year, and stripped of his licence to practise for four years.[23] A marginal note in Reid's diary indicates that he wrote to her from England ten years later, hoping to come to Canada.[24]

Following his orders, Rojas took command of the island from Portilla, a humiliation for the young governor, who had muddled through the recent troubles. A tribunal would hear submissions in the Jefetura building near the METEI camp; anyone could ask for status. Many did.

Now Alfonso Rapu emerged from hiding to present his case, and a succession of islanders came forward to state their grievances and recommendations. The famous letter with its forty signatories, which had been disseminated in Chile, was subjected to careful scrutiny. I have not

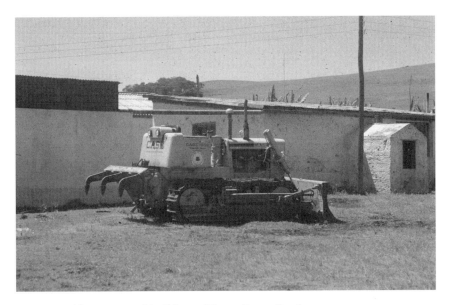

Figure 6.4 The contested bulldozer. Photo Garry Brody.

found a complete copy of this letter, but at one point it was posted near the church, and Carlotta Hacker had a copy. It was summarized in the Chilean newsmagazine *Ercilla* on 6 January with a photo of handsome Rapu on the cover. The letter complained of the lack of freedom, democracy, respect, and employment, and it described excessive punishments that included unwarranted beatings, incarceration, and the shaving of women's hair.[25] It also suggested improvements to enhance autonomy and the quality of life: an end to military rule, votes for women, a canning factory for fish and meat, a high school, and an occupational school for learning trades. The authors were adamant that they did not seek separation from Chile but justice and equality as citizens: "We ask for an end to colonialism and that we return to being the Easter Islanders that we once were, a people who could sing without being ordered to sing."[26]

The tribunal wanted to know how this letter had made its way into the Chilean press. The mechanism remained secret for a long time (see chapter 8). Some islanders disavowed any connection at all to the complaints, claiming that Rapu and his handful of associates had forged their names. The meetings continued for several days. Roberts and Skoryna were summoned to explain on what basis and by whose authority METEI was allowed to operate on Rapa Nui. We do not know their exact words, but they would have cited the Chilean permissions and argued for neutrality and the continuation of their work. During these hearings, the rehabilitated bulldozer raced up and down in front of the Jefetura, taunting the Chilean troops (figure 6.4).[27]

THE "RIOT"

At dusk on the evening of 8 January, Helen Reid was finishing up paperwork in her clinic office outside the main gate. She was tired. On that day, thirty-one examinations had been completed, including thirteen children and eight women. She heard an increasingly loud "wailing and chanting" moving toward camp. She left the clinic trailer and was caught up in a massive crowd of screaming women also heading toward the METEI compound gate. Marines wielding rifles lined up to block them. When Helen approached the gate, a soldier shoved her away with his weapon. A METEI member inside the camp opened the gate for her, and a flood of people poured in behind.

The crowd swarmed deep into the compound, pursued by the marines. In their midst was Alfonso Rapu, elegant and handsome in a glowing, white shirt. Some thought he was injured and struggling to breathe, but his distress came from the tightly encircling arms of the women who surrounded and protected him; they included his mother and aunt. The shrieking was intense. Several women lay on the ground just beyond the gate. Mesmerized by the invasion, METEI members held their breath – all except Einar Gjessing, who opened his door to complain about the noise. "How can I 'vork'?" he shouted angrily.[28] Hal Gibbs remembers being in the lab reading fecal smears with Maureen Roberts, who was examining urine samples. "We made a pair," he said. As the crowd surged into the compound past their little window, Maureen leapt up yelling in her Scottish brogue, "Douse the lights! Douse the lights!" And together they watched.

Rojas soon appeared. He spoke softly to the marines and sent them away. Especially concerned about a pregnant woman, he asked METEI doctors to examine the people lying on the ground. He addressed the crowd, "quietly and patiently" assuring them that he had no plans for arrests and told them all to go home, including Rapu. The doctors ascertained that people on the ground were unharmed. One woman insisted that she was having a heart attack. Isabel Griffiths opened the woman's blouse, patted her breast, and said, "No you're not; your heart is fine." The woman laughed and went home.[29]

Mesmerized, Hal and Maureen continued to watch as the crowd melted away. Four men brought Rapu a horse, flung a dark coat over his bright, white shirt, and put a *Cape Scott* baseball cap on his head. Like a cowboy in a Western comedy, he took a flying leap, fell short, and landed on the horse's rump. He stood, dusted himself off, shook hands with Red Lemieux and Skoryna, mounted the horse successfully, and exited through the back gate, vanishing into the night.[30]

Eyewitness accounts of this moment emphasize the high emotion, anxiety, and panic, and they praise Rojas's impressive restraint. Earlier, word had come from Maria Atán at the camp gate to Carlotta Hacker and Garry Brody that Rapu's associate Germán Hotu had been shot; then it emerged he was *going* to be shot.[31] None of it was true, although at least one shot had been fired as a warning. Was METEI finished? Would Rapu ever appear again? These questions tormented METEI that night.

Meier's diary entry about the "riot" contained the observation, repeated by many others, that people wanted to demonstrate in order to be noticed and were disappointed that nobody had taken pictures. They were "seeking asylum or something."[32] METEI members were so startled and the events unfolded so rapidly that no one had time to grab cameras – not even Mydans. Helen ended her diary entry for that night with the following: "There are elements of the comic opera, the paper revolution, the play for the press (many demonstrators asked why no pictures [were] being taken), and many wished me 'Buenas noches' ... Georgina decided that she had better go home in the middle of the excitement because she had to get up early for work tomorrow." Beyond the absurdity, Helen wrote, "some of the small scenes scattered about have pathos, fear, frustration, sorrow, hopelessness, plain for all to read."[33]

As Skoryna had insisted, Camp Hilton was not Canadian territory; no sanctuary could be found there. Yet later observers imply that the performance was deliberately calculated – as much for its content as for its audience, who would disseminate the Rapanui's grievances for "the world to see." Some go so far as to suggest that the twenty-two-year-old schoolteacher had plotted this crass "use" of METEI as a broadcast machine long before it arrived on Rapa Nui.[34] But if Rapu exploited METEI, so too did the naval administrators. Juan Atán later told Helen Reid that "the Chileans took advantage of the coming of *Cape Scott* to get along without a doctor, to [send] their products ... and the people [to Chile]. He also said that the coming of the expedition was a good thing since it brought trouble to a head, but that we [in METEI] are clueless as to what goes on. Our eyes are closed."[35] Atán must have been making this speech to anyone who would listen. It turned up in Cléopâtre's diary and (without crediting him) in Lemieux's movie.

REBELLION AFTERMATH AND ELECTIONS

Despite the gloom when they went to bed, METEI members were surprised on the following morning: Rapu returned to the Jefetura for more questioning, and a family stood waiting patiently in the reception area for the scheduled appointment. Only twenty people from three families were examined that day; however, it was much better than they had feared.

Either by Rojas's order or by an earlier order of Portilla, new elections were confirmed for Tuesday, 12 January 1965. On the 11th, a larger Chilean vessel, the supply ship *Aquila*, a substitute, dropped anchor offshore. Unlike *Yelcho*, it had taken some time to load provisions for the islanders – a soft glove approach to complement the iron fist of the marines. Those in the "Group" that Reid and Hacker identified with dissent and laziness were ecstatic to reprovision the alcohol supply. Another large *sau sau* took place. Soon, however, a different problem arose, one for which METEI was better prepared: *kokongo* (see below).

On 12 January voting took place at the school. The franchise was extended to anyone over age twenty-one, provided they could read, write, and speak Rapanui. For the first time, women would be allowed to vote, and they could participate in the procedure as witnesses and recorders. Maria Pont Hill served as a *testiga* and Maria Pate Tucki as a *vocale*. Voters declared their names before a witness who confirmed their identities and crossed them off a list based on the census. Then each voter stated his or her preferred candidate, and the vote was added to a tally on the blackboard at the front. This method did not allow for a secret ballot, but it was more democratic than the previous one, and the Rapanui took the process seriously.

The results came as predicted. With ninety-nine votes, Alfonso Rapu was again elected *alcalde*, and his councillors were the three runners up: Jorge Tepano (sixty-two votes), Germán Hotu (fifty-six votes), and Felipe Pakarati (fifty-six votes).[36] The swearing-in took place the following morning under the Chilean flag at the Jefetura; the crowd sang the national anthem, and Rojas administered the oath of allegiance (figures 6.5, 6.6, and 6.7). *Yelcho* and her troops could now make ready to leave. On 17 January, the evening before her departure, Father Sebastian delivered a scholarly lecture in English about the history of the island, possibly to emphasize justification for the new more independent order. Archie Wilkinson recorded it.[37]

The new mayor and two of his three councillors, who had not previously come for examination, now booked appointments – a welcome, if belated, endorsement of METEI. Germán Hotu, his wife, and nine

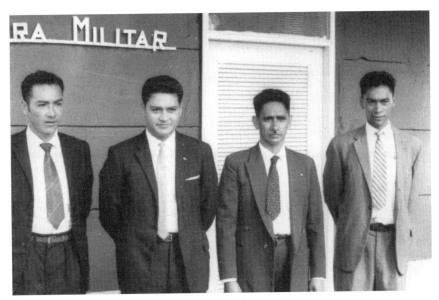

Figure 6.5 Alfonso Rapu (*2nd from left*) and his councillors, Jorge Tepano (*left*), Germán Hotu, and Felipe Pakarati (*right*) after election win, 12 January 1965. Montandon Diary.

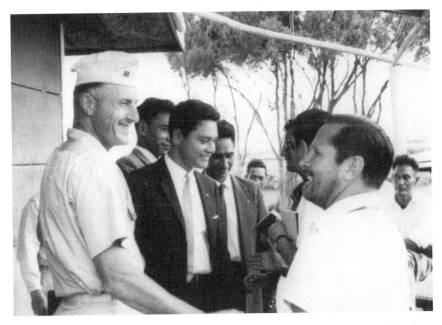

Figure 6.6 Alfonso Rapu (*centre*) with former governor John ("José") Martin (*left*) after election win, 12 January 1965. Montandon Diary.

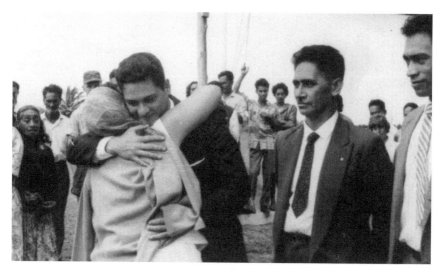

Figure 6.7 Alfonso Rapu hugged by his mother, Reina Haoa, after election win, 12 January 1965. Montandon Diary.

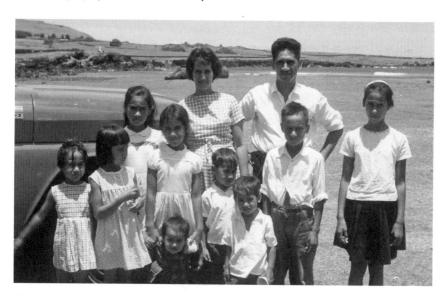

Figure 6.8 Hotu Hey family with Jeep Mea Mea: mother Maria Amalia Hey Paoa and father Germán Hotu Chavez with children Teresita (12), Maria Fatima (11), Victoria (9), Matias Aquiles (8), Maria Rubelinda (7), Melania Carolina (5), Urbano Matias (4), Pedro (3), and Sonia Margarita (18 mos). Germán was elected as a councillor with Alfonso Rapu. The family was examined a week after the election on 19 January 1965. A lying *moai* is visible behind the mother. Photo David Murphy.

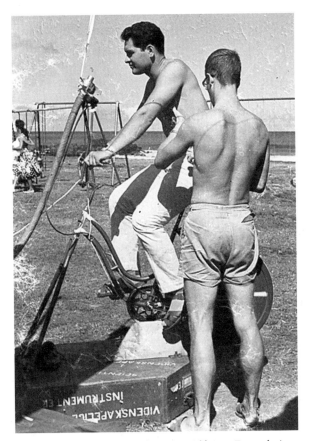

Figure 6.9 Newly elected mayor Alfonso Rapu being
tested on the bicycle ergometer by Einar Gjessing.
Note children on swings behind. Photo Helen Reid.
Originally published by Maclean's, Rogers Media
Inc., 19 June 1965.

children came on 19 January (figure 6.8). Rapu, his parents, six brothers,
and one sister appeared on 1 February, and the new mayor was tested on
the ergometer (figure 6.9). His married brother, Carlos, came two days
earlier, whereas his younger brother, Sergio, was studying in Chile.[38]
Young Felipe Pakarati, his wife, and their child had been among those
examined on New Year's Day; however, he had been the only councillor
elected from the "party" opposed to Rapu's "rebels." This exercise shows
that among the rebels, defiance against Chile may also have included
defiance against METEI.

Meanwhile, wasting no time and with *kokongo* raging, METEI doctors examined thirty-two people on election day and thirty-one the day after. The illness was directly related to the political rebellion.

KOKONGO: A POLITICAL OUTBREAK?

Kokongo was the mysterious disease that METEI had been expecting since well before its arrival. Seemingly of infectious origin and described by all the twentieth-century explorers from Katherine Routledge forward, it posed a medical challenge.[39] Virologist Armand Boudreault and microbiologist Georges Nógrády, in particular, were eager to identify the causative organism; their findings might indicate an antibiotic to treat it or a vaccine to prevent it. METEI members were relieved when *Cape Scott* did not bring *kokongo* to Rapa Nui, although several on the voyage had been ill and monitored by the scientists; however, without an outbreak, they could not investigate its nature and causes. Some islanders were explicit that friendly cooperation with the Canadian expedition was possible only because, like a good omen, METEI did not bring the disease.[40] However, the ships from Chile were a different story.

On Sunday, 10 January, Helen observed, "all during Mass, everyone is coughing, men, women, children – they come to the camp saying they have 'coconga'; they all touch the trachea and say it is sore." Some had been ill since Saturday night. On 11 January, Meier wrote, "many islanders stricken with kokongo." On that day, METEI doctors had one of their busiest days: forty-one people – twenty under age fifteen and eight women – came forward for their examinations, several complaining of *kokongo* or aggravated asthma. METEI provided cough medicines to allay the symptoms, but Helen discovered that some people, while expressing gratitude, preferred the ministrations of traditional healers.[41]

The undeniable connection between the arrival of the first Chilean ship and the onset of *kokongo* four or five days later had some METEI members wondering if it was a psychosomatic response to perceived oppression – a form of mass hysteria. Epidemiologist John Cutler visited a number of houses, unimpressed by the "vague" information. "He believes this is an act," wrote Helen.[42] Nevertheless, Cutler and Elliot Alpert took throat swabs from all the Chilean marines, who lined up dutifully for the procedure, with Rita Dwyer as translator and "petit bonhomme" Mydans, as Cléopâtre called him, "gesticulating from the roof of a jeep" and uttering Hollywood-style directions as he immortalized the scene for *Life* (figures 6.10 and 6.11).[43]

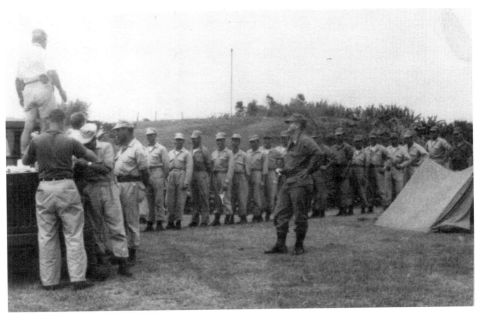

Figure 6.10 Searching for *kokongo* at Hanga Piko. Carl Mydans is standing on the jeep. Montandon Diary.

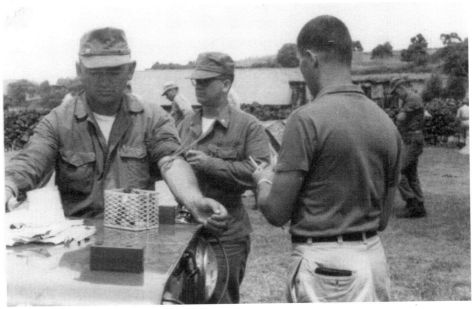

Figure 6.11 Searching for *kokongo* at Hanga Piko. Elliot Alpert is taking blood. Montandon Diary.

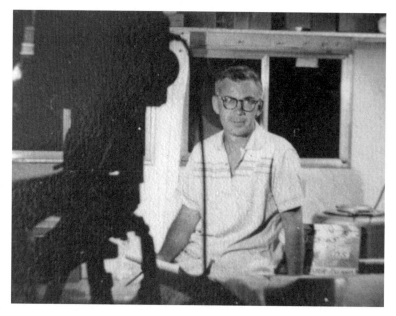

Figure 6.12 Armand Boudreault explaining his method of searching for the *kokongo* virus to CBC filmmaker Robert Williams. Photo Armand Boudreault.

Reid, however, was convinced it was a real disease entity.[44] Against the "psychosomatic" theory, even babies were sick, and several METEI members also fell ill, including herself. She described the clinical features, hour by hour: onset of headache and slight cough, which worsened to heavy coughing overnight, fever, tracheitis, aching eyes, and finally laryngitis. Some people reported diarrhea. "Imp[ression]: cocongo is an entity: virus tracheitis and N.P. [naso-pharyngitis]. Await cultures and more cases."[45] She interrogated Nógrády and Boudreault about their investigations. The former found no evidence of bacteria and decided the cause must be viral. But he offered several hypotheses as to the mechanism of its transmission, the antigenicity of the causative agent, and the ability of islanders to mount an immune response.[46] Boudreault explained his techniques to identify the viral cause, which involved taking both acute and convalescent blood samples and incubating the swabs and sera with living cells (Hela cells and K cells). He still hoped that these precious cells had not been destroyed during power interruption on the outbound journey and the hot delay while the freezers were unloaded from *Cape Scott*. The results would take at least a year (figure 6.12).[47]

Helen participated in this medical sleuthing, wondering if the difference between the Canadian and the Chilean ships had nothing to do with good political omens, personality, or psychology and everything to do with varying incubation periods subtended by the time lapsed after leaving the last port. For *Yelcho*, it had been a mere five or six days; for *Cape Scott*, it had been twelve. Could it be that the virus burned itself out on longer journeys and arrived inactive?[48] Richard Roberts accepted the plausibility of this view.[49] Boudreault continued to work on the problem for at least four years, suspicious that the culprit was an influenza virus. But the cause of this *kokongo* outbreak was never established.

MORE DISEASES:
DIARRHEA, LEPROSY, AND TUBERCULOSIS

Diarrhea was a common complaint on the island among both the Rapanui and the METEI travellers. Meier consulted Brody for medication when he was in pain with its ravages.[50] The three *campamento* toilets were "flushed" with a bucket of sea water, either from an overhead tank or directly into the bowl, but travellers remember that one or two of the toilets were often out of order.[51] When John Cutler contracted the malady himself, he took over sanitation. "This has been a revolution," wrote Helen, pleased with the changes. A hot water tank and a small sink were finally installed "one month after arrival," and water had been ordered from the governor's supply "over Easton's head," no doubt pleasing Roberts, who had argued for these amenities on *Cape Scott*. Now John also supervised the dishwashing, kept up a running commentary about "dishes, sanitation, niggers, ... [saying] 'you could do better in Georgia; Stanley should have chosen the members of the expedition better ... some interpreters have never washed dishes,' etc., etc." Helen continued, "There is a certain sick air to the whole business and an obsessive aspect that is beginning to frighten me a little. The Group drinks a good deal."[52]

Leprosy had been a problem on the island for almost a century, and the small leprosarium, or "sanitarium," where a few people were isolated was cared for by the same order of nuns who managed the school.[53] Leprosy was greatly feared on the mainland, although it was contagious only under conditions of close, prolonged contact. It was the reason – or the pretext – for denying the islanders freedom of movement and for requiring that they apply to the governor for permission to leave even the village, let alone the island. The young people who guided the ecologists, veterinarians, and other expeditionists on their outings required official passes (figure 6.13).

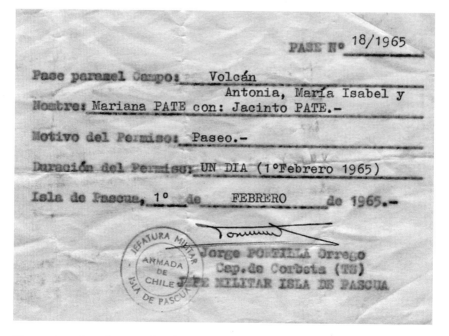

Figure 6.13 One-day pass for three sisters and their older brother to accompany the ecologists on a field trip to one of the volcanoes, signed by Governor Jorge Portilla, 1 February 1965. This was the same family as in figure 6.14. With thanks to Ian Efford.

In his lecture, Andrade had explained that "a Brazilian leprologist" came to Rapa Nui for six days in 1962 and conducted a survey involving over 4,000 nasal smears.[54] Nógrády was repeating this work.

Father Ricardo Rainer served as priest to the leprosarium, offering Mass twice a week. In the meantime, he loved to fish from a boat that he had built himself. He had been sent to help Father Sebastian Englert in the late 1950s, but the older priest "did not like" him, nor did he want anyone coming between himself and his flock. After a year, Ricardo returned to the continent but was summoned again only twelve months later when Father Sebastian fell ill in 1961. This time, he stayed, but once the old priest recovered, Ricardo was confined to ministering to people with leprosy. He mingled with METEI members soon after their arrival, and Helen Reid interviewed him at length to obtain his story and thoughts on island life and leprosy.[55]

Having never before seen the ravages of this mutilating disease, METEI doctors were interested in the people with leprosy. The six or seven people (counts vary) who lived in confinement were not allowed to come to Camp Hilton; however, on 11 January 1965, four men and one woman were examined for METEI at the leprosarium. METEI also provided these people with medical care. One day, Carlotta went along to help Peter Beighton. She was struck by the peaceful atmosphere, the garden, and the quiet life of these unfortunate human beings, whom she found friendly, cheerful, and surprisingly hopeful.[56] They were occupied with small tasks and had a treadle-operated Singer sewing machine, possibly a METEI gift, as *Cape Scott* had brought six.[57] Helen Reid noted the names of people with leprosy and their ages from seventeen to fifty-one; in addition to the six or seven in the leprosarium, twenty-one others were ambulatory, whether or not they still took treatment. She also noted the duration of the previous confinement, ranging from one to ten years for the ambulatory and up to eighteen years for those still in the leprosarium. The results of their most recent bacteriological controls showed that most were no longer infectious; however, the deformities would remain for the rest of their lives.[58] In an effort to characterize the extent of leprosy on the island, Georges Nógrády took nasal smears from 500 individuals for more detailed study back in Canada with fluorescence microscopy.

One of the men with leprosy was a gifted carver, fifty-one-year-old Gabriel Hereveri. He had been confined almost two decades; the disease had claimed both hands and both feet; his face had "caved in" grotesquely; and he was blind in one eye from the damage to his eyelids. The vision of his other eye was headed in the same direction. Carlotta was impressed that Beighton walked right up to Gabriel and shook him by his stump; Gabriel was pleased. Most members of METEI alive today – even those with no medical training – remember this man and his dreadful condition. They also remember a remarkable event.

Plastic surgeon Garry Brody studied Gabriel's eyelid and devised what he now calls a "simple" operation to transplant a part of the temporalis muscle at the side of his head to the eyelid so that Gabriel could open and close his eye in an effort to save his vision. He operated in the tiny theatre of the hospital, using instruments borrowed from *Cape Scott* and assisted – or at least witnessed – by many METEI travellers: Beighton, Alpert, Gjessing, Dwyer, and Denys Montandon. Mydans hung back taking photographs. Gjessing and Montandon were still in training; now they both wonder if this operation influenced their choice of plastic surgery.

Having stabilized Gabriel's remaining vision, Brody worried about how the man's deformity had robbed him of his craft. At first, he imagined devising a tool from a hollow piece of wood, but an islander came up with the better idea of using part of an old rubber tire that Gabriel could fit into specific grooves caused by the disease's scarring of his upper limb and manipulate to carve wood once again. For all their sophistication, numerous Rapanui, including those who helped in the laboratory, assured METEI that whatever the scientific tests might indicate, Gabriel's disease had been visited upon him by angry *aku-aku* (spirits) when he violated another family's cave.[59] Similar loss of health and *mana* (power) was said to have come to those who allowed human remains to be taken from the island.[60] A family who befriended ecologist Ian Efford explained that they all slept together – wives, husbands, children – in one room with the shutters closed for protection from the spirits. He concluded that it made "an ideal incubator" for tuberculosis.

This story of the powerful *aku-aku* needs more investigating; Pablo Seward has uncovered evidence that it was exaggerated by the islanders to dupe Thor Heyerdahl, who believed he was duping them.[61] If the tricking of Heyerdahl wasn't part of the 1955 encounter, it had become a well-established Rapanui legend by 1965. Maria Atán told Helen Reid that Heyerdahl's scorn for their carvings and his preference for the old stone statues only led the elders to make "old statues" to defraud him.[62] METEI was not immune to similar manipulation.

Tuberculosis was also a previously recognized problem on Rapa Nui. Chile had established protocols for controlling this rampant disease, which were followed by the military doctors who served at Hanga Roa.[63] Twelve islanders were known to have had the disease, but they took proper treatment and were no longer infectious. As part of his investigations and to verify numbers provided by Andrade, Nógrády did Ziehl-Neelsen (acid-fast) stains on all sputum samples, looking for activity of the causative organism, *Mycobacterium tuberculosis*. He also plated specific cultures on ready-made American Trudeau Society media, but those samples would require six weeks or more to grow – and would not be complete until the expedition was over. In their thrice weekly examinations of Archie Wilkinson's chest X-rays, METEI doctors noticed lung changes suggestive of tuberculosis in five people not previously known to have the disease. Their names were retained for follow-up on the island so that proper treatment could be given.

Control of both leprosy and tuberculosis was managed through authoritarian intervention. Rapanui were divided on whether or not they welcomed this additional Chilean incursion into their lives. It too was political.

BIRTHS AND DEATHS

Revolution or not, the cycle of life went on. The political upheaval and its resolution impacted METEI's operations. In the absence of Andrade, the Rapanui sometimes turned to METEI for care. Seven women gave birth while METEI stayed on Easter Island. For none of these mothers was it a first child. On 28 December 1964, the day the survey examinations began, a baby was born to an elder daughter – possibly her second illegitimate son. He was the first tiny infant whom METEI examined, along with the rest of his family, including grandparents, when they came for their regular appointment on 19 January 1965, a week after the election. Until that day, babies examined had been three months of age or older. METEI doctors were involved in a few of the seven deliveries. But again, it was only after the departure of the Chilean marines that the islanders turned to Camp Hilton for obstetrical help and brought their newborns for examination.

Skoryna himself attended the first METEI delivery. In the middle of the night on 23 January, he was roused by Aurelio Pont Hill, whose nineteen-year-old wife, Maria del Rosario Pate Niare, was in labour with her third baby. Helen Reid had examined her and her two daughters, aged one and two, just nine days earlier. Skoryna leapt into Jeep Mea Mea – but was warned by Aurelio that the house was a half-mile beyond a gate and down a steep track bounded by hedges and stone walls, at the bottom of which he would not be able to turn around. When Skoryna reached the gate in the dense Rapanui night, he backed the entire way down the narrow track to the house. They loaded Maria del Rosario into the truck and raced to the hospital, where her baby, a tiny girl, was born just one hour later. In the morning, Skoryna was immensely proud of his achievement, and Helen was amazed to learn that he and she were to be godparents. The child would be named Halina Irene for Skoryna's wife and Helen Reid, who, as her godmother, always called her "Mi Poki" (my child).[64]

The baptism took place on 31 January – and METEI photographers captured Stanley and Helen decked out in feather headdresses and shell necklaces (figure 6.14). Another baby girl was baptized on the same day with Rita Dwyer and Armand Boudreault as godparents; no photos of her family from that day have survived, although Rita and Armand came home with identical feathered hats.[65] METEI hosted a celebratory *sau sau* and *curando* in grand style: two cows and twenty sheep were roasted, with the entire island invited and the camp decorated with small banana trees. Exceptionally, the party began in the afternoon to please the photographers, who wanted to capture the dancers in daylight.[66] Many photos of this event show Luis Pate (later Luis Avaka), known as Papa Kiko,

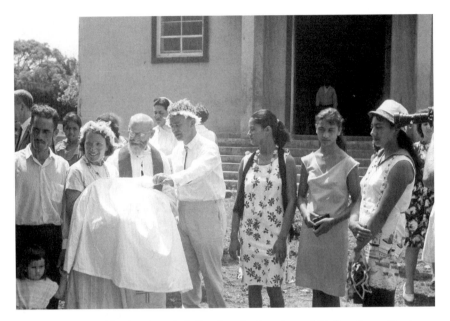

Figure 6.14 Outside the church following the baptism of Halina Irene Pont Pate ("Mi Poki"), 31 January 1965. The baby is held by Dr Helen Reid. *Also from left*, baby's father Aurelio Pont Hill and sister Ana Margarita, Father Sebastian Englert, Dr Stanley Skoryna, mother Maria del Rosario Pate Niare, and aunt Antonia Pate Niare. Photo David Murphy.

leading a performance of the beautiful, young men and women in grass skirts, feathers, and shells (figures 6.15 and 6.16).

But Stanley and Helen were disturbed that Mi Poki's father kept asking them to take his baby with them back to Canada. They were invited to a luncheon, at which they were the only ones expected to eat; and Aurelio gave Stanley a book in Spanish about leprosy, carefully inscribing it for him. Was it because Mi Poki was a girl? Was it because they were too poor to have a third child? The Canadians did not know. By all appearances, the parents adored the little mite. Aurelio was famous for having survived a journey to Tahiti with two friends in a small boat navigating "by stars," although he admitted to Helen that he had also used a map and compass.[67] From Tahiti, he joined merchant ships and went all around the world, before returning to Rapa Nui, which, he said, "is best for me." Did his world travels lead him to want the same for this daughter? Only on the voyage back to Canada did Helen connect the dots when she noticed a name from the family on the list of "ambulatory

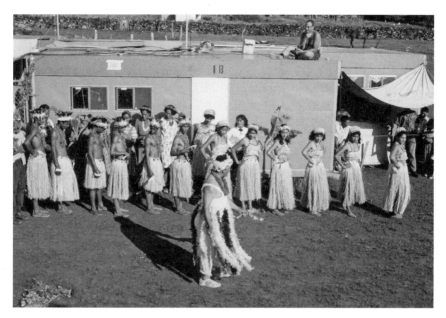

Figure 6.15 Papa Kiko – Luis Pate (later Luis Avaka) – leading dancers in reception area of *campamento*. Garry Brody is on the roof of the trailer. Photo David Murphy.

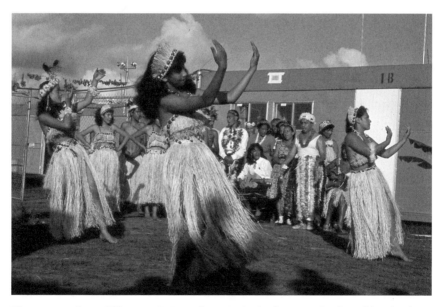

Figure 6.16 Papa Kiko – Luis Pate (later Luis Avaka) – in feathered hat leading dancers in reception area of *campamento*. Photo Ian Efford.

lepers." Why else would they have a medical tome on the disease? The desire to give away a beloved child might stem from a parental urge to protect her.[68]

On 28 January expectant father Bob Meier donated a pint of blood to a woman hemorrhaging after giving birth. "Mission accomplished," he wrote in his diary. The details of this story are best told in Isabel's words:

John [Cutler] and I (as translator) were on hospital duty; while all the other members were gone to explore the sites. A man came to the camp on a horse asking for help for his wife who was delivering a baby. We took the truck and went to their house to find a very large woman in bed with two tiny babies just born and lots of blood all over. The placenta had not been delivered. With help, we rushed her to the hospital taking the twins with us. John found a single pair of sterile gloves, gave me a can of ether and a gauze cone, and asked me to anesthetize the woman while [he introduced] his hand and arm way up into her vagina trying to dislodge the placenta, all the time warning me that if I gave too much [ether] I would kill her; too little, and she would not relax. The lady requested to speak to her husband before being put to sleep. I called him in, and they proceeded to talk in *pascuense* for, what it seemed to us, a very long time. Her request was that John tie her tubes while she was asleep. John looked at me in disbelief and retorted: "Don't say this to her, but she is lucky if she survives the day!" After that he proceeded to very gingerly remove the placenta which he said was of the consistency of cellophane paper (this was her third set of twins). After a while, I tell John that I am fainting, I don't do very well with blood – not as bad as "Doc Martin," but close. He tells me to go out for one minute and return immediately, which I did. Fortunately for the family, the lady survived the ordeal and recovered well. Three days later, however, one baby died, and that was sad.[69]

Helen Reid explained that because the twins shared a common circulation in the placenta, the weaker twin had basically transfused its sibling with its own blood.[70] The surviving child was named Maria Isabel, and Isabel and John were godparents. Lemieux captured this christening in his film and dubbed the scene "Spanish wedding," showing John with his dashing blond mustache and beard alongside Isabel with her black lace veil. A pattern was established: when METEI assisted at deliveries, babies found names and godparents.

The wide "publicity" around METEI personnel and the births had an effect on the study. Two days later, a family came for examination, bringing their three-week-old baby girl. The next day, 2 February, Mi Poki was officially examined at Camp Hilton and found to be well. But curiously enough, on that same day, four other newborns (one was only a day old) were also seen, three of them with their entire families, whereas the fourth, like Mi Poki, had been born after the rest of her family had already been examined. This clustering of the seven newborns in the two days following the *sau sau* for Mi Poki suggests that METEI had reached a new level of acceptance or trust in the eyes of the people whom it had come to observe and to help. It also suggests that Rapanui women may have been in charge.

One other death occurred besides that of the twin. Soon after their arrival, a middle-aged woman succumbed to what the METEI team believed might have been lung cancer. She had not been examined for the survey, and no autopsy was permitted.[71] Helen Reid attended the simple funeral, presided over by Father Sebastian, with burial in the little cemetery just north of the METEI camp. The islanders brought a striking matter-of-fact attitude to this rite. Heyerdahl had written something similar about stoic reactions to the tragic drownings of a teacher, a schoolboy, and the daughter of the mayor during an outing to circle the island on his ship.[72] The subtle differences in mourning hinted at deeper cultural divergences. Helen remembered that, according to Andrade, six of the seven deaths in the previous year had been of children. In this tiny population, loss of young people was a regular occurrence, less hidden than in Canada.

Animal death hinted at something unusual too. Several memoirs record the sorry state of a starving mare and her colt lurking near the Camp Hilton fence. She dwindled slowly over several days; then, on the morning of 21 January, she was dead, and the colt had disappeared.[73] The expeditionists wondered why no one would help the creature or make an end to her misery? Another shock came when, in thinking to please one of the lab girls, John Cutler gave her a living chicken. The girl seemed delighted; she whooped "weird primeval yells" and laughed, swung the hapless bird in huge arcs around her head, clipped its wings, and threw it in the air. Horrified, Cutler took it back.[74] Was this an expression of pleasure? Was it mockery? Did it hint at a mentality far beyond the ken of the scientists bent so intently on physical samples and measurements? METEI had no psychiatrist or psychologist – yet the mental adaptation of its members was just as important as the physical. Helen told Carlotta that, if nothing else, a psychologist might have helped them to understand themselves.[75]

Having come to conduct a scientific survey of Rapanui biology, METEI members found themselves in the midst of political turmoil, which, some argue, their presence had triggered. With the menacing arrival of marines, it seemed that the entire project would fail. But the eventual de-escalation of tensions and the first free election were followed by the greater acceptance of METEI by the islanders, who tended to credit the scientists for the happy outcome, whether they deserved it or not. METEI learned that island diseases – leprosy, tuberculosis, and other infections, including the mysterious *kokongo* – were both a consequence and a cause of political and social injustice. The sympathy and mutual respect that METEI members came to share with the Rapanui helped to put Stanley's dream back on track.

7

Plants, Animals, Mores, and Microbes

The Medical Expedition to Easter Island was not confined to physical examinations of people within the *campamento*, the hospital, or the leprosarium. The ecologists, veterinarians, sociologist, and microbiologist went outside the camp every day. They began their work well before the clinics and laboratories were complete, talking to the islanders, gathering specimens, and exploring the town and land. Freedom to wander meant that they enjoyed the best experiences of all (figure 7.1). The media men hovered at all times, trying to capture the essence of the mission and constantly getting in the way. From observations in homes and the store, at least one team member attempted to reconstruct the islanders' diet to compensate for the abrupt departure of the Chilean nutritionist. By the end, a more tolerant, if not amicable, peace prevailed as METEI prepared to leave.

ECOLOGISTS

Ian Efford and Jack Mathias interpreted their mandate in broad terms: study all flora and fauna and their uses. They were interested in energy flow, from the sun to plants to herbivores to carnivores, and how that might change. Easter Island's plant and animal community was "simple," like the Arctic tundra. Aware that many species had already been introduced, they tried to discover which ones and when. Prior to METEI's arrival, Efford had laid out a systematic approach to collecting plants and animals, but it had to be modified when he was confronted by the vast reality and short time.[1]

On day four, while the camp was still under construction, Efford went to the agricultural station near the sheep farm at Vaitea in the centre of the island. Mario Arévalo, who had chatted with Denys Montandon two

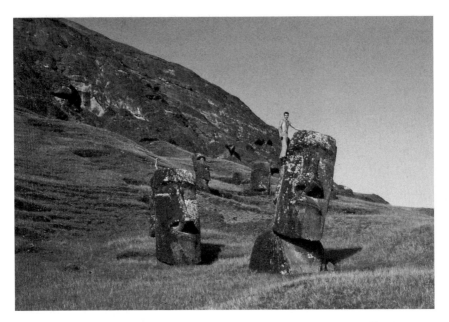

Figure 7.1 Jack Mathias atop a *moai* at Rano Raraku. Photo Ian Efford.

days earlier, gave him a lift in a Chilean jeep. Arévalo described grasses and plants imported from Australia and the fate of lemons that had flourished until 1963 when they were attacked by scale. From the station director, Karl Schantz, Efford learned that a number of other plants had been introduced, including eucalyptus, Chilean pine, and Tahitian yams. The experimental station grew crops of maize, mint, taro, and water-melon, whereas many other food and flowering plants, including coffee, were cultivated in the villagers' gardens. Schantz told him that the island had few good farmers because they were "lazy." Efford recorded all this information in his diary.[2] He also began a glossary of English, Spanish, Rapanui, and Latin names for the flora and fauna, including fish, birds, lizards, and insects. He and Jack had yet to finalize their plans for col-lecting, but for the next few days, they abandoned ecology to help set up the camp. They lobbied for a tarpaulin to create a shady space outside their trailer for handling the smelly animals, plants, and chemicals, espe-cially formaldehyde; at first, they were denied.

Two teenage boys – "Raúl and Geraldo" [Gerardo?] – adopted them and joined their searches with cheerful aplomb, eager to impart knowl-edge of the island and curious about the work (figures 7.2 and 7.3).[3] They were great swimmers and divers and, like all Rapanui children, excellent

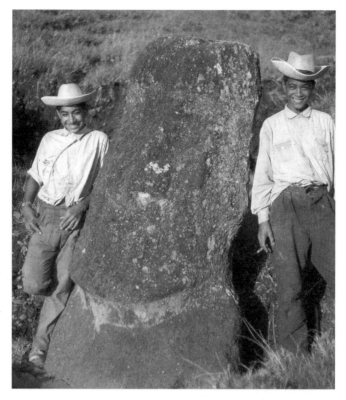

Figure 7.2 Boys who helped the ecologists. Raúl Pakarati (*left*) and Gerardo Manutomatoma Pate. Photo Ian Efford.

horseback riders. The boys were never allowed to dive alone, and Ian or Jack watched them closely from the surface. Some days the four made seventy deep dives or more. In retrospect, both Ian and Jack acknowledge how the boys' intrepid collecting skills and their ready friendship advanced their project and smoothed contacts with island families.

The ecologists' first task was to survey the island for its various "regions," aiming to collect representative samples from each. Back at camp, they dealt with the day's harvest. Plants were dried or pressed, insects were mounted, and animals were either preserved in formalin, frozen, or stuffed. The fumes and odour from organic material meant they had to work outside their trailer in the heat. The long-requested tarpaulin soon appeared, perhaps by popular demand. The shady area doubled as a METEI barbershop run by "a Scandinavian doctor" (Eivind Myhre?) in the adjoining cabin.[4]

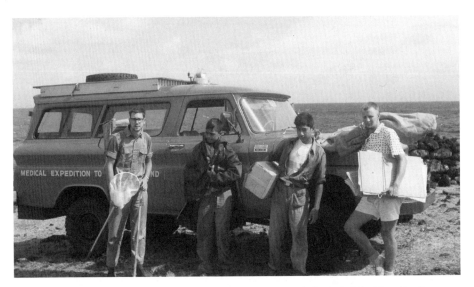

Figure 7.3 Ecology team with Jeep Mea Mea. *From left*, Jack Mathias, Raúl Pakarati, Gerardo Manutomatoma Pate, and Ian Efford. Photo David Murphy.

Efford and Mathias used two main methods for catching fish: spearing and poisoning with rotenone. But they had other strategies. As Efford's diary indicates, on 22 December 1964, they were 200 metres north of the camp and 10 to 15 metres offshore where the water was 3 to 5 metres deep; they recorded ten different species and a sea cucumber. The next day, at the same spot, they attempted a third method, setting up gill nets at right angles to the coastline; their count reached twenty-three fish species. But four days later, heavy wave action overnight twisted the gill nets into an awkward tangle.[5] Therefore, spearing and poisoning were the mainstays. Several tidal pools became favourite spots for collecting by poisoning; one they called "Ian's pool."[6]

Rapanui fishermen heard of their interest in aquatic life and began bringing presents of interesting creatures that turned up in their nets: a squid, an octopus, an eel, a large tuna. This fourth method allowed for proxy deep-sea collecting. Efford duly noted each offering in his diary. They also kept track of weather, temperature, and sightings of animals that could not be caught: a turtle and several sharks.[7] Whenever a shark appeared, collecting stopped. Once, Efford took refuge on a small rock for a long time. On another occasion, METEI doctors on horseback at Anakena Beach complimented the ecologists on daring to swim through a school of sharks; however, they had been oblivious to the danger. Efford

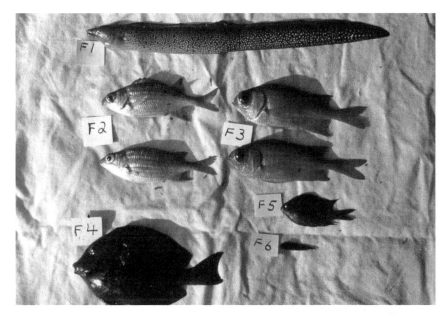

Figure 7.4 Rapanui fish. Photo Ian Efford.

noticed that Rapanui would spear fish and tie them to their waists, resulting in shark bites to their inner thighs.

In the evenings, they would set out the day's haul, organized by species, and photograph it with the Leica camera to preserve the glorious colour of the fresh specimens: blue, yellow, red, and silver (figure 7.4). Ian and Jack collected an octopus at Anakena on 21 January; the following morning, Cléopâtre Montandon was startled to find the defunct creature loitering in a bowl – an event that impressed Bob Meier enough for him to record it in his diary too.[8]

Around 1942, Chileans had introduced a small species of fish to keep down the mosquito population on the island. Called *sankua* in Spanish and *nao nao* in Rapanui, it had thrived but was considered too small to eat. Efford's informant, "Pappy," claimed that the mosquito population had declined, but, the ecologist wrote, "This needs confirmation!"[9] Father Sebastian Englert later supplied more information about this fish: the Chilean who had first brought it, in 1943 or 1944, was Germán Reigal from Valparaiso.[10] Others told Ian that a species of fish had been introduced into the crater lake in 1937 by Hugo Smith, which, Efford noted, was "different from the story of Father Sebastian."[11] The ecologist was discovering the challenges of doing history, even recent history.

Their work absorbed huge amounts of energy, as diving for a day in the cold water generated an enormous appetite. Ian remembers being hungry most of the time, although Jack does not. Nevertheless, Ian watched Jack devour a whole loaf of bread after a day spent gathering. Athlete Björn Ekblom was also hungry and lost weight. For Ian, the meals devised by McGill University's dietician were inadequate, obsessive, and boring – for example, 50 millilitres of orange juice per person per day, so much protein, so many carbohydrates, and so on – and he hated the food. The endless supply of pumpernickel was especially tedious. He remembers, "We tried to give it to the islanders by throwing it over the fence. They would throw it back."

If Ian and Jack were not collecting in the sea, they were roving over the landscape, climbing volcanoes, and descending into the craters, young helpers in tow. One memorable day was so hot that they stripped naked to work in a crater lake; nasty sunburns in unusual places added to their harvest. They had heard that one of the crater lakes was bottomless. To measure it, they brought 120 metres of rope and laughed to discover it was only 3.5 metres deep.[12]

This wide-ranging activity kept them away from Camp Hilton most of the time, and unlike some of the others, Efford does not recall much drinking in the camp for lack of alcohol. His activities on the land may have meant that he did not witness it. As HMCS *Cape Scott* left, however, they had each been given a large bottle of rum – navy rations. To make it last, Jack and Ian hid their bottles behind a row of books, laying them on their sides, one bottle atop the other. One day, Jack's hand slipped as he was replacing his bottle, which dropped, landed hard on the lower bottle, and shattered; the contents ran over the floor in a thick pool. To their horror, islanders rushed to lap it up, oblivious to the danger of broken glass.

From the beginning of their sojourn, Efford deplored the poor advanced planning. He had made lists of at least some of the known species. But with more time, a thorough search of the literature – especially the Chilean journals and reports – would have enhanced their understanding of what was already known about the flora and fauna. It also would have facilitated a more organized research plan and possibly also a reliable multilanguage dictionary. Nevertheless, like Noah with his ark, Ian and Jack did their best to gather one (or two) of everything.

An interesting challenge was posed by the plants – both cultivated and wild. One species of shrub, *Sophora toromiro* (toromiro tree), was native only to Easter Island but said to have been extinct since 1960, when the last known specimen was felled for statuettes. A few individual plants survived in Australia, and seeds, preserved by Thor Heyerdahl, were used to propagate it in botanical gardens.[13] Ian was pleased to learn from Karl Schantz that an old specimen was still growing in a Rano Kao crater and that the plant was being reintroduced at the agricultural station. The station also had a specimen of *Sophora tetraptera* (Miro Tahiti), a native of New Zealand. In the garden of islander Juan Chavez, who worked for the Chilean navy, could be found abundant coffee plants.

For their botanical work, Efford and Mathias designated four representative areas: near Hanga Roa village, at Poike headland, on the central plain near the Vaitea sheep farm, and at Motu Nui islet. They would mark off a space of 50 by 50 metres, subdivide it into plots of 0.25 by 0.25 metre, and at a certain time, gather all the contents from thirty randomly selected plots. (They had reduced the plan from an original five areas, each 100 by 100 metres, and fifty selected plots.)[14] Bob Williams's film for the Canadian Broadcasting Corporation (CBC) devoted several minutes to this botanical harvesting. Efford carefully recorded the details of the terrain and made a diagram. Plants were pulled up with their roots, stuffed into bags, and carried back to camp for processing. The number of representatives of each species was estimated and the whole plant weighed; then they determined the separate weight of various parts – roots, stems, leaves, and dead material – and they pressed the leaves. Ian was not an expert in botany. He planned to send these vegetal trophies to Harvard University.

Many other projects were part of the original, ambitious plan. Two plots of 5 by 5 metres were to be protected by fencing from sheep and other animals and examined every two weeks. The soil was to be studied too by chemical treatment, searching for microscopic soil animals. The ecologists specified how they would collect, treat, dessicate, preserve, and freeze the substrate to be taken back to Vancouver, where they would look for microarthropods. To analyze creatures that facilitated decay, twenty ground-meat samples were set out in the protected plots and inspected after one, two, and four days and, thereafter, every four days for a month.

Efford examined all the crops, those that had been introduced and those that appeared to be native. He kept track of the islanders' opinion of their value as food: corn, bananas, pineapples, peaches, lettuce, watermelons, and yams. To compensate for the extensive deforestation, alien trees had been introduced: eucalyptus, palm, bamboo, acacia, cypress, and the Miro Tahiti. Citrus trees grew on the island, but the oranges had borne no fruit for three years, and the once-thriving lemons had been attacked by parasites. A small avocado, *palto*, and a little fruit, *guyaba*, a kind of guava, were both new to him, and he had to rely on the islanders' opinions about

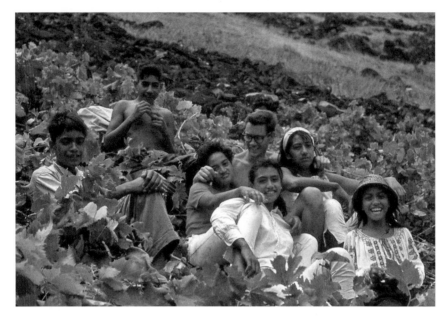

Figure 7.5 Jack Mathias with ecology helpers and family. From left, Raúl Pakarati, Gerardo Manutomatoma Pate, his sister Maria Soccoro, and their three cousins. Photo Ian Efford.

whether or not they were of typical size: a three-inch *pepino dulce* (melon pear) that he judged "large" was deemed "small" by Gerardo's older sister, Maria Soccoro (figure 7.5).[15]

The islanders brought him lizards and insects. Lizards lived inside the houses, and Rapanui were used to seeing their eggs. A man named Luis brought the team its first house lizard on 29 December. Efford described it in detail and noted its Rapanui name, "moco uru uru kahu." He kept it alive for ten days and then preserved it in formalin.[16] They also collected "field lizards," many brought in "by kids," but some were picked up by Jack or Ian on their rambles. They noted whether or not the animals had tails. On the morning of 5 January, Geraldo showed up with thirteen lizards, which he said he had caught in his house the night before.[17]

Several complained that METEI had no person assigned to handle entomology, although Ian Efford had actually been trained in the field. With their mission of documenting all the flora and fauna, Ian and Jack did the best they could. On 22 January, while plucking snails from under the leaves of young Miro Tahiti plants, they noted their relationship to aphids. Cockroaches, spiders, and beetles were abundant, and they gathered these too. Night-lights were set out to catch nocturnal flying insects. Bees had been introduced by the mayor, Juan Atán, in 1948 to satisfy the islanders fondness for sugar. At least three islanders kept hives, including Alfonso Rapu, who owned sixteen.[18] Father Ricardo Rainer explained that bed bugs had come to Rapa Nui on mattresses from Chile, but they were all killed and did not reappear.[19] No one appeared to have lice, but Hal Gibbs confirmed that 23 per cent of the children had pinworms.[20] Assassin bugs (Reduviidae) were unknown.

As for birds – hawks, sparrows, and partridges – they were shot or killed with stones and taken back to the camp to be stuffed or frozen in separate plastic bags.[21] Jack and Ian spotted hawks at the farm on 7 January. On the evening of 21 January, they watched eighteen hawks behind Mataveri. From the killed specimens, they took blood samples for Hal Gibbs to study. Mites found on a sparrow were put in a vial, also for Gibbs. The stomach contents of the preserved birds would be analyzed in Canada.

Both priests provided information about introduced animal species. Father Riccardo liked to supply specimens, particularly a fish called *conso* or *bakalao* (cod), the famous oil of which, he said, was a potent laxative.[22] Father Sebastian had been responsible for the introduction of doves in 1957, as well as some fish and plants. Carlos Rapu, brother of Alfonso, confirmed that most of the priest's doves had died but said that some had escaped and continued to live at Hanga Piko.[23]

Efford's plans included an estimate for the numbers of rats and cats on the island. On 30 December, twenty-two-year-old Jorge Pate Tuki brought him three rats and a scorpion caught that afternoon under his house. The ecologist injected the rats with formalin in the stomach and neck, and he preserved the scorpion in alcohol.[24]

Other METEI members enjoyed helping Ian and Jack by gathering odd plants and animals or by joining them for a day of exploring. On 26 December, Cléopâtre brought four plants that the islanders claimed had medicinal properties: *llerba luisa*, *puringa*, *siete vena*, and *numera*.[25] Later they received other plants purported by islanders to have unspecified healing properties: *tiapito* and *matiko* (found in the village on 4 February).[26] Possibly relying on the ecologists' findings, Helen Reid also kept a list of twenty medicinal plants and their uses.[27] John Easton provided two blue fish that he'd caught off Motu Nui on 3 January, and Jim Nielsen, who had been out with island fishermen, brought in a large tuna on 5 February. On Christmas day, Garry Brody speared a black fish off Hanga Piko. Even the austere Dr Richard Roberts remembered the ecologists while making rounds at the leprosarium and delivered a sample of a spiny plant on 23 January.[28]

Above all, Peter Beighton became a loyal helper and friend; he loved
to go out with Ian and Jack. They admired his social skills and easy
friendship with the islanders; "Beighton's corner" was a regular land-
mark in their diary. Peter remembers an exhilarating trip to Motu Nui
islet in order to look for birds and eggs. Adept with a spear, he impaled
a trigger fish on Christmas Day and both a puffer fish and a blue fish
in early January. Peter also observed fish behaviour, which Efford duly
recorded: "a pair that appeared to be courting. One fish would appear to
be picking material from the other's back and sides."[29]

Sea urchins, sponges, barnacles, and coral were scooped up and
bagged. They noted crustaceans, lobsters, and crabs, describing their
habitat and culinary qualities. But because it was impossible to collect
every animal and plant in the intertidal area, Ian and Jack concentrated
on fish. From study of the currents, climate, and their growing collection, they expected that analysis would "show that almost all the species
migrated along the chain of Pacific islands to Easter Island and few, if
any, came from South America."[30]

The ecologists believed that they had expanded, if not doubled, the
number of species known on the island, and they commented on the
origins. For example, of the fifty-three species of plants eaten as leaves,
roots, or fruits, probably forty to forty-five had been introduced by visitors since 1800. Similarly, of the seven species of terrestrial birds found,
only one had been present before 1800: the chicken. Most species of
insects had been introduced, but they were chance occurrences and not
intentional introductions.[31]

By the time METEI was ready to go back to Canada, the ecologists had
made a list of the extensive collections that would accompany them:

1 200 soil samples for invertebrate study: 120 from the research
   areas; 80 from crops.
2 whole plants from the four research areas.
3 plant collection of more than 250 species.
4 insects and terrestrial invertebrates: 150 mounted insects; many
   others in alcohol.
5 approximately 40 birds and 30 lizards.
6 approximately 2,500 fish.
7 marine algae.
8 intertidal invertebrates.
9 molluscs of the genus *Conus*.
10 zooplankton, phytoplankton, mud-dwelling organisms, and core
   samples from a crater lake.[32]

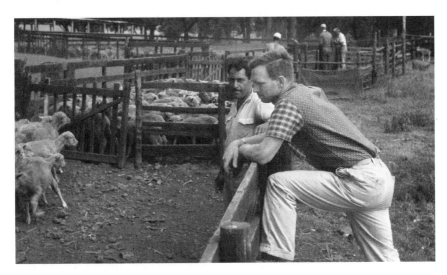

Figure 7.6 David Murphy (*right*) inspecting Rapanui sheep.
Photo David Murphy.

Efford estimated that publication would take a year, but he was already planning to return with a team of biologists to fill in the gaps that would emerge in the analysis. The next trip would not be for assessing the effects of the airport but simply to complete METEI-1.

VETERINARIANS

Although they were both homesick and worrying about their young families, David Murphy and Hal Gibbs enjoyed their task of animal examination, which took them out on the land every day. The two farms – the sheep ranch at Vaitea and the governor's farm at Mataveri – absorbed their attention. The local farmworkers readily volunteered information and helped to examine the livestock. Big, friendly Carlos Teao Ika went along with them every day as a guide and interpreter, but no one now can remember how (or if) he was paid. Their main objective was to determine the health status of the domestic animals and to document diseases. In particular, they wanted to find out if the cows had tuberculosis or brucellosis, and Gibbs was especially interested in diseases of sheep. "Where you have sheep, you have parasites," he told me fifty years later, and parasitology was his field of expertise.

The island had 40,000 sheep, 2,500 cattle, 1,500 horses, and 300 pigs. Most families had eight to ten cattle in the common pasture, but only one

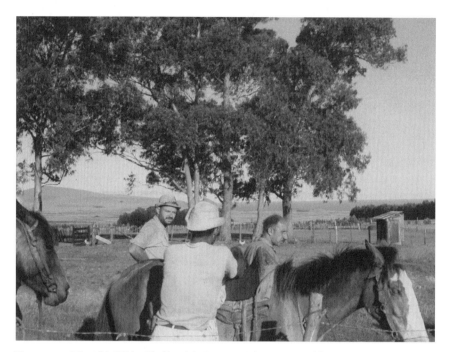

Figure 7.7 Harold Gibbs (*left*) with Rapanui farmers and horses.
Photo David Murphy.

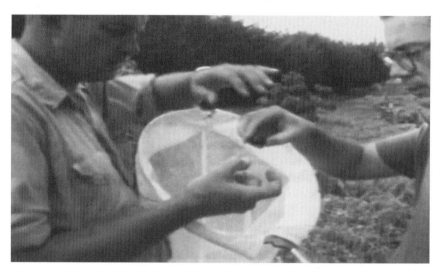

Figure 7.8 Harold Gibbs (*left*) and Armand Boudreault with interesting speci-
men from insect net. Film still from CBC, Williams. and Hrischenko, *Canadian
Expedition to Easter Island*, part 2, at 20 mins, 30 secs, with thanks to Janice
Belanger.

family in eight had a milk cow. The veterinarians tested 201 cows in the common pasture for tuberculosis by injecting tuberculin in the upper tail and returning three days later to read the result: swelling above a certain size indicated exposure (similar to a human TB skin test). They also gathered fecal material to be examined for parasites. Blood samples were taken from the jugular veins of fifty-seven cattle. With Georges Nógrády and his bacteriology lab immediately available, they took milk samples from fifteen cows under sterile conditions and cultured them in the petrie dishes prepared by Carlotta Hacker. Nógrády found that nine (60 per cent) were positive for the staphylococcus germ. The finding raised the possibility that milk products might be a source of the frequent stomach upsets and diarrhea in children, but attempting a direct correlation between the two observations was beyond the capabilities of the mission.

The thousands of sheep on the island were of the Merino breed, originally imported from Australia (figure 7.6). In Williams's CBC film, the veterinarians explain that there are 220 families on the island and that a hundred sheep are slaughtered once or twice weekly at the governor's farm, suggesting one animal per family per week (a figure that appears in the literature). They collected 150 blood samples from sheep when the animals were slaughtered at the weekly cull. Gibbs also collected some intestinal tracts, extracting and preserving the contents for later inspection. Thirteen blood samples were taken from pigs at slaughter, and they gathered samples from chickens, horses, and rats "on a limited basis."

One of the most productive aspects of their work came from "numerous trips" to the two farms, where they observed the animals and the farming practices (figure 7.7). In this way, "approximately 400 cows, 1,000 sheep and 500 horses were seen at close quarters." They had the impression that the agricultural methods were "good" and that the animals were generally healthy, with reasonable preventive measures being taken against disease; however, they wondered if the findings would have been different had they conducted their study during the rainy season, when, the ranch manager told them, pneumonia was "a very common problem."[33] In spare moments, Gibbs collected insects with the net he had been given in Montreal (figure 7.8).

David Murphy is modest about his role. "I was peripheral to the whole expedition," he now says. "The beauty of the job" was that they went out on the land every day – and could avoid the "cloying cliques" coalescing inside the camp. He contends that Gibbs, with credentials in research and parasitology, was "the bigger contributor."

Hal, too, is modest. But he worked hard. After long days chasing farm animals, he spent evenings with the monocular microscope in the Camp

Hilton lab, looking for pinworms on the patches of transparent tape that had been applied to the anuses of the human islanders under age fifteen. He also prepared the animal-blood samples by allowing them to clot for about twelve hours before separating the serum and freezing it at −70° Celsius for transport and testing in Canada. The stool specimens that METEI doctors requested from every human islander were also sent his way, although only 206 individuals from fifty-one families complied. Gibbs took a "pea-sized sample" from each specimen and preserved it in formalin for later analysis. Other scientists, including Ian Efford and Jack Mathias, consulted him about parasites and mites that they found on their wild creatures, and he often chatted with Nógrády. Hal got on well with Armand Boudreault and Archie Wilkinson, who shared a room in the next trailer. Fred Joyce also became a good friend.

THE MEDIA MEN

Murphy and Gibbs's trailer was next door to Fred Joyce, who roomed with Red Lemieux, the documentary filmmaker preparing a movie for the National Film Board (NFB). Murphy remembers Lemieux as "an obsessive kind of guy" and "fussy," always needing to have clean laundry and wearing shirts and trousers "in the best knick" – a tall order under the conditions. Others said he was "prickly." Red would tease Murphy and others: "If you aren't nice to me, I won't take your picture." It provoked some surprise a half-century later when the vets watched the resultant NFB film and saw their youthful selves exuberantly testing cows. Everyone was convinced that Cléopâtre Montandon had been deliberately left out of Red's film. Separated from his wife and children in Canada, Red had a girlfriend in New York City; however, on Rapa Nui, he was pursuing Carlotta Hacker, and she was drawn to his charisma and talent.

Bob Williams, filming for CBC, was supposed to share a room with the radio man, George Hrischenko, since they had the same employer. But in the end, Hrischenko shared with Colin Gillingham, the young cook, and Williams had another cabin-mate. METEI alumni remember that Williams was quiet and kept mostly to himself; yet he shot movie footage almost every day. His images of the medical examinations are described in chapter 5. But he also covered the ecological, veterinary, and sociological projects in careful detail, making the film one of the best sources on METEI because he invited the scientists to explain their work in person while George Hrischenko recorded their voices (figure 7.9).

With his brutal experiences in the Second World War and the Korean War, Carl Mydans had seen and documented dire hardship and disaster.

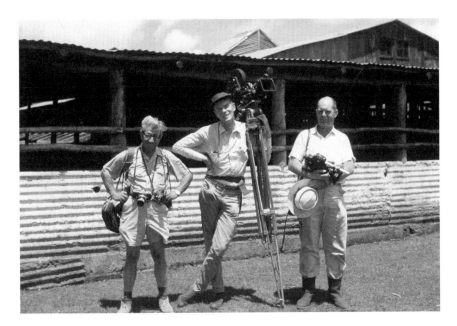

Figure 7.9 Photojournalists. *From left*, Carl Mydans of *Life*, Red Lemieux of the National Film Board, and Robert Williams of the Canadian Broadcasting Corporation. George Hrischenko is missing. Photo David Murphy.

Twenty years later, the jaunt to Easter Island was an easy gig for him. He had no patience for the members who complained about arrangements, food, or weather. At any given moment, he had three or more cameras slung around his neck and was constantly shooting pictures. Beyond the annoyance of his intrusive lens, Mydans's superiority and officious manner irritated the women expeditionists; being Scottish, English, Spanish, Greek Swiss, and Canadian, they ascribed it to his American nationality. Bob Meier witnessed an exciting moment, during *Aquila*'s visit, when Mydans slipped into the sea with three cameras.[34] Nothing daunted after his rescue, he reached into his bag and pulled out another camera. He enjoyed star status around the camp, and everyone wondered what his photographs would be like.

According to the plan, Mydans was to share a cabin with Nógrády (see appendix D, table D.3). But the photographer did not like the Hungarian microbiologist and did nothing to disguise his animus. Nógrády's obsessive preparations, the flights of fancy, the childlike enthusiasms, and the many, many hats made Georges an easy mark for Mydans's jokes. The fact that Nógrády, like so many other travellers, was taking hundreds

of photographs and making his own movie might also have annoyed
the accomplished professional. Nógrády's "adopted niece," who travelled with him often in later years, admits that he was a challenging
roommate: he snored loudly; the colossal collection of paraphernalia,
clothing, maps, books, and boxes took up space; and he had a habit of
leaping up in the middle of night to write down new ideas, increasingly
oblivious to the disturbance because of advancing deafness. I am unable
to confirm whether or not Mydans and Nógrády shared accommoda-
tions; it could be that the famous photographer and the quirky microbiologist were separated.

SOCIOLOGICAL SURVEY

Cléopâtre Montandon looks directly into Bob Williams's lens and says
that "the temptation was great to try to undertake a general study of the
Easter Island society"; however, the brief time and resources dictated a
need to focus, "restricting the study to a limited number of problems"
or "in sociological jargon, to a few hypotheses to be tested." A questionnaire was developed, "the answers to which [would] be evaluated statistically later on." In delicately accented English, she outlines two major
interests: first, to determine if the influence of "Western values" had
changed the previously documented "cooperation concepts into more
competitive ones"; and second, to assess the effects of recent population
growth on "organization, social control, education principles, desire for
children, and means of healthcare." The questions were simple in order
to encourage replies.

In a voiceover of scenes showing her smiling visits with men and
women seated outside in gardens or on doorsteps, Cléopâtre explains
that her goal is to visit every home, speaking with mothers and fathers.
She hopes for interviews with at least 80 per cent of the adult population (figure 7.10). The reaction of the islanders to her questions was
"extremely favourable." A preliminary impression was their wide acceptance of "Western medical care," although traditional practices continued in the use of certain plants and in the beliefs about causes of
disease, which were still "full of superstitious elements." Desire to leave
the island was "extremely high," although most "wish to come back and
not emigrate permanently."

Cléopâtre's questionnaire and her method of visiting islanders in their
homes and at work made her a unique member of METEI. Her increasingly obvious pregnancy also contributed to her special status with
Rapanui mothers. She asked questions about dreams, which amused

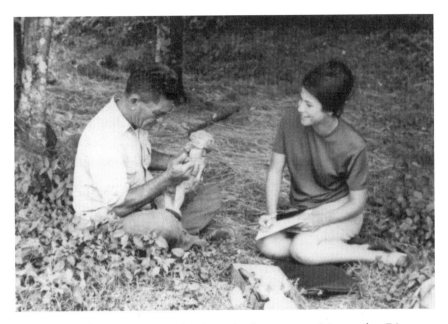

Figure 7.10 Cléopâtre Montandon interviewing a carver. Montandon Diary.

the islanders, and "Móe-v[b]arúa" (Dream) became her nickname. Her husband, Denys, also developed personal connections as he took the medical "histories," chatting with people in Spanish about their past illnesses and those of their children. Because he was so tall, the islanders nicknamed him "Poike," for their highest mountain.[35]

Possibly more than other METEI members realized, the Montandons were appreciated and included in private events; they knew the people and liked them. On the first Sunday, when they tried unsuccessfully to rent horses for an extortionist "price," two nursing aides at the hospital, "Señor Farfan" and "Niaruel," provided mounts at no cost and one of their sons as a guide.[36] Like Jim Nielsen, they were never without transportation when they had free time to explore. As they rode off on their Sunday adventures, they passed the churchgoers in their bright clothing, who waved gaily and wished them a good day.[37] Unlike many of the METEI team, Cléopâtre was an experienced rider and in spite of her "grossesse" could not resist a few gallops, earning yet more disapprobation (or envy) from her colleagues.[38] Out exploring, they encountered drenching rain, pounding heat, and kindly islanders. One day their young guide, thirteen-year-old Ana Teao, who had been desperate to accompany them, was thrown against the rocks, dislocating her elbow; surgeon Denys repaired it on the spot.[39]

Cléopâtre thought that their METEI "jobs" – conversing in a relaxed, open way – put them at a great advantage, and hers was the best task of all. She wrote in her diary,

> Sometimes I got tired of asking the same questions over and over, but I had only to stumble upon a person of great character to recover the pleasure of interesting conversation and the possibility of a discovery. I was perhaps a bit luckier than Denys because I could leave the camp to visit people in their homes. To see men pulling their boats, or children galloping on the village streets, that was all it took to reconsider things in human scale – to appreciate the importance of a gesture or a word – and to marvel that there can be tedious work in offices and factories, nuclear weapons, and racial prejudice.[40]

In the end, she had answers to her questionnaire from 206 people, 106 men, and 100 women (figure 7.11).[41]

At some point, possibly on the return voyage, Helen Reid, who had been so skeptical of Cléopâtre's youth and inexperience – not to mention the concealed pregnancy – interviewed her for the *Maclean's* magazine article. The pediatrician did not record an alteration in her opinion, but her notes seem approving of Cléopâtre's sociology work and that the questionnaire had been pilot-tested on twenty families before being employed, so far, with 145 households. Cléopâtre gave Helen information on the desire to emigrate and on attitudes to divorce, work, property, and the promised airport.[42] She also confirmed Rapanui notions, which Helen herself had explored, about causes and treatment of disease. If they had collaborated, they might have uncovered more about nutrition and living standards relevant to child health (see below).

Toward the end of the METEI sojourn, Governor Jorge Portilla asked that METEI examine the population of approximately 140 Chileans. This project had not been part of the plan, based on the erroneous proposition that the native islanders were inbred as well as isolated. Furthermore, the Chileans were transient in a way that the Rapanui were not. Being free to leave, the continentals would not be "at risk" of changes in their health status with the opening of the airport. Possibly, the Chilean citizens resented all the attention given to the "native" islanders. METEI had received good cooperation from the Chilean authorities, and the absence of a doctor on the island had affected everyone equally. Stanley Skoryna agreed to the request and assigned Denys Montandon to the task. The other METEI doctors were now more capable in Spanish than they had been – they could take the Rapanui histories; also, there were too many

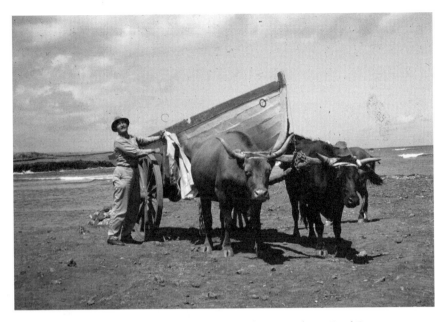

Figure 7.11 Rapanui man moving a boat with oxen. Photo Fred Joyce.

doctors in the clinic. The Chilean examinations would take place at the Hanga Roa Hospital, and Cléopâtre would help.

This unforeseen addition to the project went well. Cléopâtre wondered if the governor had come up with the idea to make himself more popular or if the people had pressured him, knowing that METEI was soon to leave, taking all the doctors along with it. The pair saw roughly the same number of people every day as the METEI team – between twenty and thirty – but the work went quickly and efficiently. Cléopâtre viewed their success in light of the optimum number of examiners needed to perform tasks, noting that at Camp Hilton this number was exceeded.[43] They tested blood for hemoglobin, and they tested urine for protein, sugar, and pH. They sent a few select cases for X-rays, but they did not perform the ancillary tests on saliva, feces, and teeth. They completed 126 examinations, leaving the charts at the island infirmary, although they took copies home.[44] In this work, Cléopâtre lost a week from her sociological study and felt guilty about it, although she reasoned that the results would scarcely have differed if she had reached Skoryna's 100 per cent instead of the final 80 per cent.[45]

This special contact with the Chilean population and their mastery of Spanish served as an entrée. Caught in the rain on one of their riding adventures, Denys and Cléopâtre were invited to wait out the storm at the home of Rodríguez, who had been directing the Vaitea sheep farm for five years. The young couple enjoyed a splendid meal and conversation, leaving with admiration for the man and his family and greater insight into the complexities of the colonial problems.[46] Remembered fondly by many, Rodríguez had a girlfriend in town and a jeep that only ran backwards; METEI members often heard him putting along, in reverse, to his evening tryst.

NUTRITIONAL STUDY

METEI keenly felt the sudden departure of Dr Gonzalo Donoso. Not only was he the sole representative of the Chilean cooperation specified in the agreements, but he was also an expert in nutrition, which was an essential ingredient for complete analysis of many other studies. For example, Björn Ekblom and Einar Gjessing wondered if the lesser fitness of the islanders, when compared to Scandinavians, was genetic, climatic, psychological, or nutritional. All the medical, dental, and physical anthropology measurements related to nutritional status too. Similarly, the small size of the children could be owing to nature or nurture – and without a reliable indicator of the nutritional value in the daily diet, the scientists would be unable to decide which factor was more important. Finally, nutrition was likely to alter dramatically with the famous "end to isolation," bringing with it more salt, fat, sugar, additives, and the so-called "diseases of civilization": high blood pressure, diabetes, heart disease, stroke, and cancer. Therefore, documenting baseline nutrition before the advent of the airport was of vital importance.

METEI had to find ways to compensate for Donoso's disappearance. The first idea entailed a questionnaire. While the medical history was being taken, Denys could ask what the family ate during the preceding twenty-four hours. Similarly, epidemiologist John Cutler, who was visiting homes as he updated the census, could inquire about diet – or ask to see supplies on the shelves. But the islanders quickly learned the "right" answers to these questions: they claimed to have breakfasted on rashers, eggs, and toast, washed down with orange juice and coffee. All these items, but eggs, were unavailable. Helen Reid paid close attention to the milk and bread offered at school and worried over the truth of the nuns' story that many children received no evening meal. She talked to islanders, like carver Juan Atán and Father Ricardo, who told her that the people did not eat fish once a week, as many claimed; once a month was more likely. They fished only a few months of the year, and their

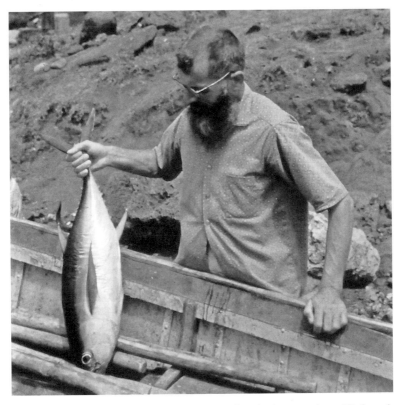

Figure 7.12 Father Ricardo Rainer, priest for the leprosarium. He loved to fish. Photo Georges Nógrády.

methods were poor. Father Ricardo would have enjoyed reorganizing their procedures for fishing (figure 7.12).[47]

METEI was never able to determine the exact quantity or frequency of the distribution of mutton and lamb, although estimates suggested roughly one animal per family per week. But among the islanders' complaints was the contention that the best animals were sent away or reserved for Chileans and that the islanders were given the weaklings.[48] Did every family receive a ration of meat on all of those days, or was it in rotation – perhaps weekly, monthly, or as needed? Beef and pork were rare delicacies for a lucky few, although everyone seemed to have chickens.

Some fruits and root vegetables grew readily, but cereal crops were nonexistent; consequently, rice and flour were among the staples that came with the annual supply ship when it remembered to appear. The ship supplied a store at discount prices: the Empresa de Comercio Agrícola (ECA). Long interested in nutrition, Reid first visited and described the ECA on 7 January. A large grey building located about a kilometre inland and uphill from Hanga Piko, it was being painted white and pink in preparation for the arrival of the supply ship *Aquila*.[49] Later she witnessed Carl Mydans's interview with the governor, who was "open" yet "evasive" about the store; he seemed anxious, stuttering with a "left facial tic" from a "masseter [muscle] twitch." The store operated on cash only or on credit against future work on the island; fifteen poor families did not pay.[50] Helen went up and down the ECA shelves examining the packages and copying the nutritive contents of items that revealed them. Mostly, however, its shelves were empty. Then, in February, she got an idea. She obtained the list of all the supplies and their quantities requested or brought by the supply ship when it last came to Rapa Nui in November 1963 with provisions for the entire year of 1964. The typewritten list was in Spanish and in alphabetical order.[51] She copied it in its entirety by hand, from *aceite comestible* (cooking oil) and *broches presien* (dome fasteners) to *marmelade damascus* (plum jam) and *zoquelles portalampanas* (stands for portable lamps). Then she set about translating the words and identifying representative foods to indicate quantities that had been consumed by the entire population of roughly a thousand people over the year. The assumption was justified by the empty shelves, which proclaimed complete consumption. How much flour per person? How much sugar? In passing, she noticed that a three-year supply of toothpaste consisted of 3,980 tubes, which she calculated to be an average of 1.4 tubes per person per year, but when children under three were eliminated it was 1.6 tubes per year; eliminating children up to age four translated into 1.72 tubes per year, which was still not enough.[52] The islanders might be blamed for not brushing their teeth, but what if they had no toothpaste?

Richard Roberts decided that Helen Reid's interest in nutrition was a waste of time. He dismissed it with a blunt statement in his shipboard preliminary report: "We found no evidence of malnutrition or avitaminosis."[53] Later he went further, snubbing Reid and claiming that the only dietary information of value came from the epidemiologists and the sociologist. He admitted that the planned nutritional study had been abandoned and that "there was controversy in our group" over quantities. In any case, he wrote, "there were excellent fish in the sea for the catching if the people had the energy to fish and the skill to get through the surf."[54]

TILTING AT MICROBES

Microbiologist and physician Georges Nógrády had been at the centre of the METEI planning since its inception; all agreed that, more than anyone else, "he had done his homework" in background reading and advance preparation for his scientific work. He wanted to document all the microbes on the island, for he believed that this aspect of the Rapa Nui biosphere was at the greatest risk of altering rapidly and dangerously with the end of isolation. He worked closely with Armand Boudreault, who was also affiliated with the Université de Montreal. They would share their results – Boudreault on viruses, Nógrády on bacteria, and both on immune status as revealed by serological studies on the blood samples.

Virologist Armand Boudreault came from a large family in the small town of Mont-Laurier in the Laurentian Mountains of Quebec. Educated at Université Laval and the Université de Montréal, he was an expert in vaccines, working with the distinguished physician-scientist Armand Frappier. Boudreault was the only French Canadian on the METEI team, and certain "diplomatic" expectations fell to him in communicating with the francophone media back in Canada or on behalf of METEI and the Canadian navy elsewhere. Erudite, quiet, and a lover of music, art, history, and culture, he had left behind his wife and five children. He largely kept to himself on the island but enjoyed philosophical conversations, made no secret of his nationalist sympathies, and welcomed the opportunity to meet the French sailors. Recruited to METEI early with a view to finding the viral cause of the *kokongo* mystery, he was also making a study on the other known viruses that afflicted the island. This work not only kept him in the camp but also kept him long hours in the laboratory trailer with Fred Joyce and their Rapanui helpers; Reid classified him as a dedicated worker.[55] He would not find the cause of *kokongo*, but later he identified a different, serious vulnerability and solved it (see chapter 11).

Georges was interested in the microbes that dwelt on humans and animals – whether or not they caused illness. To that end, he spent nights reading smears and plating cultures of the specimens taken both from people – sputum, urine, feces, hair, and the occasional pockets of pus produced by wounds – and from animals, including their excretions, hides, and milk (figures 7.13 and 7.14). Hal Gibbs's work on parasites was related. Georges made a detailed study of the flora inside Rapanui noses to look for active leprosy, and he performed special stains on sputum, looking for tuberculosis.

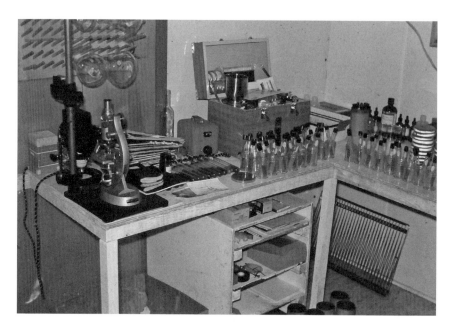

Figure 7.13 METEI laboratory. Photo Georges Nógrády.

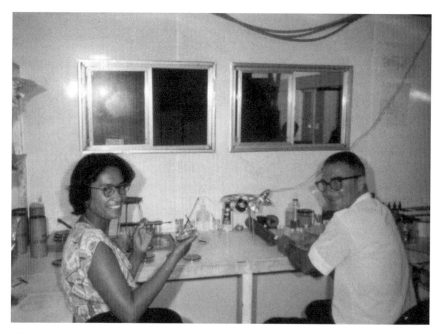

Figure 7.14 Margarita ("Uka") Tepano Kaituoe and Georges Nógrády in the METEI lab. Photo Peter Beighton.

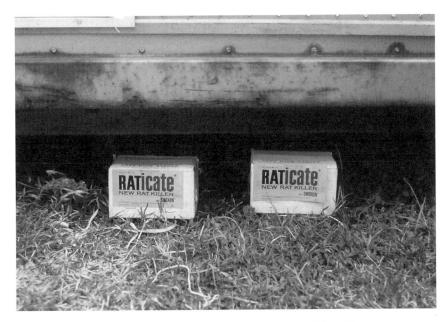

Figure 7.15 Rat killer at Camp Hilton. Photo Georges Nógrády.

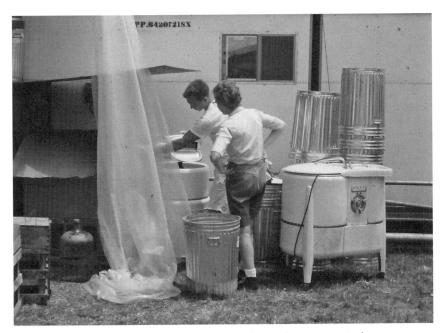

Figure 7.16 Laundry area with David Murphy and Maureen Roberts. Photo Georges Nógrády.

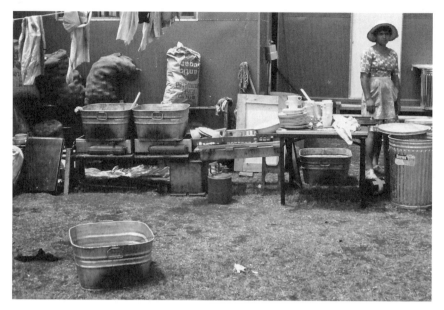

Figure 7.17 Dishwashing and food preparation with unidentified Rapanui helper. Photo Georges Nógrády.

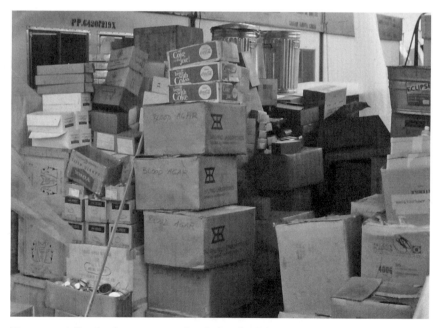

Figure 7.18 Stash of METEI supplies behind a laboratory trailer. Photo Georges Nógrády.

But Nógrády also wanted to know the identity of the organisms living in the air, soil, and waters, including crater lakes, cisterns, caves, wells, and the sea. He waged a collection campaign that covered the entire island. Obtaining a large map from the governor, he divided it into sixty-four plots of 2.6 by 2.6 kilometres and identified the exact centre by longitude and latitude.[56] From these precise spots, he would take samples and bring them to the METEI lab for initial analysis and then preparation for return to Canada. Aware of the potential for useful products coming from microorganisms, Georges also wanted to investigate caves. Stanley Skoryna had assigned epidemiologist Elliot Alpert to collect water from the cisterns used for drinking, cooking, and washing, and he passed these samples along to Georges. The CBC film shows him diligently doing so.

Like his US public health colleague, Cutler, Alpert was a member of the cynical, hard-drinking, hard-partying "Group" identified by Reid and Hacker. The Group made fun of Georges, notably his intensity, his Hungarian accent, his solemn reverence for the project, his fanatical enthusiasms, and his nearly constant grin, and they did not like him. Others were more amused than put off by his odd ways. Carlotta believed that he was the only METEI member who had missed the political upheaval, the 8 January "riot," and the election four days later.[57] The Montandons noted that he was also the only one who had failed to attend Father Sebastian's edifying lecture; Reid placed him squarely in her "oblivious" cohort of benign innocents who agreed with all sides of the personal and political strife.[58] Efford remembers him more as a devoted, eclectic "collector" than as a scientist or experimentalist. Of all the photographers, Georges Nógrády alone documented the mundane messiness of garbage, rat poison, and chaos in the *campamento* (figures 7.15, 7.16, 7.17, and 7.18).

Cléopâtre and Denys got to know Georges on *Cape Scott* when they visited his cabin. In his extensive preparations, Georges had packed attire for every occasion, including pith helmets, safari suits, jackets with dozens of pockets, and rain slickers, and he had brought mountains of equipment, from magnifying glasses, compasses, and cameras (movie and still) to sleeping bags, mosquito nets, sticking plasters, provisions for three days' survival, and a life jacket that he had designed himself. "But he is much more than all this," Cléopâtre wrote in her diary. His knowledge of history, his wartime experiences back in Hungary, his impeccable research qualifications, and his extensive knowledge from reading about Easter Island made him a remarkably "complete personality" with a special "cachet."[59] But not everyone appreciated these traits. His lengthy, illustrated talk on the ship about the geophysical properties of Easter Island had bored sailors and scientists alike.

On Rapa Nui, the Montandons sometimes explored caves with Georges. He spent many nights sleeping rough in the hills to save time and bring him closer to the targeted destinations, which is how he missed the Rapu rebellion. Back in the lab, he was grateful for the help of Carlotta Hacker and Margarita Tepano, a Rapanui seconded from the local infirmary who understood well the sterile procedures needed to make reliable stains and cultures. He also co-opted the willing adolescent girls and Jorge Ika Pakarati, respectfully keeping track of their names. He delighted in teaching young folk about the science behind their work, drawing diagrams of cell cycles and chemical equations. Hacker had been subjected to his quirky lessons on *Cape Scott*.[60] Traces of this passion for teaching remain at the library of the Université de Montreal: a 1964 annotated bibliography of films suitable for use in undergraduate education; course syllabi with detailed, engaging, and up-to-date information about microbiology; short films, which he made himself, depicting cells shrivelling under the lethal effects of the bacterial products streptomycin and staphylococcal toxin.[61] Georges loved science, he loved adventure, and he loved Rapa Nui and its people.

Like the Montandons, Reid and Hacker also appreciated Georges and wrote tender descriptions of his antics. A strong man in his mid-forties, he was in constant motion. Efford and Mathias would bring an interesting fish into camp. Georges would jump up from his lab bench, grab a camera, rush outside to examine and photograph it, and return – all in a matter of seconds. Every day before lunch, he would go for a vigorous swim, on his way bouncing a beach ball, which he would toss without warning at anyone nearby, an invitation to sport. His "wide, very sweet smile" was "as permanent a fixture on his face as his nose."[62] Georges did most of his exploring on horseback, "and the manner of his going was wonderful to behold." He refused to use reins or stirrups, although he and the horse were both "slung with gear." Under a burning sun, "he would appear in a dun-coloured version of the headgear of the French Foreign Legion, trailing a white handkerchief to protect his neck." When rain threatened, he wore "an immense cape that covered him and obscured the horse" and featured "a rubber hood with a face hole reminiscent of a Balaclava helmet." His entourage included small boys, equally laden, and sometimes an entire family on foot bearing more equipment and serving as guides.[63] Both Hacker and Reid described the occasion when Carlotta and Skoryna joined this grand procession, trudging ahead or behind Georges, who was astride his burdened horse and oblivious to its struggles as he pored over a map. The load was "so heavy that the poor beast could stand only by bracing his knees together,

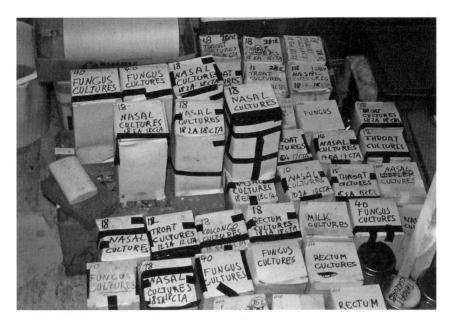

Figure 7.19 Laboratory samples packed for Canada. Photo Georges Nógrády.

his feet splayed wide for balance ... George[s]'s horse eventually decided it could go no further and gave up the effort. It slowed to a stop, and standing, dozed off, its head falling forward. You could not say that George[s] fell off, but as his mount lurched forward in sleep, he slid over its neck, landing on all fours in front of the rudely awakened animal, a clatter of cape and equipment, cameras and jars."[64] Even fifty years later, mention of Georges Nógrády prompts METEI members to invoke Dr David Livingstone, Winston Churchill, and Don Quixote.

What most angered Helen Reid about the Group was their malicious tampering with Nógrády's samples and cultures. In her estimation, Mydans participated in the Georges-baiting too, although she had inscribed his name in the "oblivious" cohort of her diary. She did not write about this criminal act in her book, nor was it explicit in the diary – which, after all, could easily have been stolen and read during the voyage. But she came home from her journey incandescent with rage over the deliberate undermining of a colleague's work – the kind of gratuitous prank that could destroy the whole point of the mission. Her grown children well remember her disgust over these "immoral" acts. Having instructed her family to buy a copy of William Golding's 1954 novel *Lord of the Flies* to illustrate the degeneracy of METEI, she explained that Nógrády was the unfortunate character "Piggy," bullied and tormented by the teasing and tampering with his work.

How much Georges was aware of the mockery is not known; however, he was aware of something. Three years after his death, his closest friend could still name his METEI enemies, but she claims that Georges took it all in stride. Given the tragedy in his past, he would not let petty behaviour spoil his zest for life and science. He brought home thousands of slides, hours of movies, many carvings, and over 5,000 cultures of bacteria and fungi for analysis (figure 7.19). The majority of his cultures were free of contamination; one resulted in the most spectacular finding of the entire expedition (see chapter 12).

WRAPPING UP

Deep into the second month of the sojourn, the personal strife seemed to wane, or at least its full dimensions were known. Trapped with people whose irritating peculiarities were consistent and no longer surprising, Helen, Cléopâtre, Carlotta – and probably others too – noticed the calmer atmosphere. Still thinking about adaptation, Helen wrote "1st month all gripes – food and sanitation; 2nd month navy out and we have progressed to the point where the vahines are in. This might be called adjustment."[65] She marvelled that the aggravating behaviours had persisted with little change since the first encounters.[66] She wondered if humans could ever learn to adapt. Both Carlotta and Cléopâtre noticed this shift too, the latter writing that "an *entente générale* has emerged – at least superficially, we are all buddy-buddy. Only Roberts and Skoryna look at each other like dog and cat," always over the matter of a 100 per cent sample. It has "caused many arguments" and "several violent eruptions that expose Roberts's lack of self-control – notwithstanding his Anglo-Saxon roots – and Skoryna's indescribable obstinacy – practically paranoid – wherein lies his strength."[67]

The examinations were winding down. The number of parties increased. On each of two Saturdays, Sergio Piñero of the Chilean air force and Governor Jorge Portilla offered meals and *sau sau* dancing for the soon-to-depart METEI team. Fairy lights, twinkling in a banana grove, illuminated an elegant meal set on the governor's terrace in what Cléopâtre called a "quasi-European atmosphere."[68] Helen Reid drew the seating plan for a T-shaped table with white linen, fine china, and cutlery, recording a menu of white wine soup, barbecued pork and mutton, hardboiled eggs, salad, fruit for dessert, and "pisco with piña" (pineapple).[69] Bob Meier told his diary about the second "party at Governor's place ... quite nice, a lot of good food, lobster, veal, beef, pork, and many vegetables and *mucho vino*."[70] Back at the *campamento*, the merriment continued with a lively "fight" that entailed tossing watermelons and pumpkins.[71]

The governor's special evening took place on 30 January, the very day that John Cutler and Isabel Griffiths had attended the parturient mother's near-death at the little hospital (see chapter 6). John was ebullient: "I saved a life today! God, it makes you feel great!" He danced wildly with Dr Maureen Roberts, making everyone laugh, including her staid husband, who slapped his knees and hooted "each time his wife was sent spinning into space."[72] Cléopâtre also described this happy evening: "We nearly died laughing ... the British rigidity in submission to the fluid Polynesian rhythms produced a letting-go that was extremely comic."[73] The jubilation was widely shared because some, like Meier, had donated blood to save that life and especially because the expedition was winding down. Colin Gillingham, the cook, was dancing the *sau sau* as if he had been to the island born. Rapanui people were grateful, but the METEI team was too.

At some point during these late days, members of the camp were brought into a huge joke at the expense of Richard Roberts. In asking islanders their age in his anglicized Spanish, he would say, "Cuantos años tiene usted?" (*lit.* how many years do you have?). The islanders, hearing him say the word "anus," would answer, "Sólo uno" (only one) and fall down laughing. The response became Roberts's nickname, although he may never have known. The joke made its way back to METEI members, many of whom still recall it; Meier recorded it in his diary.[74] It would be nice to think that the newly relaxed navy doctor enjoyed it too.

The enhanced camaraderie in anticipation of departure resulted in teasing. A married man blanched to be told that his infidelities were surely to be exposed back home because he talks in his sleep. He must be careful, he said, but the wags persisted: "subconscious tension can lead to sleep talking." Another man, longing to escape, was subjected to the prospect of a merciless (but fictitious) fundraising campaign to bring his vahine to America. John Easton lectured the "ladies" about male "locker-room" solidarity: "telling is unacceptable."[75]

Skoryna continued to obsess over his 100 per cent. Anyone on the census who was currently on the island had to come for an examination. Most people came forward without fuss, walking to the clinic or enjoying a ride in Jeep Mea Mea, with special attentions and the gift photograph at the end. METEI members wanted to include those islanders who had returned with *Aquila*. Skoryna ordered a door-to-door search to uncover who and where they were to supplement the census. A few

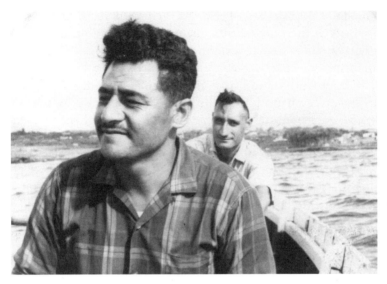

Figure 7.20 Noe Teao Riroroko, finally examined on 3 February 1965. Montandon Diary.

Rapanui determined to avoid this scrutiny, even when the new mayor gave his approval by example.

But one islander was different. Noe Teao Riroroko had not been examined because Richard Roberts refused. Noe acted as an "agent" for carvers, and many dealt with him because he drove hard bargains; however, he had been caught red-handed in "stealing" from METEI supplies. He took Bob Meier's aftershave and his steel tape measure.[76] He also took liberties; many islanders poked shoulders and chests as they spoke, but Noe would pinch female breasts, as if it were a normal cultural gesture; then he would leer.[77] Cléopâtre called him a "rascal" and pasted his photo in her scrapbook (figure 7.20).[78] For Carlotta, he was "a slick and smiling scoundrel – thoroughly unpleasant." She described the camp meeting after he'd been exposed in the act of pilfering Peter Beighton's penknife. They came to a rare, unanimous decision: Noe should be banned from camp. But Roberts wanted something more: "He is a thief ... He's outside at the moment with a complete run of the camp. I can see him from here. He's just gone into the supply trailer."[79] Roberts's refusal to sully his hands by examining Noe was a stigmatizing part of the man's punishment. The doctor's rigid resistance over this issue had the added virtue of foiling Skoryna's 100 per cent. Even today, Peter Beighton feels sadness at the memory of the shaming of Noe as a thief in the midst of the compound. Bob Meier too worried about the clash of values: "ethnographic accounts indicat[e] the Islanders did not possess a clear concept of personal ownership, and so were quite free to help themselves to any items they considered to be communal property."[80] Others agreed; for example, Reid shook down two "bulgy" tots who had loaded their pockets and underwear with dozens of toothbrushes from the box of extras in the clinic.[81] In the end, Skoryna won. Noe was examined on 3 February, Meier wrote, "but not by R. Roberts."[82]

One elderly lady failed to show up for her appointment. At eighty-five years of age, Marina Neru was said to be the oldest person on Rapa Nui and a direct descendant of the legendary king Hotu Matu'a. Skoryna tracked her down too. She made firm conditions: a ride in Jeep Mea Mea and a mouth organ. Skoryna took her in the Jeep for a picnic at Anakena and gave her a mouth organ and a cigar; she came back to Camp Hilton with him, danced the *sau sau*, played her mouth organ, and submitted to examination on 4 February.[83]

One other name was still on the list: seventeen-year-old Nelson Teao Hey, who lived in a remote house with three younger brothers, two of whom had already come to the METEI clinic. His father was dead and his mother not in evidence. Did he refuse to attend, or was he simply unaware? Skoryna sent Peter Beighton out to fetch him; quiet, confused, and painfully shy, Nelson was the only person examined on 5 February. When his physical, X-rays, and labs were complete, Skoryna assembled the medical team – Helen Reid, David Murphy, Maureen and Richard Roberts, and Peter Beighton – and summoned the photographers and Lemieux to join Stanley in shaking hands to congratulate the dazed lad: "the last one" (figure 7.21).

On 4 February, Helen Reid tape-recorded her interview with Rapu. She pointedly asked about his atheism and his politics; her notes suggest he replied with equanimity, but the recording is lost, along with two hours of movie film that she had shot on the journey. Almost as an aside, Rapu warned her that a tidal wave was expected – usually an exciting, if not dangerous, event for the Rapanui, as the withdrawal of the risen sea would leave many fish for easy gathering. But by the next day, no tidal wave had appeared. She continued her work on the island's food consumption to compensate for the lack of a nutritional survey and began packing the sculptures that she had purchased for gifts. At some point, the school gave her thirty-six students' paintings that she'd seen on her first day; she carefully slipped them into a thick envelope, where they remain to this day.[84] After two months confined with this energetic, inquisitive population, Helen saw that her opinions on morality and

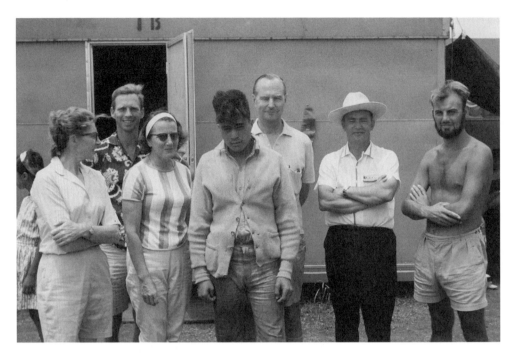

Figure 7.21 "The last patient," Nelson Teao Hey, with the doctors, 5 February 1965. *Also from left*, Maureen Roberts, David Murphy, Helen Reid, Richard Roberts, Stanley Skoryna, and Peter Beighton. Photo David Murphy.

misbehaviour had softened to a matter of perspective. She wrote, "I am too old" and "too fastidious," and she confessed her eagerness to return to hot showers and table napkins.[85]

During their time on the island, METEI members had assembled a massive quantity of data, samples, and objects, the significance of which was yet to be determined. They had also learned a great deal about themselves and how lack of preparation had hampered their work, making the very fact of their incredible journey all the more astonishing. Newly established friendships and sympathies would now confront abrupt transformation with impending separation and lack of communication. Some were longing to go home; others were already consumed with anticipatory nostalgia for a people, a place, and a way of life that they might never see again.

8

Return of HMCS *Cape Scott*

At noon on 21 December 1964, HMCS *Cape Scott* said goodbye to the Medical Expedition to Easter Island, sent the two stowaways back to shore, and set out for Valparaiso on the first leg of her goodwill tour. As she weighed anchor, she was surrounded by small boats crammed with islanders waving and singing tearful songs of farewell. In addition to her large company, she carried forty-two passengers, including twenty-six Rapanui children, three nuns, and the two doctors, Guido Andrade and Gonzalo Donoso, at least one of whom was a prisoner.

THE GOODWILL TOUR

Navy records state that the idea of a "goodwill tour" originated with Stanley Skoryna.[1] During the Cold War several such exercises in public diplomacy had attracted considerable media attention: Richard Nixon had ventured into Latin America in 1958, with painful results; Robert Kennedy had travelled in Europe and Asia in 1962; and, as vice president, Lyndon B. Johnson went to thirty-three countries, spreading what *Time* magazine called "good old Texas goodwill."[2] Canadian examples came from visits by members of the British royal family, which took place almost every year between 1958 and 1965. Indeed, in the lead up to METEI, there had been talk of a ministerial visit to Latin America, and Lester B. Pearson's government would sponsor a mining mission later in 1965.[3] Skoryna may have stumbled on the formula of the goodwill tour in these high-profile, political parallels, but his reasons for proposing it for *Cape Scott* likely stemmed from a desire to deflect scrutiny of the exorbitant costs of the project away from METEI. If *Cape Scott* made a goodwill tour, she would be doing much more than transporting the expedition: she would be helping Canada in its aspirations for trade and

Table 8.1 HMCS *Cape Scott* itinerary, Rapa Nui to Halifax, 1964–65

Date	Details
21 December	depart Hanga Roa
29 December to 8 January	Valparaiso, Chile
9–15 January	Base at Talcahuano, Bay of Concepción, Chile
18–23 January	Antofagasta, Chile
26 January to 2 February	Callao, Peru
6 February	Fire in engine room
10–12 February	Hanga Roa
15 February	Raising new flag ceremony at noon
21 February	Galapagos Islands
25–28 February	Panama City
3–7 March	Cartagena (team flown to Bogotá, 4–5 March)
17 March	Halifax

status on the world stage. Possibly, then, Canada would not object to the expense of helping METEI.

Skoryna suggested destinations along the western coast of South America, but naval concerns and contributions from the Department of External Affairs modified the plans. Guayaquil in Ecuador and Buenaventura in Colombia were dropped. The notion of shore leave in Curaçao, where fuel was "the cheapest in the world," persisted well into autumn planning until it, too, was replaced – by Cartagena and Bogotá.[4] Official reports of this goodwill tour are scant. The best sources are Commander Tony Law's candid letters to his artist wife, Jane Shaw, and the logbooks of *Cape Scott* (table 8.1).

Four days out of Hanga Roa, Christmas at sea entailed another dry Canadian pine tree, better than usual food, little gifts for the children, and lots of cake, oranges, and soft drinks, topped off by a visit from Santa Claus, who bore an uncanny resemblance to King Neptune of a mere three weeks earlier (figure 8.1). During the religious service, naval surgeon Gilbert Bérubé led the ship's choral group in a medley of carols. Alone in his cabin, Tony Law opened his present from Jane, a warm vest; he was "thrilled to death with it" and planned to "sport it" on cool evenings in South America.

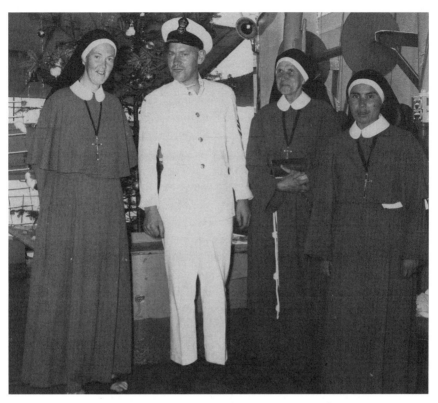

Figure 8.1 Three nuns with a chief petty officer on HMCS *Cape Scott*, Christmas 1964. Sister Esperanza (*right*). LAC, Law Scrapbook, vol. 3.

CAPE SCOTT BRINGS REBELLION TO VALPARAISO

Four days after Christmas, the sailors were ready for the mainland. But Chile was not quite ready for *Cape Scott*. No pilot boat came out to greet her when she sailed into Valparaiso on the afternoon of 29 December. Law had to turn his ship out to sea and make a second approach. This time he was met by a naval launch bearing a pilot, several marines, a lieutenant commander of the navy, and legal counsel for the Canadian embassy, Jean-Yves Grenon. The officer "ordered" Law to drop anchor, giving "the excuse that the ship was not expected until tomorrow," he told Jane. "Then the true story came out – they wanted to arrest a certain Chilean doctor from Easter Island. Mr. Grenon, typical of External Affairs, wanted to make me part of the problem by saying if the doctor resists arrest and declares asylum on Canadian territory, this will lead

to a difficult problem." But Law knew that Andrade was ready to face
his superiors. As predicted, the doctor "immediately agreed" to go along
under arrest with the marines; however, his "family broke down and
wept and [his] children were terribl[y] upset. I felt very badly for [them]."
Law heard that Andrade would be transferred to a small Chilean naval
ship, which was *Yelcho*, to be sent back to Easter Island for a "Court
of Inquiry."[5] Despite the rumours, Dr Donoso was at liberty, and *Cape
Scott*'s navigator, Charles Westropp, visited him in his Santiago home.

After the "fantastic situation" of this grudging welcome, the Chilean
pilot then directed *Cape Scott* to her berth, where the passengers dis-
embarked. Chaos ensued, with people searching for luggage, families
reuniting, young Rapanui students locating their billets, and sailors
eagerly departing for shore leave in a real city. Law was charmed by the
reaction of the "Polynesian teenagers" to their first view of the continent:
"Their eyes were popping. 'What was that that look like a very long lizard? A train. 'What was that funny looking large Jeep?' A bus. They were
am[a]zed at the high, modern buildings and the thousands of people.
What a difference from [their] quiet little island in the Pacific. This was
going to be their new life."[6]

The Canadian ambassador to Chile, G.B. Summers, a Newfoundlander,
with his "German baronette" spouse and their eleven-year-old son,
came aboard for dinner. Embarrassed and annoyed by the Chilean navy
actions, Summers apologized for the unorthodox reception, although he
admitted sending his legal counsellor, Grenon, to accompany the reception boat. Once again, the captain told Jane that he was relieved that
Rapu had been hiding back on Rapa Nui. If the governor had captured
the young rebel, pressure would have been great to transport him to
Chile, which he could not do "according to international law."

Within hours of *Cape Scott*'s arrival, details of Rapu's letter to President
Eduardo Frei Montalva had appeared in the newspapers. Because media
interest in Easter Island was high, Law was obliged to hold a press conference on board the ship; however, the diplomats and the "anxious" naval
officials cautioned him not to talk about the "delicate," political situation.
Unaware of his own role in inciting this interest, he seemed pleased that
he "managed to turn" the reporters' questions to METEI, which resulted
in some "rather nice" press about the expedition and its solar distillation
unit. But Law was vexed that a magazine printed photographs depicting
him "and the Chilean Chief of Staff with [their] hands out, and the caption
said 'Nobody knows anything' re Rapa Nui."[7] That same article listed the
Rapanui grievances and quoted Mariano Pakarati, who stated, "There is
no separation movement; we want only an end to the injustice." It also

published what it called "a curious interview" with Sister Esperanza, the nun who carried Rapu's letter. She was quoted as saying that "Alfredo [*sic*] Rapu" was an "excellent teacher," although he was an atheist. She also declared that he had been "very friendly with" and influenced by the Frenchman "Massiel [Mazière]," another "terrible atheist," who had pretended to be Catholic to ingratiate himself with the islanders.[8]

NETWORKING IN CHILE

Following the rude arrival, the Chilean officers seemed determined to make it up to Law and his crew over the next few days. They hosted a reception at the Navy Club, where artist Law admired the 7-metre ceilings of the salon, decorated in "lovely large oil paintings" of famous heroes and naval battles. "We have nothing like it in Canada," he told Jane. Then Admiral Jorge Balaresque invited the Canadians to a New Year's Eve party at the Naval Country Club. "It was out of this world." Pisco sours flowed freely alongside "wonderful Chilean wines," both red and white, and there was lively conversation. Law did not return to his ship until 6:30 a.m., blinded by the brilliant morning sun.[9]

On 3 January, Ambassador Summers and his family drove Law from Valparaiso to Santiago, stopping at the home of R.E. Gravel, the Canadian commercial counsellor, for lunch and a dip in the pool, a welcome relief from the hot, dusty drive over mountains. Law then began a round of visits with officials in Santiago: the commander-in-chief of the navy, the minister of defence, and the minister of external affairs. He was "most impressed" with these "intelligent and efficient men." Chile, he wrote, which was "well run," had begun an "all-out effort to build low-cost housing for the poor," and it boasted an "excellent police force ... similar to the RCMP [Royal Canadian Mounted Police]." The Summers family accommodated the visiting officers in their official residence and took Law and Bérubé to dine in a fine restaurant with traditional music; as the pleasant evening wore on, the French Canadian naval surgeon took to the stage to deliver an Italian aria.[10]

More visits followed to splendid private homes. They saw the sixteenth-century house of Mario Gonzalez Valdez and Ines Tonkin (now the national monument Casas de Lo Matta). They dined at splendid venues, like the Union Club, an ornate gentleman's lair with "beautiful," "romantic" paintings, chandeliers, and "the longest bar in the world ... way ahead of the Rideau Club in Ottawa."[11] While his naval visitor was making the rounds, Summers sent a "Confidential" telex back to Ottawa explaining that he had been asked by Skoryna – through Law – to support his request for a grant of $40,000 to cover the cost of the ATCO trailers and for permission to donate the three generators, belonging to the Canadian Department of Defence, to Chile. In passing along this request, Summers indicated that, personally, he did "NOT RPT NOT" support the idea of a grant. It had already been denied, and the trailers had to be left behind anyway. METEI could look for other backing; however, Summers did "strongly" recommend giving the generators to Rapa Nui.[12] Did Summers inform Law or Skoryna about his refusal to support their request?

Law was exhausted from this heavy socializing on top of the stress of his arduous journey and responsibilities. Summers insisted on driving him back to *Cape Scott*, and they took a different route through the mountains to Valparaiso, ending with a "refreshing" lunch at a "very nice little yacht club" followed by a siesta. By now the captain was drinking only wine because he'd experienced a day of diarrhea from the water. On the morning of 8 January, *Cape Scott* was set to continue her goodwill tour, but her engines failed just as a French destroyer was due at any moment to dock at the same pier. Law was reduced to begging the Chilean pilot for a tow. Drawn by a single tugboat in a glorious calm, the disabled Canadian vessel piped the French destroyer as she sailed into the vacated berth. But soon the seas were heavy, and Law had to use both anchors and buoys to avoid rocks and later make special manoeuvres to recover them and "the hose," which "came up from the bottom of the sea … like a serpent." The "fantastic operation" to restart the engines took more than six hours, and *Cape Scott* still needed to refuel.

Against a strong headwind and falling further and further behind schedule, she sailed south to Chile's main naval base at Talcahuano in the Bay of Concepción. Upon arrival, the Chilean navy had her drop anchor immediately and sent out a launch to gather the officers for Admiral Searle's welcoming reception at the Naval Country Club high on a hilltop. The party began at 11:00 p.m., with Law observing that the "Chileans love late, late parties" and that it was a "successful thrash" with a buffet, orchestra, and warm hospitality.[13]

The next morning, he brought the ship alongside her jetty and began another "terrible round of calls." During the week that the Canadians spent in the region, Law grew fond of a pair of naval commanders, Jorge Thornton and Jorge Paredes, who joked incessantly like a comedy duo of gagman and straight man. Both had been involved as naval captains in conveying scientists to Antarctica during the International Geophysical Year.[14] These "two characters" had much in common with Law, and their friendship "made my trip to Talcahuano."[15] His "most strenuous" day was 14 January. First, he and a group of officers were taken by Admiral Searle to tour a steel mill, then for a heavily libated lunch at the naval staff house, and then for "a drive" – "for an old Admiral he drives very fast." Back at the ship, Grenon, the embassy counsellor, came aboard with his daughters, wanting a tour. Immediately thereafter, Law had to rush back to shore in order to present himself at the admiral's house because Ambassador Summers had arrived, and then he went back to the ship again to change for a reception – "the usual bore" – which was followed by a splendid sit-down dinner for twenty-eight guests, after-dinner drinks with the admiral, and a nightcap on board *Cape Scott* with his new buddies, "the two Jorges." From midday, Law had been craving a siesta that never happened. On the following morning, with Jorge Thornton waving from the pier, *Cape Scott* headed north again for Antofagasta, which she reached on 18 January.[16]

Wherever they went, the Canadian naval officers were received like visiting royalty. But at Antofagasta, their hosts were coping with a recent tragedy. A ship had caught fire. While it burned, the governor of the port, Commandante Eduardo Zapata, had it towed "clear of the harbor and off to one side where it exploded and sank," with a loss of sixteen lives. Law went out in his Boston whaler to place a wreath around the mast, the only part of the ship still visible. As he returned, the intendant, Joaquin Vial, shouted across the water from the accompanying tug, "Thank you in the name of Chile!" Although they were in mourning, Zapata and his wife hosted a small reception for the visitors and extended many courtesies. A group of officers and sailors was taken by bus to Chuquicamata for a tour of the vast, open-pit copper mine, but Law took that day to paint. Zapata had him driven 24 kilometres from town to an interesting headland, where he "did two large oils and three drawings" with pleasing results. He was fascinated to find a searing-hot desert with no greenery at all. He was even more surprised at the private home of the police chief, General de Carabineros Humberto Araya Guerrero, where he discovered a lush garden irrigated through a pipe from a source "300 miles up in the Andes across the lonely desert." They dined al fresco with charming companions who spoke excellent English. At the Universidad del Norte, Law observed a number of scientific experiments that entailed distilling fresh water from salt and heating with solar energy.[17]

CANADA VISITS PERU

Cape Scott continued north for three days to Callao, the port of Lima, Peru, her last stop before returning to Easter Island. Law had been in touch with METEI by radio, and he knew that the examinations were proceeding on schedule. Whether or not he discussed the political situation or the *kokongo* outbreak is unknown. But the Andes Mountains hampered radio communication with Halifax; therefore, George Hrischenko's shack on Rapa Nui acted as a go-between for *Cape Scott* and Canada.

When Law reached Callao on 26 January, "the usual situation developed," he told Jane. "The official party with pilot were late. This meant Great Scott had to make a slow circle to kill time." Peru was in mourning for Winston Churchill, who had died on 24 January, and all official events were cancelled, except for a single reception held on board *Cape Scott*. Law began "the endless job of official calls." Here, however, he found architect Charles Fowler, a Halifax neighbour and friend, whom the navy had allowed to join the rest of the voyage as Law's guest. Fowler had been working in the Caribbean and had a great interest in pre-Columbian art.[18] They were delighted to meet the Canadian ambassador, Freeman Tovell, and his artist wife, Rosita LeSueur Tovell, whose mother was Peruvian.[19] The couple collected Canadian art, and the painter-captain and his architect friend admired their home, which was adorned with works by Tom Thompson, Lawren Harris, and Jean-Paul Riopelle. Rosita Tovell took Law, Fowler, and the "Ottawa doctor Cosseau" under her wing for a personal tour of the Rafael Larco Herrera Museum, where, Law explained to Jane, the "archeologists do not speak to each other and will not give their secrets." Nevertheless, "they are all too eager to talk to Mrs. Tovell." Consequently, she was up to date on all the latest findings. Fowler had the same memory: the archeologists' animosity extended to ignoring each other's publications. He was startled to find that he sometimes knew more than they did. The three men were shown recently acquired "naughty" clay figures, which were "too sexy" for public consumption, while their distinguished lady guide waited outside. "It appears what goes on today went on in those days regarding sex and homosexual activities of these ancient peoples ... It was very exciting."[20]

Again, officers and crew were offered an excursion, this time to the huge copper mine at Rio Blanco 80 kilometres north. Photographs of the sailors with llamas appeared in the Canadian papers. Meanwhile, Law was impressed with the parallels between the Peruvian and Chilean navies and his own. All three were roughly the same size, at 20,000 personnel. Peru had been influenced by the United States and lavished money on messes and accommodation; however, Chile, like Canada, drew upon British naval tradition and spent "all its money" trying to maintain ships. But both South American navies left Canada "far astern" when it came to "facilities ashore." Invited to lunch by Commander Boza of the ship *Villar*, Law and Fowler admired the "delightful Mess, which was designed by the President of Peru [Fernando Belaúnde Terry] ... an excellent architect with a fine feel for design together with plenty of imagination."[21]

Commander Law gathered extensive information about the navies of Chile and Peru, made many personal contacts, and absorbed numerous correctives to Canada's narrow and often smug view of itself. His interpretation of everything, from the landscape to the buildings to the people, was filtered through his artist's eyes. What the Canadian navy or the Department of Defence would do with these products of his "goodwill tour" of friendly ports was never clear. Nearing retirement, Law wanted to spend most of his time painting and quietly enjoying his afternoon aperitif. His exhausted crew members were relieved when Law secured permission for a four-day leave of absence before quitting Peru. Notwithstanding the sumptuous meals and warm welcome, they all had been biding time until they could pick up METEI and go home.

On 2 February *Cape Scott* left Callao, plying the Pacific southwest to Easter Island. Three days away from her destination, a "flash fire" broke out in the engine room, which filled with "thick, black smoke" that poured out of the skylight and the funnel. It was "brought under control quickly but was no fun while it lasted."[22] Thoughts of the recent tragedy at Antofagasta could not have been far from anyone's mind. Out in the open sea, no one would lay wreaths. At 8:00 a.m. on Wednesday, 10 February, she dropped anchor in Cook Bay off Hanga Roa for the second time.

METEI LEAVES RAPA NUI

Given his original misgivings, Law might have been surprised and gratified to be told that the mission had been a "100%" success: "the first time in history that a survey of this kind has been able to cover such a high percent." He expected to embark all the travellers and load their collections and gear, including Armand Boudreault's freezers and Mary King's telescope, within two days. The twenty-four trailers, the distillation units, the generators, Jeep Mea Mea, the X-ray equipment, and most of the lab would stay behind; the food stores were nearly depleted. The value of goods remaining was estimated at $100,000.[23] *Cape Scott* brought Chilean stamps for the postcards and a new red fender and door for the METEI Jeep, ordered by Harry Crosman through the ham radio and shipped to a port on the goodwill tour. He set about making the repairs.

Some METEI members, including dentist Al Taylor, were packed already and waiting at the harbour before the ship came into view.[24] Others had been busy making little farewell excursions to friends and favourite places. Done with measurements on the living, Bob Meier had obtained permission from Father Sebastian Englert to examine ancient skulls in his little museum. With Peter Beighton, Elliot Alpert, and Jim Nielsen, he took a boat trip to circle the island, guided by Carlos Teao Ika and Felipe Pakarati.[25] Denys and Cléopâtre Montandon walked up Rano Kao with Björn Ekblom, and they made a long-promised trip to the islet of Motu Nui in the frail fishing boat of their friend Carlos. The tiny barque was far too crowded, and "Mydans was more than tense."[26] Denys and Cléopâtre were invited for a private dinner at the governor's mansion, but Skoryna (also a guest) created awkwardness when he took the liberty of inviting notables from the village, including Rapu, without warning anyone.[27] Possibly, he thought it would help relationships.

Cape Scott's tired sailors were ready to get going. Cléopâtre noticed that they were not as accommodating as they had been earlier and that they made jokes about Skoryna and the expedition.[28] But the observed changes were mutual. Navigator Charles Westropp was surprised by the difference. He remembered, "We dropped off happy, optimistic people, eager to get on with their scientific work. When we returned, it was horrible." He asked, "Have you read *Lord of the Flies*?"

The navy crew off-loaded several tons of fertilizer as a gift for the Rapanui, and the reloading operation began in earnest.[29] At one point, a jeep heading toward the jetty lost its loaded wagon, which rolled downhill and plunged into the sea; sailors and METEI members, including Denys Montandon, had to dive into the waters to retrieve the barrels.[30] That night many travellers took up residence in their old cabins on board *Cape Scott*. Young islanders came out to the ship for a *sau sau*, although the billowing waves made dancing awkward and their return impossible; they too slept on the ship.

Archie Wilkinson sat on the seashore to tape-record his reflections on METEI in his slow, deep voice. He listed a wealth of detail about his X-ray setup in the cramped space of the ATCO trailer, the problems of troubleshooting the water supply necessary for developing films, and the complexity of using one machine for a variety of images. Conscious of METEI's connection to the World Health Organization, he hoped that these logistical details would be useful to anyone else attempting a similar radiographic survey in a remote place. A rain shower drove him inside to finish his dictation. Despite his early homesickness, his words are tinged with nostalgia and respect for the islanders.[31]

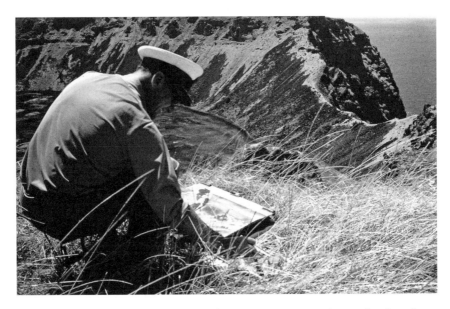

Figure 8.2 Commander Tony Law taking a moment to paint at the rim of Rano Kao crater, February 1965. Photo Fred Joyce.

The following morning, Bob Meier went around on horseback to say his goodbyes.[32] A guide saddled up with Tony Law and his friend Charles Fowler for a ride to the top of the Rano Kao volcano and the Orongo village, where Law made some paintings (figure 8.2). Then they brought Father Sebastian out to *Cape Scott* in his "fast little Boston Whaler with two outboards" for a lunch of "big lovely steaks" and beer, the priest's favourite beverage; "my, but he enjoyed himself!"[33] Carlotta Hacker felt little enthusiasm at the prospect of leaving; time was too short for goodbyes.[34] At Skoryna's suggestion, she took the excited lab girls out to *Cape Scott* as a "special treat," but their noisy laughter irritated a seaman, who yelled, "Get those natives off the boat!" Angered, she promptly set him straight about the invitation, but she was dismayed at the racism in his remark and the fact that his words had drawn her away from a newfound "colour-blind state" and back into a world of differences. But the girls had a lovely time exploring the ship, followed by Coca-Cola and ice cream in the canteen (figure 8.3).[35]

That evening Alfonso Rapu hosted a mighty *curando* of beef and mutton with another *sau sau* at the seaside with waves crashing.[36] A little ceremony at Camp Hilton in the presence of all officials entailed handing over commissioned gifts: a squat stone *moai* for Minister of Defence

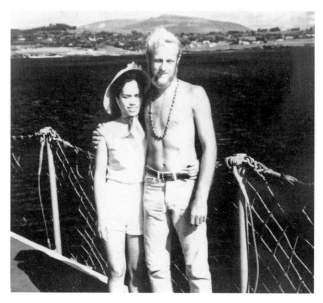

Figure 8.3 Saying goodbye. Jim Nielsen with girlfriend Margarita Huke on board HMCS *Cape Scott*, February 1965. Photo James Nielsen.

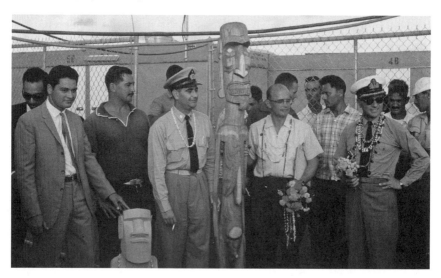

Figure 8.4 Ceremony at departure. *Front row from left*, Alfonso Rapu, Governor Jorge Portilla, Stanley Skoryna, and Commander Tony Law. METEI commissioned and paid for the gifts: the tall wooden Cava Cava Man for Prime Minister Lester B. Pearson and the small stone *moai* for Minister of Defence Paul Hellyer. Photo David Murphy.

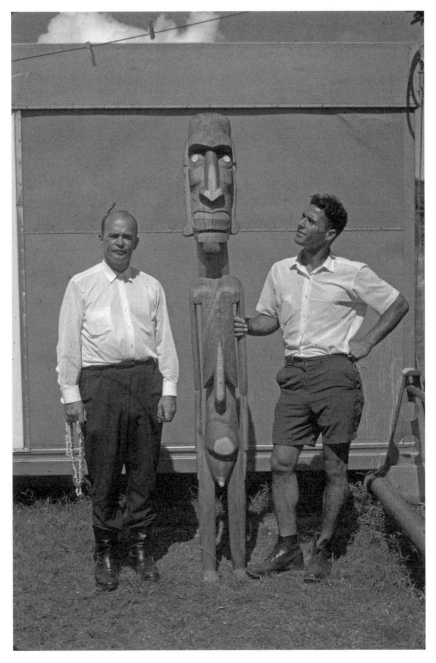

Figure 8.5 Stanley Skoryna with sculptor and the Cava Cava Man, METEI's gift to Prime Minister Lester B. Pearson. Note the fresh scraping on the chest. Photo Garry Brody.

Paul Hellyer and a giant wooden Cava Cava Man for the prime minister. Carlotta thought the Cava Cava Man was "hideous," with its ferocious scowl, hollow ribs, staring eyes, and exposed genitals. METEI members were horrified and amused, in equal parts, to see that the carver had inscribed "Lester B. Pearson" across the chest; it took serious convincing to have him remove it (figures 8.4 and 8.5).[37]

At the party, Cléopâtre noticed the subdued mood, an uncharacteristic lack of exuberance, and perhaps a sense of betrayal, as if the Rapanui knew that they were about to be abandoned and were already moving on. But the evening ended pleasantly in one of the trailers as Peter's "petite amie," Maria Teresa Ika Pakarati, sweetly sang the most beautiful island songs. Recognizing how much METEI had learned from the islanders and relied on them, Cléopâtre wondered how well these people saw through the silly, superior attitudes of the visitors.[38] Back on board, Meier gathered with a few others in Al Taylor's cabin for a post-*sau-sau sau sau*.[39] Peter Beighton was not leaving Rapa Nui, and the dentist would have the cabin to himself.

The day for departure was 12 February. Every written account and every interviewed traveller described the frosty interaction between Skoryna and Law. It shattered the team's uneasy accord so recently achieved. The former wanted the departure delayed by twenty-four hours and sent a scrawled request out to the ship;[40] the latter was firm that the ship would leave on time and that the last launch must depart Hanga Piko at 2:00 p.m. But Skoryna did not appear at the appointed time, and the "final" farewell hugs and tears on the jetty were repeated over and over, as departure was postponed hour by hour. A majority of travellers were on board the ship by 4:30 p.m., but some were missing – mostly McGill University men – as were Carlotta Hacker and Helen Reid, who stood waiting on the jetty.

Skoryna claimed that he had to complete paperwork to ensure that Peter Beighton had both a place to stay and permission to leave when a replacement physician might appear. He also needed to sign over the buildings and equipment to the governor's officials and the newly restored Jeep Mea Mea to the Rapanui people as an ambulance. He was also worried about stamps. A steady stream of activity swirled around the post office, where sailors were stamping and franking the potentially lucrative postcards to be conveyed back to Canada by *Cape Scott*. Most of all, Skoryna was determined to plant a McGill flag atop Rano Kao, and he did. Several photographs capture the moment with other McGill men – Hal Gibbs, David Murphy, and Garry Brody – while in the distance sits the tiny speck of *Cape Scott* with its invisible, fuming captain (figure 8.6). Earlier, Skoryna had tried to plant his McGill flag on the

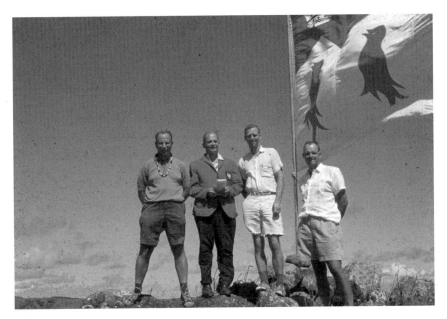

Figure 8.6 Planting the McGill flag atop Rano Kao. *From left*, Garry Brody, Stanley Skoryna, David Murphy, and Harold Gibbs. Photo David Murphy.

islet of Motu Nui, but the sea had been too rough for landing.[41] The flag raising was unfinished business.

Fifty-one years later, Isabel Griffiths (now Cutler) still marvels at Law's stiff intransigence over a few hours' delay on a journey of more than a month's duration. She sees it as some kind of power struggle, similar to the strife between Richard Roberts and Skoryna – military man versus dreamer.

Helen Reid described the last, frustrating hours in her diary:

The tensions on the ship are enormous; for the past two days, they mount. The sea is flat, the loading is complete in one day. The navy is weary of its wanderings and yearning to be homeward bound. Small irritations are near the surface.

Stanley wishes sailing delayed 1 day. The captain is adamant. Stanley has sent a note aboard that they must wait one day to settle Peter Beighton as doctor ... the Chilean government has not given him guarantees of passage home. The captain comes ashore with witnesses (1st officer) to say to Stanley he must sail at 6. I ask to have 2 min[utes] with Stanley first. I find him distributing food from our

stores and I tell him the captain wishes to speak with him and that I
believe the ship must sail. He says that he is not ready and if the ship
sails, he will stay. I say I think the navy has been extremely cooperative and we must go. He says the stamps are not complete. Then
we meet the captain. It is a matter of *ultimata*. I then drive with the
captain to the post office where two sailors are working on stamps.
They are at maximum [speed] since there is only one franking device.
The captain offers Sergio help with sticking the stamps on. He says it
is not necessary. They are averaging 3000 an hour [figure 8.7].

I blow the whistle at 4 and at 5 – the tension mounts. The officers
must get the ship under weigh [*sic*]. Reports are that Stanley has gone
to Orongo [on Rano Kao] to plant the McGill flag ... that he has gone
to help Beighton settle in, etc, etc. 10 personnel are still not aboard.

[inserted] 5 p.m. Father Sebastian comes aboard to say goodbye to METEI. In a scholarly moving message he thanks us all and
quotes from Julius Caesar "farewell forever and if not forever when
we will meet again, we will smile, etc?["] He says he will remember
us in his prayers. We weep a little, some with our eyes and some
with our hearts.

At 6 p.m. sailing time the Governor's launch comes alongside.
Stanley and the others board with garlands and flowers and a few
pascuense. The Captain suggests a whiskey sour. Half an hour later
Alfonso Rapu comes up the side splashed and immaculate, he is
taken to the Captain too. It is 40 minutes before they all leave with
tears and kisses.

We weigh anchor and sail. As the night falls quickly bonfires flare
on the shore, lights wink on and off. We fire a display of verey lights
[flares] from the bridge. We are going home.[42]

As the ship slowly sailed off, the gorgeous sunset faded, giving way
to a clear, moonlit sky. Meier wrote, "I must admit I had some regret
about leaving. The island had become a friendly place and the people
old friends."[43]

Carlotta found the flower-bedecked Stanley Skoryna in tears as he
stood at the rail and waved to the small boats of islanders, who were
singing and calling out "Eskoryna! Eskoryna!" Oblivious to the "slight
chill" in the officers' reception, he was heady with emotion. "For this,"
she admitted, "was probably the greatest moment in his life ... The dream,
his dream, had become reality." He spoiled the effect by stating, "This is
only the second time I have wept since I was a child."[44] Cléopâtre and
Denys watched as the Rapanui fires grew smaller, "seeming as inaccessible

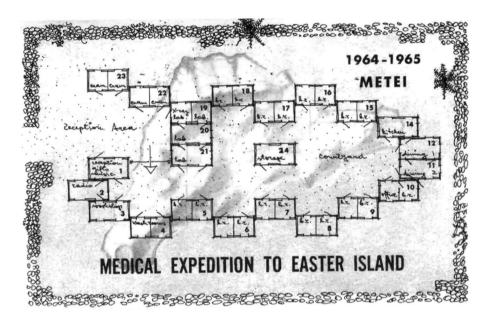

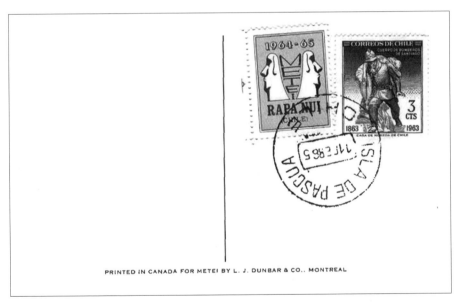

Figure 8.7 Both sides of an unused METEI postcard stamped and franked at the Easter Island post office. It featured a map of Rapa Nui superimposed with an architectural plan of the camp. The small break between trailers 18 and 19 is missing, and trailer 24 was not in the centre but on the upper left as the third clinic trailer. Note the METEI seal. Wilkinson Papers.

as the stars," until they vanished. "Had they been extinguished, or could we no longer see them?"[45]

Law told Jane about how "much trouble" he had in trying to get Skoryna aboard: "The man was so tired that he had lost control of his judgment and was no longer rational ... Everyone will agree [he] is a[n] impossible man to work with. Many fights broke out during the two months on the island ... personality clashes and changes of allegiance and the camp was a shambles." But Law credited Skoryna, for all his foibles, with having done "an excellent job" in making the expedition a "great success" and for building a "wonderful relationship between the members of the expedition and the islanders." His task had not been easy, he wrote, because the Chileans were "not popular" with the Rapanui; he could risk offending no one and managed to "steer a safe course between the two political factions."[46] Skoryna collapsed with a severe cold and exhaustion. Law ordered him to bed for a few days. "He is a man who cannot delegate authorities and has to do everything himself. Well, he fell flat on his face ... He was a different man after his rest."[47]

On the first night out, Law hosted a dinner for the Montandons, John Easton, Helen Reid, and his architect friend, Charles Fowler, who was now sharing Easton's cabin. The conversation turned to "over-developed societies." Fowler opined that the Incas had been hoist by their own exaggerated zest for organization; parallels with METEI lurked unstated. Cléopâtre was astonished to hear Law criticize Skoryna; she confided to her journal that their McGill leader seemed to have been demoted to a second-class citizen and a small, airless cabin. While he lay ill, sailors and expedition members "reproached his lack of organization, his promises made of air, his exaggerated diplomacy."[48] Fowler remembers that Skoryna had wanted to seem "a bigger man than he was," allowing the islanders to perceive METEI's leavings as his personal benefaction, not that of Canada. It did not help that Stanley was no longer seen aboard. Cléopâtre wondered if his ailment was truly just a cold or something far more serious.[49]

SAILING HOME

Weeks of travel still lay ahead. Once he felt better, Skoryna emerged to encourage METEI members to begin composing their preliminary reports (figure 8.8). Most of the scientists and doctors wrote by hand for Isabel Griffiths and Ana Maria Eccles to type, sometimes in multiple drafts. The long days aboard allowed for reflection on what had worked, what had not, and what needed to be done to leverage the results into useable data and publications. Poring over her extensive notes, Helen Reid realized

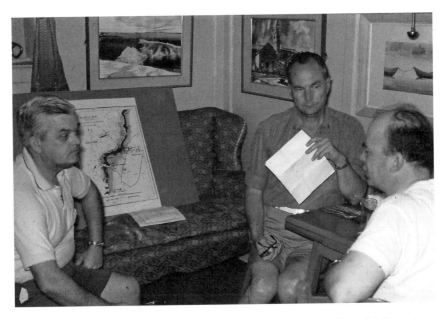

Figure 8.8 Shipboard meeting in Commander Tony Law's cabin with his paintings on the wall and Hanga Roa map on the setee. *From left*, Air Vice Marshal John Easton, Richard Roberts, and Stanley Skoryna. Photo Georges Nógrády.

that her "impression" of Rapanui children being "small" had no meaning without a comparison group. She developed the idea of examining 500 Canadian children in the same manner.[50] Similarly, her admittedly limited efforts to sort out the nutrition status would also need some kind of comparison. She continued calculations, relying on information from David Murphy that 549 sheep were consumed each month by the 923 people (338 as gifts and 211 as wages). With an average dressed weight of 10 kilograms, or 22.5 pounds, per sheep, each person enjoyed 13.3 pounds of meat, including bones, every month; if the 140 Chileans were included, the amount dropped to 11.7 pounds per person, or roughly half a pound daily.[51] These were not starvation rations. Thinking of her promised article for *Maclean's* magazine, she developed a questionnaire and interviewed fellow travellers to learn more of their research, credentials, prior experiences, perceived accomplishments, and recommendations for future expeditions: Hal Gibbs, Ian Efford, Eivind Myhre, Bob Meier, Armand Boudreault, David Murphy, Georges Nógrády, and even Cléopâtre Montandon. She did not interview Richard and Maureen Roberts.

Fresh from the trenches, the travellers made initial recommendations that were consistent and clear. Everyone emphasized the need for greater advance planning, possibly a "dry run" visit, and better financial security. The projects should have been shared and vetted among the team before the journey. A master plan of mundane duties, a division of labour, and more liaison would have avoided grumbling and perceived injustices. Boudreault was reminded of Jean de la Fontaine's fable about the wolf who envied a dog, learning that easy food came with an unwelcome collar. "One man cannot do it all," said Myhre. Most would take more technologists and fewer doctors or scientists; a doctorate is not needed for many skilled tasks. Efford longed for a botanist and expert divers. Gibbs thought that things would have been better with a "good deputy" in case of "failure of the leader" and perhaps an "executive council" to avoid discussing problems in open meetings. Everyone complained about the constant intrusions of the "media men," who "interfered" and "caused difficulties." Gibbs said, "a person does not work well under such intense scrutiny," but he realized that the pressure for publicity stemmed from the inadequate funding. Finally, no one should be on the expedition who did not *want* to be there.[52] None of these oft-repeated recommendations, recorded by Dr Reid, were included in Skoryna's preliminary report.

The Easter Island census also needed work. It was important to establish an accurate list of all the people examined and those who had been absent, connecting them with the assigned identification numbers and clarifying their relationships with each other. Some of this information would apply to the genetic studies promised by Maureen Roberts, although, from the earliest days, most travellers despaired of ever obtaining accurate information on the biological relationships. John Cutler went over the census, comparing the numbers with names on the examination sheets and the X-rays, and Isabel typed many drafts. Months after the return, the census was still not complete.

Skoryna's flu spread around the ship, but sympathy was strained. Einar Gjessing remembers lying in his bunk and feeling ill with a bad headache, while unwelcome music blared from an overhead speaker. He asked for it to be turned off but was denied. Undaunted, he found a way to disconnect the source and did so, only to be chastised by Commander Law, who threatened him with punishment for not respecting the crew's need for entertainment. Law's intemperate outbursts were familiar to the "lower" members of the team, although the leaders were sheltered. Einar remembers that Helen Reid tried to interview him and asked if he had a girlfriend. Not inclined to reveal that someone special waited back home, he said "no."

The movies and talent shows of the outward journey resumed. Bob Meier and Cléopâtre found the journey tedious, with all the days similar and nothing much to do – sunbathing, laundry, reading, playing bridge or chess, and a bit of work. On 14 February the lonely Bob wrote, "Happy Valentine's to My Girls back home." He was a regular at the evening films, and his journal lists the nautical, Cold War fare: *Fail Safe*, *Robin and the 7 Hoods*, *633 Squadron*, *From Russia with Love*, *Stitch in Time*, and *Cruel Seas*.[53]

RAISING THE FLAG

At noon on 15 February 1965, the third day at sea, an unforgettable ceremony took place. On that day, Canada officially proclaimed its own flag. After considerable controversy, the flag project had been one of the cornerstones of Prime Minister Lester B. Pearson's national plan to raise the country's profile, promote unity, and celebrate its distinct identity. Various designs came and went, but the red and white version of historian and soldier George Stanley became the special committee's final selection, approved by the government in December 1964 to take effect on 15 February 1965. During the course of the "flag debates," Skoryna had been sending encouragement and praise to Pearson in letters and telegrams, expressing his hope that the new flag would be approved and that METEI would be able to fly it; the prime minister's office even replied to one of these ingratiating missives.[54] Much of the decision making had occurred while METEI was out of the country, far from newspapers and television; however, verbal descriptions of the design were not lacking. Once again, the signalmen of *Cape Scott* got busy and stitched two flags with the new design, overseen by Tony Law and Charles Fowler, just as the "ladies" had done for METEI's own banner three months earlier. Law's flag went on the masthead and Fowler's at the stern.

The crew relished enacting this symbolic ritual, unique among the many ceremonies that the navy always performed so well – rituals that now seemed threatened by the impending merger of the armed forces. With their cameras ready, METEI members – especially the Canadians – were dazzled by the seamen, who were standing at attention, resplendent under the South Sea glare in their brilliant, white uniforms, which Charles Westropp called "ice-cream suits." The four-page order of service to mark the moment is kept with Law's papers in the national archives, and a copy was sent to the prime minister.[55] The same rite was taking place on all the nation's ships stationed around the world (figure 8.9).[56]

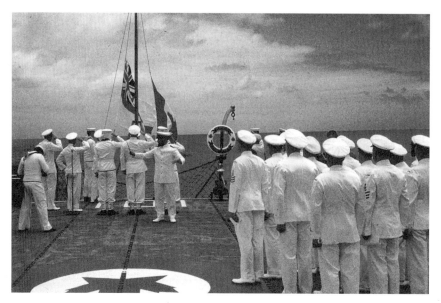

Figure 8.9 Singing "O Canada" as the White Ensign is lowered and the new flag is raised on board HMCS *Cape Scott*, 15 February 1965.
Photo Archibald Wilkinson.

After inspecting his men, Commander Law read the proclamation. The piper played "Cock o' the North" as the colour party moved forward with the new flag, giving it to the captain. He passed it on to the yeoman, who secured it to the halyard and announced, "One minute to colours, sir." And then, "Twelve o'clock, sir." The captain ordered, "Make it so!" The boatswain's mate struck eight bells over more piping. Then, as the White Ensign was slowly lowered, the new flag was raised to the singing of "God Save the Queen." At the end of the first verse, the two flags met on the pole; the "wind blows and for a moment the two banners stream together." The anthem changed to "O Canada" in English and then in French as the new flag rose. The retired ensign was folded and passed to the captain. A bilingual prayer followed, and then the colour party marched the old flag off to the bridge as the pipes played "Flowers of the Forest," an ancient tune used traditionally to honour those fallen in war.[57]

Helen Reid noted a "catch" in Law's voice. She wrote, "There is a sadness as they bear the limp ensign away." But she looked "hard at the new flag. It is mine and Canada's, and I shall learn my new love and love my old."[58] Young Jack Mathias was deeply moved. A half-century

later, he said, "It was a gorgeous, brilliant, rough day ... I felt so proud."
Having witnessed this remarkable ceremony through her European eyes,
Cléopâtre wrote that it was "a small blow against the British Empire,
and a little victory for French Canada and Canadian nationalists." But,
she added, for the navy, "that little red maple leaf would always be under
the English crown," and the royal portraits were not about to disappear
from the canteen.[59]

ACCORD AND DISCORD

The torpor that had infused the journey until this moment seemed to lift.
On 18 February, METEI members formed the Rapa Nui Science Club –
with its own "Charter," signed by both Law and Skoryna – promising to
keep an accurate mailing list, produce a newsletter, promote the fortunes
of Rapa Nui, and communicate results of the analyses that had yet to
come (figure 8.10).[60] Meanwhile, Red Lemieux continued his pursuit
of Carlotta Hacker. The sailors spied on the couple with night-vision
binoculars and swore that they saw "something consummated" at the
back of the ship. This romance may explain why she ends her book with
METEI's departure from Rapa Nui. As another sign of the happier mood,
the ship's company began preparing a talent show to mock METEI, the
navy, and themselves.

But Richard Roberts and Stanley Skoryna continued their tedious
bickering. A few dull meetings took place, wrote Cléopâtre, "to say the
same things over and over again and to watch [them] argue with each
other."[61] Helen marvelled at their mutual antagonism. On 19 February
she described the ambience of a meeting in which Roberts adopted
the uncompromising stance that "he would disassociate himself from
Stanley if the figure 100% was used." She continued,

> If it were used at a press conference [Roberts] would feel bound to
> state he did not concur. He quotes the fact that there was one chart
> – a 20-month-old child Dec 28th – who did not have a physical
> examination. He says Fred Joyce did not take blood tests and this
> chart cannot be considered to be examined. He further says we do
> not know who came on the *Aquila* and hence cannot say we exam-
> ined everyone. Stanley replies that he went to all the houses with
> Elliot in the last three days and got the remaining 12 who had not
> been examined. There is much embittered passage. Richard says we
> cannot claim 100% scientifically. Stanley says we can.[62]

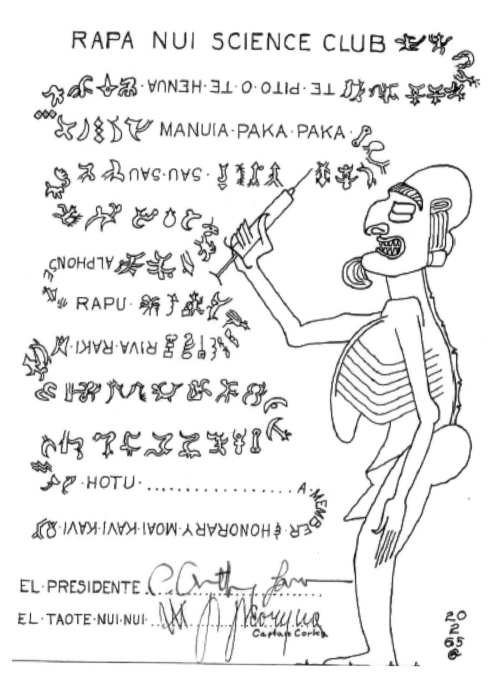

Figure 8.10 Rapa Nui Science Club charter. Signed C. Anthony Law and S. Skoryna, 20 February 1965. Montandon Diary.

Helen analyzed their animus within the context of an extended, ship-board discussion on the concept of morality that she had been conducting with Commissioned Officer James R. Barlow. His "system" of universal "forgiveness," she said, was merely "comfortable." He disagreed with her view that "people do what they want to do, that having made the choice, they cannot expect gratitude or commendation." In the case of Roberts, she decided, "He is right, but immoral." She wrote,

He could have been both right and moral if he had taken the imper-fections he found privately to Stanley and attempted to work out a solution with him which would correct these imperfections. Several possibilities are open. He might have searched to find other areas in which the examination was [in]complete, called up Peter Beighton and had him complete the exams, etc. to make up the deficiencies. To attempt deliberately to destroy another's reputation or work is immoral. To do it in the name of one's own personal integrity is a sin.

This aspect of the expedition presents great possibilities – the struggle of the two personalities the one imaginative, flexible, practi-cal; the other a rigid perfectionist who is indeed usually right.

The clashes, which occurred in the camp, were inevitable. The two persons were confined and forced into a constant dialogue. The very perfectionist qualities of the one led to the aggrandizement of the other, which was intolerable.

Isolation prevented the escape of the one from the other. The dreamer struggled for his goal of 100%; the perfectionist wanted less, demanded less, and tried to produce less but at a superior level – less quantity and more quality by follow up. At the denou[e]ment, I predict that the perfectionist will destroy himself on his own integrity and, in the classical Greek sense of tragedy, it will be because he is right.[63]

Little did Helen or anyone else know that Roberts was furiously typ-ing with two fingers a scathing report for his surgeon general that would condemn METEI, Skoryna, and many of their colleagues (see chapter 10).

GALAPAGOS

Ten days out, on Sunday 21 February, the ship stopped for eleven hours in the Galapagos at Santa Cruz Island (also called Indefatigable). They went to the Charles Darwin Research Station and saw giant turtles and several kinds of finches. Given advance notice by radio, the Hotel Nelson prepared a lunch for METEI travellers and let them swim in the pool. Cléopâtre noticed how the impenetrable, lush vegetation contrasted sharply with Rapa Nui. She was disappointed to realize that they would see little beyond the station and its fearless birds and amphibians; however, the English director and the Belgian administrator intrigued her: people who accept jobs in such isolation are always "des types assez spéciaux."

But this most exotic destination held little interest for the weary, homesick (and seasick) travellers, who were sensitized to the tragedy of "spoiled" environments. A few thought that they could detect evidence of the nefarious influences that would soon be visited upon Rapa Nui when its airport opened. Commander Law wrote to Jane, "The Galapagos Island was a disappointment ... uninteresting people [who] did not talk to each other as each considered themselves superior to the other ... Even the children were solemn and did not smile like the young *pascuenses*." Nevertheless, hindered by the tremendous heat (42° Celsius) and the dank smell of the jungle, the captain "saw everything one could see." He chatted with Dr Roger Perry, the English director of the biological station, who had known Peter Scott, the famous British conservationist, artist, and naval officer.[64] Bob Meier thought that the town was "rather poor looking."[65] Archie Wilkinson shot 30 metres of film and many photos but was eager to be off. Even George Hrischenko – ever so keen on Charles Darwin, Thor Heyerdahl, and discovery of lost worlds – said, "Once you've seen one turtle, you've seen 'em all." METEI travellers were missing Rapa Nui almost as much as they missed home.

A surprising encounter with a Swiss woman who had recently settled in the Galapagos caused Cléopâtre and Denys to overlook the last call for return to *Cape Scott*. Panic set in for a few moments, but many volunteers came forward with motorboats ready to help. They accepted a ride from the island's young German dentist, who exuded "the air of a juvenile delinquent." As they raced across the waves, they met Leading Seaman Thomas Picco returning in the landing craft to look for them. Skoryna was angry, and they received a severe scolding from Lieutenant Commander Ross Thompson. "Ah ces anglosaxons!" Cléopâtre wrote.[66]

The next day, METEI members, especially the hard-partying "Group" identified by Reid and Hacker, made radio contact with Peter Beighton back on Rapa Nui, exchanging greetings and asking for updates on their friends. One of the Rapanui "girls" was pregnant, and the Group reported that "Peter really wants a child." Helen duly recorded this news in her diary.[67] While still on the journey, Garry Brody quietly took Maureen Roberts aside and warned her "about not telling on the boys"

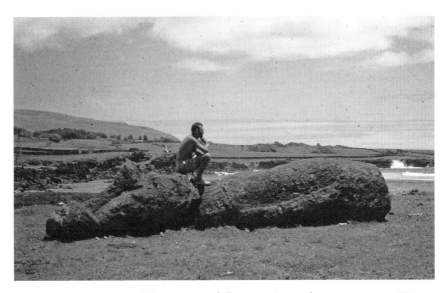

Figure 8.11 Dr Peter Beighton atop a fallen *moai* near the *campamento*. He remained on Rapa Nui when HMCS *Cape Scott* left for Halifax.
Photo Fred Joyce.

and asking her to pass the message on to Helen. The latter wrote, "He was sure we were old enough and sensible enough to close our eyes."[68]

Now the solitary physician, Peter was managing well (figure 8.11). No severe illnesses arose during his sojourn, although as a budding internist, he was alarmed when a woman developed acute cholecystitis. He wondered if he would have to play surgeon and remove the last remaining gallbladder on the island. But to his immense relief, she recovered spontaneously. A woman with leprosy had an acute inflammatory episode that settled with steroids, and an old man died of tuberculosis. Beighton pronounced him dead but did not attend the funeral. His girlfriend, Maria Teresa Ika Pakarati – "the Mrs." – and her warm family looked after him. As he later wrote to Jim Nielsen, she "managed [his] home with great skill, even entertaining the governor to a formal meal." In spare moments, he continued his exploration of the island, visiting favourite haunts, Motu Nui, many caves, volcanoes, and a sunken ship.[69]

All contemporary sources agree that Peter was absolutely the best person to stay behind given his experience in tropical medicine, mastery of Spanish, smattering of Rapanui, and comfort with the locals and their ways. He defended the parting agreements and made sure that Jeep Mea Mea stayed on the island for the people, not the military (figure 8.12).[70]

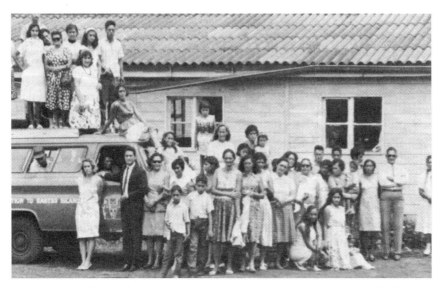

Figure 8.12 Alfonso Rapu (*dark suit*) with METEI's Jeep Mea Mea, which was given to the people to serve as an ambulance. Photo Peter Beighton. Originally published in Hacker, "Aku-Aku and Medicine Men."

Some "admired his sacrifice," but Helen was skeptical; if she had been younger, less homesick, and less fastidious, she might have envied the adventure of being left behind with a complete clinic, a laboratory, and a case of wine.[71] Eventually, a Chilean supply ship brought a new doctor, and Peter left with it on 3 April 1965. Before flying home to England, he travelled through Chile and Peru, with military officer status granted by the Chilean authorities because of his previous service with British forces and the United Nations.

On 23 February the crew members staged their satirical review "South Pacific Fiasco." In drama, song, and dance, they mocked METEI and its scientists. At one point, a sailor was reduced to wearing nothing but a box, having traded all his clothing for statues. The inseparable Montandons were imitated "à deux" by two men, one doing his best to be a blushing lady in the family way. The "Saga of Easter Island" and the "Ballad of *Cape Scott*" were joined by the songs that Law had been carrying since the farewell party in Halifax, including "Disenchanted Island." At this event, the travellers were awarded their "shellback certificates" for crossing the equator (twice). The certificate included a map, but it was incorrect, having been printed in advance with the goodwill destinations that were eventually cancelled (figure 8.13).[72]

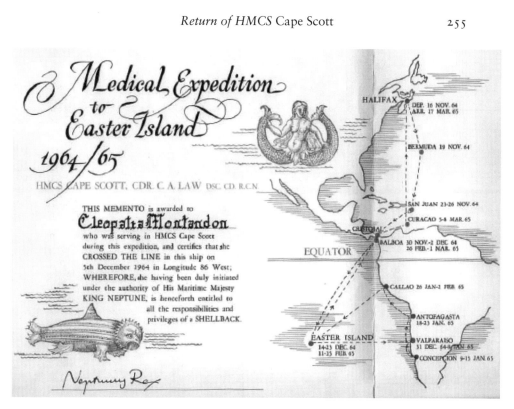

Figure 8.13 Certificate presented to every "tadpole" turned "shellback" for crossing the equator. Montandon Diary.

DISPERSAL AND COLOMBIAN DISSEMINATION

At Panama, the team began to disperse (figure 8.14). After a final get-to-gether in a Balboa bar, Bob Meier and David Murphy flew home, eager to see their wives and children. Ian Efford left too, wanting to see his family and get started on studying and distributing all the samples that he and Jack Mathias had gathered. Ekblom, Cutler, and Alpert also went home. Garry Brody's wife, Sonia, met him in Panama, and the wives of Eivind Myhre and Carl Mydans flew to Cartagena, Colombia, turning their long-awaited reunions into little holidays à deux before going home. McGill's Al Tunis flew out to Cartagena too. Obliged to remain with his team, Stanley Skoryna asked that his wife, Halina, be allowed to join *Cape Scott* at Cartagena for the final leg of its journey. After all, Commander Law had enjoyed the company of his friend Charles Fowler since Peru, and the Montandons and the Robertses had had each other all along. The request did not seem unreasonable. But

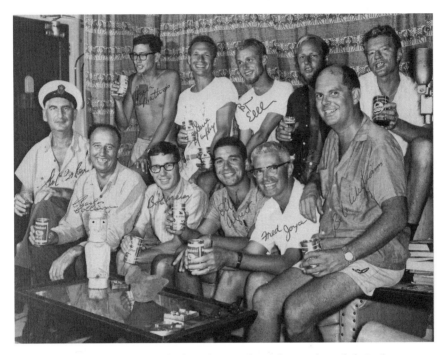

Figure 8.14 Shipboard party before dispersal. *Back row from left*, Jack Mathias, David Murphy, Björn Ekblom, Jim Nielsen, and Red Lemieux. *Front row from left*, illegible [Cohen?], Charles Collinson, Robert Meier, Elliot Alpert, Fred Joyce, and Robert Williams. Murphy Papers.

having made exceptions for the eight METEI women, the nuns, and the Rapanui mothers, the Canadian navy was done with special favours for seafaring females. His request was denied.[73]

METEI's re-entry was marked by receptions and parties, an extension of *Cape Scott*'s goodwill tour, and a "shore-leave" moment for the travellers. The Montandons first stop was a bank to reimburse Skoryna for their camera purchases. There, the Canadian ambassador to Costa Rica threw a reception for all the Canadian vessels in port; their first contact with so-called "civilization" after many weeks of exile was at an "ultra chic golf club" with officers in dazzling uniforms (figure 8.15).[74] In Panama City, it was Carnival time, and the travellers strolled the old streets, stumbling on pockets of dancers and musicians in brilliant traditional costumes. Several found themselves "the only gringos" in a huge crowd that was throbbing "as one" to the music – impossible not to dance, and if you fainted, you would not fall down.[75]

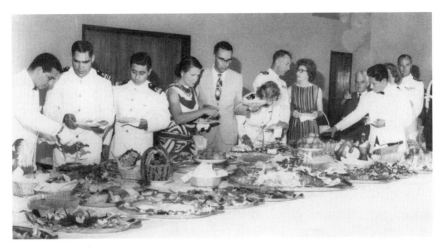

Figure 8.15 After three months of hard rations, pumpernickel, and navy fare, HMCS *Cape Scott* passengers enjoyed fabulous receptions thrown by ambassadors in Panama and Colombia. Lieutenant Commander Alfred Shaw (*2nd from left*), Dr Helen Reid (*4th*), Lieutenant Mary King (*6th, bending over*), Lieutenant Commander Duff Pennie (*7th*), Dr Maureen Roberts (*8th*), John Easton (*9th*), and Dr Richard Roberts (*12th*). Unidentified photo. Reid Papers, file 22.

At a cocktail party for METEI, hosted by the British ambassador, Helen Reid met accountant Betty Bryan, whose husband was Rear Admiral Boyd Bryan, commander of the United States Navy in South America and the Caribbean. They spent a relaxing day together and remained epistolic friends for some time.[76] Betty took Helen to visit American archeologist Bob Turner, who gave her a pre-Columbian Chiriqui bowl for her anthropologist daughter, Judith. They also attended to repairing the eye glasses of Margarita Tepano, who had helped in METEI's lab. Helen was relieved that they would be taken back to her via diplomatic pouch by the American navy and the Chilean supply ship *Antofagasta*.[77]

Before he left, Ian Efford had told the Montandons about Barro Colorado Island in Gatun Lake in the middle of the Panama Canal; the island was affiliated with the Smithsonian Institute and would soon become its Tropical Research Institute. With Georges Nógrády, Hal Gibbs, and a petty officer, they went there by train and boat and met the director, Dr A. Stanley Rand, who provided a map of the trails. The group spent a wonderful day wandering the jungle and admiring the wildlife.

At the diplomatic gatherings, the formal attire, ladies' cosmetics, fine meals, elegant table settings, and general pomposity seemed strangely artificial, often absurd, and the necessity of these occasions was a burdensome delay. Although Helen was tempted to fly home (as her husband was urging), she thought it was important to stay on the ship to support Skoryna and the navy, but she recognized that her loyalty stemmed from "guilt complexes."[78] Armand Boudreault had also planned to fly home, but Skoryna asked him to stay on too to maintain a French Canadian presence.[79]

Cape Scott cleared the canal on 1 March and headed for Cartagena, which she reached on 3 March. The Canadian ambassador handed them each an envelope with details about invitations and excursions. The following morning, the remaining METEI members, plus seven officers and the captain, were flown by the Colombian navy's elderly Douglas DC-4 the 700 kilometres to Bogotá for a twenty-four-hour visit. The purpose was to "debrief" about their expedition at a press conference and a seminar held in the Faculty of Medicine at the Universidad Nacional de Colombia. "Bogotá will be hell!" wrote Helen to her husband – a "meeting of scientific minds." "There are 41 professors from 3 Universities and the school of Tropical Medicine – anthropologists, microbiologists, Deans ... My god we'll be over our depth!"[80]

An hour after they landed, Ambassador Ormond Dier hosted a glittering reception for 300 people at the beautiful Canadian embassy.[81] That night, they were billeted with Canadian families. The following morning, 5 March, they were bussed to the university for the dreaded press conference and seminar, followed by a luncheon and more receptions, one in honour of Commander Law. But the seminar was a surprising success, with interesting questions, many of a sociological nature, and "la petite sociologue enceinte" had to stand several times to respond. "What a difference from those idiotic press conferences!" Cléopâtre wrote. She kept the list of distinguished attendees in her scrapbook.[82] Helen understood that the seminar was a "big thing for the navy" and the nation, which wanted to "show the new Canadian flag," and that all the lavish fuss – notwithstanding its scientific merit – was related to ongoing "trade talks" with Colombia and conveniently timed after most American members had left METEI to go home.[83]

Following the seminar, METEI members were offered another formal luncheon and reception; Cléopâtre and Jim Nielsen kept their embossed invitations. But Helen skipped that event and asked instead to tour Parque el Canada, an education project for 75 to 100 disadvantaged schoolchildren in the poor neighbourhood of Barrio Santa Inés.

Supported by Canadian charities, diplomats, and visitors without government help, the school taught kindergarten to grade 3 or 4. New buildings had been completed in 1963, and it was hoping to expand.[84] She grilled the teachers about clothing, food, supplies, and medical attention. So impressed was she with this project and its potential that she convinced her colleagues and Tony Law to leave one of *Cape Scott*'s newly stitched flags with the ambassador for the school.[85] METEI members flew back to Cartagena and their ship that same evening.

But the two youngest members, Jim Nielsen (alias Kon-Tiki-Iti-Iti) and Jack Mathias (alias Santiago), left the group in Bogotá and set out together on a wild ramble. As they exited the plane, they were greeted by a huge crowd and many journalists; their pictures graced the front page of a local paper, which claimed that they were part of an unrelated story – yet another instance of mistaken identity, Nielsen's trademark all along. A professor of protozoology, Roberto Galán, whom they met at a cocktail party, put them up for several days, loaning them his silk shirts for parties. At the suggestion of his neighbour, anthropology professor Gerardo Reichel-Dolmatoff, they went down the Magdalena River in a dugout canoe with two Indigenous paddlers to Puerto Nare. Then they made their way overland across the mountains by taxi and train, travelling through Colombia and Venezuela en route to Trinidad. As they slept on a beach at Güiria, they were arrested by "a belligerent crowd of one mayor, thirty villagers, and three soldiers, heavily armed with a rifle each."[86] Letters of recommendation that they carried from the Colombian police and professors did not constitute the "get-out-of-jail-free cards" that they had anticipated.[87] They were held in the small prison for three days and then driven six hours in a paddy wagon to Cumana, where their papers were inspected, and from there overnight to Caracas. Then their captors quietly released them, simply by leaving the truck unattended and its back door open. With American embassy help, they reached Jamaica and then flew to Florida. Jack crossed North America driving a new Lincoln Continental for delivery to its purchaser in Vancouver. Jim went home to start medical school in New York City.

Everyone else carried on to Halifax. This time, the Atlantic journey was uneventful. Both Helen and Cléopâtre commented on the improved shipboard atmosphere with the Panamanian departures.[88] Helen was "thrilled" to learn that her husband was to become dean and, in advance, would enjoy a travelling professorship around the world as a sabbatical.[89] But feeling old, outclassed, and thwarted, she pleaded with him for a position or a title: "Can't you get me an appointment of some kind at the hospital? ... no remuneration or anything. It sounds dreadful and distresses me that when the press and everyone [asks] where do you come from, I will have to say 'nowhere,' and they always ask too ... Come on now, just one year, honorary and I will sign something when I get home."[90] She reminded him that she expected to complete a scholarly study of the Easter Island children. Her family insists that Dr Reid would have understood that her husband had been joking when he replied that his secretary was leaving, "so I'll be in the market for another secretary – why don't you apply?"[91]

CANADA AGAIN

Al Tunis had been orchestrating a splendid dockside reception with dense media coverage at Halifax. Dignitaries on hand to greet *Cape Scott* included the unofficial head of the navy, Flag Officer Atlantic Coast Rear Admiral Landymore; Nova Scotia's lieutenant governor, Henry Poole McKeen; Mrs Gerd Hurum of the METEI Foundation; and Member of Parliament Dr Stanley Haidasz, who had hitched a ride on an air force plane. Regrets came from the Chilean ambassador and Dr Ray Farquharson, head of the Medical Research Council. Hundreds assembled at the jetty, including many family members of the crew.[92]

The whole event went off perfectly. *Cape Scott* docked around 9:00 a.m. on 17 March. A press conference took place in her wardroom with standing room only. Commander Law presided, introducing the speakers. Tunis's program notes have Skoryna's name added with an annotation as an afterthought.[93] Both Law and Skoryna spoke for ten minutes, and then Helen Reid, Al Taylor, Georges Nógrády, Armand Boudreault, and Hal Gibbs each had five minutes before the session opened for questions. Law ended the event with a flourish by throwing open the bar. Forty people enjoyed a delicious lunch ashore at Admiralty House. Lieutenant Governor McKeen wrote to McGill principal Rocke Robertson on 19 March to assure him that all was well.[94] A truck was loaded with the luggage of those going on by train. Wags aboard *Cape Scott* sent delivery instructions by telex in verse.[95]

When the travellers reached Montreal on 19 March, they held another news conference in the train station; a photo of Boudreault, Nógrády, and Skoryna – all wearing hats and holding a wooden Rapanui sword – graced the write-up.[96] Two weeks later, Skoryna told the Canadian Club about his bid to have Chile change the name of Motu Nui (without a flag) to "McGill Island."[97] On the evening of Wednesday, 7 April, he gave a public lecture in the Leacock Building at McGill for the Faculty of Graduate Studies and Research.[98] The newspapers reported for many

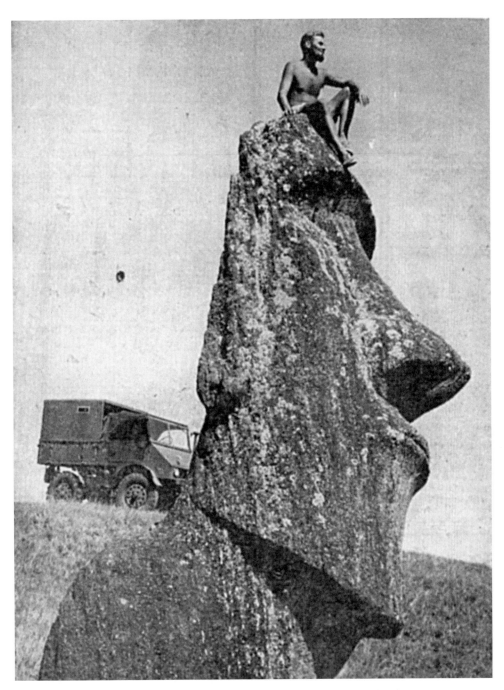

Figure 8.16 Dr Peter Beighton atop a moai. Macfarlane, "Most Islanders Free,"
sec. 4, 1.

days, and David Macfarlane wrote articles for *McGill News* and the *Montreal Star*, keeping some personal interest stories in reserve until June. Jane Shaw, Sally Archer, and the parents of Archie Wilkinson, David Murphy, and Jim Nielsen had been clipping all the items that they could find. One lavishly illustrated story featured a big photo of Peter Beighton atop a *moai* – appropriately so, as the English doctor was still on Rapa Nui (figure 8.16).[99]

With *Cape Scott*'s safe return and the journey complete, many seemed to think that that was the end of METEI. But much more was to come. Bills had to be paid. Skoryna began combining the draft reports typed on *Cape Scott* into his formal "Preliminary Report," full of pride and promise and devoid of recommendations. Law contributed a short report and Isabel Griffiths and Anna Maria Eccles did more typing. John Cutler kept working on the census. The research materials and results had to be analyzed and reported in the scientific literature before Skoryna could write a final synthesis. Slipping beneath the radar at this time of relief and homecoming was the crucial question of when and how to launch the second half of the project – the return journey for METEI-2 – in order to study the changes wrought by the forthcoming airport.

Stanley's dream may have become "reality," as Carlotta Hacker said, but it was far from over. Fed up with the constant squabbling and skeptical about the worth of what they had done, METEI team members had been surprised and buoyed up by the keen interest of scientists in the Bogotá seminar. It reminded them how their journey had been a unique privilege; it proclaimed the precious value of the information and materials that they had gathered; and it demonstrated their collective responsibility to have the results published. Notwithstanding Stanley's grandiose assertions of a "complete success," by March 1965, METEI had reached somewhat less than 50 per cent of its mandate.

PART THREE

The Products of METEI, March 1965 to 2017

9

Personal and Popular Results

The multiple independent draft reports composed on HMCS *Cape Scott* were typed by Isabel Griffiths and Anna Maria Eccles and assembled into a "Preliminary Report" of some seventy-five double-spaced, typewritten pages.[1] Stanley Skoryna excluded many of the travellers' recommendations and Denys Montandon's report on the health of the Chileans. By 23 March he was distributing it widely to, among others, Prime Minister Lester B. Pearson, Minister of Defence Paul Hellyer, McGill University principal Rocke Robertson, politician and champion of the Medical Expedition to Easter Island Dr Stanley Haidasz, the Medical Research Council, Chilean and Canadian diplomats, and probably the World Health Organization. Each METEI traveller and many *Cape Scott* sailors received a copy too.

But a final report never appeared. This chapter and the next four serve as a stand-in for that nonexistent document by tracking the more than 130 popular and scientific publications and unpublished research papers that resulted from the METEI work (see appendix A). They also explore the reasons why a final report was not written. I begin with the popular accounts, which appeared quickly, and in the next chapters move on to the scientific papers, which came more slowly, if they were published at all.

PERSONAL CHANGES

The Rapa Nui Science Club, formed with nostalgic ceremony aboard *Cape Scott* on 18 February 1965, was gently nurtured by Carlotta Hacker and Isabel Griffiths. They composed sporadic issues of the club's *Newsletter* from 28 April 1965 to 28 August 1967, bringing updates from Easter Island and the travellers, along with revised address lists.[2] Jokes, crossword puzzles, and thinly veiled satire permeated the prose:

canned meat on pumpernickel, silly raffles for stamped METEI postcards, and "100%" everything. They sent out an all-points bulletin searching for Peter Beighton. Having left Easter Island on 3 April, he turned up on a five-week expedition with the British army in the Sahara Desert in August.[3]

By August 1965, Richard and Maureen Roberts had moved to Ottawa for Richard to take up a position at National Defence Headquarters. Under the heading of "Births, Engagements, and Infections," Carlotta and Isabel announced the arrival of the Montandons' daughter, Lydia Ariane, and of Bob Meier's baby boy, "to be named 'Scott' for a certain ship"; and they described the strange *kokong-algia* that afflicted returnees. Occasional METEI reunions with the energetic consumption of "pisco sours" were duly noted.[4]

Rapa Nui exerted its romantic effect on travellers, leading some to alter their états civils. Colin Gillingham was engaged by late 1965, and a photo of him with his fiancé, Françoise, made the rounds. Charles Westropp was presented as an eligible young man to the Roberts's daughter, Susan, but "it didn't take." He soon found a "more suitable" bride, and Tony Law gave the happy couple one of his Rapa Nui paintings, still cherished in their family home. Even quiet Archie Wilkinson reversed his comfortable bachelor status in October 1965 by marrying Sally Archer, the pretty X-ray technologist, twenty years his junior, who had presided over the Royal Victoria Hospital's radiology unit during his absence. Sally helped Archie prepare the 3,450 Rapanui X-ray films for reporting. Before the journey, she had been fond of him and he knew it; however, he had resisted the idea of marriage because of the age gap. Easter Island changed his mind.

To Carlotta's disappointment, filmmaker Red Lemieux dropped his New York City girlfriend and went back to his wife and children. Compounding her misery, Carlotta slipped on the Montreal ice and fractured her leg. She returned to England in late 1965, but she was back in Canada by mid-1966. She began dating various eligible young men, but none really pleased her, although she confided in Helen Reid that she had a hankering to marry.[5]

THE POPULAR ACCOUNTS

The first publications emerging from METEI served a public eager to read stories about the mysterious island. On 1 May 1965, David Macfarlane's big cover story with colour photographs appeared in *Weekend Magazine*, a weekly syndicated in forty-one newspapers with a readership of over

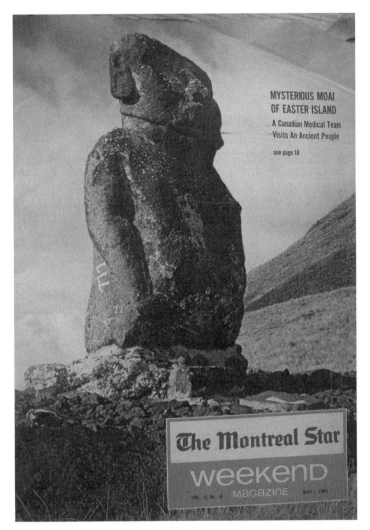

Figure 9.1 *Moai* on cover of *Weekend Magazine*, story by David B. Macfarlane, 1 May 1965. This *moai* was erected by Rapanui for Thor Heyerdahl at Anakena. Murphy Papers.

2 million across Canada. Macfarlane's title might not have pleased Skoryna, but it attracted attention: "Mysterious Moai of Easter Island: A Canadian Medical Team Visits an Ancient People" (figure 9.1).[6] Helen Reid published her long-planned illustrated account for *Maclean's* magazine in the issue of 19 June 1965.[7] She corresponded with Skoryna and Carlotta Hacker in Montreal, looking for pictures of people at work; in

reply, Hacker sent the most "suitable" of the images taken by Isabel and Skoryna, but they had few photos of people working. Through Carlotta, Stanley asked that she return them quickly, as he had a talk to give soon. He urged her to find a picture of Camp Hilton with the ATCO name visible to allay hard feelings over the $50,000 debt. At the very least, could she please mention ATCO in the text "favorably of course!"[8] In her *Maclean's* article, Reid acknowledged the Canadian navy, government, and industries, but did not name ATCO; however, her personal papers show that the article had already gone to press by the time she received Skoryna's request.[9] The article provoked a flood of congratulations from METEI members and questions from unknown readers who wanted to join the promised follow-up expedition. Many questions also came in response to her atmospheric and anonymous phrase about "couples slipping into the night." Unapologetic, Reid thought she had handled the matter "delicately"; "if it is alright, correct and proper to behave in a certain way, then why are you ashamed to have it told?"[10]

Simultaneous with Reid's account, the French-language version of *Maclean's* published Armand Boudreault's own story of the journey, featuring a photograph of him in his lab. He too described the expedition, the work, and the promise of a return visit, and he delved into the political unrest and election of Alfonso Rapu.[11]

Skoryna published next to nothing on METEI. All along he had made it clear that he was not conducting research himself; rather, he was fostering the conditions that would permit others to do so. Always attentive to influential people and the optics of good publicity, he began pestering the prime minister's office for an appointment to deliver the Easter Island gifts. Pearson annotated an internal reminder that people are waiting for a rendezvous to give over the gifts: "First I ever heard of it. Who *are* these people?" His secretary reminded him of METEI, his support, and the earlier requests, but now the file was lost. After days of scrambling between Pearson's office and his aides Jim Coutts and Jules Pelletier, Skoryna was told that he would hear soon about an appointment.[12] When he finally obtained the coveted invitation, Skoryna leaned on Tony Law to join him for the little ceremony at 24 Sussex Drive, Ottawa. Law obliged, and the newspapers and photojournalists captured them presenting Prime Minister Pearson with the large Cava Cava Man carving, shell necklaces, and a grass skirt – gifts of the islanders – on Friday, 16 July 1965 (figure 9.2).[13]

On 27 June a small delegation had presented Defence Minister Paul Hellyer with the stone carving. Press photos show "the man who sent the ship" smiling with Helen Reid and Richard and Maureen Roberts as

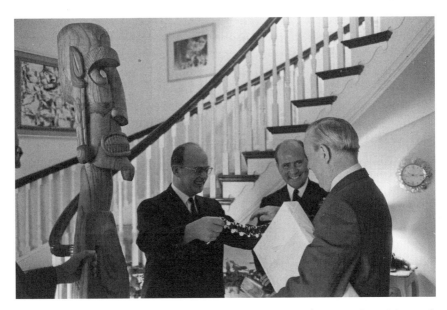

Figure 9.2 Stanley Skoryna (*left*) and Tony Law present the Cava Cava Man and other gifts to Prime Minister Lester B. Pearson at 22 Sussex Drive, 16 July 1965. LAC, Photograph Room, file 28, box 03764.1, negative sleeve 10385, July 1965.

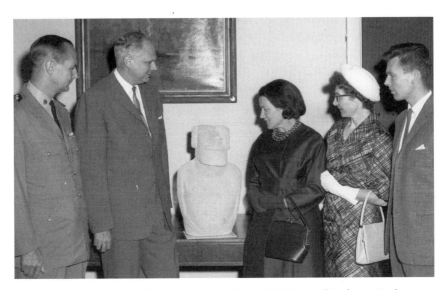

Figure 9.3 Presentation of stone moai carving to Minister of Defence Paul Hellyer. *From left*, Richard Roberts, Paul Hellyer, Helen Reid, Maureen Roberts, and unknown, 27 June 1965. National Defence Photograph. Reid Papers, file 1.

they admire the squat *moai*.[14] The ladies are gloved and holding purses; Maureen wears a hat (figure 9.3). But Hellyer's smile would fade when the auditor general's report of February 1966 deemed the $215,000 cost of the navy's contribution to be a "questionable" use of defence funds.[15] Members of Parliament demanded answers in the House of Commons, both during and after the expedition, about the government's contribution. The minister was embarrassed; he replied that he did not know the cost, as METEI was not under the auspices of the navy.[16] This scrutiny did not help the problem of METEI's debt, and it guaranteed that no financial relief would come from the government.

In August 1965, Carlotta Hacker described the expedition and political upheaval in a newspaper report and in a bilingual article for *Canadian Nurse*, later confessing to Helen her disappointment that the journal offered no honorarium.[17] Everyone was eager to see what Carl Mydans would produce for *Life* and anxious for the lifting of the publication embargo on everyone else. The promised date was September or October 1965.

Serving those hungry readers around the world, some METEI travellers succumbed to requests from newspapers and magazines in their home countries. Cléopâtre Montandon wrote a general interest article in Greek, her mother tongue, about METEI and Easter Island. Respecting the *Life* embargo, it appeared in the April 1966 issue of a popular newsmagazine out of Athens.[18] The numerous illustrations were photographs that she and Denys had taken while on the island. Björn Ekblom and Einar Gjessing also published articles in their native Sweden and Norway; but to Einar's dismay, the publishers sent them to press sooner than the embargo allowed.[19] In Oslo, Eivind Myhre invited Thor Heyerdahl to dinner for a personal update on Rapa Nui. He received visits from Chilean ex-governor John Martin and later from *Cape Scott* navigator Charles Westropp, who came to Norway aboard the aircraft carrier HMCS *Bonaventure*.

The illustrated slide talk was a common practice for METEI returnees. Although they may not have resulted in scholarly publications, these events usually received wide coverage in local media, testifying to the early 1960s popularity of the "travelogue." Richard and Maureen Roberts, Eivind Myhre, John Easton, David Murphy, George Hrischenko, Helen Reid, Georges Nógrády, and Stanley Skoryna were called upon often to describe the adventure, drawing on their extensive personal slide collections. Isabel was broadcast in Spanish to South America. The navy personnel were popular speakers too, including Fred Joyce, Mary King, and Chief Petty Officer Harry Crosman, who alone had delivered thirty lectures by May 1965.[20] With his deep voice and dry sense of humour, Archie Wilkinson also received many invitations to describe METEI to Rotary Clubs, church groups, and radiography technologists in Montreal, Maine, and along the upper St Lawrence River, near Prescott, where he and Sally moved after he retired. Archie screened an 8-millimetre film and showed his 35-millimetre slides, which he kept in carousels, always ready for the next appearance; his collection featured portraits of Rapanui people and their X-rays, a form of radiographic storytelling. Local papers would describe his talks both before and after they took place. Ian Efford and Jack Mathias sometimes performed as a duet. Once with his back to the screen, Ian was perplexed when his audience suddenly exploded in laughter. Jack had "sabotaged" the slides by inserting an image of the speaker, nude but for a champagne bottle positioned strategically.

Helen Reid addressed the Royal Canadian Institute in Convocation Hall at the University of Toronto and a pediatrics conference in Vermont, but she had to decline requests to publish or "digest" her *Maclean's* article for American journals, explicitly blaming her refusal on Carl Mydans and the *Life* contract imposed on METEI by Skoryna. In early December 1965, she spoke at the annual meeting of the Laboratory Section of the Canadian Public Health Association. Identified, once again, as "the wife of A.L. Chute," she delivered an "entertaining" luncheon speech, illustrated with "abundant" and "excellent" coloured slides.[21]

HELEN REID'S BOOK

By May 1965, possibly earlier, Ryerson Press had approached Reid about writing a popular book in time for Christmas sales. Her detailed diary and the notes from her interviews meant that she had plenty of material to draw on. She wrote to Skoryna about the opportunity, still uncertain it would be realized; she asked him to keep it quiet, signing her missive, "Love, Helen."[22] The affection would soon evaporate. She began asking her friends among the fellow travellers for photographs, especially of people at work. Because of the *Life* embargo, she asked for another "release" form, like the statement Skoryna had signed for her *Maclean's* essay; helpfully, she supplied a draft statement and asked for its return with his signature. She expected the book to coincide with, or follow, Mydans's *Life* article (still anticipated for October 1965); its timing would honour the spirit of the agreement. In any case, Ryerson was a *Canadian* publisher and the contract did permit publishing in Canada. During the ensuing silence, Carlotta alerted Helen that Skoryna did not wish to sign. When pushed, he claimed that he did not have "author-ity" and that she needed to appeal to lawyer R.F. Laing and the Easter Island Expedition Society. For his part, Laing claimed that he did not have "authority" with Skoryna out of town, and the indebted society demanded any proceeds that her book might earn.[23]

Reid was aghast. She fired off a blistering letter, tracing the history of her involvement with METEI: how Skoryna had engaged her *for* her writing, how she had served METEI by gathering donations in excess of $4,000, how she had supplied all her own medical equipment and covered all her own expenses, including trips to Ottawa and Montreal to meet with Hellyer and Skoryna both before and after the expedition. (She did not know that Skoryna had paid for Maureen's visit to New York City.) She reminded him that while on the island, most METEI scientists had enjoyed the support and salaries of home institutions, whereas she had worked unremunerated the entire time. After the deduction of her expenses, little would remain from the hypothetical royalties. Furthermore, because of the rules about children and women, and because Maureen and Richard Roberts had both refused to work overtime, she had worked harder and done more physical examinations than any other medical member.[24] She also reminded the METEI leaders that there would have been no *Cape Scott* and no expedition without her.[25]

Goaded by fury and humiliation, she finished the book in just six weeks. In late June 1965 she brought the entire 200-page manuscript to Montreal and sat silently in Laing's outer office while Skoryna and Laing read it and what she suspected was a tape recorder hissed nearby.[26] At first, they wanted her to delay publication until Skoryna's own final report had appeared. Then they agreed to publication simultaneous with Mydans's article but demanded that she give half her royalties to the indebted expedition.[27] Ryerson Press needed her to sign the contract expeditiously in order to publish by Christmas.

Helen offered Laing a $300 flat fee for release from all obligations. She pointed out that the work was not scientific but a "chatty," "feminine" memoir aimed at general readers – and, again, noted that Ryerson was a *Canadian* press, one unaffected by the embargo.[28] It was baffling. Skoryna had been eager for publicity to prompt donors. Why would he oppose this book? The original "approved" manuscript now lies in an envelope, on which she scrawled, "S-the bastard, I should have let him sue me."[29]

Helen complained about her legal travails to other METEI alumni with whom she corresponded about images for her book. They replied with sympathy and accounts of their own frustrations with Skoryna. Mary King reported that he had instructed her to "hang on to the

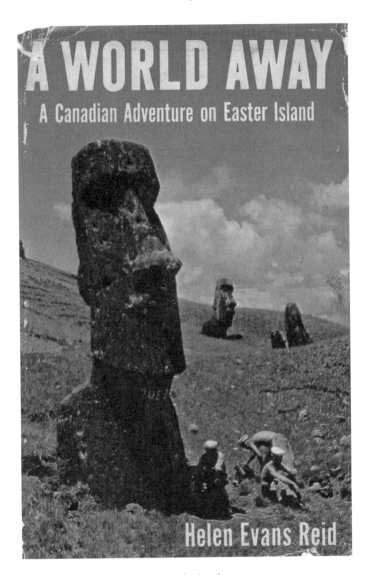

Figure 9.4 Cover of Helen Reid's book, 1965.

portraits" and her other photographs: "He doesn't want anyone to have anything."[30] Armand Boudreault released the first of several impressive scientific papers quickly (see chapter 11). He told Helen that he did not bother to ask for permission; he simply published as he wished and sent Stanley a reprint.[31] Perhaps she was being overly scrupulous in seeking the signed release. But well before the journey, Skoryna had engaged her *as a writer* on advice from seasoned editors, and she had warned him long ago about the risks of signing away world rights. She was annoyed.

A World Away was released in late November 1965 and advertised as an ideal Christmas gift at $4.95 (figure 9.4). To her enormous surprise and vindication, it proved popular in Canada, Australia, and New Zealand and went into a second Toronto printing two years later. The lure of Rapa Nui and Reid's well-written prose, with humour and human interest, no doubt enhanced sales. It still commands respectable prices in the used-book trade and is frequently cited by scholars of the political history of Rapa Nui as a key source on Rapu's rebellion. Historians tend to overlook her chapter "In Defence of Chile," in which she tried to explain the difficulties and expenses of maintaining the health and education of the islanders. Some writers help themselves to Reid's photographs without credit. The women's section of a Melbourne newspaper marvelled how "Mrs. A.L. Chute" could produce a book in six weeks. She explained that she had been under pressure to have the book ready to coincide with Carl Mydans's anticipated article in *Life* magazine.[32] But Reid's success was not popular with METEI leaders in Montreal; they retaliated with pettiness and petulance. Skoryna refused to place flyers for her book at a McGill open house with a session devoted to METEI.[33]

MORE PUBLICATIONS: MYDANS AND HACKER

As it turned out, Reid beat Mydans. His long-anticipated article did not appear in *Life* until 4 February 1966, beautifully illustrated with his excellent photographs. He had prepared it quickly; however, editorial decisions beyond his control had bumped it to the end of a series about science. He confided to Tony Law that Skoryna was "upset" by the delay because he had been hoping that the article would leverage more funds for the nagging debt.[34] Given that the *Life* magazine contract had forbidden any METEI reporting outside Canada, the delay was particularly galling to the Montreal organizers and other METEI members.[35] *Life* may also have tried to restrict publication within Canada, but with two Canadian filmmakers and a journalist travelling with METEI, their costs paid by the Canadian Broadcasting Corporation (CBC), the National Film Board (NFB), and a newspaper, the magazine backed down. According to agreements signed at departure, Canadian photographers and journalists were permitted to distribute their material only in Canada. *Life* retained the world rights to everything else.

After the appearance of Mydans's article, Al Tunis wrote to inquire if his many *unused* images would be available. Mydans refused, blaming the magazine.[36] Whether it was his doing or not, the embargo, the delay, and the lack of generosity garnered even more enemies for the famous photographer among the METEI alumni, who had put up with what they felt was his superior attitude and constant intrusion into their work. Many of his unused photographs can now been seen on the *Life* website. They are indeed beautiful – but few METEI members ever saw these wonderful pictures of themselves; those who did see them waited half a century.[37]

Carlotta Hacker in Montreal was well aware of the parlous state of METEI's books, and initially she defended the official stance. She chastised Helen for being unkind in her book to navy doctor Richard Roberts, whose stiff rigidity and military formality (you could "never" call him "Dick") Helen had contrasted with Stanley's creativity and utter imprecision.[38] "Dick!" Carlotta wrote.[39] The Robertses' daughter, Susan, remembers that her father so hated the book that he refused to have it in the house. Drawing attention to the fragile finances, Carlotta also worried that auditors would find fault with her inexpert accounting of the "blasted books."[40] By late 1965, however, she revealed her own disgust with the whole business. She had been "ghostwriting" Skoryna's book, which may have been a popular account or "final report"; we do not know. Here, then, was another reason why Stanley opposed Helen's book and the sharing of METEI memories. But Carlotta was exasperated because Stanley was writing "fiction." For example, he claimed that the virtuous expedition had not "corrupted" the islanders by bringing alcohol. "Firstly, we did take alcohol, and secondly they had it anyway and drank with discretion." She removed the false passages, but Skoryna put them back. She quit her job and announced her return to England. Now, she claimed, she had joined the ranks of those about whom Skoryna spread lies: he began criticizing her writing abilities to anyone who would listen.[41] Ironically, Carlotta is well known as a gifted, insightful writer, editor, and historian.

Hacker would publish her own popular book about the journey and her adventures masquerading as an indefatigable research assistant. *And Christmas Day on Easter Island* appeared in London, England, in 1968 (figure 9.5). She described her two restless *wanderjahrs*, from Karachi to Australia to Rapa Nui, and her shameless lobbying of Stanley Skoryna for inclusion in his expedition. METEI occupies the last third of the narrative. Thin on names, it is nevertheless one of the best-written sources about the ambience of the political situation and about social life on the ship and in the *campamento*. Together with Reid's *A World Away*, it remains a popular travel book.

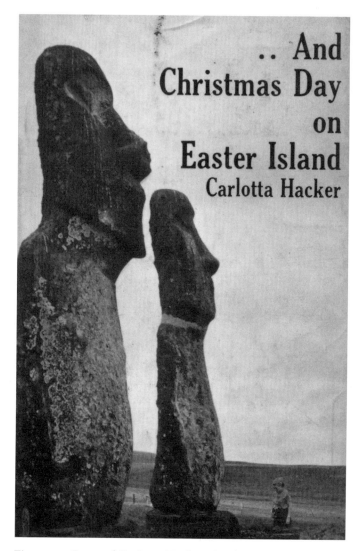

.. And Christmas Day on Easter Island
Carlotta Hacker

Figure 9.5 Cover of Carlotta Hacker's book, 1968. Dr Reid at Ahu Akivi.

With their gentle humility over the encounter with a "colonial frontier," both books correspond well to the genre of scientific and sentimental travel writing described by Mary Louise Pratt as a "large-scale effort to decolonize knowledge."[42] Because METEI's final report never appeared, their scientific content, small though it was, loomed larger than planned.

METEI'S DEBT

In October 1965, capitalizing on his July meeting, Skoryna wrote a "personal and confidential" letter to Prime Minister Pearson that claimed he had been contacted by the new governor; he asked "for Canadian assistance to Easter Islanders ... to purchase surplus goods, which could be useful and improve conditions." He wanted a prime ministerial referral to the Crown Assets Disposal Agency. His letter was forwarded, but no funds emerged.[43] Skoryna made appearances at a few symposia, organized by others, where he would outline the objectives and tout the "100 per cent success" of METEI. He spent three weeks giving lectures on gastric ulcer disease in Chile and Argentina and was decorated with the Order of Bernardo O'Higgins, the highest civilian honour accorded to non-Chileans. Meanwhile, the postcards and stamps failed to sell, accumulating in the travellers' papers.[44] During 1965, 1966, and well into 1967, Skoryna went on numerous junkets, speaking about METEI and raising funds for his debt; he appeared at the Canadian Club of Montreal and at the Royal Military College in St Jean, Quebec, and he presented to groups of McGill alumni in Ottawa, Hartford, New York City, Minneapolis, Rochester in Minnesota, Port Arthur in Ontario – and probably elsewhere too.[45] On 6 April 1966, he delivered a speech in Montreal on the "Contributions of Industry" to METEI at a reception to honour travellers and thank (unpaid) "donors," basically indicating which invoices had not been (and would not be) paid.[46] He urged Law to attend that event too.[47]

Also in 1966, possibly by invitation, Skoryna composed a five-page essay for the glossy magazine *Abbottempo*, published by Abbott Laboratories pharmaceutical company.[48] Featuring medicine, science, and culture, *Abbottempo* was not a peer-reviewed journal; however, it had attracted contributions from several medical luminaries, including Sheila Sherlock, Wilhem J. Kolff, and Kurt Isselbacher. It is possible that these articles generated large honoraria for their authors from the drug company. The reprint made a handy, colourful item to leave with potential donors. Every METEI member was sent one or more copies. Only in comparing the photographs in that journal with the slides of the travellers does it become clear that Skoryna had "doctored" some images to imply that a large sign in recognition of the Canadian company Alcan had graced one of the laboratory trailers (figure 9.6). The sign might have been added in late January. In Helen Reid's papers is another more obviously doctored photograph showing ATCO-style trailers under construction in a suburban lot with the names "Merck Sharp & Dohme"

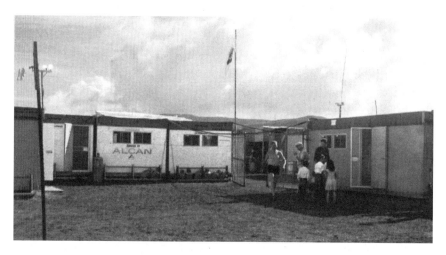

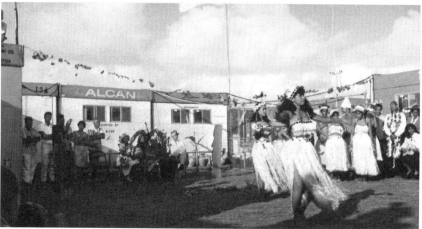

Figure 9.6 Stanley Skoryna's "doctored" photos showing varying Alcan labels on a laboratory trailer, with a *sau sau* following baptism (*above*). Compare figure 5.2, where the trailor has no sign at all. Skoryna, "Operation METEI," 1966.

and "Mead Johnson & Company" inscribed on their roofs in ballpoint pen (figure 9.7).[49] Tiny stencilled acknowledgments to Merck and two other companies (unreadable) appear in photos of the three examination trailers but never with the prominence donors had been promised.

Always looking for strategies to raise funds, Skoryna advertised a raffle in journals and announced it at the close of his speech to 600 McGill alumni gathered in Ottawa (figure 9.8).[50] Purchasers of a ticket stood a chance to win a free trip for two to Easter Island. When psychologist June

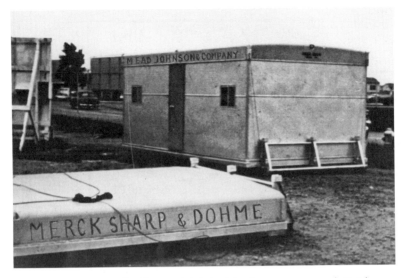

Figure 9.7 "Doctored" photo with inked-in donor names, nd. Reid Papers, file 11.

Pimm heard this surprise announcement, she said to a friend, "I hope Gordon has enough sense not to buy a ticket." But her husband, Gordon Pimm, was president of the local McGill Alumni Association, and having organized the Ottawa event, he felt obliged to purchase a ticket. News reports suggest that the Chilean ambassador pulled Pimm's name "at random" out of a hat.[51] But now both June and Gordon wonder if Stanley had rigged the result. June was a doctoral candidate in psychology "addicted to research." Upon first meeting her, Skoryna expressed regret that METEI had taken no psychologist. Notwithstanding her fear of flying, June saw a golden opportunity to turn her husband's windfall into a fascinating adventure, and Skoryna imagined yet more publicity. The scientific results of their lottery journey appear in chapter 11.

Skoryna did not pay METEI bills unless he had to. He maintained a list of accounts that, he decided, could be ignored, hoping the creditors might forget about them.[52] He staged "thank you" receptions to those who forgave debts and used them to curry media attention, which he applied to convincing others to do the same. He sent a personal bill for $936 to filmmaker Bob Williams for the cost of accommodating and feeding him on the island, but the CBC refused to pay, and Stanley was "furious."[53] Skoryna leaned on Charles Fowler to drop in on Ron Southern at ATCO in Calgary when he happened to be in Alberta to ask that the large debt

> **FREE TRIP TO EASTER ISLAND !**
>
> To pay for the trailers, which were given to the Pascuenses as hospital facilities, the Easter Island Expedition is offering the two following opportunities:
>
> **Free Return Trip to Easter Island**
>
> By becoming an Associate of the Easter Island Expedition Society, at the cost of $1.00, you stand a chance of being the lucky person to go to Easter Island next year. This entails a flight to Chile for two people, via Canadian Pacific Airways and then a short voyage on the supply ship. All arrangements will be made by the Society. If you don't want to go all the way to the island, you can remain in Chile for your holiday.
>
> Applications should be made to:
>
> Medical Expedition to Easter Island,
> Donner Building,
> 3640 University Street,
> Montreal 2, Quebec.
>
> A self-addressed stamped envelope should be enclosed.
>
> **Special Souvenir Postcards**
>
> A limited supply of special Expedition postcards is still available. Each bears an Expedition seal in addition to the Chilean postage stamp. The cards are the first ever to be cancelled on Easter Island, and may be obtained by sending one dollar, plus six cents postage, to the above address.

Figure 9.8 "Free Trip to Easter Island,"
Canadian Nurse 61 (August 1965): 640.

be forgiven. Fowler had the impression that Southern thought repayment was hopeless, although the company did not want to give up.

Skoryna never paid the promised stipends, nor did he reimburse expenses of the students and trainees who had joined METEI as researchers. Einar Gjessing still needed to complete his medical education and had borrowed from his father, but the promised $2,000 to support his travel and time on Easter Island failed to appear. Isabel Griffiths quietly arranged to send Einar $500 from the dwindling coffers in Montreal, a fraction of what he was owed but for which he is still very grateful. Björn Ekblom never received a penny. Peter Beighton had similar problems. He wrote to Jim Nielsen, "That bastard Skoryna still hasn't come round with my money. I write weekly using increasingly forceful and derogatory language, so far without effect! I hope you are having better luck."[54] Eventually, Beighton was reimbursed for the cost of his journey home but not for his time.

Finally, an audit on 14 November 1966 by Touche, Ross, Bailey, and Smart indicated that the METEI's debt to the ATCO company for the twenty-four trailers had been discharged by a large donation from the McConnell Foundation.[55] In the meantime, Skoryna had returned to his clinical work and his lab at St Mary's Hospital, where he continued to explore the role of trace elements in health and disease. Stanley's widow, Jane, recalls that "he had to earn a living," and his METEI performances were exhausting. He was relieved when they could stop, but he was proud that "100 per cent" of his bills were paid.

THE FILMS

Two films came out of the expedition. The first, *Canadian Expedition to Easter Island*, in black and white and an hour long, was completed for the CBC by Bob Williams, with sound by George Hrischenko.[56] The second, *Island Observed*, in colour and a half-hour long, was filmed and directed by Red Lemieux for the NFB.

Williams's film aired in the summer of 1965 and received a nasty review for not being romantic enough by Roy Shields, television critic of the *Toronto Star*. Nevertheless, offers to purchase it came from McGill, the British Broadcasting Corporation, the Australian Broadcasting Corporation, and the Educational Television Network. As described in chapters 5 and 7, Richard Roberts stands stiffly as the uneasy "MC" in the centre of Camp Hilton, trying not to read from his script as he introduces his colleagues. Williams himself was "not overly happy" with his work: he told Helen Reid that the sound could have been better and that it was "too technical or medical with not enough travelogue or pretty pictures," although that was what he had been charged to create.[57] This film has the tremendous advantage of documenting the scientists' accounts of their work in their own voices in situ, and it was extremely useful for this book.

Lemieux's film, in contrast, is very different: colourful, romantic, aspirational, and inspirational. He did not have a sound crew. In fact, every sound – scratching, typing, animal noises, the clinking of laboratory glassware, and music of guitar and accordion – was added post hoc behind an authoritative male voiceover.[58] When it was nearing completion in the fall of 1965, Skoryna, Isabel, and Carlotta were invited to a private viewing at the NFB office. Still bruised from Red's decision to return to his family, Carlotta asked if he would be present and was assured that he was "away in Lebanon." In a hilarious letter, she described the day for Helen Reid. Carlotta wore a dress that she'd made of red fabric, originally purchased, but deemed "too good," for a bedspread; the considerable leftovers she had passed on to Isabel. Of course, they both appeared clad in the same red bedspread, and the absurdity sent them into hysterics. The NFB editor apologized "in a jolly way" that unfortunately Carlotta had been cut out of the film "over the weekend." She responded in a "jolly way," but was "wild" with anger. Then halfway through the viewing, Lemieux slipped into the theatre and sat directly behind her. Everyone, including Skoryna, was now watching Carlotta, who vacillated between laughter and fury. "It is frightfully annoying to be cut out of a film 'over the weekend'!! 'We had to take you out last week' doesn't sound so insulting!!" But despite her vexation, she had to admit that it was a very good film.[59] Lemieux relented. The final version was revised to add a few seconds' close-up of a mirthful, unidentified Carlotta working in the lab. Release was set for March 1966, and it was shown across Canada on 30 September 1966.[60]

But the differences between these two films run much deeper than tone, colour, length, and sound. They codify the tensions in the camp by selective inclusions of whom they portray and name, although only the travellers were likely to notice. Both address *kokongo*, but only Lemieux includes the rebellion, the Chilean marines, and images of Rapu walking in a crowd of women. Carlotta told Helen that, in addition to herself, only Cléopâtre was excluded from Red's film: "it can't be accidental." Indeed, just as he had threatened on the island, Lemieux settled some scores. His narrator identified by name only John Cutler, Stanley Skoryna, Helen Reid, Denys Montandon, Maureen Roberts, Peter Beighton, Isabel Griffiths, Armand Boudreault, Björn Ekblom, and Ian Efford. Unidentified glimpses appeared of Georges Nógrády, Einar Gjessing, Tony Law, Garry Brody, David Murphy, Eivind Myhre, Fred Joyce, Hal Gibbs, Richard Roberts, Elliot Alpert, Gonzalo Donoso, Rita Dwyer, Al Taylor, possibly Jim Nielsen, and later Carlotta Hacker. Completely absent from the film was Cléopâtre Montandon, as Carlotta noticed, but also Jack Mathias, John Easton, Ana Maria Eccles, most navy personnel (Harry Crosman, Robert Fulton, and Mary King), and his media rivals, Carl Mydans, George Hrischenko, and Bob Williams. Red's friends John Cutler and Isabel Griffiths appear multiple times – in fact, Cutler seems to be the leader, and Lemieux opens with him, "a doctor from California" conducting his census. From the splendid baptismal scene of the handsome godparents, bearded John with Isabel in black lace, Red later produced the still image that he called "the Spanish wedding."

In Lemieux's film, Skoryna, Nógrády, Reid, and the unnamed Richard Roberts look ridiculous. Reid is identified, looking lost, as she wanders the camp opening doors, seeking (but not finding) some unknown person or thing. Following the baptism scene of John and Isabel, Skoryna is shown in his little feather headdress without Helen Reid, but the identical reason – godparents at an *earlier* baptism – is distorted and situated in the *next* week, although Skoryna and Reid's baptismal event had preceded theirs. Nógrády (unnamed) stumbles into the sea wearing his pith helmet. Unidentified Roberts – leader of the medical examinations – is seen rolling his tongue and encouraging a patient to do the same in examining the cranial nerves, while the narrator explains that, to the islanders, some things seemed "silly." In closing, the narrator suggested that METEI might return in three years and spoke of "mysteries giving way to the probing eye of science" – with findings that "may be less melodramatic, but in the end, more useful to mankind."

Not only did Williams include scenes with all the scientific and navy team members, most identified by name, but he also had ambient sound and allowed fifteen of the travellers to speak for themselves on Hrischenko's recording, while images portrayed them or their colleagues performing the work. He deferred to Roberts, given centre stage, and Skoryna. He allowed the latter to summarize what he thought were the benefits of METEI, capturing for posterity the claim of "100 per cent," the methodological lessons, and the future biological station. A two-minute scene with Father Sebastian Englert includes the priest's concerns over the islanders clinging to pagan "belief in spirits" and "ancestral instincts," such as the "lascivious behaviour" of its young people. Williams's film closes with a statement acknowledging the ongoing controversy over the island's prehistory but recognizing that its current history – its *medical history* – is now one of the best documented in the world "thanks to the imagination and persistence of a Canadian" and his METEI colleagues. In places, it is difficult to believe that the filmmakers had been on the same journey.

By 1967 many METEI articles had appeared in the popular press of
North America and Europe, and its alumni were busy responding to
multiple requests for public talks, a demand magnified by broadcast of
the two films. Skoryna still had to wrestle with the unpaid bills, currying
potential donors. The generous government backing, which he had been
counting on for a future METEI-2, was discredited and collapsed. His
"Preliminary Report" appeared within a month of METEI's return, but
it had merely summarized the work on Rapa Nui, describing the collections and emphasizing the need for analysis and interpretation. Scientific
publications were needed to establish the credibility of METEI and reas-
sure its supporters. A "final report" would rely on their results, which he
estimated would take "at least six months." Publications began to trickle
in slowly over a decade, but the final report would never appear.

The Scientific Papers Begin

Stanley Skoryna's "Preliminary Report" of March 1965, compiled from the shipboard accounts, explained succinctly the numbers of examinations, interviews, electrocardiograms, and samples of blood, urine, fingerprints, soil, fish, plants, and bacteria that had been gathered. The Medical Expedition to Easter Island expanded its team to involve dozens of other experts, including specialists from the list of honorary consultants and beyond, who would use their skills and computers to assist in the interpretation. Skoryna probably never knew who they all were, a situation that posed another obstacle to his final report. Despite his optimistic prediction of "at least six months" for the analysis, he never failed to emphasize that the research would not be complete until it was repeated in its entirety some years after the opening of the airport. Nevertheless, scientific papers slowly appeared.

Peter Beighton spoke about METEI by invitation at a meeting of the Royal Geographical Society in London on 6 February 1966. His talk resulted in one of the first scientific articles to emerge from the expedition, published in the *Geographical Journal* of the following September. He traced the history and human geography of the island, relying on the observations of Father Sebastian Englert, and described current health and sociological conditions. In attendance and invited to comment was Joseph S. Weiner, one of the originators of the International Biological Programme (IBP) and the head of its Human Adaptability (HA) section. Beighton described METEI as Canada's contribution to that initiative.[1] A year earlier, while METEI was still on Easter Island, Weiner had briefly mentioned it in an IBP report as one of two ongoing projects that were testing the feasibility of HA designs for the IBP; the other was the 1964 Cambridge summer expedition to the "hairy Ainu" of Hokkaido.[2]

Therefore, Weiner would have been especially interested in the results; however, it was still too early for Beighton to provide significant data.

FISH, PLANTS, INSECTS, AND FUNGI

Ian Efford set about sending his carefully preserved sea snails, filefish, coral, sea urchins, sand dollars, and ants to respective experts. The beetles went to a specialist in Chile. The plants went to Harvard University. But Efford could not ask these distinguished outsiders to drop everything else in order to study his creatures. Nor could he expect that, having looked at them, they would deem them worthy of comment. Worse, mould infected some of the plants, and the entire botanical collection that he and Jack had gathered with such care had to be thrown away. The lexicon of traditional healing plants that they had been building with Cléopâtre Montandon vanished. It was not until 1992 that David K. Holdsworth, unaware of their work, published an inventory of twenty-five plants, with their Rapanui names and uses, in what he believed "to be the first such record."[3] Convinced that the collecting could be done better, Efford devoted many hours to planning a return journey for 1967 (see chapter 11).

As director of the large Marion Lake freshwater project, which formed part of Canada's contribution to the IBP, Efford moved on to other ecological research, always focused on crabs. In 2015 Efford had no idea that METEI had once been touted as another part of that same initiative. Consequently, having placed his products in the custody of experts and turned to other work, he published nothing on Rapa Nui. Nevertheless, the collections that he and Jack Mathias had gathered are acknowledged in at least fifteen peer-reviewed biological publications from 1967 to 1978; they may have contributed to many other papers without recognition. Those reports identified at least four new species and updated descriptions of many others.[4] His Easter Island fish – 384 specimens representing 64 species – still reside in the Beaty Biodiversity Museum at the University of British Columbia.[5] Indexed under "Chile," they are recorded in the online database FishBase.

Some METEI scientists published their results quickly, often in Canadian journals. Armand Boudreault's work is discussed in chapter 11. Hal Gibbs summarized the incidence of enteric parasites in children in the May 1966 issue of the *Canadian Journal of Public Health*. Based on his readings of the anus tests using transparent tape, which had so amused the islanders, he showed that 23 per cent of the 307 children so examined were infected with pinworms (*Enterobious vermicularis*);

the incidence increased with age and with the numbers of children in each family.[6] The evidence of infections in the hundreds of blood specimens that Gibbs and David Murphy had collected from cattle and sheep were described in April 1968 in the *Canadian Journal of Comparative Medicine*. Both cattle and sheep had been exposed to ornithosis and sheep to toxoplasmosis, but tests for other organisms were negative or negligible. They emphasized that serology is only one indication of infection.[7] The work on intestinal parasites in human fecal samples was later expanded with Gibbs's colleague Eugene Meerovitch and published in a British tropical medicine journal. Of 206 individual fecal specimens examined (from both adults and children), 76 per cent had evidence of parasites, the most common being round worm (*Trichuris trichiura*) at 43 per cent, followed by amoeba at 24 per cent, and giardia at 7 per cent. Some specimens displayed multiple infestations in single individuals, with up to seven different parasites.[8]

Prompted by the head of entomology at McGill University's Macdonald College, D. Keith McE. Kevan, Gibbs had also collected insects. Before departure, Kevan had supplied equipment, including an insect net, and urged him to look for grasshoppers, which were Kevan's specialty. Gibbs duly returned with a number of grasshoppers, spiders, wasps, dragonflies, and roaches, which still reside in the Lyman Museum in Montreal.[9] Kevan soon produced a paper about the collection that acknowledges Gibbs, Efford, and Mathias but opens with the testy (and erroneous) observation that "for some unknown reason no entomologist had been included" on the voyage.[10] Efford was an entomologist. Kevan described small and giant cockroaches, crickets, web spinners, and earwigs, claiming that four of the species had not previously been reported on Rapa Nui. In particular, he noted a small brown cockroach, *Blatella germanica*, otherwise widespread in the Pacific. Gibbs well remembers that HMCS Cape Scott was infested with that cockroach, raising the uncomfortable possibility that METEI had introduced it (see chapter 12). Two other papers based on the same collection appeared in the *Canadian Entomologist* in 1967 (on a leaf miner) and 1974 (on a parasitic wasp).[11] In 1972 Edward Mockford published on Efford's barklice, which he then deposited in the US National Museum in Washington. The following year, Edward O. Wilson of Harvard published an article on Efford's ants, bringing to at least five the entomological products of the expedition with no entomologist.[12]

In 1972 Elliot Alpert co-authored an article about keratophilic fungi in Easter Island soil with renowned mycologist Libero Ajello of the Centers for Disease Control; they identified seven species in five genera from forty-four samples collected by Alpert himself as he surveyed the island. They claimed it was the first such report for Easter Island; METEI was mentioned with no names.[13]

DENTISTRY

Having written about METEI for navy dentists, Al Taylor published his scientific findings in the May 1966 issue of the *Journal of the Canadian Dental Association*. Based on his visual inspection of the mouths of 236 islanders aged eighteen to seventy-nine and the 650 "bite-wing" X-rays taken by Archie Wilkinson, he concluded that they suffered considerable decay due to poor oral hygiene and a largely carbohydrate diet. On average, Rapanui each had a total of twelve missing teeth and only 1.4 fillings. The data had been transferred to computer punch cards and analyzed by the Bureau of Dental Health of the State of New York Health Department. METEI had distributed the more than 3,000 toothbrushes, which Reid had gathered from donor Warner Lambert. Taylor hoped that the toothbrushes would serve to raise awareness about dental health. He admitted, however, that without a permanent program, the benefits would be minimal and temporary. He did not comment on the inadequate supply of toothpaste.[14]

Taylor had also made impressions – "casts" – of some islanders' teeth, but he made no mention of them in this article. It was Roy Ellis, dean of the University of Toronto's dental school, who had requested the impressions. In fact, Ellis had supplied the materials and recruited Taylor. Without Ellis's special interest in obtaining dental casts, Reid explained, "no dentist would have been on the journey." Two years later, the impressions had failed to arrive in Toronto, although Dean Ellis had sent many inquiries. He appealed to Helen Reid to help locate them. Only then did they discover that Taylor, with the help of Bob Meier, had sent the casts to dental anthropologist Christy Turner at Arizona State University, where they still reside.[15] Turner got around to analyzing 175 of Taylor's casts of 97 males and 78 females for a report published twelve years later in 1977. He also mentioned Skoryna, Meier, Taylor, and the casts in a memoir published in 2013.[16] By May 1966 Al Taylor had already moved to Chevy Chase, Maryland, and would later move to Chilliwack, British Columbia.

WORK PHYSIOLOGY

Björn Ekblom and Einar Gjessing went back to Sweden and Norway and got busy writing about their diligent investigation of work capacity and oxygen consumption. Ekblom presented their results at a symposium in

1966, and Karl Lange Andersen, as organizer and editor, published his paper in the proceedings.[17] Little did Björn and Einar know that their supervisor, Andersen, had also published some of their results in March 1967 in the *Canadian Medical Association Journal* (CMAJ). Andersen acknowledged METEI without naming Ekblom or Gjessing, who had done all the work.[18]

In fairness, omission of the researchers' names might not have been Andersen's fault. He had been invited to read two papers at a Toronto symposium on cardiovascular health through his involvement with the IBP's work physiology arm, for which he was "theme coordinator." The event took place in October 1966 at the splendid, new suburban hotel Inn on the Park. In keeping with the athletic focus, entertainment included a relay sponsored by the YMCA: ten middle-aged businessmen, bearing the flags of the nine participating nations, raced from central Toronto to the hotel – a distance of almost 13 kilometres – uphill. The proceedings appeared in a single issue of the CMAJ, edited by Canadian exercise physiologist Roy J. Shephard.[19]

Ekblom and Gjessing published their results in 1968 in the prestigious *Journal of Applied Physiology*; they included studies of 57 females and 121 males aged nine to sixty. The article contained useful graphic information on Rapanui height and weight by age and compared with Scandinavians. Maximum heart rate and oxygen consumption for males and females were presented by age. Occupation-related data on eight selected individuals were included: housewives, fishermen, and outdoor labourers. The study revealed lower maximum oxygen uptake compared to Europeans, suggesting that Rapanui were less fit; however, in the discussion, the authors speculated on the heat and lifestyle, which did not require heavy work.[20] They acknowledged Skoryna and METEI, but did not cite Andersen's earlier use of their own material because they did not know about it. Jim Nielsen was not mentioned in any of the physiology papers. METEI travellers remember his greater interest (and success) in exploring the charms of the landscape and its female inhabitants. Nielsen remembers that too, although he has not forgotten the long, hot hours spent in the lab with the oxygen machine.

A decade later, the physiology work on Easter Island was cited and situated in a global context in the synthetic work of Roy J. Shephard, who remained heavily involved in the Canadian IBP effort until the project came to a close in 1974. Weiner's foreword for the 1978 book stated, "Physical activity and capacity for work are such fundamental determinants of human survival that it may come as a surprise that their exact measurement on a population scale has only been achieved

quite recently." He complimented both Shephard and Andersen for
their many contributions to this aspect of the Human Adaptability section of the IBP.[21]

FINALIZING THE CENSUS

The medical reports on humans were delayed by ongoing corrections
to the census of Rapa Nui's people that had been provided by Chilean
authorities on the outward journey. The two epidemiologists, John Cutler
and Elliot Alpert, had to keep revising it. They had been door-to-door,
confirming the presence and size of each family and the absence of forty-four families and a few individuals who were residing in Chile. Absent
parties should not be held against Skoryna's 100 per cent. Cutler then
used punch cards to computerize the information from the examinations
so that it could be correlated and cross-referenced. He was still tweaking
the data in 1966, but he had many other responsibilities. In May 1967
Skoryna sent Carlotta Hacker out to California, where she spent three
weeks living with the Cutlers and working on the census with an updated
copy that she had collected on Rapa Nui (see chapter 11). Copies of this
final "programmed" census were sent to all METEI scientists and those
helping them, but it was never published in its entirety. Cutler, especially,
seems to have been disappointed that no articles emerged from all their
hard work on the island and beyond.

Toward the end of Carlotta's stay in San Francisco, Red Lemieux
showed up – as if inadvertently; however, he'd been summoned by John,
who knew that the filmmaker's marriage was failing and decided that
the pair should see each other again. Carlotta was at first annoyed and
then pleased to see Lemieux; they planned to marry in early 1968 as
soon as his divorce was finalized. "I just happen to have been in love for
three years with a screwed-up film maker," she wrote to Helen Reid. She
also expressed her joy and feelings of guilt, selfishness, and immorality,
as well as her gratitude to the "loyal" friend who "only ever really liked
anything in Red because I liked him."[22]

X-RAY RUCKUS AND CHILD HEALTH

As soon as Helen Reid finished her popular book manuscript in July
1965, she launched into the scientific analysis of the data from the physical examinations of Easter Island youth. Her plan to recruit 500 children in Montreal and Toronto as a cohort for comparison seems to have
fallen by the wayside. For her study, she needed the "bone-age" X-rays

of hands and wrists taken by Archie Wilkinson of 480 youth under age eighteen. But painful confusion arose over who had custody of these films and who would interpret them.

Reid repeatedly wrote to "Dear Arch" in Montreal asking him to pack up the films in two lots and send them to Toronto. When she first asked, Archie responded, on 18 April 1965, that his boss, radiologist Dr Robert G. Fraser, was too busy to do the readings, but he did not send the films. When the X-rays did not appear, she wrote again in July and again in September. During this strife and with his wedding looming, Archie also made arrangements to donate the grass skirt that he had purchased on Rapa Nui to McGill's Redpath Museum, where it still resides.[23]

Then, on 29 October 1965, Reid turned to Fraser himself. Her exasperation is plain: the films "were taken at my request, for me, as an integral part of the study ... which I had planned." Archie was still away on his honeymoon. Fraser replied, "It is indeed possible and in fact probable that this was part of your programme." He continued, "It is true, however, that when the original radiographic survey was planned with Mr. Wilkinson and myself (as Consultant Radiologist to the expedition), [we] included ... the assessment of skeletal maturation." In any case, Fraser wrote, he and his staff had just finished interpreting all the films. He would leave it to her to decide what to do. If she wanted to repeat the interpretive exercise, it might be "interesting" to compare the "independent" results between the two departments in Toronto and Montreal. A dare! Had Reid's repeated requests goaded Fraser into conducting the interpretation after all, simply to avoid passing the project on to a rival university?

Fraser displayed massive ambivalence over the entire mission and possibly some snide resentment over his technologist's role. When Wilkinson was invited to give a one-hour presentation on METEI before a large audience in their own hospital, Fraser refused to allow the ten to fifteen of his radiology staffers (Archie's colleagues) to attend. He scheduled a meeting at the same time and notified the executive director of the hospital that he would appear simply to introduce Archie and then leave.[24] Later, in granting permission for Archie, whom Fraser always addressed as "Mr. Wilkinson," to speak at an international meeting of radiologists and technologists in Maine, he wrote, "You seem to be spreading far and wide the beauties of Easter Island; I trust that you give some attention in your many speeches to the beauties and efficiencies of the Hospital to which you belong."[25] Ouch!

Bob Williams's film for the Canadian Broadcasting Corporation (CBC) reveals the impending jurisdictional argument between Fraser and Reid as an accident waiting to happen: in part 1 Archie takes X-rays of hands and wrists "for Dr Reid's study," and in part 2 we learn that "all the films will be taken back to Montreal for interpretation by Dr Fraser."[26] Likely, no one anticipated the problem until they were back in Canada. Archie was probably caught in the middle. Reid's mollified response included an apology but also a detailed description of who said what, when, and where (between Puerto Rico and Panama), along with a reminder that Archie had told her back in April that Fraser was too busy. She "made nice," appealing to Fraser's expertise in asking for his opinion on two specific cases. She wished him well for his own publication of the data and told him how fond she was of Archie and glad that he'd married. Fraser ignored her and delegated Archie to respond. In December the films on the 480 youthful subjects were finally bundled up and sent to Toronto. Mutually reassuring letters passed between Helen and Archie. They both blamed the "confusion abounding" that was METEI. "I am wearied of the chaos," Helen wrote. "The same thing happened with the bloods that were due to come here," she said. "It will just have to be sorted out ... Now that Stan is back, this may be easier – or then again, it may be more difficult."[27]

Fraser published nothing from his readings of the X-rays, nor did his technologist, Wilkinson; however, Archie (bless him!) kept the detailed, fifty-eight-page, typewritten manuscript of the McGill interpretation of all the X-rays of adults and children – hands and wrists, chests, and skulls – linked by number to every person in the census.[28] A short preface indicated that nine different (but unnamed) radiologists had participated in reading the films, without clarifying who read what, nor were any references given for the standards used to determine bone age. No copy of this report can be found in Helen Reid's papers, so it may never have been sent to her, meaning that she would have needed to interpret them again herself. One copy went to Richard Roberts, who was supposed to be coordinating the final medical report.[29]

By the time the films finally arrived in Toronto, Helen was leaving with her husband for a round-the-world tour as part of the prestigious Sims Professorship awarded to Laurie Chute in advance of his becoming medical dean. She would not be able to work on the X-rays until after their return in late 1967. Relying on a published method for establishing bone age on a total possible score of 32, she read the films of hands and wrists all over again, twice: first, arranged by chronological age; second, arranged randomly by file number. The majority (63 per cent) of the double readings were identical, but when discrepancies arose, she took an average. The exercise took her "hundreds of hours" and revealed a few height and weight inconsistencies in the census, which she tried to clarify in letters to Cutler and Roberts for fixing the census but without success.[30] She also corresponded with the authors of the 1959 method, which she had selected to calculate bone age.[31]

Reid's original readings of bone age still exist, and it is now possible to compare her readings in Toronto with those of Fraser in Montreal – his cheeky suggestion that Helen had ignored.[32] Perfect correlation between the two institutions occurred in only 119 of 419 films (28 per cent), but the differences were not great: in general, Helen's analysis placed the bone age slightly older than Fraser's at McGill by an average of 3.5 months. It is impossible to determine the source of the discrepancy. Was it differing methods or the fact that McGill's reading entailed nine different radiologists and Reid's only one?

Helen's study of growth and development finally appeared in the March 1968 issue of the *Canadian Medical Association Journal*.[33] Gone were the made-in-Canada comparators. Instead, she juxtaposed the stature of Easter Island children with that of a cohort from Boston, amplified by some British and Polish data. Rapanui youth were "generally healthy," smaller at ages twelve to thirteen, and slower to mature – all impressions she had observed while on the island and could now confirm with evidence. She described weaning practices and the use of powdered milk, but abandoned making a firm statement about menarche, although she had tried to collect ages at onset of menstruation while on the island.[34] With the help of a Toronto nutritionist, she attempted to analyze their diet based on her detailed observations of food supplies and rates of consumption, concluding that it was low in protein. METEI still sorely felt the absence of Chilean nutritionist Gonzalo Donoso, who had fled the project as it began. In concluding, Reid emphasized the overall goal, in keeping with the IBP: "to lay a foundation for a continuing study in human adaptability before the construction of an international airport ended isolation forever." Archie Wilkinson was warmly thanked in the acknowledgments.

Soon after, Richard Roberts sourly observed to John Cutler that Helen Reid's paper was "probably factual." He was "glad to see that she [had] considerably watered down her opinions about malnutrition among the children." He "would have been much happier if Archie Wilkinson had been a co-author after all the work he did," but, Roberts admitted, she might have asked Archie.[35] Being caught in the middle, Archie may have declined.

RICHARD ROBERTS AND THE METEI SILENCE

Roberts published nothing from his METEI experience; and that too is another METEI mystery. Like the other travellers, he received many invitations to speak about the journey and the research in Canada and beyond. He addressed a "Canadian/US army medical group" serving in Germany as part of NATO. Yet he was unable, or unwilling, to transform these presentations into print. He invited John Cutler to Ottawa to talk about his research on stroke in late May 1968 and mulled over John's suggestion that they write some articles together. Roberts confessed that he had "tried to give some time and intelligent interest" to the idea "but without much success." He suggested that an "intelligent discussion" take place when they met in person. "I would like to produce a paper with you, ... if we can come to a satisfactory decision about it."[36]

Maureen Roberts also delivered many speeches about the travels. Her good humour and Scottish wit made her a favourite of the travellers and colleagues back home. She addressed the Canadian Medical Association (CMA) in Halifax in 1965, but its journal did not describe her speech, of which no trace remains. She also delivered a slide-illustrated talk at some point in "London" (England or Ontario?); its existence is recorded in sketchy, handwritten notes on pink paper and a heavily annotated typescript of the final three pages of a seven-page text.[37] Like Helen Reid, Maureen was an object of curiosity for the women's pages: one item featured a photograph of her "at home" wearing shell necklaces and holding carvings. It opened this way: "'Easter Island? Where shall I begin?' Dr. Maureen Roberts slipped off her shoes, wriggled her toes, took a deep breath, and started in."[38] She had set up a chromosome laboratory at Dalhousie University and joined the expedition to cover genetics and hereditary diseases.[39] But she too, like her husband, published nothing on METEI.

The closest we have to Richard Roberts's views on the scientific "results" of METEI is the manuscript text of a speech that he delivered to the annual meeting of the CMA in June 1966. Having few data himself because products had been "farmed out" to others, he appealed for help in preparation. John Cutler had the punch cards and Archie Wilkinson had the X-rays; they both scrambled to send him some information.[40]

Roberts opened by saying that he would expand on Maureen's presentation from a year earlier and on the "Preliminary Report." He stated that he had "personally examined the results from 312 adults" and was having the data entered onto computer punch cards. He told of the appearance of "the general good health of the islanders" and cited their size (small), skin colour (coffee), and epicanthal folds (rare) as indicators of "racial type" and hence possible geographic origin. Hypertension and heart disease were "rare," but Archie's 2,800 X-rays revealed "much old and some new" tuberculosis in sixty-six people and numerous straight spines. Fifteen people were known to have leprosy. Many bore operative scars on their face or abdomen, which Roberts blamed on the surgical proclivities of the former "Island doctor" – Guido Andrade, unnamed – who had loved to perform skin biopsies for leprosy and to remove gallbladders (at least sixty-four). The poor dentition, described by Al Taylor, set Roberts musing about how things had changed since Jacob Roggeveen's eighteenth-century observation that the islanders had "wonderful, white teeth."[41]

In a rare foray into medical analysis, Roberts speculated on the quantities of calcium and fluoride in the rocky terrain of the island and the origins of the relatively frequent attacks of asthma and bronchospasm. The latter he connected to similar reports from Tristan da Cunha in the South Atlantic. He cited a 1963 *British Medical Journal* article and had corresponded with its authors.[42] Surmising that no genetic relationship existed between those islanders and the Rapanui, he opted for environment and the soil and said, "I cannot but wonder whether asthma is perhaps one of the penalties of living on a dusty, windy volcanic island." Roberts also mentioned the anthropological and sociological studies still to be completed. He acknowledged Skoryna, crediting him for the "happy liaison" that had permitted the research, and he closed with humility: "The Islanders regarded our scientific activities with tolerant amusement and were pathetically grateful for the small things we were able to do for them ... They rapidly became – and have remained – our friends. We hope that what we did may bring them some lasting benefit."[43]

More telling, perhaps, of Roberts's anxiety about the METEI results is his strong letter to the CMA public relations officer with his refusal to provide an advance copy of his speech to the media. Apparently, the embargo that he had placed on another of his CMA talks in 1958 had been broken by an "unscrupulous reporter." At that time, it resulted in a heated exchange with the secretariat, copies of which he also forwarded with the letter in 1966.[44] He was not about to have that happen again; his Easter Island paper – vague though it was – must not be published.

The mid-June meeting in Edmonton where Roberts spoke enjoyed the presence of famous Americans Richard C. Lillehei and William B. Bean. His cautious METEI presentation was tucked into an afternoon session on Wednesday, 15 June. Reporters wrote that the CMA delegates viewed Roberts's speech about "the world's loneliest outpost" as "a welcome

respite for the speed of modern developments." Using Roberts's own
words, they duly noted that most expedition members had been "on
loan from other universities" and that "no member had been able to
devote full time to the analysis." Delegates seemed surprised by the delay
but impressed with the effort: "even some 15 months after the expedition, only a part of the work has been completed." The report continued,
echoing the speaker's observation that "with a population of only 950
inhabitants, the group was too small for any very valid statistical deductions to be made ... No very startling results have come to light as yet,
but the analysis of results is still incomplete."[45]

Roberts had failed to appreciate, or communicate, the significance of
Skoryna's 100 per cent, which he had described as "all but about eight
Islanders – an incredible sample of over 99%." On a complete sample of
100 per cent, no "statistical deductions," as Roberts called them, were
needed for validity! Nor did he seem to realize that *absence* of illness
and significant risk factors constituted a crucial finding and important
baseline, especially with the looming end to isolation and the promised
repeat study. Furthermore, perhaps because of the language barrier, or
because he had not asked, Roberts was unaware of the alarming significance of results flowing from Boudreault's lab, although he had mentioned virology in his speech (see chapter 11). Even more surprising, he
did not mention the World Health Organization (WHO), the IBP, or that
METEI had been timed to happen before the airport "ended isolation forever," as Helen Reid had put it.[46] The words "ecology" and "veterinary
survey" appeared only as handwritten reminders in the margins.

Roberts's relative silence about the massive effort, of which he ostensibly had been a director, demands an explanation. After all, he was
in charge of the "medical" in METEI. The differences with Skoryna –
personality clash and management styles – were evident on the journey and the island (see chapters 3, 5, and 8). Many other clues can be
found in the fulsome private report that he prepared for his superiors
while still aboard *Cape Scott* and mailed from Balboa. The main thrust
of that screed was an outright condemnation of Skoryna, whose woe-
ful leadership skills Roberts blamed for the poor preparation, the lack
of information and structure, the personal insults, the disorganization
and inefficiencies, and the many frustrations and missed opportunities.
Roberts wrote that Skoryna was "indecisive," at times "pigheaded to the
point of stubbornness," and "bewitched by the idea of a 100% sample
to be achieved by all means fair or foul." Inflamed by the unreasonable workload and expectations, Roberts may also have felt narcissistic
injury. Skoryna "never delegated any authority to me, rarely took my

advice, and was in fact violently and publicly in conflict with my suggestions on several occasions. It now seems quite clear that I was asked to be Deputy Director purely as a public gesture to acknowledge Naval support and that he never had any intention that my position would be anything other than nominal." "In no circumstances would I go on any similar venture under his direction." Roberts may have been right about the token "gesture," as Skoryna had also quietly told Garry Brody that he would be the deputy director.

Roberts's scathing criticisms extended to the inexperienced cook, the "boring" food, the questionable hygiene, the "uncouth" ham radio operator who "played favorites," Carlotta Hacker's "total lack of science training," the fatigue and disinterest of John Easton, who was "too old" and "fell down completely on the job," resulting in domestic arrangements that were "lamentably wrong." Al Taylor, Carl Mydans, and Roberts himself were all experienced at living "in the field," and they knew things could have been much better.[47]

For his Edmonton audience, Roberts avoided these opinions and stuck to the highroad of propriety and promise. But with limited access to results and less comprehension of those available, he had little else to say. In April 1966 Cutler had hastened to provide some preliminary data on adults, explaining how the codes and tabulations worked and offering to help in "finding certain combinations ... for instance we might correlate body build with blood pressure ... there are innumerable possibilities."[48] Roberts seemed incapable of finding any value in reporting the results – especially if they were normal. He told his navy bosses that he wanted to distance himself from Skoryna's claim of 100 per cent: "I pointed out to him that I would not be associated with such a claim in any press release and certainly not in a scientific report." Roberts was also dismayed, if not embarrassed, by the shocking lack of a prior literature review – and the surprise of genetic diversity. A simple advance visit by two or three travellers using the Chilean supply ship to reconnoiter the situation would have avoided so many errors.

Rancour pervaded Roberts's island memories. He was bitterly disappointed that the absent literature review had left the team unaware of useful contemporary comparisons, especially those in the data collected by the Chilean team in the spring of 1963.[49] His temper and undisguised scorn for Skoryna and METEI may have inhibited other travellers from communicating their findings to him. His angry outbursts were unforgettable even a half-century later.

On the surface, relations were pleasant; Richard and Maureen hosted several small reunions in their new Ottawa home, inviting nearby

Montrealers, including Skoryna, whenever more distant METEI alumni appeared. But his mischievous family could tease him into a rage by reading Helen Reid's description of his prickly behaviour. With a military passion for precision, he was quick to decry others' misdemeanours. This trait, coupled with his increasing responsibilities in the armed forces, the painful past, the exposure of inadequate planning, and the discovery of the islanders' relatively good health, may have conspired to kill all desire to revisit the work for publication. Roberts also seemed to misunderstand the purpose of METEI and to have forgotten about the airport, the impending contact with the world, the WHO, and the IBP. He saw little point in describing a relatively healthy population of diverse genetic stock.

This silence is truly unfortunate because the "*almost* 100% study" of the islanders' blood pressure, cholesterol, glucose levels, and hematological results would have helped researchers of the future by providing a 1964–65 baseline – a reliable baseline because few studies ever manage to capture the entire population. Roberts's failure to publish METEI's extensive data meant that they were excluded from all other subsequent reviews of biomedical research on Rapa Nui. No one knew about them. The results are reported here for the first time (see below and appendix B).

TEST RESULTS:

ELECTROCARDIOGRAMS, URINE, AND BLOOD GROUPS

Electrocardiograms were performed on sixty-five Easter Islanders. John Cutler engaged in a correspondence with Henry Blackburn of the University of Minnesota about their interpretation. An expert in cardiac epidemiology, Blackburn found "one clear infarct" and strips that contained "enough suggestions that the population is unusual." He continued, "it is very sad there wasn't a sample of all people."[50] Knowing that he had failed to perform at least thirteen promised cardiograms, that comment probably grated on Roberts's frazzled nerves.

The urine tests of Easter Islanders were mostly normal (see appendix B, table B.1). The results – for protein, glucose, pH, and microscopy – were read on the island for later entry on the computer punch cards in Cutler's care. Remembering that the specimen cups had been vanishing, many being used for "drinking glasses," Helen Reid found a list of 300 urinalysis results pertaining to all but six people examined after 11 January 1965, possibly the date when she noticed the neglect of samples. They came in chronological order by the date of collection, a presentation that would have made data entry by census number very cumbersome and potentially erroneous. None were positive for glucose, only four people had protein greater than "trace or +," and one twenty-nine-year-old woman had signs of a bladder infection. More than a year after the journey, on 30 May 1966, Reid sent this typewritten list of urine results to Roberts and Cutler, who were still wondering what had become of the earlier tests. She referred again to her dispute with Roberts and Brody or Myhre over whether or not some islanders had enlarged thyroid glands, contending that they did and citing a reference to the classification system on which she based her opinion.[51] Nothing about urine or thyroids ever appeared in print.

Blood was another problem hampering production of a final report. Armand Boudreault and Hal Gibbs had quickly analyzed serum samples and published. But other blood results were slower to come. Forty millilitres had been collected from people over age seven, and lesser amounts and fingers pricks had been taken from those younger. If a sufficiently large sample had been collected, it was sent for chemical analysis – including glucose, urea nitrogen, and cholesterol – and it was tested for blood groups and "genetics." Only blood groups could be finalized on Rapa Nui.

The scientific world was especially interested in the geographic origins of the peoples of the earth. Comparing genetics – or DNA – promised to be a good way to analyze the problem. The general public had been fascinated by the early 1950s discovery of James Watson and Francis Crick, who had drawn on the crystallography work of Rosalind Franklin to determine the structure of that molecule common to us all. For their work, they won the Nobel Prize in 1962. In 1965 genetics was a "hot topic"; however, although people could see chromosomes – the large bundles of genetic material inside dividing cells – no one could yet measure or characterize DNA molecules in individuals. Those techniques came much later. Nevertheless, they could use substitutes.[52] Everything in the human body is determined by genes: eye and hair colour, tissues, structures, and chemistry. Therefore, blood groups and variations in types of body chemicals – including enzymes and proteins, such as haptoglobin and hemoglobin – reflect DNA. Proxy parameters like these substances had already been applied to studies of the inhabitants of the Arctic and their origins. Had North American Inuit travelled across the Bering Strait? Did the first *Homo sapiens* reside in the fertile crescent or in Africa? Because Thor Heyerdahl had raised a conflicting view on the geographic origins of South Sea islanders, the genetics of the Rapanui cried out for attention. Although "origins" was not its main purpose, METEI was on the case too, seemingly unaware that others were well ahead of them.[53]

METEI's real interest in genetics stemmed from the notion that proof of inbreeding would suggest vulnerability to disease.

Recall that, at the outset, Skoryna and many organizers had assumed that the Islanders, being isolated, *must be* inbred. They touted this characteristic in numerous press releases before and after their journey. But they were wrong. Long before METEI, several scientific observers, as well as Heyerdahl, had made the case that the islanders were genetically diverse.[54] In 1940 Harry L. Shapiro travelled to Easter Island on the yacht *Zaca* and wrote of "the paucity of pure natives." His twenty-one samples were analyzed by the ship surgeon, George Lyman.[55] Similarly, in 1957 an Australian team analyzed blood samples collected by Dr Emil Gjessing on Heyerdahl's 1955 expedition, claiming that it was difficult to find any Polynesians of "unmixed blood."[56] Like Eivind Myhre, they relied on Father Sebastian's lists, but they tested only the fifty-one islanders deemed by the priest to be the least mixed.

Skoryna's team realized their error of inbreeding as soon as they arrived, simply by observing the beautiful, varied people and their social and cultural practices. Far from being "inbred," the islanders were, as ecologist Ian Efford put it, "aggressively outbred." The genetic studies were not going to live up to expectations. In particular, they would not show the anticipated homogeneity and vulnerability to the threat of increased contact. Here was yet another disappointment to inhibit Skoryna's final report. If his inbreeding premise was wrong, perhaps *all* the genetic work was invalid. Some METEI scientists, like Bob Meier, were prepared to deal with that mixity, knowing that gene flow from outside sources had been going on for at least 150 years. The geographic isolation was far more important, and the greatest impacts of increased contact would be felt in community and personal health, including immunity. Scientists everywhere else were waiting to hear what they had found.

Like his fellow Scandinavians, Myhre got on promptly with his work on blood groups. While still on the island, the Norwegian pathologist analyzed the ABO and Rh status of 905 islanders, including the smallest children, whose tiny fingers had been pricked for drops of blood. Only a few samples were spoiled, making his by "far the largest group" of islanders ever studied. He used "Eldon cards," which were not as sophisticated as newer, more complicated methods; however, he wrote, "due to unforeseen changes in plans of the expedition," the simple test "had to be adopted." With Father Sebastian's help, Myhre had also tried to sort the samples into three cohorts according to presumed genealogical origins: sixty-nine Rapanui viewed as "short-ear" Easter Islanders; sixty-three whose roots were "mixed" with other Polynesians; and twenty-three whose ancestry was mixed with the more ancient "long-ear" stock. These "long-ears" were likely the same families that the priest had indicated to Dr Emil Gjessing in 1955;[57] they were identical to, or relatives of, the same cohort that Chileans had examined in 1963.[58] Myhre did not explain how Father Sebastian made these determinations, although Rapanui families kept track of their genealogies and the priest listened to them. Myhre found a high frequency of blood group A and Rh positivity and a very low frequency of blood group B, confirming what others had already reported using better tests but on much smaller samples. He compared his results with predecessors, including Gjessing's fifty-one samples. Although he referred to the 1963 Chilean expedition's blood work on 162 Rapanui, he missed the Chilean team's more detailed results on a sample of 233 islanders published in *Nature* in 1967.[59] In the slight variation between the three "racially" selected groups, he perceived support for Thor Heyerdahl's theory about the South American origins, something Heyerdahl had maintained from the blood taken on his own expedition.[60] Myhre published in English in the January 1969 issue of a German anthropology journal, acknowledging a grant from the Kon Tiki Museum in Oslo.[61]

MORE STUDIES ON BLOOD: SERUM ENZYMES AND GENETICS

Maureen Roberts brought back a few hundred frozen or refrigerated serum samples that she planned to examine for other genetic proxies. Because of her husband's abrupt transfer to Ottawa, she lost both her job and her lab and had to appeal to others for help. Dr Nancy Simpson, geneticist at Queen's University, had just moved from Toronto, where she completed her doctoral work on classifying enzymes as a reflection of genetic status. "I wanted to go on that trip!" she told me fifty years later. "I never understood how Maureen got to go. My research was on exactly that problem. This was the kind of work I did." The women knew and liked each other; however, Nancy was the researcher, and Maureen was not. Nancy admitted that Maureen might have enjoyed the inside edge because her husband was going anyway as a "contribution" from the Canadian armed forces. Independent of genetics, Skoryna had first suggested to Richard Roberts that his pediatrician spouse join the expedition to examine children.[62]

When Maureen returned, she found a letter waiting from Nancy: "I am definitely counting on receiving any samples you were able to obtain."[63] She also asked for information on the genealogical relationships – as

rarities run in families. Maureen attempted to untangle the genealogical connections, but her notes on index cards are covered in messy
lines, showing how the high incidence of adoption and "out of wed-
lock" births defeated her.[64] She never reported on the topic. But she duly
shipped the serum off to Nancy, who analyzed the enzymes contained in
497 samples. She communicated her "rather dull" findings to Maureen
by letter on 12 December 1966 "as a jolly Christmas present," offering
to do further testing, as needed, on the stored frozen specimens.[65]

Simpson published the Easter Island enzyme results in early 1968 as
part of her review article in the prestigious *Annals of the New York
Academy of Science.*[66] She was particularly interested in variant cholin-
esterases – mutations that occurred with differing frequencies in different
populations – since peoples with similar frequencies of rare mutations
might be related. She identified these changes through starch-gel electrophoresis. This relatively new technique entailed applying an electric
current that caused molecules to separate as they migrated across a gel
field at varying speeds depending on their size and electrical charge. For
comparators, Simpson referred to her own unpublished studies on Thais
and on Canadian Cree. I asked her what happened to the serum samples
because they could have been used for other tests. "I don't remember,"
the vivacious nonagenarian replied, gazing thoughtfully out the window.
"If I kept them, they must still be kicking around in a freezer somewhere
here in Kingston. No one would throw away my samples without asking
me first!" Dr Simpson and I have searched through the labs at Queen's
University for more than two years, but we have yet to find them.

Not all of Maureen's samples went to Simpson. Geneticist Alexander
G. Bearn of the Rockefeller University in New York City, an honorary
consultant to the expedition, had asked for serum samples from Easter
Island to analyze for transferrin, haptoglobin, and group-specific components – more proxy DNA. Williams' CBC film shows Fred Joyce in
the METEI lab dropping serum into tiny tubes labelled "Bearn." Soon
after her return, Maureen sent 450 serum samples in 5-millilitre vials
to Montreal with Georges Nógrády, refrigerated at 4° Celsius as per
instructions. They were forwarded to New York.

Using these samples, Bearn and his associate Kari Berg discovered a
new X-linked serum system marker, which they named Xm, providing
evidence for its existence in four unrelated populations: Norwegians,
whites and African Americans from Georgia, and eighty-three Easter
Islanders. The results were considered important enough to be published
in two scientific journals, both in 1966.[67] On 4 April 1966 Berg wrote to
thank Maureen, enclosing a reprint and asking if it was possible that a

little girl – whose system was "negative" but whose father was "positive" – might be "illegitimate."[68] We do not have the reply, but surely Maureen said, "yes."

Here again, confusion and embarrassment arose. To sort out the relationship between this child and her father, Bearn wanted not serum but red blood cell samples to do ABO and Rh blood grouping. Myhre's paper – which had yet to be published – dealt only with large groups; however, his raw data were still available. Bearn wanted to know the combined Xm status and blood groups of these two individuals and others. He was concerned about illegitimacy only in so far as its *absence* in this pair would seriously confound the significance of his discovery. Illegitimacy was a strong possibility in Easter Island families. For her own genetic study, Maureen Roberts had failed to unravel these relationships and Carlotta's census work had shown that the METEI cohort of islanders contained 166 children for whom one or both of the home "parents" were not the biological parents.[69]

As for the haptoglobin and transferrin tests that Bearn had promised, no publication has been found. Nevertheless, haptoglobins and milk precipitins were indeed measured at the Ottawa General Hospital by the head of pediatrics, Dominick J. Conway, and biochemist Elena Ross. The undated list of these results was sent to Maureen Roberts, but she did not analyze or publish it (see appendix B, tables B.2 and B.3).[70]

THE WANDERING RED BLOOD CELLS

Goaded by Bearn's request about family relationships, Maureen wrote to hematologist Dr Ronald Denton at Montreal Children's Hospital, one of the honorary consultants who had dropped out of METEI travel.[71] She asked if the frozen red-cell samples that METEI had passed on to him could be used for Bearn's purpose of identifying blood groups as well as his own. As a teaser, she suggested that Bearn might be motivated to do all the blood group testing for them on his sophisticated equipment. It seems neither Maureen nor Denton thought to ask Eivind Myhre in Norway, who had *already* done the blood group testing on Rapa Nui! If he had kept his Eldon card data on individuals, he could have answered the paternity question with ease.

A week later, Denton wrote to Bearn.[72] He was still planning to study the hemoglobin inside the red blood cells through electrophoresis. Hemoglobin was another of those proxy stand-ins for DNA. Some variants of hemoglobin – like sickle cell – could be dangerous. But many were subtle and of little consequence for health, although they could be yet another way of conducting genetic studies. New hemoglobins were being discovered all the time. For these tests, scientists needed the red-cell part of blood in the solids that are separated from liquid plasma or serum. But Denton's lab was for hospital service, not research, and he had not yet been able to "assign staff" to the task. Moreover, he was worried that the "150 samples stored at minus 60C" could not be thawed twice. He apologized if his reservations seemed like "obstacles in your way" and offered to send the blood to Bearn if he would hemolyze it, use it, and send it back prepared for hemoglobin electrophoresis. He enclosed the instructions used in his lab for preparing the samples. I do not know if Bearn ever received the red cells.

The blood problems did not end here. In addition to all his measurements of fingers, skulls, noses, lips, eyes, hair, fingerprints, and hand-prints, the young anthropologist Bob Meier had been hoping to examine blood groups connecting them to genealogical data (similar to the work of Eivind Myhre). He knew that Denton's planned electrophoretic study of hemoglobin inside the red blood cells would also be useful. But now those particular samples were lost, and no one knew where to find them.

Eager to finish his dissertation and include the blood studies, Bob Meier began looking for the red cells. He wrote to Roberts, who wrote to Skoryna. The latter replied cordially on 27 February 1967 and offered to contact Dr Bearn in New York City asking him to forward the samples – if he still had them (or ever had them) – to Bob in Wisconsin.[73] Bearn did not have the red cells. Either Denton's suggestions for sharing and preparing the samples had been too daunting or Bearn had already used the samples and returned them. Finally, they were located in Denton's own lab – possibly where they had been all along.

In May 1967 Carlotta Hacker was dispatched to Madison with the frozen blood samples from Denton's lab.[74] But they were not tested and were returned the next day. More than a year later, the disappointed Meier explained the reason: "someone" had decided that Wisconsin would analyze the plasma and prepare the cells for hemoglobin testing back in Montreal – the technique that Denton had requested of Bearn. Meier and the lab director agreed that this was not a good plan: one lab should not perform part of a test for another. Therefore, it was best not to thaw any of the specimens (because of the risk of cell lysis) and to send them all back, still frozen, to Montreal. There "went my hope of getting gene frequencies done for the Easter Islanders," Meier wrote.[75]

When Ronald Denton received the frozen samples back from Wisconsin in May 1967, he learned that the Madison laboratory had actually tried to thaw a couple specimens. But the cells had burst, releasing their hemoglobin contents into the plasma (hemolysis). This phenomenon had made them back off and was yet another reason why they returned the blood. Denton could not figure out what had happened, unless the cells had perhaps been frozen in anticoagulant without the usual glycol needed to stabilize them. He and his associates "tried many different stunts," attempting to extract intact red blood cells and hemoglobin-free plasma. Then he realized that he could still perform the hemoglobin electrophoresis using the dilute, hemolyzed samples. "All is not lost," he wrote to Maureen on 7 November 1968; "to date we have done about 50 and will continue to do them as our crowded schedule permits." So far, after a single "false alarm" hinting at a new type of hemoglobin, nothing unusual had appeared; the Rapanui hemoglobins seemed "to conform with those of the usual white population."[76] Denton wrote no more and did not publish. The fifty completed analyses are missing, and this paragraph is the first publication of his results.

Like Bob Meier, Denton apologized to Maureen for his long silence on the matter. He had wanted "to avoid any recriminations or embarrassment to anyone." Quick to take umbrage, Richard Roberts – writing to one Dr Roberts clearly entailed addressing the other – was "astonished" by Denton's reply: first, because he had not been informed of these difficulties at the time when they occurred; and second, because they implied that the intrepid and highly competent navy man, Fred Joyce, had made an error when preparing the blood for the freezer. He hastened to write to Joyce before responding to Denton, looking for other explanations. Carlotta Hacker and Georges Nógrády had been to visit the previous weekend, and they reminded the Robertses of the freezer that had been wrongly connected in the ship's hold and left on deck, allowing its temperature to rise. Roberts "did not know this" – yet another reason for outrage – or, he admitted lamely, he "had forgotten."[77] The multiplicity of problems that were hidden from Roberts's view may have had something to do with his short temper. Joyce reassured him that he had followed the proper method.[78]

Some tests on red blood cells were done well but kept secret and not correlated with other relevant data. Others were done but also kept secret, possibly because of doubts about their accuracy. Some were not done at all because the samples were ruined. How could Denton publish his data on hemoglobins when he had followed an unorthodox procedure? The fact that no intriguing discoveries seemed to be emerging from the studies was all the more reason to keep his head down, avoiding criticism for the exploded cells and renegade method. The tyranny of negative results is a well-known damper to scientific publication.

BLOOD CHEMISTRY:
CHOLESTEROL, GLUCOSE, AND BUN

Like genetics, cholesterol was a hot topic in the mid-1960s. Researchers were exploring its connection to high blood pressure and heart disease, both now recognized as leading causes of death. In 1958 Ancel Keys of Minnesota had launched a study comparing diet and cholesterol in seven countries. By 1961 this lipid, which accumulated on the inner walls of arteries, was considered a serious risk factor for heart disease. The famous Canadian researcher Fraser Mustard wanted to compare cholesterol levels around the world, and he was eager to know what would happen to Rapanui cholesterol when isolation ended. Before the expedition, he had been recruited as an honorary consultant when William Harding Le Riche dropped out. Through a special grant from the Atkinson Foundation, Mustard provided METEI with test tubes for collecting his samples. Upon its return, he was eager to receive his specimens, or at least reliable data that he hoped to correlate with the islanders' blood pressure and electrocardiograms. But two years later, despite repeated requests, nothing had arrived – no serum, no blood pressures, no results.

In June 1967 Mustard wrote to Richard Roberts. But Roberts replied testily that the data were "in a miscellany of computer print-outs with a lot of other information" and that he did "not have the time or the secretarial assistance to make a transcript." He would refer the request to John Cutler, who had the punch cards in California.[79] The same day, Roberts wrote to Cutler, reminding him that Mustard had provided the team with specimen tubes for cholesterol results, "but whether we used these – or left them on the jetty in San Juan – I cannot say." Almost as a warning, he continued, "In any case, he is a very serious investigator with much work on atherogenesis to his credit."[80] Five days later, Mustard kept up the pressure, politely thanking Roberts for outlining the "plans for providing us with the data. We are very grateful for your help."[81] A month later, Cutler wrote to Mustard, thanking him for his interest in METEI, explaining that the cholesterol results were "fairly low," and promising a publication soon with a reprint, of course. He added a note to the bottom of Roberts's copy: "Richard I hope this seems adequate to you. I really thought he asked for quite a bit."[82]

Finally, in exasperation, Mustard appealed to Helen Reid. She complained on his behalf to no less a person than Dr Rocke Robertson, principal of McGill and Skoryna's ultimate boss. She pointed out that, just as in the case of the dental impressions, Skoryna had been no help at all and was not responding to letters. She demanded that Robertson communicate with Skoryna so that these scientists could finally obtain the material that they had requested and made possible.[83]

Robertson did as he was told. Skoryna replied in writing on 8 December 1967. Abrogating any continuing responsibility for METEI and cloaking himself in the ethics of academic freedom, he declared that he "made a practice of not interfering with the distribution of material and the private arrangements of scientists."[84] Two more months passed before Robertson finally got around to relaying this information back to Dr Reid. He explained that the reasons why the METEI dentist, Al Taylor, had handed over the Toronto material to Arizona scientists were unknown; however, he could not see how McGill could force the Americans to give it back. Dean Roy Ellis of Toronto's dental school should communicate with Taylor directly. Skoryna claimed that the data for serum chemistry, including cholesterol, were in Berkeley with John Cutler, who had already collated the results. Skoryna had told Robertson that Mustard had "originally planned to send one of his assistants [likely Michael F.X. Glynn]," but "that plan was withdrawn at the last minute." Robertson omitted that victim-blaming recrimination from his reply to Helen. Instead, he suggested that Mustard contact Cutler directly – something he had already done.[85] A vicious circle! Neither Mustard nor Cutler ever published on Rapanui cholesterol.

The only "public" dissemination of these chemical test results that I have found came in Roberts's 1966 speech to the CMA – the text that he refused to publish:

· The blood urea nitrogen (BUN) results were "not remarkable."
· The blood glucose results from tests performed on 243 individuals one hour after a sugar drink were "abnormally low"; however, he suspected that they were invalid owing to a problem with method.
· The 252 cholesterol results, he said, were "low by North American standards, all under 270 mgm% with a mean of 170 mgm% (S.D. 34.06) – only 50 were over 200 mgm%." Cholesterol levels rose with age.[86]

Most of the vague figures Roberts offered in that speech would eventually prove to be incorrect. In particular, he minimized the total number of tests completed, although the general good health of the islanders was never in dispute.

RAPANUI HEALTH STATUS – AT LAST!

In early 1968 John Cutler sent Roberts computerized tabulations of all the results of weight, height, blood pressure, pulse, blood glucose, blood urea nitrogen, and cholesterol with cover letters urging a publication (see appendix B, figures B.1, B.2, B.3, B.4, B.5, B.6, and B.7).[87] He also included electrocardiogram results and the chest expansions and outlined five possible articles that could come out of these data: one or two with Richard Roberts; one or two with Maureen, possibly helped by Meier on demographics and genetics; and a final paper on nutrition, using information that he had collected with Isabel Griffiths (and ignoring Reid). He thought it was important to point out whether or not the islanders were inbred.[88] To encourage an article, he even sent sample graphs comparing Rapanui weight, height, blood pressure, cholesterol, and ponderal index with that of Californians (see appendix B, figures B.8, B.9, B.10, B.11, B.12, and B.13). The Rapanui were healthier.

In the same letter, Cutler said that he'd heard nothing from either Elliot Alpert or Stanley Skoryna and that he had no data from them; he assumed that "the idea of a book [final report] has died." Despite Cutler's hard work and constant urging, the articles never appeared, and the tabulated results were never cross-referenced as he had proposed. In other words, they did not uncover relationships between cholesterol and blood pressure or between blood pressure and BUN (a measure of kidney function).

These computer "print-outs" are now with Roberts's papers in Library and Archives Canada. Consequently, we can recreate the never-published data graphically in appendix B. Documenting the near total absence of diabetes, hyperlipidemia, hypertension, and obesity would have been a boon to the health researchers who followed METEI and were forced to rely on far less thorough and less reliable comparators.

Twenty years later, in June 1984, Roberts was invited to address the annual conference of the Canadian Federation of Medical Students, which was featuring military medicine as the theme. In his thirty-minute speech, he described METEI and its problems as "an exercise in specialized medical logistics."[89] For all his sophistication as a clinician and medical leader, once again, there was no IBP, no WHO, no ecology, no airport, and no real science. Nor did he appear to wonder if the cholesterol levels of the Easter Islanders had risen in the intervening twenty years.

SOCIAL SCIENCE

The social scientists on the journey pursued their work, but it was slow, a normal delay that exemplifies why Skoryna's estimate of six months for a final summary was unrealistic. Meier read a progress report on his physical anthropology work at a conference in 1967, mentioning the skulls that Father Sebastian had allowed him to examine in the museum. He successfully defended his dissertation on 9 January 1969. That same year, he reviewed a 1968 book by Rupert I. Murrill, who had analyzed the skeletal material collected by Heyerdahl.[90] Meier maintained a life-long interest in what could be learned from prints of fingers and palms, as well as from their relationship between other body measurements. Between 1975 and 1987, he published six more articles on Easter Island and its dermatoglyphics.[91] Considered an expert in the genetics of evolutionary biology, he has also conducted research on Natives of Alaska and holds the status of Chancellor's Professor Emeritus at Indiana University, Bloomington. In late 2015 he was pleased to finally have an explanation for what had happened to those frozen blood samples that he was never able to incorporate into his thesis.

METEI sociologist Cléopâtre Montandon returned to Montreal in March 1965, and by June she was the mother of a little girl. She had mountains of data from the families that she had interviewed. Fortunately, the questionnaire meant that her data was easily sorted into categories for analysis and could be set aside for later. After the May 1967 appeal sent by Carlotta and fulfilling the promise of her journey, she prepared a 100-page manuscript in French about her sociological research on Easter Island and dutifully sent it to Richard Roberts for inclusion in the "Final report." But she never had a response. The paper is in the national archives.[92]

Denys Montandon decided to leave Montreal and move to Columbia University in New York City to continue his surgical training. He too specialized in plastic surgery, and like Einar Gjessing, he never forgot Garry Brody's operation on Gabriel Hereveri's eye. Cléopâtre persisted in her desire to study sociology and enrolled in Columbia's doctoral program, successfully defending her dissertation in 1973. The topic was not Easter Island, although she had presented a paper on the subject while still a graduate student. Instead, for her thesis, Cléopâtre conducted a historical case study of the eighteenth- and nineteenth-century scientific community of Geneva – an "epistemic-community" topic that was truly ahead of the wave for social studies of science.[93] A son was born too.

The Montandon family returned to Geneva, where Cléopâtre was appointed a professor at the Université de Genève, becoming an expert on the sociology of childhood and education. Back in Switzerland and now with a job, she could return to the Easter Island data. Her thirty-eight-page English-language paper on the sociology, beliefs, dreams, work, leisure, and aspirations of the people finally appeared in a Swiss ethnology journal in 1978. Emphasizing that it was a "case of social change," she traced the history, politics, and culture; then she laid out the hypotheses that had governed her questions, anchored in the scholarly literature, and described the results derived from interviews with 206 individuals (106 men and 100 women) from 129 households representing 82 per cent of the families on the island.[94] She now claims that she would not do the study in the same way and that in 1965 she was "not well prepared" in terms of theory and method. Considering her youth and inexperience, and how rapidly she assimilated the relevant background to put together her questionnaire, the article is a remarkable achievement, documenting that moment in time. It deserves wider visibility.

Cléopâtre was also credited, with Elliot Alpert and Georges Nógrády, for the sampling maps, which had been essential to the census and her work on identifying family groups.[95]

The scientific publications that emerged from METEI were slower but far more numerous than Skoryna expected or likely ever knew. Plagued by the personal acrimony, paltry advance preparation, and confusion over roles and responsibilities, METEI's aftermath lurched from problem to problem. Well-intentioned researchers grew angry. Some gave up in frustration; others simply polished off their papers and sent them to scattered but respectable journals, doubting that a synthetic final report would appear. Fortunately, the work on human health status was preserved in the national archives, allowing us now to perceive the baseline that had been promised. Meanwhile, Armand Boudreault published his meticulous studies on viruses, with a startling discovery that prompted the first of the Rapa Nui returns (see chapter 11), and Georges Nógrády began sharing his extensive collections, which led to METEI's greatest discovery of all (see chapter 12).

Virology, Psychology, and Return Visits

Stanley Skoryna's dream included a return visit to Rapa Nui to repeat investigations. METEI-1 would not be complete without METEI-2. Several travellers began plotting the work that they would do if and when they could go back. But none of those trips took place. Only three alumni of the Medical Expedition to Easter Island ever saw Rapa Nui again. Sometimes, friends and colleagues went as tourists and reported on changes or performed favours, delivering gifts and letters. This chapter describes the unrealized plans for return, the three visits, and the remarkable results of Armand Boudreault's research, which have previously been overlooked.

BEIGHTON'S IDEA, *LIFE* MAGAZINE, AND MONA WILSON'S REPORT

Back in his residency training at Hillingdon Hospital in Uxbridge, England, Peter Beighton wrote to Roberts with a few follow-up ideas. On his way home through Santiago, he "had a long chat with the Minister of Health, about many matters, including the medical status of the Islanders, of whom there are about 300 ... living in Chile." He continued, "I would be most interested to examine them and compare them, as a group, with their relatives on the Island. For instance, what is their instance of cholecystitis, what are their serum cholesterol levels, and is there any evidence of atherosclerosis? ... Do you think METEI would rise to a follow up of this nature?"[1]

Beighton's proposal anticipated Skoryna's repeat study but with a new twist. Rather than returning to the island in some ill-defined future, Easter Islanders living in Chile could be examined for the same parameters; differences between them and their relatives back home could be

related to the length of time they had been away. Did life on the mainland and in its cities expose the Rapanui to new risks and the diseases of
affluence or alter their physiology? Rather than fretting about the infections that had originally motivated METEI, Beighton was contemplating
the "pathologies of progress."[2] This project would have been much easier to conduct than another expedition on a navy ship. It also displays
Beighton's flare for scientific inquiry, which, he now claims, was first
kindled on Easter Island. To be valid, however, his study would have to
be done quickly so that the data from the two groups – on the island and
off – would be nearly contemporaneous. Roberts ignored the suggestion,
and Beighton's idea was not pursued.

A year after METEI's return, Canadian nurse Mona Wilson booked a
South Pacific cruise on the ship *Bergensfjord*. Internationally known for
her work in public health, Mona was seeking to ease the misery of her
forced retirement in 1961. She knew Richard Roberts from their previous
connections to navy medicine, and she had followed the press reports of
METEI from her home on Prince Edward Island. She wrote to Roberts,
offering to carry messages or gifts and to gather any information needed
for their research. Richard and Maureen Roberts took her up on the
offer and sent gifts for individuals and poor families. They also put her
in touch with Carl Mydans, whose *Life* magazine article was just about
to be released. Mydans arranged for a big bundle of fresh copies to reach
her on board the ship. Mona spent only one day on Rapa Nui in March
1966, but her reporting letter to Roberts and Mydans fills three densely
written pages.

Father Sebastian Englert came aboard, and Mona "presented him
with the book, letters, and envelope with *Life*. "When I told him who
they were from, his face lighted up with surprise and delight – as if
he just couldn't believe his eyes and ears. That moment was worth all
the time that everyone had spent to round up the gifts – and I wish
you could have been there to experience it – a moment of sheer joy
and utter amazement." Mona went on to describe her day: a trip with
Alfonso Rapu in Jeep Mea Mea to visit statues; a tour of the "hospital,"
where both Roberts's and Skoryna's offices were preserved unchanged;
a drop-in at the expanding school; and a jaunt to the church and priest's
home to make sure that the three cartons of gifts had safely arrived from
Bergensfjord. "Appalled at the number of cartons of cigarettes that went
ashore," she also conveyed the sad news that Father Ricardo had died of
cancer in May 1965.[3]

EFFORD'S EFFORT TO RETURN

Back in Vancouver, Ian Efford devoted much thought and energy to trying to assemble a Rapa Nui return for ecological work. He still had many intriguing questions and hoped to seize the momentum of METEI-1 for a second expedition to complete the collections gathered on the first. He told Helen Reid that the group of twenty biologists would leave in March 1967.[4] His "original intent had been to put together a three-volume book on the flora and the fauna of the island with a review of its biological history."[5] That the plant material had reached Harvard University damaged and infested with mould meant that it could not be identified, making a good reason for another trip all by itself. The names and topics of his targeted scientists appear in the document "Easter Island Manuscript," now in the University of British Columbia (UBC) Archives; he viewed this write-up as a "first step."[6] Some of these people did eventually produce articles on the material that he had sent to them – or they forwarded it to others, who ignored it. But several things conspired to defeat his plan, and eventually he lost contact with the experts and abandoned both the return journey and the book project.

Nevertheless, Ian went on a "world tour of museums" to speak with their directors about his Rapa Nui findings and ideas. He corresponded with Skoryna and John E. Randall at the University of Hawaii about the proposed "second expedition." They were supportive but sympathized with the challenge of fundraising and the complexities of dealing with Chilean authorities.[7] The idea of appealing to the American branch of the International Biological Programme (IBP) emerged, only to be rejected because Efford had heard that its budget in Washington had been "cut significantly (to 30% of that asked)." By April 1968 he was directing a Canadian IBP project at Marion Lake and could not take on another, although he remained ready to help anyone else who would. Efford never went back to Rapa Nui. He deposited all his METEI papers in the UBC Archives in 1977 when he left to work for the federal government on energy and environmental policies, the beginning of what he calls "intellectual wandering" in Europe and Africa.

BOUDREAULT, VIRUSES, AND *KOKONGO*

Boudreault's serum samples survived the troubles with his freezers (see chapters 3 and 4), as did some viral cultures. He quickly analyzed them for antibody evidence of measles, polio, and other infections. With colleagues at the Université de Montréal, he published the results on

Rapanui antibodies against polio and measles in two French-language articles for the July and December 1966 issues of the *Canadian Journal of Public Health*.[8] These studies revealed levels of immunity to various viruses according to age. Articles on rubella soon followed.[9]

In late spring 1968, he published a lengthy article for the *Bulletin of the World Health Organization* that opened with the reminder that METEI had been carried out under that organization's auspices.[10] The paper included results for evidence of other infections, including influenza, parainfluenza, respiratory syncytial virus, mumps, herpes, and mycoplasma pneumoniae. From 1,500 tissue cultures, Boudreault's team had also isolated eighty enteroviruses, none pathogenic. For their interpretation, they had adopted the latest, elegant methods in virology and serology: antibody inhibition, hemagglutination, and complement fixation. With these tests, the relative resistance to various infectious agents could be determined by the levels of antibodies in people of different ages. The goal of this work, they emphasized, was to highlight possible dangers for the islanders when they come into more frequent contact with the outside world; however, warnings about potential vulnerabilities to infections were "probabilities," not certainties. This method also allowed a tracing of the history of various epidemics on the island: those people exposed would have antibodies; those born later would not. Their conclusions were hampered by the restriction on sampling, which meant that the virologists had "not a drop of blood" from children under age seven; and for those between ages eight and nine, the volume of blood was often insufficient to perform all tests.

Boudreault shared his samples with Juan A. Embil, a microbiologist at Dalhousie University in Halifax, who was working with Dr Vanora Haldane, a younger sister of Maureen Roberts. During 1969–70 their team, supported by a grant from the Canadian Public Health Association, produced three articles on the comparative prevalence of cytomegalovirus on Rapa Nui.[11] Since the late nineteenth century, cytomegalovirus had been the object of microbiological study for its appearance as "inclusion bodies" in cells; however, recent findings had enhanced interest: the virus was named in 1960 as scientists were grappling with its frightening capacity to harm babies in utero, provoking physical and intellectual birth defects.[12] Consequently, this novel work also pointed to another potential danger for the islanders: birth defects from viral invaders. But surprisingly, in comparison with eight other geographical locations, Easter Island had the *highest* titre of cytomegalovirus antibodies, and it occurred in younger children, meaning that most Rapanui women had likely contracted the infection by the time they reached fertility. The authors related these high titres to poor socio-economic conditions and crowding.

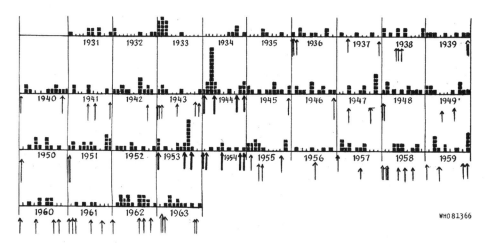

Figure 11.1 Mortality linked to arrival of ships, Easter Island, 1931–63. Each arrow represents a ship, and each small square records a death. Boudreault and Pavilanis, "Epidémiologie des infections virales," 395. By permission of Armand Boudreault and the WHO.

Boudreault also discovered reduced immunity to measles in children aged seven to twelve, leading him to suspect even less protection in younger children. Older people displayed more antibodies. He related this situation to a severe epidemic of measles in 1953 that had likely spread from Chile and provoked seven deaths. His team also studied the incidence of rubella on Easter Island and compared it to that in another isolated island community, Quebec's Iles de la Madeleine. Knowing that medical examiners had documented a high frequency of respiratory infections and asthma, he worried about a contrast between levels of influenza A and B in people under age twenty compared to those who were older. Furthermore, only 12 per cent of Rapanui had any antibodies to influenza A.

With his graphs of Easter Island immunity according to age, Boudreault also printed an interesting – and disturbing – chart, drawn by hand, that linked the number of deaths on Rapa Nui to arrivals of boats for each month in the thirty-two years between 1931 and 1963 (figure 11.1). The year of the 1953 measles epidemic stood out, as did 1944, when a widespread respiratory infection followed the arrival of a ship from Valparaiso, leaving thirteen dead. Boudreault wondered if *kokongo* had been influenza.

In his paper, Boudreault described the *kokongo* outbreak five days after the arrival of *Yelcho* and the collecting of serum samples, both acute and convalescent, and the throat swabs from islanders and marines. He promised a future report on the findings, but that paper never appeared. Those carefully nurtured cells, transported from Montreal to Hanga Roa and back, had died. Although he had success in isolating the eighty innocuous enteroviruses, nothing in the *kokongo* samples would grow. Some blamed the long, hot delay in moving the unplugged freezer from HMCS *Cape Scott* to the shore. Boudreault is more inclined to blame it on the error during the outbound voyage, when the freezer was attached to the wrong voltage and the temperature fell. He made the discovery only one or two days from Halifax and had it corrected immediately, but he spent the rest of the expedition wondering if all the work on viral cultures would be wasted.[13]

The identity of the *kokongo* virus was and still is unknown, although Boudreault continued to suspect that it was a form of influenza until his death in 2018. Endorsing his suspicions and METEI fears, the World Health Organization (WHO) reported an Easter Island epidemic of a respiratory infection, with a "severe clinical picture" affecting almost the entire population, that began in March 1968. "Serological evidence of infection with influenza virus A2 was obtained in a large proportion of the blood specimens."[14] The outbreak started on mainland Chile in January; the airport had been open less than a year.

THE POLIO SAGA AND BOUDREAULT'S GIFT

Well before his articles appeared in print, Boudreault realized that most people on Rapa Nui had no immunity to type 1 poliovirus: only two young adults displayed any antibodies at all. This lack of immunity was seemingly backed up by the medical examinations, which found "no cases of apparent sequelae of polio, such as paralysis." He also wrote that the island's doctor, Guido Andrade, did not recall ever seeing a single case of polio in the two years that he served there. However, Helen Reid, in her 1968 article, wrote of a three-year-old child, likely a girl, with "partial paralysis suggesting that he [*sic*] had previously had poliomyelitis."[15] Peter Beighton also remembers (and can name) a three-year-old girl "with flaccid paralysis" – possibly the same child because at that time the masculine personal pronoun stood for all in "neutral" reporting. Boudreault did not know about the paralyzed child(ren). In any case, the cause of paralysis in this one (or these two) three-year-old(s) is unknown because the blood of children under age seven was not tested. Given the serological results, if the child had suffered and survived polio, the virus would likely have been type 2 or type 3, against which moderate to high antibody concentrations had been identified in 38 and 68 per cent of seven-year-olds respectively.

Easter Islanders may not have been homogeneous from a genetic perspective, but they were uniformly isolated. Furthermore, despite great personal cleanliness, their living conditions facilitated airborne and, especially, fecal-oral transmission of disease (common to polio). They were vulnerable to death from any new infectious agents, and their innate resistance would be sorely tested when the new airport opened. Several hundred Rapanui lived in Chile, Boudreault wrote; they would be able to return for visits more easily and more frequently. Added to this strong probability was the absolute certainty that tourists from all over the world "would take advantage of the new destination to visit this paradise peopled with giant, mysterious statues."[16] Something needed to be done.

Boudreault determined to send polio vaccine to Easter Island as soon as possible. The thought of urging plans on public health authorities in another country, in another language, and waiting for their response did not appeal. The idea that the expedition itself might have left behind some nasty viruses was yet another incentive for action. METEI had relied on Rapanui cooperation to define the risks; it should do everything possible to eliminate or reduce them. He had Skoryna generate a formal request to Armand Frappier at the Institut de Microbiologie et d'Hygiène de Montréal. The vaccine was released on 1 March 1967.[17] Boudreault assembled the supply of trivalent Sabin oral polio vaccine to be carried to the island. He also recommended that virology studies be repeated *every year* following the opening of the airport.

Sabin polio vaccine was first licensed in the United States in 1960 with action against type 1 poliovirus. By 1963 it contained live attenuated viruses of all three types. It was a new and effective way to help people build resistance to any type of polio because it exposed them to a living but harmless form of the virus. It did not need to be injected; it could be swallowed.

What about measles and rubella? Measles vaccine was first licensed in Canada and the United States in 1963. But between 1959 and 1968, at least in Canada, measles was not a reportable disease; aggressive programs for vaccination would not appear until 1970.[18] Boudreault's team did not gather measles vaccine, but in their 1968 article, they strongly recommended that it be sent to Easter Island as soon as possible. As for rubella, the vaccine was still in development; it would receive its first licence in 1969, with Canadian programs beginning only in the 1970s.[19] Those vaccines were not available.

Readers who reliably get their annual "flu shots" might also be wondering why Boudreault did not also gather influenza vaccine. This virus had a long history of research that had entailed growing it in culture and creating vaccines; however, by 1958, scientists understood that it mutated quickly. To be effective, different vaccines were needed for each year and place. Furthermore, it was not until 1973 that the WHO began recommending at-risk individuals receive yearly multivalent vaccines based on surveillance of what viral strains would next appear. Boudreault was caught in that "in-between" period. Any influenza vaccine that he might locate in Canada – and even that was not obvious – would likely be useless on Easter Island.

So polio vaccine it was. But how to get it there? Completion of the new airport loomed, somewhat behind schedule, for March or April 1967, and regular flights were not yet established. Although air travel would be easier and faster, Boudreault aimed to get the vaccine to the island *before* many planes had landed. Therefore, on 1 March 1967, Isabel Griffiths and Carlotta Hacker were dispatched by air to Chile and from there by sea to Rapa Nui.[20] They were laden with gifts, a large bronze plaque, and "25 pounds" of Sabin oral polio vaccine – enough to immunize the entire Rapanui population.

FUNEI: THE RETURN OF GRIFFITHS AND HACKER

Skoryna was delighted that METEI alumni were going back to Rapa Nui. With the debt discharged, he wanted to lay claim to the legacy of the ATCO trailers for the Donner Biological Station. Word had come from Mona Wilson and others that most of the buildings were being used as a hospital and medical clinic. The plaque would identify them as gifts of Canada and McGill University, and it would help to keep the focus on international research, as well as clinical care. Some trailers were to be used for labs and temporary shelter for visiting scientists, whereas the remainder served as a health facility.

Other agendas emerged as the trip was planned. Legal arrangements were still needed to establish ownership for Jeep Mea Mea and the trailers to keep them on Rapa Nui. Scientists, including Boudreault and John Cutler, wanted updates on demographic changes, illnesses, deaths, births, and ship arrivals. METEI had left behind a distillation unit with the permission of its owners in New Orleans; however, those owners later changed their minds. Skoryna had eventually arranged for its return through the Chilean navy. After more delays caused by Chilean customs, the unit was finally returned to the United States but without its expensive compressors.[21] If that missing equipment could be found, the travellers were to ship it back to New Orleans.

Since February 1965, some administrative changes had taken place in consequence of the "rebellion" that METEI had witnessed. Governor Jorge Portilla had been recalled in 1966, replaced by the first civilian governor, Enrique Rogers Sotomayor. Rapanui were now free to move and travel, and they had become Chilean citizens in 1966. The new Easter Island Law (Ley 16,441) of February 1966 established the island as a department of Valparaiso with its own council. The first citizen chosen by Alfonso Rapu to receive her Chilean identity card was the oldest woman on the island, Sofía Hei (Marina Neru having died), followed by Rapu, Manuel Tuki, and his son, Alfredo, who had been on the mainland during the expedition.[22] However, the new governor was not an improvement and "did everything but please the Rapanui."[23] As he came ashore at Hanga Piko, a crowd of angry women hurled insults and stones; forty *carabinieros* rushed to protect him, and the women were beaten with batons – an unprecedented event that deepened ethnic tensions.[24]

The other big change was the arrival of the American air force, committed to developing a "top secret" satellite tracking station for spying on Russia but ostensibly devoted to atmospheric studies. Located at Mataveri, the airmen mingled happily with the population and would stay until the election of Salvador Allende in 1970, leaving behind a lot of equipment, some improvements to infrastructure for water, and several children.[25] Their presence was felt by the time Carlotta and Isabel set out on their second METEI expedition. It is best described in their own words, printed four months after their return in the August 1967 issue of the Rapa Nui Science Club's *Newsletter* – nostalgia and diplomacy liberally mixed with honour, humour, and horror.

```
FUNEI
```

```
The First Unorganized Nonmedical Expedition to Easter Island,
F.U.N.E.I. (pronounced "funny") took place in March and April
this year. The members were Isabel Griffiths and Carlotta Hacker.
Due to pressure of work (etc.), we regret that this expedition
to Easter Island has not been reported earlier. However, we are
happy to announce that it was a Hundred Per Cent Success.
   The members and their undetected excess baggage (one large
bronze plaque, 25 lb. of polio vaccine, one heavy microscope, one
typewriter, a reasonable amount of reading matter, two overnight
bags containing over-year clothing for the Pascuenses, and various
```

other trifles) flew as far as Chile and then boarded the <u>Navarino</u>
for Pascua. The ship was only twelve hours late in leaving.

On arrival at the island, the ship anchored off Vinapu, on
account of rough weather, but even so the entire population of
Rapa Nui — with flowers, babies, and horses — gave the returning expeditioners a true Pascuense welcome. Under a scorching
sun (257°F), the entire company and luggage then <u>walked</u> to Hanga
Roa. Isabel and Carlotta knew they had come home.

Because of the diphtheria epidemic, it was impossible to stay
in the trailer-hospital so FUNEI made its headquarters at the
house of the doctor Jaime Cruz. This made life a little complicated, since Jaime was not only anti-governor and anti-pas-
cuense, but also anti-American and very anti-FUNEI.

To give readers some slight idea of the vigorous activities of
FUNEI during its two weeks on Rapa Nui, here follows an extract
from the diary of Isabel and Carlotta.

DIARY (typical day)

8:00 a.m. Breakfast at doctor's. Isabel discussing Chilean politics with doctor's wife. Carlotta saying "si," "claro," and
  "no," generally at the wrong moments.
8:30 a.m. Walk to notary's office to check births, marriages, and
  deaths since METEI left. Find that half the records we need
  are kept in other files in other parts of the island.
9:00 a.m. Call at governor's office to get permission for ceremony inaugurating plaque. Find governor doesn't start his day
  till 2:30 p.m. Make appointment for 2:30 and look through his
  files in his absence to find shipping records. His pascuense
  secretary most helpful.
9:30 a.m. Set out to walk to Hanga Piko.
9:35 a.m. Two Pascuense on horses pass and give us a lift,
  Pascuense style.
9:45 a.m. Arrive Hanga Piko. Surprise! Surprise! A launch is
  just about to leave and take us to Navarino.
10:15 a.m. Arrive Navarino to collect frozen vaccine from frig.
10:17 a.m. Find it's cleaning day for refrigerators and we can't
  get out the vaccine.
10:18 a.m. Carlotta gives way to brief seizure of temper.
10:20 a.m. Are told no launch will be returning to Hanga Piko
  until 3:30 p.m. because it takes that long to load it.
10:21 a.m. Another slight seizure.
10:25 a.m. Isabel finds CHARMING Pascuense who has a boat.

Pascuense found to be not so charming when he charges $20 for trip to the shore. Eventually settles for 20 Escudos.

10:45 a.m. Leave on boat belonging to another Pascuense who charges nothing and gives us a lobster each into the bargain.

11:14 a.m. Swim.

12:00 [p.m.] Walk to Rapu's.

12:10 p.m. Lunch at Rapu's and we admire plaque which he and Jorge Paté have placed on a wooden board which they have painted white with much loving care.

2:30 p.m. Meet with governor. Tell him what a great guy Rapu is. Get permission for plaque ceremony and discuss legal arrangements for establishment of Donner Biological Station.

3:30 p.m. Call at Rapu's to tell him what a great guy governor is and how cooperative.

4:0[0] p.m. Run to doctor's for "once" (Chilean tea). Find doctor is opposed to plaque ceremony and he insists on phoning Chile for official permission (in other words, to get authorities to say "NO").

4:30 p.m. See Fr. Sebastian in church to ask him to officiate at plaque ceremony. Thereby avoiding offending

    the governor (if Rapu or doctor does ceremony)

    the doctor and Rapu (if governor does it)

    the whole island (if doctor does it)

      etc. etc. etc.

    Fr. Sebastian delighted to do it and starts composing his speech.

5:00 p.m. Run to telephone shack because Rapa Nui secret service tells us that doctor has gone there to talk to Chile.

5:15 p.m. Arrive at telephone shack in time to overhear doctor's conversation, only to learn that the radio is burnt out — so conversation with Chile is impossible.

5:17 p.m. Sigh.

5:30 p.m. Fifteenth frantic search in hospital for spare parts of distillation unit (which were sent to Pascua after METEI left and are worth $3000).

6:00 p.m. Invited to "inspect" the hospital and by mistake find ourselves inspecting, at close range, a small boy with diphtheria.

6:01 p.m. Isabel develops sore throat.

6:30 p.m. FIND spare parts in a trailer.

7:00 p.m. Approaching Plaza Hotu Matua and see old lady who was proved by expedition results to be syphilitic.

Isabel (to Carlotta): "Don't allow her to kiss you. She may be infectious."

Old lady (from afar): "ISABEL! MI AMIGA!" (Runs towards Isabel arms wide and clinches her in a ten-minute embrace.)

7:10 p.m. Isabel's sore throat gets worse.

7:15 p.m. Swim.

8:00 p.m. Visit to American ionospheric camp (at the foot of Rano Kao) in search of antibiotics. Are supplied with assurance and alcohol which proves just as healing. Americans agree to transport spare parts gratis. Also agree to copy latest census for us on their machine.

9:00 p.m. Dinner with governor.

10:30 p.m. Call at Rapu's for after-dinner drinks. Alfonso agrees to hand over Jeep Mea-Mea to hospital. Arrange for public handing-over ceremony of Jeep so that the whole island will realize that the Chileans are not taking it from islanders.

10:45 p.m. Dinner at Atans. Lobster.

11:45 p.m. See notary to arrange METEI wagons to be given to farming cooperative (fortunately there are only two cooperatives, since there are only two wagons).

11:55 p.m. Lift in American jeep (thank goodness) to Icka's.

12:00 [a.m.] Lights go out.

12:10 [a.m.] Rather late for Icka's sau-sau.

1:00 [a.m.] Start walking back from Icka's.

1:45 [a.m.] Enter doctor's house, knocking over and breaking ornament. Baby wakes and cries.

1:55 [a.m.] Wash feet.

2:15 [a.m.] Plan schedule for tomorrow.

2:30 [a.m.] Cock crows.

2:45 [a.m.] Candles expire and so do we.

The achievements of FUNEI are as follows:

1. The trailers were officially inaugurated by Fr. Sebastian in a beautiful ceremony that took place on Sunday March 19. Everyone attended, and it was the first time that the governor the doctor, Fr. Sebastian and Rapu had all been present together in public and had actually smiled at each other and shaken hands [figure 11.2].

2. Legal arrangements for the future of the trailers have been made through the Island notary. When FUNEI arrived, half the trailers were serving as a hospital and were being very well looked after, but the other half were being used as a housing estate for arriving Chileans. The negotiations with the notary (with the approval of governor and doctor) specified that all

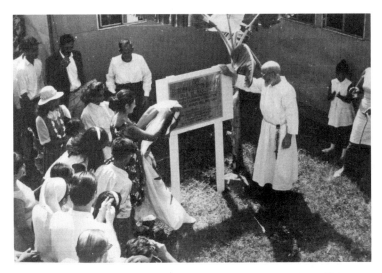

Figure 11.2 *Above*: Father Sebastian Englert and Isabel Griffiths
(*with sheet*) unveiling the plaque to signify that the METEI *campa-
mento* is a gift of the Donner Foundation. Photo Boudreault papers.
Below: Plaque of the Donner Biological Station transported by
Isabel Griffiths and Carlotta Hacker and mounted by the islanders.
Photo June and Gordon Pimm, December 1967.

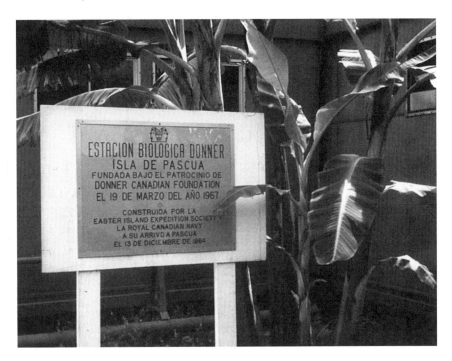

Chileans would leave their trailers on May 1st and that hence-
forward, although still belonging to METEI, the trailers would
be place[d] "in usofructo" to the National Health Service of
Chile to be used as a hospital for Pascua. A similar document
was signed concerning the function of the Jeep Mea-Mea.

A clause was added that visiting scientists could stay in a
maximum of ten trailers — provided they have written permission
to do so from METEI. If anyone wishes to stay in the trailers,
it would also be preferable to write to the governor or doctor,
in advance, advising him of this.
3. The anti-polio vaccine, supplied by Armand Boudreault, has
been safely placed in the hospital refrigerators. There is
enough vaccine to immunize the whole population against polio.
4. The spare parts of the distillation unit were safely shipped
to New Orleans.
5. Up to date records of all ships calling at the island since
1965, of population changes, births, deaths, marriages, and epidemics, as well as related information on immunization etc. This
information may be obtained from John Cutler, who is comparing
it with his census data.
6. As a result of two weeks' propaganda by FUNEI in Chile, Dr.
Jaime Cruz has been removed from Easter Island. This must be a
joy to the Pascuenses, since at least ten of them could be said
to have died through his negligence.

PROGRESS ON PASCUA
Rapa Nui had changed considerably in two years, while retaining its very Rapa Nui character. There is now a bank (no more
bartering sessions) where you can change dollars for escudos;
main roads are being tarred; water is being piped to all houses,
and 24-hour electricity should have been installed by now. And
of course, there is the airport. But we will leave a detailed
description of modern Rapa Nui for Fr. Sebastian's visit [planned
for October]. In the meantime, if anyone requires specific information, please write to Carlotta c/o METEI, Donner Building.

CLM and MIG[26]

Isabel now insists that it was witty Carlotta who composed that only
mildly fictitious essay. In late April the *Montreal Gazette* interviewed
them both. The reporter focused on their interesting personal stories and

seemed to miss the scientific agenda of the long, expensive journey. They had been "lucky" to represent Canada at a dedication ceremony, the journalist wrote; it "fulfilled life-long dreams." Rapanui women were interested in hearing about the new fashions; they asked the Canadian visitors to cut their hair in the latest styles and show them "how to use make up." Polio vaccine was ignored.[27]

FUNEI AFTERMATH: THE FIRST AIRPORT INFECTIONS

If the *Montreal Gazette* wasn't interested in the polio vaccine, did the Chilean health service also ignore the precious gift? Armand Boudreault closed his article by noting that trivalent Sabin vaccine had been given to the island's medical authorities in April 1967.[28] Was it administered to the people? Did the unpopular doctor, Jaime Cruz, arrange to vaccinate all the Islanders before he was sent home? Or was his animus against the Canadian intruders so great that he neglected the task? Did his successor accomplish it instead? Did that successor even know about the vaccine sleeping in the Rapanui hospital freezer? And what was the subsequent incidence of polio on Rapa Nui? Boudreault does not know.

Thanks to those vaccines used elsewhere, the incidence of polio was already declining globally and in Chile.[29] Consequently – and mercifully – the risk of imported polio was also on the wane. Perhaps Boudreault's anxiety had been misplaced. Isabel recalls that Skoryna focused far more on the Donner Biological Station, the plaque, the compressors, and signing the legal papers. Polio vaccine was part of their journey as an add-on.

But what must have been far more concerning to Boudreault was the news of "diphtheria." Caused by a bacterium, not a virus, immunity to that deadly scourge had not been part of his research. Diphtheria had long been a killer of little children, yet it had been moderately well controlled by antitoxin since the 1890s and by vaccine since 1923. In fact, the first Nobel Prize in Medicine went to Emil von Behring for his discovery of that antitoxin in 1901. Georges Nógrády, relying on information provided by Chile, stated that it was "never reported" on the island.[30] Had diphtheria been the first gift of the new airport? How many were afflicted? Was it *really* diphtheria? Had Chilean health authorities not thought to bring reliable vaccines before sending work crews and bulldozers for the airport? The outbreak served as a sobering reminder of exactly the kind of tragedy that "civilization" might bring to the island paradise – the very challenge to human adaptability that Skoryna and Nógrády had imagined in their earliest plans.

METEI'S PSYCHOLOGY ARM

The airport received its first commercial flight on 3 April 1967 (soon after the visit of Isabel and Carlotta).[31] But regular flights were infrequent. At first, Chile's LAN Airlines established a monthly service, which had increased to twice monthly by January 1969.[32] The winners of Skoryna's lottery (see chapter 9), Gordon Pimm of Ottawa and his psychologist spouse, June Pimm, came to Rapa Nui in December 1967 on one of the early LAN flights. An issue of the Rapa Nui Science Club's *Newsletter* had identified them as "the lucky associate members" of METEI who had been "selected" by the Chilean ambassador to Canada, Fausto Soto.[33] Both were McGill grads, and she had been a school psychologist and was pursuing a doctorate at Carleton University. Although the lottery win had been intended as a holiday adventure, the Pimms planned to spend a week on Rapa Nui conducting psychological tests on ninety islanders, both adults and, especially, children. A McGill press release before their departure reported that the airport was still "under construction" but noted that the island now had four "visits" each year by supply ship. In addition to the psychology research, the travellers were to investigate recent changes and "attitudes to the construction of the airport." Their work was said to be "under the auspices of the continuing expedition."[34]

The Pimms had planned to take the supply ship, but the interval between the win and their departure made it possible to fly. They travelled on Canadian Pacific Air via Mexico and Lima to Santiago. Skoryna had notified his contacts in Lima and Santiago, who received them warmly; however, they were dismayed to discover that their hosts thought that they had won this "lottery" because of their superior knowledge of South America. Nevertheless, the Spanish-speaking wife of the Canadian ambassador to Chile was an enthusiastic guide; she would be leading a group of elite tourists on the LAN flight from Santiago to Rapa Nui. A large marching band gave the plane a resounding send-off, but a certain tension filled the cabin on the long flight. A German navigator helped the Chilean pilots – and when the island finally came into view, a crew member was so excited (or relieved) that he ran up and down the aisle announcing their arrival.

Gordon and June lived in an ATCO trailer among the small cluster of the newly inaugurated Donner Biological Station. Comparing their late 1967 photographs with those taken in 1965 reveals that most of the trailers in the Camp Hilton arrangement had already been dragged away in the few months since Isabel and Carlotta's visit (figure 11.3). To June's horror, their abode was swarming with cockroaches. The

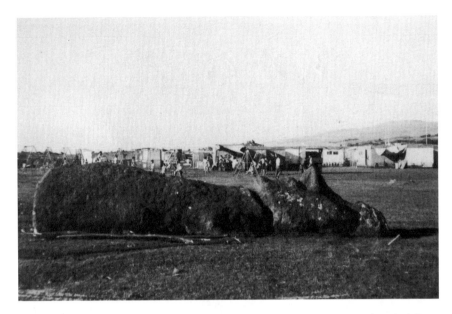

Figure 11.3 *Above*: METEI's Camp Hilton and children's playground with fallen *moai*, early 1965. Photo Armand Boudreault. *Below*: June Pimm seated on fallen *moai*, December 1967. Most of Camp Hilton has already vanished. Photo Gordon Pimm.

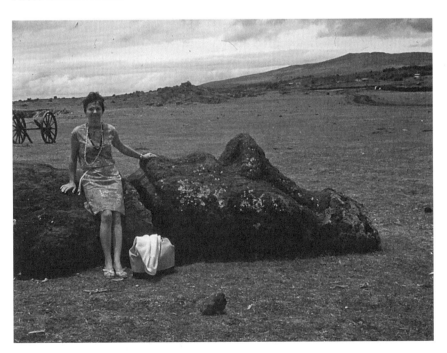

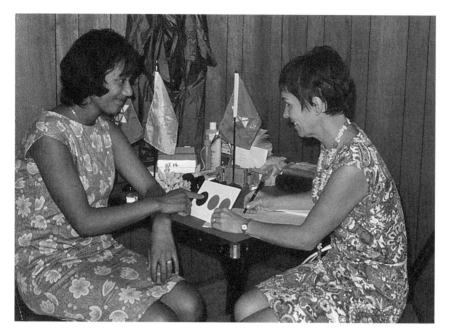

Figure 11.4 June Pimm (*right*) at work performing psychological tests on Rapa Nui, December 1967. Photo Gordon Pimm.

ever-resourceful Gordon produced a spray can of insect repellent and thoroughly soaked the bed and its environs. No one had warned them that the island still lacked hotels, stores, and restaurants, and no provisions had been made for their meals. On the first morning, thoughtful Rapanui left fruit and milk at their door, and they were invited for a meal in a private home. Sometimes, for a hefty price, they joined the elite tourists who were lodged in a tent city nearby, having brought all their supplies along. The Pimms also took note of Americans doing "top secret" work.

Skoryna's good reputation and his advance planning on June's behalf meant that people came voluntarily to the old hospital for her research (figure 11.4). They used a metal gurney as a desk and parked it outside to avoid cockroaches. At the end of a week, they had tested ninety individuals – half male and half female – with fifteen of each sex in three age groups: five to eleven, twelve to twenty, and twenty-one to seventy-two. They used the Goodenough Draw-a-Man test to explore IQ – a test that was said to be without cultural bias, for it did not depend on language or calculation. The resultant IQs were average compared to developed nations. They went on to investigate two variables: preference for delayed versus immediate reward; and colour-form preference.

The test for "delayed gratification" had been inspired by the Stanford University "marshmallow experiments" of Walter Mischel, who hypothesized that children capable of delaying gratification did better in school and in life than those who could not. He had also implied that there were ethnic differences: but no one knew if these differences were innate or learned. The Pimms found that the islanders preferred to wait for a delayed but larger reward, and this outcome was independent of IQ. One could not help but speculate on whether this behaviour was due to their longstanding relationship to the often-tardy supply ship.

The colour-form variable was also a product of the recent theorizing of Norman L. Corah, who had shown that roughly between ages three and six, children prefer colour to form, whereas after age six, they revert to form – the "more mature" choice. The Pimms found that all age groups displayed a strong preference for colour over form. They compared their findings to other groups reported in the literature from Canada and elsewhere.

No publication emerged from this research. In retrospect, Dr June Pimm realizes that the topic was remote from that of her still incomplete dissertation, and it drew on theories that were unpopular with her supervisors. Nevertheless, she prepared a scholarly paper that was accepted through peer review for a psychology conference in Sao Paulo, Brazil, in April 1973.[35]

The Pimms gave a debriefing presentation at McGill during the weekend of 19–22 January 1968. METEI alumnus David Macfarlane was in attendance and reported in the *Montreal Star*.[36] Skoryna had also summoned a television crew, and June recalls that he was coaching her "from the wings." Many improvements had appeared on Rapa Nui, to which Canada had "contributed tremendously," although the (unmentioned) American base had done its part. Macfarlane stopped short of attributing all benefits directly to METEI; however, the tone of his story was boosterish: the islanders "think of B.C. as 'Before Canada.'" In late December 1967, the attitudes on the island to Canada, to METEI, and especially to Skoryna were positive. Macfarlane also reported on the anticipated return journey to be led by Ian Efford. At that time and even fifty years later, the Pimms were unaware of Alfonso Rapu and his rebellion. Things were calm.

MORE RETURNS:
MOAI RAISING AND DR BRODY'S SECOND VISIT

The airport was opening up archeological and anthropological activity. In 1967–68 another *moai* was raised and crowned with a red topknot with French funding and the help of Rapanui carvers, American air force personnel, a mechanized crane, and possibly also the famous bulldozer. Enticing more tourists, the event was covered in *Paris Match* magazine with lavish illustrations depicting Father Sebastian, Alfonso Rapu, and the Rapanui team. Tragically, the journalist and photographer perished in a plane crash at Guadeloupe on their way home before their article had appeared.[37]

Father Sebastian had helped this team, just as he had helped METEI and many of the other researchers over the years. He now had contacts all around the world and set out to use them to raise awareness of the plight of his island and its antiquities. Although he was frail and well on in years, he twice made the long journey to North America, giving lectures and meeting with old friends. In early October 1967, he spoke in Montreal, renewing contact with METEI alumni over dinner at the McGill Faculty Club. On a second visit in January 1969, he died suddenly in New Orleans; his body was returned by air to Rapa Nui, an emotional event with "heartbreaking singing" witnessed by the visiting American writer John Dos Passos.[38]

Dr Garry Brody had hosted the travelling Father Sebastian in his home, and soon afterward he became the third original METEI member to return to Rapa Nui. Upon arriving, he was saddened to learn of the death of Gabriel Hereveri, for whom he had performed the eyelid operation and devised an adapted carving tool. Brody remembers that at least some of Camp Hilton was still standing as the Donner Biological Station. Once again, he was needed as a surgeon. On 18 January 2016 he wrote this account of his family's 1970 vacation:

I had a meeting in Australia and decided to take the opportunity to show my family Easter [Island] by tracing the ... Heyerdahl migration routes. This led us first to Samoa and then to Easter, ending in Machu Picchu. We had one suitcase filled with textbooks, so the kids wouldn't miss too much school. As we approached the Island [runway], we noted construction at one end and we were told they were lengthening it, as it was too short for jets like ours! Fortunately, we made a safe landing.

We were housed with one of the Pasquenses ... Amenities were challenging to say the least. There were a number of tourists, but [it was] not crowded. The flights were weekly, so we had lots of time to roam around. One day, a boy fell off of a horse and had left upper quadrant pain. The doctor was on vacation in Chile, so I was asked to see him. Also on the Island were a pediatrician and a University of Texas anesthesiologist. We all agreed that the boy could [have] ruptured his spleen. Without such things as MRI and blood banks, [we knew that] his life [could be] in danger. So we all agreed that it was better to look and see, rather than wait and see. The only anesthesia available was ether.

... [W]e took him to surgery, with the pediatrician as assistant. And indeed, [the spleen] was ruptured. I removed it and stopped the bleeding. As I was working, I looked up at the anesthesiologist. He would repeatedly give the boy 2 drops of the ether and then take one for himself. However, fortunately, all went well.

As we were finishing, I was shown a man with 3rd degree burns on his leg that needed skin grafting. The anesthesiologist decided to give him a spinal block – thus he didn't need to share the ether.[39]

Brody completed that procedure too.

By 1970 METEI members believed that Skoryna would never produce the final report of their expedition, but they could not understand why. The physicians were puzzled by Richard Roberts's reticence to leverage their data into papers, and the other scientists simply got on with their work and their lives. Boudreault's lab generated several important articles about the immune status of islanders, including their past exposure and continued vulnerability to infections, especially polio. Skoryna was always happy to "spin" about METEI and Canada, hoping that it would allay the bad feelings and encourage donors. In that context, the return visit of Isabel Griffiths and Carlotta Hacker was to tie up loose ends; however, Boudreault seized it as an opportunity to provide vital polio vaccine only days before the airport would open. But we do not know if the vaccine was given. Similarly, June and Gordon Pimm were sent to correct a defect by establishing a METEI psychology arm. Meanwhile, the idea of that essential return expedition had died. Individual articles continued to be published wherever they could find a home, scattered and unrecognized as the fruits of METEI. One person alone tried to keep track, circulating updated bibliographies of all the speeches, abstracts, posters, and articles that he could locate: Georges Nógrády.

Nógrády's Legacy and a Wonder Drug

The last research product stemming from the Medical Expedition to Easter Island was the surprising achievement of microbiologist Georges Nógrády. The much-maligned bacteriologist had diligently gathered more than 5,000 specimens, mostly bacterial cultures and soil samples, from his carefully determined points across the entire island. Many were plated and grown in the lab on Rapa Nui. Carlotta Hacker told Helen Reid that one of her best days was when she found "little black things on red," referring to bacterial colonies on blood agar.[1] But many other samples had to be taken to Canada for further analysis. Given his diligence in gathering material, publications should have flowed from his lab; however, one is hard-pressed to find a single peer-reviewed publication stemming from his work. In fact, Nógrády published very little over his entire university career, which ended with his death in 2013. A total of six peer-reviewed publications from 1959 to 1976 are listed in the online Web of Science database. Nógrády imagined that his task was to gather, document, and share. Ian Efford's observation that he was a "compiler" rather than a scientist seems apt, for Georges plunged into sharing his material with others and organizing speeches and symposia to discuss what they had found.

Nógrády's own papers, like Stanley Skoryna's, are gone. We find the ideas of this naive but ever-so-enthusiastic man in his letters that others kept and in the traces of the scientific events that he organized. One can imagine that he spoke often with Skoryna; they both lived in Montreal and had conjured the dream together. Little remains to reflect those conversations, if indeed they ever took place. For all the work that he accomplished and all the material he amassed, Georges published only one peer-reviewed paper on the Easter Island work: a two-page 1976 article addressing the archeological subject of stone basins.[2] Nevertheless, Nógrády's legacy is the greatest of all.

GEORGES STARTS TALKING AND SHARING

Like the biologists, *micro*biologists (bacteriologists) were interested in identifying previously unknown species, whether or not they were harmful to humans. They were equally interested in the properties of these bugs. In order to protect themselves in their natural habitats, some bacteria were tiny factories of complex substances that could kill other living organisms, such as enemy bacteria and fungi. Soil bacteria had produced streptomycin, the first drug known to have specific activity against tuberculosis – an achievement that garnered the 1952 Nobel Prize in Medicine for American Selman Waksman. The award provoked a great deal of controversy over who really deserved the honour: the scientist or his angry graduate student Albert Schatz. This much-publicized discovery also meant that pharmaceutical companies could imagine untold riches lurking in the earth of unexplored lands. Georges had included a search for antibiotics in the soil samples from caves, and while still on Rapa Nui, he had told Helen Reid that Ayerst Pharmaceuticals in Montreal was interested in this work.[3]

Nógrády fell in love with Easter Island. He adored all aspects of its people, history, geology, anthropology, archeology, mythology, and culture. He tried to decipher its runes and explored their interconnections with writing from other places. He cherished the publications of his fellow travellers, maintaining a bibliographical list, which he distributed with updates to Richard Roberts, Reid, and others.[4] It included speeches, posters, abstracts, and manuscript reports, as well as published articles. Assuming everyone shared his passions, he wrote to his METEI friends Richard and Maureen Roberts, Tony Law, Helen Reid, and Denys and Cléopâtre Montandon, enclosing clippings from newspapers and magazines and notifying them of Rapanui news, gleaned from his reading, radio, and television. He was surprised and charmed by Helen Reid's tender description of him in her book and wrote to tell her so.[5] Some missives were typewritten, crawling with mistakes and corrections; others were handwritten, often on scraps of torn paper and signed with "Warm regards," even "Love." When a colleague visited Easter Island in May 1972, Nógrády quoted this letter to Tony Law: "The Donner Biological Station has been swollowed [*sic*] up by the hospital and only exists as a sign ... Everyone's ambition is to build a bigger house so that they can welcome tourists ... Their notions about acquiring goods resemble remarkably your average suburbanite. There are over sixty private vehicles on the island ... and another 10 private ones are expected on the next boat."[6] Things were changing rapidly.

Georges also wrote to the Robertses about the similarities he had observed between the Rapanui language and Hungarian: "at first I thought I was hallucinating," he said. But he found a scholarly treatise to back up the observation.[7] In another handwritten letter to the Robertses from 1978, he numbered ten exciting and eclectic topics of interest, including Easter Island news, Hungarian poetry, recent conferences, physiognomy, and reviews of Australian Nobel laureate Frank Macfarlane Burnet's "controversial book" on "the future of the human race."[8] If he was aware of the opprobrium that had been heaped upon him during METEI, no trace appears in this florid correspondence.

Like all the other travellers, Georges was often invited to speak about the voyage, and we have the impression that he readily volunteered to do so. On his list of METEI products, we find seminars that he delivered in Montreal. In 1966 there were four: one to his own department, another to the pediatric branch of the Med Chi Society of McGill University, a third to the Société de Microbiologie de la Province de Québec, and the fourth, with colleague R. Toutant, at the annual conference of the Association canadienne-française pour l'avancement des sciences (ACFAS). The first three of these presentations were tailored overviews of METEI work, skewed for the audience. A ten-page typescript by Nógrády in Richard Roberts's papers may have formed their basis.[9] The fourth, in French, was the only 1966 paper that delved into what could be called "research results." It concerned the demonstration of antibiotic properties in staphylococci taken from the mouths of the islanders. These oral bacteria might have displayed an inhibitory (or killing) effect on streptococci, which is the bacterial cause of "strep throat," scarlatina, and erysipelas. The only thing we know about that paper is its title.[10]

In 1967 three more Nógrády communications appear on his list. He spoke, *en français*, about the problems of Rapanui teeth at the Université de Montréal's dental school. Presumably he relied heavily on Al Taylor's newly published article, although he may well have included his own findings about the "protective" staphylococcal bacteria in the mouths of the islanders. He addressed the Ottawa Valley chapter of the Biological Photographic Association on "photography and cinematography for documentary and scientific purposes." For these two talks, again, we have only their titles. Although photography seems to be a leap in subject matter for the microbiologist, Nógrády was no stranger to cameras. He had made two short films for teaching purposes at the Université de Montréal: one featured the inhibiting effect of streptomycin on *E. coli* bacteria; the other featured the lethal action of a toxin from staphylococci on a chicken embryo. He had also produced an annotated bibliography of microbiological films ranging in length from two minutes to an hour.[11] And Georges took hundreds of slides and photographs and shot many metres of movie film on Rapa Nui.

For the third 1967 communication, an abstract resides in the national archives.[12] It simply states that Nógrády had given a set of his soil samples to Professor Paul Hauduroy, director of Lausanne's International Center for Information on and Distribution of Type-Cultures, affiliated with the World Health Organization (WHO). We do not know if Georges travelled to Lausanne to meet Hauduroy and deliver his samples or if he relied on the mails. Here at least was one dutiful return on the original WHO investment.

Hauduroy was a distinguished bacteriologist with a Lausanne professorship and more than a hundred postwar publications to his credit.[13] He was instrumental in creating the first international initiative for sharing information around microbiological culture collections. Since the late nineteenth century, various institutions had established bacteria collections: the oldest are in Louvain, Belgium (1894), and Utrecht, Netherlands (1906). Hauduroy's centre began in 1946.[14] By August 1962, the first international conference on culture collections was held in Ottawa: 266 scientists from twenty-eight countries were in attendance. They recommended that a special section for collections be created within the International Association of Microbiological Societies. That section was launched the next year, and by 1970 it had become the World Federation of Culture Collections, which still coordinates myriad collections around the globe. Among delegates at the original Ottawa conference, two years before METEI, were Georges Nógrády and his Université de Montréal colleague Claude Vézina (see below).[15]

Hauduroy's personal area of interest and expertise, like that of Armand Frappier in Canada, was mycobacteria, the type of germs that cause tuberculosis and leprosy. Mycobacteria were known to be sensitive to the antibiotic derivatives of soil bacteria, including Waksman's Nobel Prize–winning streptomycin and rifamycin; rifampin, a later derivative of rifamycin, is still a mainstay in tuberculosis treatment. In 1950, reflecting his personal, lengthy combat against tuberculosis, Hauduroy nominated French veterinary bacteriologist Camille Guérin for a Nobel Prize for his role in the development of Bacille Calmette-Guérin (BCG).[16] An attenuated form of mycobacterium, much like Sabin's living poliovirus, BCG was intended to provoke immunity to tuberculosis without causing disease. It had been widely promoted in the second third of the twentieth century. In 1963 Hauduroy and colleagues published on methods for determining the sensitivity and resistance of mycobacteria to new chemotherapeutic agents.[17]

These pharmaceutical fruits of the earth and the evidence of tuber-culosis on Easter Island became major preoccupations for Nógrády. In January 1968 he submitted a detailed progress report to distinguished chemist Roger Gaudry, who had been appointed rector of the Université de Montréal in 1965 following a decade as research director at Ayerst Pharmaceuticals. Nógrády reported on aspects of the expedition that concerned him: "mycology, bacteriology, immunology, dental caries, and sample preservation." Like Efford, Nógrády had given many of his sam-ples into the hands of colleagues at laboratories in Canada, England, France, Germany, Hungary, Sweden, Switzerland, and the United States. He described a total of forty-two different METEI-generated "projects" with names of collaborators, twenty-five of them marked "finished," some of which can now be traced to subsequent publications. Several others were "in progress," with reports expected in one to twelve months. But for a few – in particular, those of Elliot Alpert on histoplasma and Richard Roberts on the medical examinations – no report had appeared; reminders were sent.[18] Nógrády was keeping track of METEI's scientific results far more closely than Skoryna.

By 1969 Nógrády was immersed in tuberculosis identification and treatment. He travelled to Kalamazoo to read a paper on "Easter Island and Its Medical Problems" for the American Chemical Society and the Upjohn Company.[19] The manufacturer had a deep interest in poten-tial new drugs from biological sources. Since at least 1946, it had been bringing forward its own versions of several bacteria-derived products, including albamycin, clindamycin, erythromycin, neomycin, streptomy-cin, tetracycline, and its neomycin-containing compound for topical use Mycitracin.[20] Vancomycin had famously been isolated in 1953 by Eli Lilly and Company from soil collected by a missionary in the jungles of Borneo.[21] Equally mysterious and tantalizing, surely Rapa Nui's earth contained a wonder drug.

THE 1969 SYMPOSIUM, TORONTO

Nógrády's big event in 1969 was a Toronto symposium about Easter Island, organized as part of the fifth annual meeting of the Canadian Society of Chemotherapy. ("Chemotherapy" did not imply cancer treatment, as it does today, but referred to all drug treatments for any disease, as opposed to diet, exercise, surgery, or radiation.) One of the society's founders was Dr K.J.R. ("Kajer") Wightman, chief of medi-cine and holder of the University of Toronto's prestigious Eaton Chair.[22] Perhaps the Toronto location was Wightman's doing. With a cluster of other organizations, the society sponsored its own *International Journal of Clinical Pharmacology, Therapy and Toxicology*. All that remain of the symposium are the program and the slim pocketbook of abstracts.[23]

The symposium took place on 16 April 1969 at the Park Plaza Hotel in downtown Toronto. The papers were to be ten minutes long, but because of some dropouts, Nógrády had extended their time to a quarter-hour each.[24] He induced both Skoryna and Roberts to attend. In summarizing the purpose of METEI, Skoryna reverted to his tired (and tiring) leitmotiv: "All objectives of the Expedition, have been fulfilled, and the total sampling of the population as well as the environment (animals, plant life, ecology) have been obtained. These will likely be particularly valuable in view of the fact that isolation of the island has ended with the construction of the airport."[25]

These triumphant words probably set Roberts's teeth on edge. Speaking next, the latter gave a shortened version of his 1966 speech on health and hygiene to the Canadian Medical Association, supplemented with slides and reference to Armand Boudreault's articles and Helen Reid's paper of the previous year in the *Canadian Medical Association Journal*, although she was not on the program.[26] Where *was* Helen? The symposium was taking place only a pleasant, fifteen-minute stroll from her hospital. Was she invited to speak? Did she decline? She told Boudreault, who had hoped to see her, that she could not attend because she was "on call" for children recovering from surgery for cleft lip.[27] This eminently moveable duty could easily have been switched with a colleague; however, it offered an excuse (or a pretext) for avoiding people she did not wish to see, especially those who had slighted her research.

A featured guest was Chilean physician Israel Drapkin, founding director of the Institute of Criminology at the Hebrew University of Jerusalem. Early in his career as a physician and criminal anthropologist trained in the "Italian tradition," he had begun studying socially marginalized peoples, starting with leprosy on Easter Island. Participating in the "Franco-Belge" expedition of 1934–35, Drapkin had offered medical care as needed to its 456 inhabitants. His Toronto paper summarized the health findings that he had gathered three decades before METEI. It would have been a useful comparator for Skoryna's never-written final report. Drapkin recalled that the "totality of the population" had suffered from scabies and gonorrhea of a mild variety but no other venereal disease. He described "a kind of grippe ... exacerbated by the arrival of ships," the *kokongo* of his day. "Everybody received smallpox vaccination," said Drapkin; however, his preoccupation, then and later, was to determine physical "types" of criminals and marginalized peoples from careful measurement of their bodies through a "traditional" approach soon deemed passé. He was working on an edited volume about "victi-mology." Loyal to the method, for a series on great figures in Judaism, he authored a 1977 Spanish-language biography of Cesare Lombroso – "the creator of modern scientific criminology."[28]

Another distinguished visitor was the Danish physician, paleopathol-ogist, and leprosy expert Vilhelm Möller-Christensen, director of the Medical History Museum in Copenhagen. In 1973 he would take up a position with the WHO Institute for the History of Leprology. He had studied skulls in the catacombs of Paris and at the anatomy museum in Edinburgh. From the abstract of his Toronto presentation, it appears that he summarized previously published work and referred to his newly completed research on the signs of leprosy in 650 well-preserved skele-tons from a medieval burial site in Denmark. It is not clear that he had seen any of the same Easter Island skulls examined by METEI, although he had studied human remains in India, Malaysia, and Thailand. Because leprosy was a health problem on Rapa Nui and often affected the face, he emphasized the diagnostic significance of loosened incisors early in the clinical course.[29]

How Drapkin and Möller-Christensen were known to the METEI alumni is yet another mystery. Delegates to the chemotherapy society meeting might have been wondering why history, anthropology, and clinical signs were relevant to their interest in drug innovation.

Two symposium papers were products from Nógrády's own sam-ples. For the first, he spoke about how he had executed his "antibio-sis" project to gather sixty-eight soil samples, with forty-seven more from water and five from caves.[30] For the second, two colleagues joined him in reporting on his mycobacterial research, seeking evidence of the leprosy germ in swabs taken from the noses of the islanders. The usual techniques to diagnose leprosy – skin biopsy, animal inoculation, and tissue culture – were impractical on the island. METEI scientists resorted to rubbing the nasal mucosa of islanders with cotton swabs that were immediately smeared on glass slides for later staining and examination by microscope for *Mycobacterium leprae*. Only one of the 485 smears thus examined displayed the organism. In addition, Nógrády's little team reported that 458 samples of blood serum had been frozen for later testing for antibodies against various mycobacte-ria. They also informed the audience that a complete series of smears and serum samples had been sent – like his soil samples – to Hauduroy's Center for Type-Cultures in Lausanne.[31] Nógrády was a collector and a disseminator par excellence.

The remarkable Dr Edith Mankiewicz (née Meyer) presented the mycobacterium antibody results from Nógrády's 458 serum samples. A physician and microbiologist at the Royal Edward Chest Hospital in Montreal, she was Jewish, born in Leipzig, and had twice suffered from tuberculosis herself. Her husband was a judge whose 1930s decisions against Nazi supporters put their lives in grave danger, notwithstanding their conversion to Roman Catholicism. They escaped to Paris before the war; however, during the German occupation of France, they had to flee again, this time to Shanghai. At the end of the war, they settled in Canada. At each stop, they were obliged to learn new languages and repeat qualifying examinations, but they always found work.[32] They were Nógrády's kind of people.

Mankiewicz discovered that sixty-three (13.8 per cent) of the Rapa Nui serum samples were positive for antibodies to typical or atypical mycobacteria and that sixteen (3.5 per cent) were strongly positive to typical human tuberculosis. For three of these patients, she confirmed active disease using Archie Wilkinson's chest X-rays. As for leprosy antibodies, the scientists had collected enough serum from only one of the people known to have the disease. The sample was strongly positive for *Mycobacterium fortuitum*, a rapidly growing variant, capable of causing skin and lung infections, although it was not deemed responsible for either tuberculosis or leprosy. Eight other samples from apparently healthy people were also positive for the same germ. This paragraph is the first publication of these results.[33]

The only other woman scientist on the program was Sigyn Magnusson from the virology lab of Erik Lycke in Gothenburg, Sweden. She compared the virus-inactivating capacity of twelve samples of Rapanui seawater to that of the Baltic and North Seas. Since some viruses, like polio, were known to thrive and spread aquatically, scientists were interested in their relative survival in different types and temperatures of water. Lycke and Magnusson had noticed that viruses grew less well in natural seawater than they did in laboratory salt water of the same salt concentration (salinity) and pH (acidity). Given that bacteria were known to produce substances against other bacteria and fungi, was it possible that microorganisms living in the sea were responsible for this effect? If so, could discovery of their identity be leveraged as treatment for viral infections or as a means of attenuating viruses to make vaccines – like Sabin polio vaccine? The study presented in Toronto claimed that Rapa Nui's seawater did indeed inactivate enteric viruses – specified in the abstract as nine "DNA or RNA animal viruses and one bacteriophage" – and that it did so just as well as the Nordic waters. Heating for only one hour at

45° Celsius destroyed the inhibitory activity in most samples, tending to suggest that the antiviral effect came from something "alive" or organic that had been killed or denatured by heating. From the seawater, she isolated a type of *Pseudomonas* bacterium that might have been responsible. She noticed, however, that two of the Easter Island samples were not sensitive to heat, as they continued to inhibit the growth of viruses. This observation led her to wonder if their effects were the result of a chemical secretion or a toxin.[34] Into the future, only a handful papers would pursue the intriguing idea of seawater antivirals. The last work on the subject appeared in a Canadian journal in 1982, citing Magnusson and Lycke but not Easter Island.[35]

One final paper in the symposium was an analysis of bacteria in the soil samples that Nógrády had collected on the island. The speaker was a university colleague of Nógrády, microbiologist Claude Vézina, who had been in the loop of the 1967 correspondence over polio vaccine with Armand Frappier and was also affiliated with the laboratories of Ayerst Pharmaceuticals in Montreal. Since completing his 1956 doctorate at the University of Wisconsin–Madison, Vézina had been active internationally, specializing in fermentation processes for industry; he would eventually serve as the president of the Canadian Society of Microbiologists for 1978–79. Nógrády probably knew him through the microbiology department at the Université de Montréal, where Vézina had been teaching courses and supervising students since 1960, the same year that he also joined Ayerst.[36] Vézina forwarded seventy-three of Nógrády's soil samples to his contacts at Ayerst to be examined for bacteria and fungi. Nógrády could grow the organisms in his lab, but he did not have facilities for gathering their secretions – nor would he be able to test them in comparison with many different antibiotics, other than the small panel of already known drugs. Industry could perform these tests on a large scale. Georges gave the samples to his colleague.

By the time Vézina went to the Toronto symposium, his team had examined fourteen surface samples and one taken from a cave, from which they had isolated 403 different organisms. About 8 per cent of these microbes (approximately thirty-two) displayed activity against various bacteria and fungi. Those active only against "gram-positive bacteria" were set aside; the others with activity against gram-negative bacteria or fungi, or both, were being mass cultivated in "shake flasks" for further investigation.[37] This short paper about Vézina's incomplete work was the beginning of a blockbuster discovery, although no one, except perhaps Vézina and his team, realized it at the time.

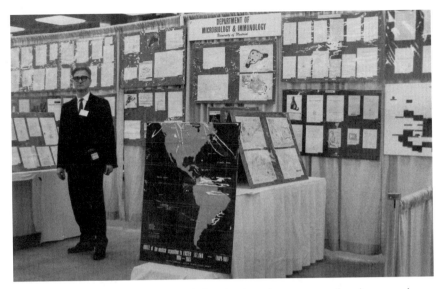

Figure 12.1 Georges Nógrády with his display about METEI for the annual conference of the American Society for Microbiology, Boston, April 1970. LAC, Roberts Papers, vol. 1, file 6.

Richard Roberts received a thank-you letter from psychiatrist Heinz Lehmann of the Douglas Hospital in Montreal in his capacity as president of the Canadian Society of Chemotherapy. German-born and Jewish, like his fellow Montrealer Edith Mankiewicz, Lehmann had been a pioneer in testing the effects of the drug chlorprozamine on people with mental illness during the 1950s. Having attended Nógrády's symposium, he wrote that all the Easter Island papers had been "well received, highly interesting, and of great informative value," although he was sorry for the small turnout. Lehmann also expressed his appreciation for an exhibit that had remained up for the entire meeting and for a film (unspecified), which was shown three times.[38]

Nógrády was delighted. His samples of earth, water, and blood were attracting the attention of distinguished colleagues all around the world, and they were stimulating novel ways of thinking about humans and other organisms. He sent the booklet of abstracts to METEI alumni. What did the audience members of the chemotherapy society really think of the symposium? Despite Lehmann's prediction, none of the papers appeared in the society's *International Journal of Clinical Pharmacology, Therapy and Toxicology*. Perhaps the delegates had enjoyed hearing about the logistics, anthropology, sociology, and health conditions on Rapa Nui as diversions from their main agenda. But Vézina's paper and possibly also that of Magnusson were right up their alley: these papers hinted at future drugs.

A year later, in April 1970, Nógrády attended the annual conference of the American Society for Microbiology (ASM) in Boston, where he mounted a multipanelled poster about METEI – possibly the same exhibit that he had presented in Toronto. A large black and white photo shows him standing solemnly in front of his display (figure 12.1).[39] Avid for new ideas, Nógrády was probably a regular at these meetings. The following year, he described the 1971 ASM meeting in Minneapolis for the Montandons, and in 1981 he gave Richard Roberts a description of his presentation on isolating the *Pseudomonas* germ from contaminated samples at the ASM meeting in Dallas.[40]

THE 1971 SYMPOSIUM, MONTREAL

In April 1971, one year after the Boston meeting, Nógrády hosted a three-day international symposium at the Université de Montréal. The task was to present the fungi and bacteria uncovered by METEI in the soil and water of Easter Island, as well as the relevant immunology. Stanley Skoryna made introductory remarks, once again claiming that the expedition had "totally fulfilled its objectives."

Nógrády's breathless, eight-page letter to Denys and Cléopâtre Montandon describes the three-day symposium, his lonely efforts to run all aspects by himself, the inevitable dropouts, the grandiose assumptions of some delegates, and the myriad last-minute headaches of local arrangements.[41] He wrote about the naysayers who rose "like sharks" to predict "disaster," "failure," and "scandal" – and about the insulting boycott by microbiologists from Montreal universities and hospitals. His wife, Bernadette, feared that he would have a heart attack from the enormous stress. But Nógrády prevailed. "Perhaps the genetic message of my *condottieri* ancestor, or the systematic training of my father to forget weakness in an emergency, helped me in those critical moments ... I felt this is an important moment of my [career], which needs the maximum output of energy." Kind people appeared to help at the last minute: a disabled secretary, his adopted niece, and the adolescent children of a neighbour. "I am convinced enthusiasm is an infectious disease," wrote the microbiologist.[42]

After the first successful day of papers with "high professional standards," the enemy voices fell to a whisper and then to silence. Evening receptions raised the spirits of the 120 scientists; one featured Skoryna, and all boasted plentiful food, Rapanui music, Rapanui gifts, and Rapanui movies – including Red Lemieux's *Island Observed* and another about the Franco-Belgian expedition. Some guests attended the add-on lecture about the "Iconography of Leprosy" through the history of art, and they viewed Nógrády's restaged exhibit. Georges heard many compliments about how it was the "best organized meeting ever," but he had to hide "in the toilette" to compose himself before his "emotion-laden" closing remarks. "I remembered the saying of my father 'one can pray even on a garbage heap.' This was true in that moment." At the end of the meeting, Armand Boudreault was ready for more roundtable discussion, but they all went to "a cozy cellar" for drinks, followed by dinner at an "elegant restaurant in Old Montreal," where Georges projected three of his own 8-millimetre Easter Island films on the wall, attracting the attention of other diners and waiters. "It was sweet," he wrote of the helpful neighbour children, "when at the end one of them – Yvette – came to me and said, 'Uncle Georges ... what is MICROBIOLOGY?'"[43]

NÓGRÁDY'S BOOK, VOLUME ONE

Now Nógrády had to face the utter lack of funding for the publication of his proceedings. He was pleased by offers of help from distinguished scientists, including William A. Clark of the American Type Culture Collection. "All contributors ... left like one big family without regard to nationality, religion, or political opinion. This was my biggest contribution – I feel so. Their entire confidence towards me put high moral responsibility to arrange the publication as good as possible."[44]

The incomplete product of this meeting took three years to produce. Georges had assembled an editorial board, and he was looking for a scholarly press, but that was not to be. Perhaps the prominent role of the Université de Montréal or Skoryna's many enemies had disqualified it from rival McGill's university press. Eventually, Georges settled on Sovereign Press in Oakville, Ontario, publisher of tabloids and little more than a vanity press for Hungarian and Ukrainian poets. The result was a 300-page mimeographed tome edited by Nógrády and supported by funds from the Easter Island Expedition Foundation: *The Microbiology of Easter Island*, volume 1 (1974). Although Georges and his team scrutinized the contributions, it was not peer-reviewed. The contributors' countries of residence included Hungary (1), Germany (1), the United Kingdom (2), the United States (3, all from Madison), Israel (1, Drapkin), Switzerland (1, John Cutler, who had recently moved to Geneva), and Canada (10, including Nógrády, Skoryna, and Richard Roberts). Volume 2 never appeared.[45]

Nógrády's decision to feature staphylococci in volume 1 over other organisms needs some explaining, especially since his research had demonstrated tuberculosis and leprosy on Rapa Nui, with staphylococcal infections not particularly noticeable. First, it is clear that he planned a second volume to cover other microbes, although it was never finished. Second, some strains of staphylococci had proven stubbornly resistant to the first generation of antibiotics and were therefore "sore spots" for clinicians. Scientists were interested in the molecular mechanisms of how these germs managed to mutate and generate that invulnerability, among them Sorin Sonea, who was the head of Nógrády's department. Discoveries in this realm, which dealt with cell walls and cell contents, could potentially have wide applications. As a testament to the draconian and persistent reputation of *Staphylococcus aureus* in the early 1970s, it still was under investigation in 2017 in a Canadian laboratory (among others) as the bioweapon that might have been used to assassinate the beloved Chilean poet and Nobel laureate Pablo Neruda for his opposition to the Augusto Pinochet coup in Chile in 1973.[46] Strains are now known as multi-drug-resistant superbugs.

Third, a few new types of antibiotics – derived from microbes – were coming along to vanquish infections caused by staphylococci; for example, gentamicin had been discovered in 1963. Fourth, Nógrády's friends at Ayerst had set aside the gram-positive bacteria, which included staphylococci; therefore, in choosing that microbe, he would not be intruding on its research-in-progress while mopping up work on an important group of organisms.

The published papers of volume 1 were grouped in five parts. The first dealt with Easter Island staphylococci, including the methods of collection and the human and animal types, with a focus on their production of penicillinase (an enzyme that made them resistant to antibiotics) as well as their toxins, genetics, phage types, and serology. Drapkin and Roberts compared the staphylococcus infections that they had seen, as clinicians, on their respective expeditions separated by thirty years. The second part contained a single paper, devoted to antibodies to staphylococci in the blood serum of the islanders. The third and fourth parts, provided by Nógrády and Cutler, related strains of the bacteria to anonymous families in the Easter Island census. Part five contained suggestions for future studies on Rapanui blood samples. Five more parts were appendices: maps, the route of HMCS *Cape Scott*, and abstracts of the papers in English, French, and German.

Nógrády dedicated the work to his late first wife, Ilona, and decorated the title page with the METEI logo and Rapanui motto: "Ina Ka Hoa"

(Don't give up the ship). In his preface, dated December 1973, he thanked Helen Reid, Armand Frappier, Leslie Eidus, and several other Montreal colleagues and secretaries. He also thanked the Chilean authorities and the people of Rapa Nui. Remarkably, he named every Rapanui citizen who had helped with the laboratory and the collecting, even the teenage girls. He concluded, "Hopefully all the efforts embodied in these results will alleviate the tragic mistakes committed by the white man against Oceanians, who are among the noblest members of the great human family."

THE MISSING VOLUME TWO

The second volume preoccupied Georges for years; it would contain the remainder of the papers delivered in April 1971. In late 1975 he wrote to Tony Law, asking him to check the English of his commentary on Easter Island cockroaches. At that time, he claimed, volume 2 was "about 80% ready" and had been held up by a mail strike. The cockroach paper in question would go in the forthcoming "chapter on entomomicrobiological studies." It was a response to the distinguished, versifying entomologist D. Keith McE. Kevan of McGill's Macdonald College in Montreal, who had accused METEI of introducing to the island a small species of yellowish brown cockroach, "*Blatt[ell]a germanica.*"[47] In his paper sent to Law, Nógrády admitted that the roach could have arrived via *Cape Scott*, picked up either in Halifax or a port of call, especially San Juan, where they took on board a lot of material. But large cockroaches were already well known on Easter Island and figured in the accounts of Thor Heyerdahl and all earlier travellers, including Katherine Routledge, who suggested heraldry for the island depicting "two cockroaches rampant."[48] Nógrády also pointed out that other ships had visited the island during the same period, including the French navy frigate, the Chilean gunboat, and the supply ship; all but the first unloaded "significant amounts of cargo." Nógrády described how he had collected a few insects, referred to Hal Gibbs's studies, recommended that an entomologist be included in future expeditions, and concluded that the new pest "could not be attributed solely to the METEI visit."[49]

In his boundless joy, Nógrády branched into anthropology – or he borrowed from Bob Meier's thesis – to present a poster on the "facial reconstruction of an Easter Island man" at the Hungarian Medical Association of America in Toronto in May 1981 and at a Kentucky speleology conference in July. Father Sebastian granted him access to a skull that he had found in a *hare moa* ("chicken house," or mound of stones). The practice of putting bones in these structures had been observed by Routledge and

Alfred Métraux, and it constitutes still another Rapanui puzzle: islanders believed that skulls increased the fertility of chickens; or possibly chickens entered and occupied the stone burial sites in pursuit of calcium.[50] On the basis of a plastic replica made by expert caster Luke McCarthy under the supervision of anthropologist Jerome Cybulski of Ottawa, Nógrády commissioned Hungarian sculptor Károly Arpás to recreate two versions of the head in bronze. Nógrády later sent the finished heads to the Hungarian National Museum, where they still reside (figure 12.2).[51] Arpás had prior experience in this technique, which is still used in physical and forensic anthropology and continues to fascinate scientists and an avid public through museums and documentaries.[52] At the Hungarian gathering, Nógrády also read a paper on *Pseudomonas* bacteria in hospital infections and in nature, possibly the same paper that he had read in Dallas earlier that year, which may have been slotted for volume 2.[53]

In early March 1981, Nógrády had asked for a short "slow down" (sabbatical) to devote time to editing volume 2.[54] He wanted to include a broad report on the medical findings from Richard Roberts. The two-page squibs that he had inveigled from Drapkin and Roberts for volume 1 were insufficient, having dealt only with a single infectious agent. Finally, in desperation or exasperation, he drafted Roberts's article himself, weaving together the two papers that the navy doctor had previously read in Toronto and Montreal. This exercise left Nógrády with a long list of well-defined questions, gaps, and editorial concerns, including a need for references. He sent the list to Roberts, asking for his input on the draft and for help with its numerous outstanding problems.[55]

Roberts's reply was cool. He and Maureen were leaving for a month in Austria. He noticed that, in Nógrády's toiling on the second volume of the "magnum opus," he had blended Roberts's two papers into a "composite." But the navy physician was not content with this solution and would need time to evaluate the synthesis for "balance." In particular, he thought that the "slides" (probably tables or graphs) did not correspond properly with the text. In any case, he had put those slides away "with all the others" and could not "readily identify the actual slides presented." Georges could "come and look through" them if he wanted; "as always," he "would be most welcome." He closed by asking Georges for advice on a camera. Nógrády responded quickly, wishing them both "excellent holidays," promising to come to Ottawa to sort through the slides, and endorsing Roberts's leading choice of camera; he signed the handwritten missive on pink airmail paper, "Love, Georges."[56] Again, seventeen years after the expedition, it seems that Roberts was still actively resisting any report.

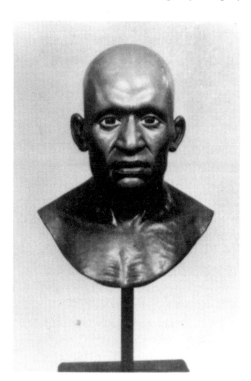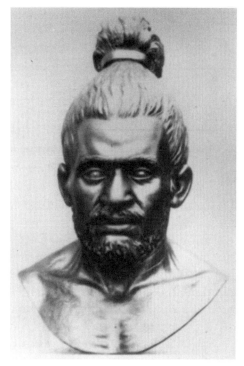

Figure 12.2 Reconstructed heads made by sculptor Károly Arpás from Luke McCarthy and Jerome Cybulski's plastic cast of a Rapanui skull, Hungarian National Museum, Budapest. Nógrády, "Facial Reconstruction."

Georges lost his beloved wife, Bernadette, in 1986, and at some point, he gave up on volume 2. Did he destroy the manuscript that he had once claimed was 80 per cent complete? It has not been found; however, in my searching for it, I found some other surprising things that he had hoarded (see chapter 13). Nevertheless, a few undated, mostly bilingual abstracts with Roberts's papers seem to represent some of the intended content of volume 2, which can therefore be partially reconstructed.[57] Three numbered abstracts and short papers by Roberts in his file labelled "speeches" may also have been part of the plan; they deal with bacterial infections, tuberculosis, leprosy, and *kokongo*.[58] Nógrády's volume 2 may not have been for microbiology alone. For example, Israel Zipkin presented a detailed analysis of the fluoride content of Nógrády's forty-seven Rapanui water samples by geographic location; he also speculated on the dental health benefit of pineapple juice, the fluoride content of which he also measured.[59] The contribution by soil scientists J.E. Brydon and A.J. MacLean was a complete essay with tables of the minerals, chemicals, and nutrients in Nógrády's sixty-seven soil samples, again by geographic location. Roberts kept their paper in a separate file.[60] None of this meticulous research was ever published.

RAPAMYCIN

Notwithstanding the frustration over publishing, Nógrády's natural ardour never diminished. While in Dallas in 1981, he had connected with the "research director" of Ayerst Pharmaceuticals. METEI alumni, especially Georges, had already been aware for some time that at least two of his soil samples had yielded promising results against microorganisms, as heralded by Vézina's paper in 1969. He was pleased, if not astonished, to hear that one bacterial substance was "under study" with the National Cancer Institute in Washington. "It stirred sensation that this antibiotic has – at least in experimental condition[s] – effect on solid tumours."[61] Named for its island home, it was called rapamycin.

Rapamycin (sirolimus) is celebrated as the discovery of Ayerst microbiologist- pharmacologist Surendra Nath Sehgal. It is a natural secretion of the bacterium *Streptomyces hygroscopicus*, which was unknown until Georges Nógrády brought it back to Canada from Easter Island, said to be its only natural home. It was initially thought to have strong activity against fungi, such as *Candida*, as Vézina had reported for Nógrády in 1969; however, at that time, its isolation and structure had yet to be worked out.

Sehgal came from a small village in present-day Pakistan.[62] With a special interest in medicinal plants, he had studied pharmacology in Varanasi, India, followed by a doctorate in Bristol, England, in 1957. He came to Ottawa on a National Research Council postdoctoral fellowship in 1958. Between 1960 and 1962, he published several research papers with Norman E. Gibbons, who would soon serve as the chair of the Canadian Committee for the International Biological Programme.[63] Sehgal was lured to the well-developed pharmaceutical industry in Montreal by Ayerst's research director, chemist Roger Gaudry, who became rector of the Université de Montréal in 1965. Since 1943 Ayerst had been a Canadian affiliate of Wyeth Pharmaceuticals, which had been producing vaccines at its Montreal plant since 1883. The Ayerst lab, therefore, was a logical workplace for an inquisitive, young scientist keen on the search for antibiotics. Giant fermenters meant that interesting microorganisms could be grown in huge quantities.

Sehgal and Vézina were great friends and remained close for years. Since 1962 they had prepared dozens of articles and conference papers together, and by the time of METEI, they already held five patents. With technologist

Teodora M. Blazecovic, they filed for a patent for rapamycin synthesis and preparation in late 1974; by 1978 it had been issued in nineteen countries around the world.[64] In 1975, a whole decade after METEI, they published the first of their papers on rapamycin – already so named – as a two-part article.[65] They stated that the source organism, *Streptomyces hygroscopicus*, had been "isolated from an Easter Island soil sample" and that rapamycin was its product. Other publications fixed the date of its isolation as 1972.[66] They mentioned neither METEI nor Nógrády.

Vézina and Sehgal continued to study the antifungal antibiotic properties of their new drug and its mechanism of action, producing parts 3 and 4 of their work in 1978 and 1979 respectively.[67] Their results were sufficiently interesting that they wanted to know the chemical structure of the drug. They donated crystalline rapamycin to John A. Findlay's laboratory at the University of New Brunswick in Fredericton. Findlay used X-ray crystallography to reveal its structure: a "completely new type of macrolide antibiotic."[68] Two years later, working with a colleague from Hungary, Findlay used a visiting professorship in Rome to further investigate its structure, now using the relatively new technique of carbon-13 nuclear magnetic resonance.[69]

Meanwhile, other colleagues at Ayerst began studying rapamycin's effects as an immunosuppressive that operated on the lymphatic system of the rat; it stood up well to comparator drugs cyclophosphamide and methotrexate.[70] This inhibition of immune cells meant that it could be applied clinically to autoimmune diseases, such as rheumatoid arthritis and lupus, and to organ transplantation in dealing with the side effects of graft rejection. Inhibition of immune cells also implied that the drug might inhibit other cells, such as cancer.

Sehgal sent a sample to the American National Cancer Institute "for testing." He later said, "They found absolutely fantastic activity of the drug against almost all solid tumors ... the anti-cancer effect was absolutely astonishing ... It was a totally new class of anti-cancer agents ... cytostatic [whereas] to that point they were all cytotoxic."[71] The first papers on rapamycin's anti-cancer effects – about which Georges had heard in Dallas in 1981 – appeared in print in 1983.[72] Another article came from Sehgal and Vézina a year later, describing rapamycin's effect on human tumours transplanted to mice.[73]

Here was an exciting new drug, with a novel structure and action against three different biological realms: anti-biotic, anti-immune, and anti-cancer. But in 1983 Wyeth-Ayerst Laboratories closed its Montreal lab and moved operations to Princeton, New Jersey. Sehgal was invited to move with the company, but Vézina was let go along with many others. He stayed behind in Montreal, where he was hired in 1983 as "directeur adjoint" at the INRS-Institut Armand-Frappier, where Boudreault worked too.[74]

Despite its tremendous promise, rapamycin was "not a company priority," and the owners ordered the destruction of all "non-viable" compounds. Sehgal just couldn't do it. In anticipation of losing access to his giant fermenters, he whipped up a large batch to take along and "squirreled a few vials of *Streptomyces hygroscopicus* into his freezer at home."[75] Finally, in 1987, Wyeth bought out Ayerst completely, and Sehgal was able to convince the new management to reconsider.

In the twenty-three years since Nógrády had scooped Easter Island dirt into his little tubes, rapamycin had been the subject of fewer than ten articles indexed in the Medline database. But in the next decade, from 1988 to 1998, it generated more than 1,500 research papers, more than forty of which were written by Suren Sehgal as he sought to uncover how the drug worked in animals. Clinical trials on humans soon analyzed its effect as an immunosuppressant to prevent rejection of transplanted organs. By 1996 positive results had begun appearing from randomized, double-blind, placebo-controlled phase 1 studies on patients with kidney transplants. In September 1999, the US Food and Drug Administration granted Wyeth a licence for rapamycin, called "Rapamune," to prevent rejection in renal transplantation. Johnson and Johnson received a licence to use it for coating prosthetics, such as stents, in patients undergoing surgery on the heart and other organs. These studies showed that rapamycin could be used, safely and synergistically, in combination with other drugs, a technique that was also incorporated into its early applications in cancer. When the drug was released, plastic surgeon and METEI alumnus Garry Brody was intrigued by the name and called the manufacturer, asking to speak to the scientist-developer. A startled "gentleman in the bowels of the company" said that he had been "a student of Nógrády" and that the drug was derived from bacteria collected on Rapa Nui.[76] Was this man Suren Sehgal?

Having been diagnosed with stage-4 colon cancer in 1998, Sehgal retired, although he continued as a consultant for the drug company. Wyeth officials made a trip to Rapa Nui in 2001, led by Bernard Le Duc, and they invited the ailing Suren to join them, but he was obliged to decline. During his final illness, he even experimented on himself, believing that his own discovery had controlled his liver metastases and added almost five more years to his life. He died in 2003.

Beyond its specific effects, rapamycin gave rise to an entirely new class of drugs based on its mechanism of action. At the end of his career, Sehgal explained: "The molecular mechanism underlying the antifungal, antiproliferative, and immunosuppressive activities of sirolimus is the same."[77] And that unique mechanism – just like the unique bacterial source and the unique chemical structure – was entirely new to the science world. It was elucidated in 1991 for yeast and in 1994 for human liver cells, T-cells, and bone cancer in two short reports that have now been cited by other scientists more than a thousand times each.[78] As Sehgal explained, the drug interferes with the G1 phase of the cell cycle by binding to a "mammalian FKBP-rapamycin-associated protein." This protein or kinase is now called "mTOR" for "mammalian Target Of Rapamycin."[79] Drugs that act upon it are known as "mTOR inhibitors."

These novel molecular medicines are widely discussed in cancer care; however, few oncologists know that the familiar acronym "mTOR" refers to rapamycin; fewer still know of its embedded reference to Easter Island. Thus added to its many other unique characteristics, rapamycin was the beginning of an entirely new class of treatments. Some now tout it as a potential source of longevity, an elixir of eternal youth;[80] however, in 2013 its manufacturer was fined almost $500 million for marketing it for unapproved or "off-label" uses.[81]

By the time of Sehgal's death in 2003, rapamycin was worth billions. Six years later, Pfizer bought Wyeth for US$68 billion.[82] To date, more than 40,000 articles have been published about rapamycin in the peer-reviewed literature, and mTOR inhibition has become an equally important topic, with over 4,000 articles appearing in 2018 alone (figure 12.3). As its derivatives are now applied to malignancies and immune therapies around the world, rapamycin's miracles continue, and they hit ever closer to home. We use its derivatives in the cancer clinic where I work, and while I was writing this book, rapamycin became the "wonder drug and life line" of a young physician with the lethal, rare condition lymphangioleiomyomatosis: brilliant, beautiful, and alive, Dr Lyndsay Hoy is the daughter of my Toronto medical-school classmate Dr Fred Hoy.[83]

Not to take anything away from Sehgal's genius and persistence in this discovery, Nógrády's contribution, through collecting *and sharing*, was crucial. It is not known if the two men ever met, although they had both lived in Montreal, worked with the same colleagues, and attended meetings of the American Society for Microbiology.[84] Aside from the fact that the first rapamycin publications came from scientists based in Canada, the METEI connection was all but lost. Sehgal's son, Ajai, corrected the record in a website dedicated to his father: "In 1964, a Canadian scientific expedition traveled to Easter Island (or Rapa Nui, as it is known by locals) to gather plant and soil samples. The expedition shared their soil samples with scientists at Ayerst's research laboratories in Montreal."[85] Indeed.

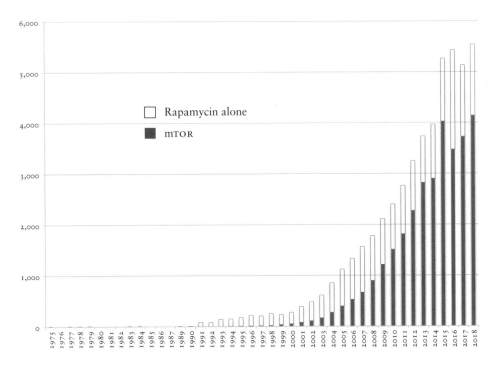

Figure 12.3 Numbers of articles on rapamycin and mTOR inhibition since 1975. Notice mTOR publications begin in 1994 and overtake those devoted to rapamycin alone by 2009. Calculated from Medline database.

Little troubled by the ridicule on the expedition, Nógrády carried on collecting and disseminating information and materials. He organized METEI's only scientific conferences and, after many difficulties, managed to publish some papers in proceedings, although volume 1 of *The Microbiology of Easter Island* is little known. With his trademark enthusiasm, he kept his fellow travellers apprised of new work, confident that they shared his passion for the island and its people. His microbiological samples resulted in the spectacular discovery of the important drug rapamycin and a new class of therapeutic agents. But Nógrády's role and that of METEI had been lost – until now.

13

Forgetting METEI and the IBP

In 1981, sixteen years after the Medical Expedition to Easter Island, Canada's ambassador in Santiago asked Allan Gotlieb in the Department of External Affairs for a copy of the final report because Chilean authorities were still waiting to have the results.[1] If his request was forwarded to Stanley Skoryna, we do not know. From chapters 9 to 12, it should be evident that Stanley Skoryna had no shortage of material for compiling a final report. Yet he failed to do it. Such a document would have made the research accessible to other scholars, and it might have prevented the utter oblivion that has engulfed METEI for most of the past half-century. This chapter addresses the possible reasons why that report does not exist, recognizing that the travellers themselves never forgot their journey or its heady promise to Rapa Nui. The reasons lie in METEI's nagging debt, its baffling disappearance from the Canadian International Biological Programme (IBP), political changes in Chile, and Stanley himself.

WITHER THE IBP?

While planning his expedition, Skoryna and his supporters at McGill University, including Principal Rocke Robertson and Al Tunis, made much of METEI as one of Canada's contributions to the International Biological Programme. The $5,000 seed money, awarded in 1963 by the World Health Organization (WHO), was linked to the forthcoming international endeavour. Indeed, the earliest press releases refer to METEI in the context of the International Biological *Year* – which by 1962 had already become a *Programme* (see chapter 1).[2] Consequently, the language of the METEI press releases changed "year" to "programme" to correspond to the new plans.

From the outset, several Canadians participated in the IBP's Human Adaptability (HA) section, and they knew of METEI. When Joseph S. Weiner hosted his HA symposium in Austria in June and July 1964, Canadian Jack A. Hildes contributed a paper on circumpolar peoples that appeared in the resultant volume (see chapter 1).[3] Later that same July, when the first general assembly took place in Paris, Canadian Arctic researcher J. Sandy Hart chaired the international committee to receive and coordinate the HA proposals. Norwegian physiologist Karl Lange Andersen, who headed up the work physiology theme for HA, also attended both meetings; he would recruit Björn Ekblom, Einar Gjessing, and Jim Nielsen for METEI. Andersen collaborated with Toronto physiologist Roy J. Shephard in research and on an IBP teaching initiative concerning methods for measuring work capacity (see chapters 2 and 10).[4]

As "World Convener" of the HA section, Weiner wrote about METEI as a "pilot" project for the 1965 IBP newsletter while Skoryna's team was still on Easter Island.[5] He also attended and commented on Peter Beighton's paper about METEI delivered to the Royal Geographical Society in London in February 1966; the paper was published in September, noting the IBP and Weiner's presence.[6] This attention to METEI from the top echelon of the international bureaucracy seems to have meant very little to the Canadians in charge at home.

METEI appears in none of the archival documents pertaining to the Canadian Committee for the International Biological Programme (CCIBP). After HMCS *Cape Scott* returned, even the people at McGill stopped referring to the IBP connection in their letters and press releases. Only the Canadian auditor general referred to it in 1966, condemning the entire mission as an inappropriate expense (see chapter 9). The slim annual reports of the CCIBP number the projects in each section. Ian Efford's work on Marion Lake is always listed as "PF 1" in the section on "Productivity of Freshwater." However, there are numerical gaps in the HA section, to which Skoryna had always claimed METEI would belong: the CCIBP printed annual updates for projects HA-1, HA-3, HA-5, HA-6, and HA-7, but the missing projects HA-2 and HA-4 are never identified, nor are "three other projects already in existence before IBP started but which had applied for IBP recognition."[7] Was METEI one of these? Was it actually rejected, or was it simply ignored?

At first, I thought that perhaps METEI was "done" too soon – in the sense that the expedition had returned to Halifax before the CCIBP was fully formed. But with its extensive advance billing, WHO funding, and broad scientific scope, METEI was glamorous and hard to ignore. It met many IBP goals: an isolated population, international collaboration, and an emphasis on adaptability and ecology. Furthermore, as seen in the previous chapters, its research products took many years to appear. As the CCIBP got underway, METEI scientists were only just beginning to analyze and publish their results. METEI was not "done" but continued in parallel with the CCIBP.

Then I wondered if the people who served on the administration of the CCIBP came along too late and from fields unrelated to METEI concerns. They might have overlooked METEI as a function of timing or of differing research priorities. But as my work progressed, I discovered that many connections could be found between those directors and METEI, implicit rather than explicit but undeniable.

The first Canadian IBP director was F.R. Hayes, a fish biologist and oceanographer who served just one year and resigned in the spring of 1964, when he became chair of the Fisheries Research Board. He had strong opinions about the inadequacy of Canadian policies on spending for research in science.[8] Efford would publish several articles in the *Journal of the Fisheries Research Board of Canada* between 1967 and 1975. Hayes's successor, bacteriologist Norman E. Gibbons, had served as the Canadian delegate to that first international meeting in Paris in July 1964 when the basic structure of IBP was laid out. He would have met Georges Nógrády at least by the time that they both attended the 1962 Ottawa meeting on culture collections (see chapter 12). Gibbons certainly knew Claude Vézina and Surendra Nath Sehgal, the latter having been his postdoctoral fellow and collaborator at the National Research Council (NRC) between 1958 and 1962. But Gibbons returned from Paris, believing that he was not the right person to lead Canada's IBP; he recommended that the CCIBP be disbanded and reformed.[9] He seems to have absorbed the idea that human physiology was more important to the IBP than bench work in microbiology. Gibbons continued to serve but not as chair.

The next two CCIBP directors were from McGill, and no one at McGill could pretend ignorance of METEI. Physiologist Frank ("Hank") Campbell Macintosh replaced Gibbons as chair, serving for three years until 1967. He was succeeded by veterinary parasitologist Thomas Wright Moir Cameron, a much-honoured emeritus professor and the country's leading expert on parasites. Furthermore, Cameron had been Hal Gibbs's supervisor for his doctoral work on hookworm in dogs and wolves. Gibbs admired Cameron for his many achievements; however, they had had a falling out around 1959 when the old mentor disapproved of his former student – now a young father with a freshly minted doctorate – taking a better (and better paying) job with the Animal

Disease Research Institute. Gibbs also had the impression that Cameron had been annoyed when METEI failed to consult him about who (if not himself) should represent parasitology on the expedition. This sentiment may have been shared with his Macdonald College colleague D. Keith McE. Kevan, who reported on the METEI insects (see chapter 10). In the years following METEI, Cameron spoke to Gibbs only once: at a conference, he said, "Hello."

Toronto physiologist Roy J. Shephard served the CCIBP in numerous ways, especially in leading an HA project. He invited Karl Lange Andersen to Toronto for a physiology meeting in October 1966 (see chapter 10). One of Andersen's two papers there relied on results gathered by the researchers whom he had sent to Easter Island; Shephard edited it for the *Canadian Medical Association Journal*. Deepening the mystery around what happened to METEI and the CCIBP connection, the commentator on Andersen's Norwegian paper was J.S. Hart, physiologist with the NRC in Ottawa, and physician-physiologist Jack A. Hildes of Winnipeg also attended, commenting on the METEI results. Both Hart and Hildes were prominent in the reformulated CCIBP and had been engaged with the IBP's HA section since its inception, as explained above. Through the IBP, they met with Americans who shared their interests. Furthermore, Hart chaired the HA subcommittee, he had co-authored several research papers with Andersen, and he had served on a team to study caribou with METEI parasitologist Hal Gibbs. Therefore, although their own interests were in adaptation to cold and Arctic populations, Hart and Hildes could not deny knowledge of METEI. Their failure to mention it in any of the Canadian IBP reports is puzzling and seems deliberate.

When the IBP came to an end in 1974, a series of "synthesis volumes" collected the state of work conducted under each IBP theme. Shephard wrote the volume on work physiology. He cited the CCIBP, especially on Arctic peoples, and he included "Easter Island" in his index, referring to the article of Ekblom and Gjessing, although he did not mention METEI.[10] Given his close connection to Andersen, Shephard may not have realized that Canada had had anything to do with this apparently Scandinavian project. Shephard's many contributions to the IBP are celebrated at the University of Toronto, and he too knew of METEI; however, fifty years later, he did not remember that it had ever been part of the IBP.[11]

Hart died in 1973 and was replaced as chair of the HA subsection by geneticist Nancy E. Simpson. She knew about METEI long before it left Halifax and felt slighted to have been excluded. She had published on METEI serum samples in 1968 (see chapter 10).[12] Her article, comparing

298 Igloolik Inuit with other groups from Canada and elsewhere, was included in the assembled products of the CCIBP.[13] She was acquainted with its leaders, Hart and Hildes, who had heard Andersen's METEI paper in Toronto in 1966. Not once in the long decade of her service to the CCIBP did she hear of METEI's connection to the IBP. In 2015 she and Ian Efford were both surprised to learn that METEI had once been touted as a Canadian contribution to the IBP. Efford and Simpson participated in both METEI and the IBP; yet, like Shephard, they were unaware of any connection between them.

It seems, then, that knowledge of METEI as a CCIBP prospect was once held at the top – Weiner, Macintosh, Cameron, Hart, Hildes, and Shephard – but it did not trickle down. Only five Canadian HA projects are named in Kenneth Collins and Weiner's official IBP history of adaptability research.[14]

Three reasons may explain METEI's expulsion from the IBP. The first is money. All those who have written about the IBP refer to its unwieldy mechanics both *within* countries, as IBP projects cut across many different departments, and *outside* countries, as scientists, accustomed to working on small projects in their own labs, were suddenly expected to find collaborators across borders and oceans with little or no financial support. Ministers were pleased to make optimistic pronouncements about the benefits of ecological collaboration, but no one wanted to face bills for new projects that would squeeze already tight budgets. Just as the expense of *Cape Scott* had been an embarrassment for Minister of Defence Paul Hellyer, the outstanding bill for the ATCO trailers was a huge burden for METEI. The "questionable" expenditure absorbed by the taxpayer was more than $200,000; the unpaid ATCO bill was almost $50,000. Skoryna had collected $5,000 from WHO and $10,000 from the Medical Research Council (MRC). In contrast, Canada's annual dues to the IBP amounted to only $2,500 for the entire country, and they were not paid at all until 1966.[15] Furthermore, the CCIBP was underfunded: volunteer contributions consumed "900 man years" of work at an estimate of $15,000 per "man" per year; HA received one-eighth of this amount, roughly 46 per cent of which came from the NRC, with the remainder, in declining amounts, coming from universities, governments, and private foundations.[16] Significantly, however, Ian Efford recalls no shortage of funding for his IBP work on Marion Lake, which was part of the Freshwater Productivity section and not HA. Given Skoryna's endless attempts at fundraising, the METEI debt was no secret, especially at McGill, home of both CCIBP leaders Macintosh and Cameron. Embracing METEI might mean embracing its large debt – and neither professor was willing to sacrifice future projects for a cause that had been launched by others without their input, especially not at the expense of the taxpayer.

The second reason for METEI to be expelled from the CCIBP could be priorities of philosophy. In both the United States and Canada, the HA section of the IBP enjoyed less support than other sections. Consequently, according to historian Toby Appel, it focused on "simpler social systems in which genealogical, cultural, linguistic and nutritional patterns have been maintained."[17] Small, local projects were to replace grand, holistic ones. This shift in attitude may have prompted Gibbons's early withdrawal as chair. An echo of that shift appears in a CCIBP report summarizing its first six years and citing a recommendation to "favour large integrated research projects within Canadian interests and capabilities rather than a thinly scattered effort over time."[18] This language seems to deliberately exclude METEI. With its emphasis on "Canadian capabilities," the recommendation also rejected the IBP desideratum of international collaboration.

The third reason is Skoryna. As Robin Strachan, the editor of McGill University Press, once told Richard Roberts, Skoryna had "deadly enemies" on campus.[19] As an upstart, a dreamer, and an "operator" who espoused wild, ecological notions of humans and their diseases and made endless pronouncements on stochastic causation, he and his work stood far outside the mainstream of academic medicine. His involvement with teaching was remote – confined only to residents who rotated to St Mary's Hospital or were sent to do research projects. Nevertheless, he fearlessly approached people whom others deemed far above him: Ray Farquharson at the MRC, the presidents of universities, governors general, and prime ministers. Insubordinate, inappropriate, and arrogant, Skoryna insisted on explaining his views about the nature of research and his visions for the future to political and academic leaders. That he came from eastern Europe would not have helped. He likely suffered the same parochial scorn that was heaped upon Hungarian Georges Nógrády on Easter Island and in Montreal.

Even though Canadians rejected METEI as an IBP project, it fit the bill for the IBP in many ways, and, as shown in the previous chapters, its scientific output was considerable – probably far greater than Skoryna ever realized and far greater than any other CCIBP project. Rather than dwelling on the unknowable reasons why the CCIBP decided not to recognize METEI, it is instructive to examine what the CCIBP *did* recognize as its Human Adaptability work. This exercise offers further clues as to why METEI did not belong.

CANADA'S IBP IN GENERAL

With Thomas Cameron as one of the editors, the CCIBP leaders published a summary of their achievements in a 1975 volume tellingly entitled *Energy Flow: Its Biological Dimensions.*[20] Ian Efford's co-authored report on Marion Lake formed chapter 11 within the Freshwater Productivity section. The Human Adaptability section was reduced to two chapters: one on Igloolik and the other on a comparison of growth in Canadian children of different ethnicities. METEI was not mentioned, even in the list of projects registered but unreported.[21]

At the outset, the CCIBP had contemplated a massive five-volume treatise of all the publications. Every author was to submit a copy of any manuscript sent to a publisher. But organizers quickly realized that it would be expensive and unwieldy to print them all – especially if the papers were to be published in scientific journals anyway. Instead, they insisted that reprints of all publications be sent to the NRC. Consequently, the National Science Library (formerly the Canadian Institute for Scientific and Technical Information) in Ottawa holds a multivolume set of fat binders that assemble reprints or photocopies of the papers that had emerged from the nation's IBP adventure by 1975. Every reprint was assigned a number stamped on the first page that corresponded roughly to its date of publication or to the date it was received at the NRC. It appears that all IBP papers from every subcommittee were treated the same way, being assigned a number as soon as they arrived. Volume 5, the binder for Human Adaptability, contains a total of thirty-four papers, whose numbers are not consecutive.[22] Project HA-1 was a multidisciplinary study in Igloolik, from which twenty papers had appeared by 1975, thirteen of which were authored by the Toronto team of physiologist Roy J. Shephard. They examined work capacity, oxygen consumption, cardiac output, and oxygen intake in "the Eskimo." One of these was co-authored with Karl Lange Andersen of Norway. Another five papers within HA-1 concerned the dentition of "Eskimo" children and the effects of diet, published by Toronto dental anthropologist John T. Mayhall and colleagues. Nancy Simpson's work on the genetics of enzymes in Igloolik people was also included in HA-1.

The smaller projects HA-3, on isolated French communities, and HA-5, on child development, both came from the Université de Montréal, and HA-6, on child fitness, was conducted out of the University of Saskatchewan. These projects were considered part of the IBP, but the budget shows that they had no CCIBP funding; instead, they relied on universities, foundations, and provincial governments.[23] By 1975 this research had resulted in two papers for HA-3, twelve for HA-5, authored by the team of Arto Demirjian and Milos Jenicek, and none for HA-6 or HA-7. All but two of these fourteen papers were published in French. Projects HA-2 and HA-4 were still unaccounted for.

This list of publications shows that the CCIBP's Human Adaptability projects were tightly focused on specific groups of Canadians and their specific problems: the teeth of francophone youth, the exercise tolerance of Saskatchewan schoolchildren, and especially the diet, exercise tolerance, and genetics of the Inuit. The task was to push the envelope beyond the vagaries of qualitative work in previous ecological studies. Outspoken American ecologists had criticized the IBP for being a "boondoggle," for producing "some pretty crappy stuff," and for funding projects when peers had recommended rejection.[24] In contrast, these well-focused, rigorous studies were to generate quantitative data in small nuggets. Piecing all these reliable nuggets together was supposed to build a mosaic of human ecology on a global scale. Their authorship reveals that the Canadian approach to the IBP, especially its HA section, did not value (or could not afford) collaboration across borders, not even provincial borders. It could also be that no resources were available to support it, so researchers simply fell back on their usual patterns. If this collection defines the goals of the CCIBP, then METEI was far too diffuse, too geographically remote, and too eclectic – rather like Stanley Skoryna.

THE IBP AND HUMAN ADAPTABILITY BEYOND CANADA

We might also ask if the Canadian IBP output differed in any way from that of other countries. In their 1977 history of the HA section of the IBP, Kenneth Collins and Joseph S. Weiner provided a 300-page compendium of all 232 known Human Adaptability projects emerging from forty-four different countries, cross-referenced for the twelve related HA themes.[25] Some were brief entries, naming titles and leaders; others submitted detailed methods and results equivalent to a final report. Of these, 212 entries were replete with resultant publications or reports. Although the Collins and Weiner volume may not cover all the projects once associated with the HA initiative, it gives a good indication of the types of projects that "counted," where they were conducted, and how many were truly international, collaborative, and multidisciplinary (table 13.1). It includes five of the Canadian HA projects, described above, although the HA numbers differ, and it mentions Canada collaborating in one other. Weiner himself was in charge of a UK project, Karl Lange Andersen was

Table 13.1 Number of IBP Human Adaptability projects and proportion in foreign countries

Country	Projects	Foreign country (%)
Argentina	1	0
Australia	8	87.5
Austria	1	0
Belgium	2	100
Brazil	12	8.3
Burma	1	0
Bulgaria	3	0
Canada	6	0
Chile	2	0
Czechoslovakia	9	22.2
Denmark	1	0
East Germany	9	0
Finland	1	0
France	5	100
Ghana	1	0
Greece	2	0
Guatemala	2	0
Hungary	2	0
India	8	25
Indonesia	1	0
Israel	6	0
Italy	5	60
Japan	9	22.2
Korea	6	0
Malawi	2	0
Malaysia	4	0
Mozambique	1	0
Netherlands	12	66.7
New Zealand	6	66.7
Nigeria	1	0
Norway	2	0
Poland	18	5.5
Roumania	3	0
Singapore	1	0
South Africa	8	0
Soviet Union	10	10

Country	Projects	Foreign country (%)
Spain	2	0
Sweden	2	0
Switzerland	1	0
United Kingdom	24	83.3
United States	21	71.4
Venezuela	2	0
West Germany	5	100
Yugoslavia	8	0

Source: Derived from Collins and Weiner, *Human Adaptability*.

leader of both projects emerging from Norway, and an essay by Björn Ekblom (not about Rapa Nui) is cited as a result from one of the two Swedish projects.

The IBP's HA work was interpreted by most countries – twenty-nine of forty-four (66 per cent) – as something to be done at home, usually on specific ethnic groups. For example, all eight of South Africa's HA projects focused on "Bantu" or "negro" peoples within its borders. Eleven studies involved comparison of the researchers' homeland with another locale; only two of the latter were collaborative.

A quarter of the projects – sixty-six (28 per cent) – were conducted in locations outside the home country of the researcher. Three countries conducted all projects outside their own borders: Belgium, West Germany, and France. Similarly, Australia, Italy, Netherlands, New Zealand, United Kingdom, and the United States conducted the majority of their projects offshore. Did researchers in these privileged countries imagine that no human adaptability issues could pertain to their own citizens? Or did they view IBP initiatives as an opportunity to conduct expensive work elsewhere that would otherwise be difficult to fund?

Collins and Weiner classified the resultant work within the twelve defined "themes" that represented Human Adaptability projects rather than by the specific scientific disciplines used to study them. These were the "practical problems" that had been determined somewhat controversially at the outset in 1964 (see chapter 1) and grouped according to "worldwide" or "regional" research topics. Again, from their book, we can identify the most heavily studied themes. Most projects entailed more than one theme: two studies (Australia, HA-2 and HA-9) combined

Table 13.2 IBP Human Adaptability projects by numbers of countries, collaborations, and single themes

Worldwide themes	Projects	Countries	Collaborations	Single themes
1 Human growth and development	86	30	6	0
2 Physique and body composition	87	32	8	2
3 Physical fitness	61	27	7	4
4 Climatic tolerance	43	14	5	2
5 Genetic constitution	111	34	9	34
6 Nutritional studies	74	31	9	9
Regional themes				
7 High altitudes	27	12	3	1
8 Circumpolar and other cold climates	13	9	1	0
9 Tropical and desert climates	23	13	3	1
10 Islands and isolates	32	17	3	0
11 Migrant and hybrid populations	21	12	3	0
12 Urban and rural populations	50	20	3	5

Source: Derived from Collins and Weiner, Human Adaptability.

nine of the twelve themes; and three studies (the United Kingdom, HA-3, and the United States, HA-5 and HA-9) combined eight themes. But a sizable minority (26.4 per cent) addressed only one theme as the sole topic (table 13.2).

The majority of the 232 HA projects were small, focused studies equivalent to one or two of the METEI publications. For example, four different studies targeted the prevalence of the phenylthiocarbamide (PTC) taster gene, and three from eastern Europe determined age at menarche. Only six included the word "multidisciplinary" in the title, and only one included the word "international" (Canada's study of the Inuit). Many researchers identified the Human Adaptability handbooks as a source for their methods – which shows that, if nothing else, the IBP helped to standardize methods for biological investigation and served to promote sharing and communication of information between nations. The IBP also prompted the 1971 formation of UNESCO's Man and the Biosphere Programme, which continues today with more than 660 collaborative projects between scientific experts and local volunteers in

120 countries around the world.[26] Many of its ongoing studies focus on islands, sustainable development, and peoples living within their cultural and natural environments. For these projects, the results and logistics of long-forgotten METEI might have been useful in addressing the social determinants of health and sustainable development goals of today, now that the limitations of the disease-eradication model are understood.[27]

One striking fact about this review of the IBP's HA projects is the near total absence of interest in infectious disease: the words "infection," "bacteria," "microbiology," "tuberculosis," "malaria," and "communicable" appear in no titles, and "virus/viral" appears in only one. This one project (New Zealand, HA-8) analyzed the serological levels against rubella and respiratory infections in 500 people living on Fiji. Armand Boudreault's work would have been an excellent comparator, but the authors did not cite him.[28] Indeed, the word "disease" itself appears in only five titles: two concerned with heart disease and aging, two about genetics, and one on mental illness. "Epidemiology/ical" appears in just two titles, both also using the word "disease": one about coronary heart disease and the other on mental illness.

Clearly and surprisingly, the entire Human Adaptability section of the IBP eschewed medicine, microbiology, and infectious diseases – possibly another reason why Gibbons felt he should step down as leader of the CCIBP. It exemplifies the naive, triumphalist notion of false security that pervaded mid-twentieth-century medicine, prompted by vaccines and the advent of ever more powerful antibiotics. In a world that had yet to confront AIDS, Ebola, SARS, and Zika, infectious diseases as serious threats to human adaptability were passé.[29]

COULD METEI HAVE BELONGED TO THE IBP?

Where would METEI have fit in this ensemble? Six projects focused on peoples in Polynesia and ten in New Guinea, but none addressed Easter Island. If we were to classify METEI within the HA projects, it would conform to themes 1, 2, 3, 5, 6, 9, and 10 (table 13.2). No project in the Collins and Weiner volume displayed exactly the same profile. Four correspond most closely with the goals of METEI: two Australian studies and two American. Both Australian studies (HA-2 and HA-5) concentrated on the human biology and epidemiology of specific populations in New Guinea; conducted from 1968–71 and 1966–74 respectively, they had produced a combined total of nineteen publications between 1970 and 1974. The first American study (HA-27), entitled "Medical Anthropological Studies in the Solomon Islands," was based on fieldwork conducted by the

Peabody Museum; it produced thirty-five publications on a wide range of topics between 1968 and 1977. The second American study (HA-3) also concerned New Guinea and was entitled "Child Growth, Development, Behavior, Learning and Disease Patterns in Primitive Cultures." Its leader was D. Carleton Gajdusek, who was awarded the Nobel Prize in 1976 but was disgraced and convicted of child molestation two decades later.[30] His 1977 report in Collins and Weiner includes twenty-two references published between 1964 and 1975, but the first few articles relate to his earlier work on kuru and rely on research conducted in the late 1950s – well before the IBP was created. Five studies on "Eskimos" from Canada, France, and the United States and three studies on Lapps from Finland, Sweden, and the Soviet Union aspire to the same "total" assessment of an isolated group and share up to six of the themes with METEI, despite the geographic and climatic differences.

This exercise is not to argue for the retrospective inclusion or celebration of METEI as an unsung IBP achievement but rather to "test" it and demonstrate that its preoccupations, methods, and findings correspond well to the concerns of that giant multinational endeavour. Therefore, with the one possible exception being its inclusion of "outmoded" bacteriology, parasitology, and virology, no argument can be found in METEI's composition to have caused the CCIBP to reject it. Well situated in its scientific context, METEI used current theory and method. Sadly, its products were never available for comparison and contextualization by others.

Similarly, the early start date for METEI is not a sufficient criterion for its exclusion. Several of the IBP's HA projects from other countries began well before the IBP and continued to gather data and publish during the IBP period. For example, a New Zealand study (HA-3) on the acculturation of Maori people began data collection in 1962; a Polish study (HA-15) on growth and development began in 1959; a Yugoslavian study (HA-4) on development of university students began in 1954; and an American study (HA-15) on the anthropology of aging began in 1949. In one aspect, METEI might have been *too* early – premature, if not prescient. By at least 1962, Skoryna and Nógrády had grown worried about the impact of international air travel in spreading infectious disease; however, it was not until 1968 that a WHO leader thought to warn of a recrudescence of those passé "old plagues in the jet age."[31]

Finally, it must be remembered that although METEI was originally touted as one of Canada's contributions to the IBP's Human Adaptability section, its numerous publications on the biological status of land, lakes, and sea ended up relating to four *other* sections of the IBP:

Terrestrial Productivity, Marine Productivity, Freshwater Productivity, and Physiology and Energy Transfer. A similar study of the "synthesis volumes" for these sections would identify other parallels between METEI and these IBP goals.[32] Nevertheless, despite its perceived flaws, METEI resulted in many more publications than all of the Canadian HA panels combined and most other HA projects from around the world. But without a final report, it was impossible to identify its published and unpublished achievements. Even the archives of the WHO, the body that had awarded the original $5,000 grant, could trace only three resulting articles, one of which was a news item.[33] No Canadian project connected better to IBP goals or produced more publications.

REMEMBERING METEI: WHAT HAPPENED TO THE ALUMNI?

For his 1992 article in the *Rapa Nui Journal*, navy historian Jim Boutilier interviewed Skoryna and navy personnel Tony Law, Fred Joyce, Rita Dwyer, and Richard and Maureen Roberts. He had also communicated with Helen Reid. Richard Roberts eventually rose to serve as surgeon general at National Defence Headquarters in Ottawa, and Maureen built a career in clinical genetics in pediatrics, which continued at the Children's Hospital of Eastern Ontario when it opened in 1974. Helen Reid worked clinically at Toronto's Hospital for Sick Children and kept up her writing.

By the time I began this research (with Boutilier's blessing) in January 2014, all these people had died, as had Harry Crosman, John Cutler, John Easton, Ana Maria Eccles, Colin Gillingham, Mary King, Red Lemieux, Carl Mydans, Eivind Myhre, Georges Nógrády, Al Taylor, Archie Wilkinson, and Bob Williams – some only months before I began looking. Every obituary mentioned the Easter Island journey as a career highlight. It took three years to find seventeen of the still-living METEI members and the families of ten of the deceased. One tremendous advantage was the Internet, but two of the total are still missing: Robert Fulton and Elliot Alpert.[34]

The younger METEI alumni never forgot their journey or its purpose. Many had been graduate students or still in residency training. They got on with their lives and work, wondering what had happened to the final report but scarcely in a position to do anything about it. The data were in the hands of leaders or outside experts.

For the medical examinations, Cutler had done most of the computer analysis and sent it to Roberts, who – inexplicably – simply sat on it (see chapter 10). Cutler's marriage soon ended in divorce, and in 1969 he married Isabel Griffiths (now Cutler), who, having left her own unhappy marriage with a McGill professor, became stepmother to his teenage children. John left the Public Health Service, moving first to San Francisco; then the couple went to Geneva, where he worked with the World Health Organization. John used his medical and epidemiological skills on a wide array of problems in Ghana, Senegal, New Zealand, North Africa, and the former Yugoslavia. The Cutlers returned to the United States, both working in Washington, DC, Connecticut, and Massachusetts, before retiring to Maine in 1988. He died of lung cancer at age sixty in 1992. They carted around the computer punch cards of METEI data for many years until it became obvious that no one would ever ask for them; however, they could not write the final report alone. Nevertheless, as translator and secretary, with an intimate view of the planning, execution, and aftermath of METEI, Isabel's insightful memories have been an indispensable source for this book.

Now a retired professor of sociology at Geneva University, Cléopâtre Montandon has at least ten books and almost one hundred scholarly articles to her credit. As a distinguished plastic surgeon, Denys Montandon is also affiliated with the university and deeply involved with research and philanthropic work, especially on noma, a disfiguring disease of children. A prolific author on these topics and on medical history, he left the writing about Easter Island to his spouse. When John and Isabel Cutler moved to Geneva, the couples saw a great deal of each other, even spending a holiday together cruising off Greece. Stanley Skoryna would also visit the Montandons when he came to Europe, and Georges Nógrády occasionally sent long, loving messages. The Montandons helped me to find Isabel, who summers in Maine and winters in Florida.

Isabel is still friendly with Carlotta Hacker, who lives in London, Ontario. Carlotta went on to write about making films with Red Lemieux and their travels in Africa, as well as many books for young adults on Nobel laureates, women doctors, scientists, and explorers. As Carlotta Lemieux, she is well known as an excellent copy editor in the Canadian publishing world, and for historians of medicine, her prosopography of Canada's early women doctors is a classic. She declined to be interviewed but sent greetings and encouragement through Isabel.

By 1970 Peter Beighton had married nurse, collaborator, and soulmate Greta Winch; they went to South Africa to conduct a genetics research project for just one year and never left. From the University of Cape Town, they made many contributions to the scientific literature, and like Denys, Peter has published scholarly works in medical history. During the writing of this book, his brilliant career was the subject of a fest-schrift, for which I was invited to provide a short essay about his Rapa Nui sojourn.[35] The festschrift release resulted in kudos for him from many METEI alumni. Peter was easily located through the website of his university, and our many Skype chats were made joyful by his palpable verve, intelligent honesty, and delightful sense of humour.

The members of the work physiology team are also very much alive. Einar Gjessing soon finished medical school, married his sweetheart, started a family, and specialized in plastic surgery in Bergen. Like many of the travellers, he never forgot Garry Brody's operation on the eyelid of Gabriel Heriveri. Did it influence his choice of plastics? He does not know. Reflecting on the difficulties with the bicycle ergometer on Rapa Nui, Gjessing went on to invent a new ergometer based on rowing. A Norwegian national champion, he later told me that the main objective of his invention was to help train the rowers of Norway – where rivers and lakes are frozen for half the year. However, his patented machine "took off" in physiological research, and many scientific articles refer to the "Gjessing ergometer," although they have nothing to do with Easter Island. Isabel and Einar staged a reunion on the Canary Islands in 2016. He is still grateful for her kindness in sending him some of the promised stipend back in 1965.

For his part, Björn Ekblom completed his doctorate under the supervision of Per Olaf Åstrand in 1969 and became an exercise physiology "superstar," with more than 200 publications and multiple international invitations, including a visiting professorship at Harvard University. He met his wife, Ulla Ohlsson, "by accident" – like his recruitment to METEI – when she set a record in long jump at a track event. They have three children and eight grandchildren. He still works at the prestigious Karolinksa Institute in Stockholm and often cycles the 18 kilometres to his lab.[36]

Jim Nielsen survived his odyssey with Jack Mathias, made it into and through medical school, and is an ophthalmologist in Florida. All three "physiologists" were students at the time of METEI and in no position to force a final report out of their bosses. But they willingly spoke to me of their Rapa Nui experiences, sending messages, photographs, and even Rapanui carvings and shell jewelry.

The "veterinarians," Harold Gibbs, in Maine, and David Murphy, in Nova Scotia, are still friends, but neither work as vets. Parasitologist Hal accepted an academic position at the University of Maine, Orono. His wife, Elizabeth, who had cared for their four children while he was on Rapa Nui, completed her own doctorate in entomology, "for revenge"; she also joined the university. They both have made many contributions to science; she authored a biography of Edith Patch, an important American entomologist. Murphy completed his surgical residency, specializing in the heart disease of children and becoming a professor in Dalhousie University's medical school. Following his early retirement, he pursued a graduate degree in fine art and, with his surgeon's dexterity, is now a noted sculptor. His daughter, born while he was at sea, is now fifty-four years old and still has not forgiven him for leaving his wife, Sonia Salisbury, alone. David often bumps into *Cape Scott* navigator, Charles Westropp, in the Halifax liquor store and put me in touch. As the youngest officer on the voyage, Westropp's unique perspective bridged the gulf between the navy and the scientists, and he readily responded to my queries, even from his own beloved boat.

The ecologists, Ian Efford and Jack Mathias, are also in touch with each other. It was Efford's papers in the University of British Columbia Archives that launched my research, and he was the first to respond to my request for an interview, making him the "patron saint" of my project. Mathias went on to complete his doctorate, but they both left academia to pursue their ecological concerns through government; most of their research is found in reports. Both have retired, are grandfathers, and live in British Columbia. Efford recently published a book on rhododendrons and is working on the evolutionary relationship between those plants and bumblebees.

Some METEI travellers wrote stories of the journey many years after it happened. In response to Jim Boutilier's two-part article in the *Rapa Nui Journal* in 1992, Skoryna sent a short essay that added details, corrected impressions, and emphasized his "100 per cent." Plastic surgeon and METEI "chauffeur" Garry Brody also published in that journal, describing the causes of the "rebellion" linking them to custody of the bulldozer. Now one of the most prominent plastic surgeons in the United States, Brody has maintained a life-long interest in the island and, like Denys Montandon, has served on many philanthropic missions from his base at the University of Southern California. At the time of writing, he is composing another article on Gabriel and the tool that he devised from an old tire to allow the man with no hands to return to carving. Garry too has been supportive of this book, sending photos, memories, and special artifacts from his collection.

In 2014 and 2015, the ham radio operator, George Hrischenko, published an excellent account of the communications issues on the journey and another on his impressions of the Galapagos Islands for TCA, the magazine of the Radio Amateurs of Canada. He left the Canadian Broadcasting Corporation and ended his career in a rewarding position teaching electronics at Sheridan College. A fly on the wall for the radio calls to families and offices, he has an incisive understanding of the personal stresses and class hierarchy that contributed to tensions in the camp.

Bob Meier completed his doctorate in physical anthropology and joined Indiana University in Bloomington. He is an expert on the microevolutionary aspects of human populations, having conducted fieldwork in the Arctic, with Native Americans, and with twins. He is now retired as Chancellor's Professor Emeritus. I have relied on his expertise, patience, and kindness in trying to unravel many complexities. Although he managed to gather all his own Rapanui results in a complete, open-access thesis, he too was in no position to comment on the scientific work of others and spent half a century wondering what had happened to the final report.

Armand Boudreault was the last alumnus to be found in January 2017. Retired from his career on the international virology stage, he was living in an elegant apartment on Ile des Soeurs featuring exquisite, cherished art from Easter Island and a breathtaking view of "le tout Montréal." He shrugged with modesty at the memory of returning polio vaccine to Rapa Nui; it was "normale." But he still regretted the death of his tissue-culture cells. Having quickly published all his own data, Armand had no idea what happened to the final report. He was the first to read the entire manuscript of this book in draft, and I will always be grateful. He died in October 2018.

METEI alumni have had remarkable careers, and, at first, I wondered if they had been inspired to greatness by their Rapanui adventures. But it is now obvious that they were already remarkable people to have wanted to embark on the journey in the first place. The family members and descendants – widows, children, and friends of the deceased – concur. An extraordinary group of accomplished people in themselves, they readily shared what they could of the unusual adventure, which was always remembered in their homes, although it was forgotten everywhere else, and about which they have always been curious (see Acknowledgments).

In my search for Nógrády's volume 2, I learned that after the loss of his wife, the childless Georges was plagued by intermittent depression, advancing deafness, and later blindness, but he continued to collect and protect. He died in 2013. Judith Hermann, his adopted Hungarian-born "niece," became his executrix and had to clean out his cluttered apartment. For years, she had heard Georges wax eloquent on the METEI journey, his concern for the well-being of the islanders, and his passion for new discoveries about its health and its past. She could not keep everything. She carefully digitized 400 of his slides, which, unlike all the others, included images of messiness, garbage, and rain. She cannot now recall seeing a manuscript

Table 13.3 Location of the material products of METEI

Found	Location
Carvings in stone and wood	METEI alumni and families
Cava Cava Man wooden statue	Museum of History, Ottawa
Dental impressions	University of Arizona
Face masks (7)	Smithsonian Institute (NT20653-NT20660)
Facial reconstruction	Hungarian National Museum, Budapest
Fish	Beaty Museum, University of British Columbia
Grass skirt and accessories	Redpath Museum, Montreal
Human skull	Being repatriated by Chile
Insects	Lyman Museum, Montreal
Lab values	Library and Archives Canada, Roberts Papers
Records of physical examinations	Hanga Roa and Santiago, Chile, and Queen's University
Stone tools	Museum of Anthropology, Vancouver
X-ray results	Wilkinson Papers
Not found	
Plants	Harvard University (destroyed)
Serum samples	Last seen in Kingston and Ottawa
Microbes from soil and water	Sent to Lausanne

for his missing volume 2, although she knew about volume 1; as a writer herself, she would have recognized it as something special to preserve. But she found other papers that she could tell were documents of scientific interest as well as the poster of his "facial reconstruction." These items could not be thrown away. At first, Nógrády's papers went to the offices of the Hungarian-Canadian Society in Toronto, but when that organization closed and its building was sold, they went to another Hungarian friend, retired music teacher George Demmer of Ottawa. Hermann and Demmer believed that the scientific documents belonged to Chile and the people of Rapa Nui, and after many telephone calls, an official from the Chilean embassy came to collect them.

That is where on 23 August 2016, in my ongoing quest for volume 2, I was astonished to find all the paper records of METEI's physical examinations, complete with a black and white polaroid photograph of each person as taken by Mary King. They were in twenty-one filing boxes, marked on the outside and grouped by the METEI census numbers from 00101 to 23101. The diplomats were not sure what they represented, but I provided them with an explanation of METEI and a complete index. This research had been funded by the Canadian taxpayer, and the copyright belongs to those who wrote them – the doctors – for fifty years after death. But METEI alumni and their families agreed that they should be protected and made available to the people of Rapa Nui, whose medical and cultural past they represent. Through kindness of officials at the Chilean embassy in Ottawa, their superiors in Santiago, and a grant from Associated Medical Services, we have had them digitized and returned, making them available for future analysis by qualified investigators. A celebration of their repatriation took place 1 February 2018.[37]

The discovery of the medical examination records saved by Georges Nógrády (see chapter 12) prompted me to take stock of the material products of METEI. Many objects have been located in museums across North America. Some are still missing (table 13.3). During the proofing of this book, the cranium used for Nógrády's reconstruction was identified; following consultation with the Ontario coroner, Chile is in the process of repatriating it. Its 1965 removal raises questions about the alleged "theft" by Mazière of the skull of Hotu Matu'a.

WHAT HAPPENED TO STANLEY SKORYNA?

As originally planned, METEI was only half done in 1965. Were Skoryna and Roberts waiting for that follow-up study planned for a few years after the opening of the airport? The lack of IBP support, the debt, the embarrassment over the navy costs, and the animosity within the team probably meant that the prospect of a return journey grew ever more remote.

As the years rolled on, yet another factor obliterated any idea of a METEI-2. In September 1973, Augusto Pinochet seized power, murdered Salvador Allende, and set up a violent dictatorship that resorted to torture, imprisonment, sexual abuse, and executions. Canadian diplomats hid sixteen refugees in the embassy, and in the years of the junta, they helped 6,000 migrants flee the brutality of his regime.[38] Until the restoration of democracy in 1990, Canadian scientific collaboration was just as unthinkable as trade. Both continued to be sensitive topics even beyond 1990 for lasting concerns over human rights abuses, which the recent presidents – physician Michelle Bachelet and her successor, Sebastián Piñera, elected in December 2017 – have been trying to correct.

Skoryna seems to have lost all interest in METEI, possibly defeated by the strained relationships, the slow pace of research, and the disparate network of scientists, which made identifying published results difficult. He was distracted too. The 1967 World's Fair, Expo 67, was coming to Montreal as part of Canada's centennial celebration, and it was much in the minds of Canadians, especially the people in Montreal. Using his new connection to Chile, while METEI was still on its return journey in 1965, McGill principal Rocke Robertson, perhaps goaded by Skoryna, wrote to Chilean president Eduardo Frei Montalva, asking for the loan of an Easter Island statue for one of the pavilions.[39] By 29 October 1966 – and before his METEI debt had been discharged – Skoryna was once again leaning on Robertson. This time, his goal was to apply for $75,000 through the Donner Foundation to encourage Expo 67 organizers to convert the soon-to-be-opened American pavilion – a geodesic dome designed by Buckminster Fuller – into an international biological centre for gathering and disseminating scientific data.[40] I do not know Skoryna's role in (or reaction to) that request and the eventual use of the American pavilion dome (after a fire) as the Biosphere, an interactive museum for biology. Nor do I know about his relationship, if any, to the concrete replica taken from an original Easter Island *moai* that still resides in Jean Drapeau Park, site of Expo 67.

In August 1967 Skoryna chaired the organization of McGill's international conference on the risks of environmental radiation, editing the proceedings as the first set of *Guidelines to Radiological Health* and managing to insert a few of his ideas about multifactorial, stochastic causation in its preface.[41] Later, he again began goading Member of Parliament Stanley Haidasz for help in obtaining charitable status for the Rideau Institute of Advanced Research, founded by Skoryna basically as a way to render tax deductible his own support for projects that could not otherwise find funding. Haidasz took on this task with the same eager dedication that he had taken on his tasks respecting METEI and the navy ship.[42] Alas, the products of Skoryna's Rideau Institute are slim and difficult to find.[43]

Yet another – and perhaps the greatest – inhibition to Skoryna's output was the tragic loss of his fifty-year-old wife, Halina Irene (née Grygowicz). In mid-February 1969, she was killed in a house fire that had ignited while she was asleep. Until the funeral on 18 February, her body lay "in state" at St Michael and the Archangel Church; news of her death and the fire was drowned in the flood of reporting on the student riots and the aftermath of the 11 February destruction of a computer at Sir George Williams University (now Concordia). Halina was buried near their country home in Elgin, Ontario.[44] June Pimm remembers that Stanley could never speak of her without tears. Skoryna received a letter of condolence from the new prime minister, Pierre Elliott Trudeau, who had likely been alerted by Stanley Haidasz. Never one to let an opportunity go by, the bereaved Stanley replied to Trudeau. He explained how much his late wife had admired the young leader, reminded him that he had been the director of METEI, and asked for a private meeting to discuss the future of scientific research in Canada.[45] The missing final report was not mentioned.

Nevertheless, a handwritten note, dated November 1970, on a McGill copy of his "Preliminary Report" indicates that Stanley had not forgotten the unfinished work, even if he had yet to write it: "Dr. Skoryna says he is looking for a publisher for his final report." That exercise should not have been necessary. Was he dissembling? METEI had already agreed that McGill University Press (amalgamated with Queen's University in 1969) would be the logical publisher for that book. But publication would not be automatic. Peer review stood in the way. Back in 1968, Carlotta Hacker had urged Richard Roberts to meet with McGill's editor, Robin Strachan, who told Roberts that Skoryna's "deadly enemies" among members of the press's board would "do their damnedest to stop publication." But Strachan also claimed that Stanley had "numerous influential friends in the University." Roberts wrote to Cutler, "Well he must have, mustn't he? How else can one explain his success?" Not the least of these friends, the editor told Roberts, was Principal Rocke Robertson. Roberts reminded Cutler that the head of McGill was "an MD and an eminent surgeon [who] must have something in common with Stan though at the moment I am not sure what this can be." Roberts went on to lament, once again, the lack of advance preparation. He kept finding articles with information that they should have known before they set out.[46] Even if Skoryna could find a publisher, he would have great difficulties marshalling a motivated team of writers, and their work might not pass the scrutiny of peer review. METEI slipped into oblivion.

Skoryna married again. His new wife was Jane Polud (Paludkiewicz), the effervescent Polish-born executive with the Purina feed company who had helped obtain Chilean approval for METEI and served the mission as an honorary consultant (see chapter 2). They adopted a daughter,

Elizabeth, and a son, Richard. He also kept up with his and Halina's son, Christopher, and family. Stanley's grandchildren adored his visits for his antics, imagination, and affection, but they also recognized his foibles of easy distraction, exaggeration, and fabulation that veered into mendacity. He took to wearing a toupee and tolerated their hilarity when it fell into his breakfast cereal. Later, Skoryna would pen a folk ballet, *Rideau Lakes* (1983), and two novels, *Inside Mara* (1982) and *Atlanta on My Mind* (1996), twice relying on a body-voyaging device with giant aliens who come to earth with severe gut problems.[47] His aim was to educate children – including his own, who figure in the books (as well as himself) – about the peculiar combination of history, ecology, and physiology and about the fascination of trace elements. Under the name "Stan Constantine," he composed several pieces of music, some of which were copyrighted and recorded for a 1981 album called *Dreamland*. Skoryna had moved on. He wrote no final report, but he never stopped dreaming.

The CCIBP dropped METEI from its purview without explanation. Delving into its products and that of other nations deepens the mystery because METEI and its products corresponded well to the overarching goals of the IBP. It also reveals troubles with financing and philosophy that were common to IBP projects in other nations. Possibly aware that he was part of the problem, Skoryna did little to amend the situation, while his team members got on with their lives and work, some becoming prominent in their research fields. Therefore, METEI's exclusion from Canada's IBP projects seems to be best explained by concerns about money or by the personal animus that seemed to track Stanley Skoryna in all his activities. I have placed a new binder in the Queen's University Library containing paper copies of the METEI publications that I have found, a disc with available digital copies, and a complete list of references, as it appears in appendix A and on my website. These small gestures help to restore METEI to the IBP, and they recompense the support given to Stanley Skoryna and his expedition by the World Health Organization, the Medical Research Council of Canada, Canadian taxpayers, and the Rapanui people.

METEI alumni and their family members kept urging me to go to Easter Island in order to find out what had happened to the *campamento* and its laboratories, identify the post-airport changes that the second expedition had been intended to uncover, and probe the memories of the Rapanui. Did they remember METEI? And had they loved it as much as METEI members had loved them?

METEI 2017

As the jumbo jet slowly descended in a dull grey light, gaps in the ragged clouds offered fleeting glimpses of deep-green land pockmarked by little volcanic cones and craters. Having traversed the island, it continued a long way out to sea and then turned almost 180 degrees, aiming for the famous 3.4-kilometre runway fit for a space shuttle. The houses, hotels, and roads of Hanga Roa swept into view on the left, with the Rano Kao volcano on the right, and the six-hour flight from Santiago de Chile over a vast, empty ocean ended gently to the enthusiastic applause of passengers. With my old friend and colleague Ana Cecilia Rodríguez de Romo and my husband, Robert David Wolfe, we had come to Rapa Nui bearing a few long-overdue "gifts" and seeking answers to three big questions about the Medical Expedition to Easter Island:

1 What had become of METEI's Camp Hilton trailers, laboratory, and X-ray equipment? Was the Donner Biological Station still a reality? No one had been able to tell us.
2 What were the Rapanui's memories of METEI? The expeditionists had taken away the impression of friendship and gratitude. Could that have been a self-congratulatory notion born of wishful thinking and the islanders' politeness? Was METEI resented for failing to keep its promise of return or for exploiting the islanders' trust? Would the Rapanui even talk to us? Those who had any memories would be sixty years old or more. We had heard that they were tired of Eurocentric researchers coming to investigate the remote past and disturbing or carting off artwork and human remains for selfish scientific ends without any regard for the people who live there now.[1] A repatriation movement was underway with the support of Professor Jacinta Arthur of the Universidad Católica de Chile.[2]

3 What is the health status of the Islanders now? Had the airport brought the predicted changes? Had they adapted? Could we determine how the prevalent diseases had changed, without repeating the physical and laboratory examinations? Perhaps tracking the causes of death over the past fifty years would provide a reasonable stand-in for the never-conducted METEI-2 and thereby turn a bit more of Stanley Skoryna's dream into a reality.

ADVANCE PLANNING

For guidance on seeking answers to these questions, I had written to the offices of the appointed governor and of the elected mayor well in advance of the journey. I had also contacted a number of scholars – anthropologists, archeologists, historians, and librarians – who are familiar with today's Rapa Nui and its ways. Most had vaguely heard of METEI and were eager to know more, especially because they knew that it had coincided with Alfonso Rapu's rebellion. They responded kindly with suggestions, advice, and contact information for islanders who might help, and some made phone calls on our behalf. The governor's office did not reply, but just two days before we left home, I heard from Marcos Astete Paoa, an agronomist in the mayor's office. He and his colleagues Claudia Tuki and Vanessa Gomez urged us to get in touch as soon as we arrived.

The original METEI travellers had also encouraged this journey. Nostalgic for the simplicity and hospitality that had greeted them half a century earlier, they were curious to know how island life had changed. Only Carlotta Hacker, Isabel Cutler (formerly Griffiths), and Garry Brody had ever been back, all before 1971. Björn Ekblom and Nancy Simpson both considered joining us – but the timing was not right. The eleven-hour flight from Toronto to Santiago was another inhibition. Several METEI alumni provided letters for us to give to friends and former girlfriends. Helen Reid's son and daughter wrote to her godchild, Halina Irene Pont Pate ("Mi Poki"), born in January 1965. We had no idea if we would be able to find any of these people or even if they were still alive.

Originally, I had planned to hire a local translator. But in thinking about the love affairs, the political strife, and the contentious problems with Chile, it seemed better to turn to a hispanophone who was not of the island as a way to protect the privacy of our conversations. Ana Cecilia was perfect for the task. She had completed her medical degree in Mexico City and her doctorate at the Sorbonne in Paris, where we had met as graduate students working with the same supervisor. At that time, she was the mother of a small boy the same age as my son, and we took turns watching our children play while the other studied. Like me, she went back to her home country, where she became the history of medicine professor in the local medical school and served her national society for the history of medicine as president. Over the years, we had visited each other as guest speakers, and we became grandmothers on the same day. Although we did not get together often, we were close. Her medical training, her experience with Latin American bureaucracy, her previous trips to Chile, and her no-nonsense, maternal disposition would be invaluable assets. The university kindly granted her a leave of absence. She read a draft of this book before meeting up with us in Santiago for the LAN Airlines flight.

Our "gifts" for the Rapanui – digital and paper – were a product of the METEI scientists' generosity and my research: a copy of Skoryna's unpublished "Preliminary Report" of March 1965; a bibliographical list of 125 publications that had eventually emerged from the METEI research; an illustrated, forty-page update about the METEI team members; and more than 1,000 images from their personal collections of photographs and slides, digitized by them, their families, or me. These things were destined for the William Mulloy Library and the Secretaría Técnica del Patrimonio Rapa Nui, run by the Chilean Ministry of Education, where they could be made available to anyone with an interest.

Other scholars who had worked on the island also asked us to take along messages and photographs, which we were happy to do. On the advice of Chilean diplomats in Ottawa, we also carried a letter of introduction signed by my dean in both English and Spanish, translated first by Ana Cecilia and again by an official private translator when the Canadian government rejected her version because they did not know her. The letter had been endorsed with seals and stamps by the Canadian Department of Global Affairs and by the Chilean consulate.

RAPA NUI TODAY

Easter Island is greatly changed. The air is still soft, warm, and humid. The rollers are still massive, with flamboyant plumes of spray, and when it rains heavily, the roads melt into slippery red mud. But the population has grown from 1,000 to about 7,000 permanent residents, and hundreds of tourists – 80,000 in a year – arrive on the two daily flights to stay an average of three days. Sometimes, these numbers swell with the denizens of giant cruise ships, whose stops are brief. Instead of the few military vehicles that greeted METEI, at least 2,000 registered cars, trucks, and vans ply the roads, together with many more unregistered vehicles. Traffic jams occur near the old Camp Hilton site. Horses and cattle still roam free outside town, but the Vaitea farm and its sheep are gone, replaced by a vast, eucalyptus plantation and an interpretive centre. The island is being reforested. A remarkable botanical garden and greenhouse cultivate native plants for island gardens and nurture a single spindly, but deeply cherished, toromiro tree, grown from rescued seeds. The leprosarium closed long ago and was torn down in 2000, its site now occupied by one of six schools on the island. Rapanui youth can now complete high school at home, although they go to mainland Chile for college. Near the town centre is a large arena, gymnasium, and sports field, where soccer is played late into the night. In high summer, dozens of surfers ride the waves, defying the jagged chunks of volcanic rock still lining the shore. Restaurants, bars, hotels, and shops are numerous, and many homes offer bed and breakfast. A new hospital opened in 2012. Rapa Nui has Internet, ATM machines, satellite dishes, and a radio station, but no traffic lights, no McDonald's, and no Starbucks – at least not yet.

In METEI's time, a few *moai* were upright, but only one prehistoric site had been reconstructed. Raising the seven *moai* of Ahu Akivi in 1960 was the work of American anthropologist William Mulloy, who died in 1978 and is buried on the island. With the exception of Rano Raraku, where vertical statues were sunk deep in the earth, most *moai* had been toppled and lay whole or broken on the ground. The lone *moai* that Thor Heyerdahl had goaded the Rapanui into raising near his camp still looks out over Anakena Beach, and the unusual statue that he had excavated still kneels on the slope of Rano Raraku. The Easter Island Foundation hosts themed academic conferences every three years with published proceedings, and since 1986 the *Rapa Nui Journal* has published scholarly articles on a wide range of topics, now completely online. New books on expeditions and paleontology appear often.[3] Many sites have since been reconstructed, including the monumental Tongariki, with its line of fifteen gigantic *moai*, and Rapa Nui is still the subject of intense archeological work, notably through the Easter Island Statue Project, led by Jo Anne Van Tilburg.[4] Almost the entire island is a national park and a UNESCO World Heritage site. Every tourist must pay US$80 on arrival for a park pass, which lasts ten days; however, the two principal volcanic sites may be visited only once: the reconstructed village of Orongo, on the lip of Rano Kao; and Rano Raraku, with its many scattered and incomplete *moai* on the inner and outer slopes of its crater. We saw bitterly disappointed tourists who had not understood this rule being shooed away, their visits incomplete, because they had arrived too near the 6:00 p.m. closing time. Many Rapanui find work as private tour guides or as park officials, who randomly check the passes of visitors from tiny thatched huts at the entrance to the sites. We discovered some resentment among the islanders that the US$80 park fee goes to Chile, although the schools, roads, park employees, and hospital display the money that Chile spends on Rapa Nui.

DAY ONE

We were met at the airport by Leo Pakarati, from our hotel. He is a filmmaker who knew of METEI and had used clips from Red Lemieux's film *Island Observed* for his own documentary *Te Kuhane o Te Tupuna* (The Spirit of the Ancestors). Pakarati's film explores lost *mana* (power) and repatriation through a journey he took to England; travelling, like Aeneas, with his father and his daughter, Leo went to visit Hoa Hakananai'a, the famous *moai* taken from the island in 1868 and now in the British Museum. The islanders want it back. He took us for a quick tour of Hanga Roa town, pointing out the *moai* at Plaza Hotu Matu'a and giving us a summary of Rapanui history, including the decline of health and quality of life and the loss of *mana* since the coming of tourism and money. Our hotel, Aukara B and B, is a tranquil cluster of cabins in a shady floral garden where hens and their chicks roam free. The owners are the gifted sculptor and tour guide Bene Tuki Pate, his partner, Ana Maria Arredondo, who is a retired teacher, historian, and writer, and her daughter, Paola Rossetti, who is Leo's partner. They were curious about our project and made helpful suggestions. Bene remembered METEI examining him as a child. Since it was Thursday and we had heard from the mayor's office, they urged us to go there right away, warning us that, in addition to the weekend's closings, the whole island was preparing for the big Tapati festival celebrating cultural heritage. People might be too preoccupied to help.

I was most concerned about access to the civil register because the governor's office had been silent. Several scholars assured us that it existed on the island and should be publicly available. It had been cited for causes of death in the excellent article by Clara García-Moro and colleagues describing the change in islanders' health up to 1996.[5] We had written to its Spanish authors for advice but received no reply. At the municipal compound, we found Claudia Tuki outside her office in a little blue house, which we came to call the *casa azul* in honour of Mexico's Frida Kahlo, an artist favoured by Ana Cecilia and me. Claudia listened politely to our explanations but did not think that we would be able to

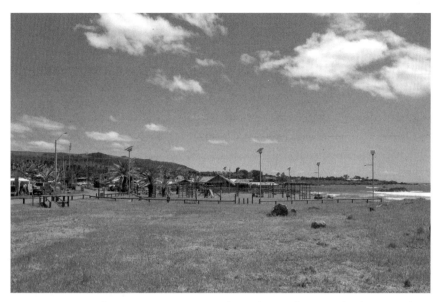

Figure 14.1 Site of METEI's *campamento* from the northeast with playground and restaurants (*middle distance*) and Rano Kao (*background*), January 2017. Compare with figure 4.14. Photo author.

see the death records. She doubted that the governor would permit it and said that we should have written in advance. We protested that we *had* written to the governor *months* in advance but received no reply. She took us to the arena where the mayor was at a sporting event – and too busy to talk to us. Next, she led us to another office, which turned out to be the Secretaría Técnica del Patrimonio, where we were surprised to find Camila Zurob and Jacinta Arthur, with whom we had been corresponding and were to meet the following morning. Camila insisted that the civil register should be open and available for consultation. Claudia still looked doubtful and continued to insist that we must seek permission from both the governor and the mayor. We would have to wait until Monday for appointments. Clearly, my requests raised some tension. I began to despair. Claudia told us to come back to her little blue house the next morning at 9:00 a.m. sharp. We felt very disappointed.

We went off to look for the Camp Hilton site just beyond Plaza Hotu Matu'a (figure 14.1). Nothing remains of the METEI compound. But that was not surprising: in 1972, Georges Nógrády had written to Tony Law to convey a visitor's report that the Donner Biological Station existed "only as a sign."[6] The site, which borders the seashore, is now engulfed by the

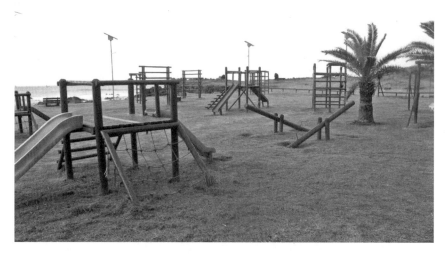

Figure 14.2 Plaza Hai Mahatu playground, formerly the site of METEI's *campamento*, from the southwest. Compare with figures 5.19 and 11.3. Photo author.

town. The little hill to the northeast, where so many METEI scientists stood to take their camp photos, is now recognized as an as-yet-unreconstructed *ahu* (platform), and it is forbidden to walk on it. A paved road lined with houses runs along the inland side of the METEI site, heading north to the cemetery and the library and museum beyond. An excellent restaurant sits on the southwest corner, and a small ditch drains water running down the main road from the church into the sea. But the METEI space is still a grassy field that – poignantly – holds a beautiful children's playground: Plaza Hai Mahatu (figure 14.2). This function was determined by the swings and slides that METEI had established in 1964 to keep little people happy while waiting for their family examination; the playground was left behind. The sign in Spanish and Rapanui makes no mention of METEI. It declares that Rapa Nui culture is based on "The Family" and that the park is a place "where grandparents and parents can transmit their experiences, values, and wisdom to the new generation in a natural, playful, and blessed environment in the constant breeze of the sea." What had become of the ATCO trailers and the laboratories? None were in sight. Over the course of the next ten days, we would uncover five different, and not entirely incompatible, answers.

We continued north along the shore, went past the huge Tapati festival stage, under construction, and arrived at the cemetery, much expanded but still in the same place and still carefully maintained with its low wall and bright flowers – just as Helen Reid had seen it from the deck of HMCS *Cape Scott* a half-century earlier. Several reconstructed seaside *ahus* and *hare moas* ("chicken houses," or mounds of stones) lay further to the north near the Tahai complex, where William Mulloy is buried. We wandered the cemetery and I began to recognize names from the METEI census; some markers gave dates of birth and death. The tomb of master carver Juan Tuki explained that he had died in 1997 at age eighty-three. I would have to pass Bob Meier's letter for Juan and his family to a descendant. Perhaps by collecting all the inscriptions, we could at least determine the age at death of the people whom METEI had examined. Would there be enough information to stratify age at death by early or late dates of birth? In other words, might the cemetery compensate for the seemingly forbidden civil register if only to help determine whether Rapanui were living longer or shorter lives? Sensing my anxiety and disappointment over the register, Ana Cecilia and David leapt to action and began taking photographs of every marker. But it was starting to rain, and only some gravestones provided the birth or death information. I could feel a destructive desire welling up for 100 per cent or nothing, bringing an existential appreciation of Skoryna's obsession.

We went to La Kaleta, a little bistro at the far end of tiny Pea Harbor with its colourful fishing boats bobbing under the gaze of the stubby *moai* at Plaza Hotu Matu'a. From its sheltered terrace, we sipped pisco sours and stared at the surfers and the former Camp Hilton site with its vacant playground. It became our favourite restaurant. Boats still drop anchor in Cook Bay, where *Cape Scott* had bided her time during the setup and shutdown of METEI's camp. Two ships were waiting patiently there either to unload or for their crews to take leave, perhaps both, and a half-dozen identical sailboats floated offshore. At nightfall, a jet passed overhead, went far out to sea, turned almost 180 degrees, and headed straight toward us with landing lights blazing as it completed its long slow descent to Mataveri International Airport at Hanga Roa. It was the second plane of the day.

Exhausted, Ana Cecilia went to bed, and David and I found sustenance in spicy empanadas with a Rapanui brew around the corner from Aukara B and B.

DAY TWO

In Hanga Roa roosters begin their uninterrupted crowing well before dawn. At 8:00 a.m. the church bells play a daily carillon rendition of "Angels from the Realms of Glory." After a delicious breakfast, with pats of butter shaped as *moai* statues, we set out for our two meetings: Claudia at 9:00 a.m. and, one hour later, Camila Zurob, Jacinta Arthur, and the team at the Secretaría Técnica del Patrimonio. We stood waiting in the muddy, rutted parking lot at the *casa azul* for a half-hour, growing anxious that we would end up missing both meetings. Had we come all this way for nothing?

Suddenly, Claudia rattled up in a truck and jumped out, smiling triumphantly and waving several large binders; she invited us inside, and we met Marcos Astete Paoa (figure 14.3). Were these binders the civil register? Claudia's partner, Raúl, waited quietly while she showed off the treasure. The civil register is overseen by the national authorities, but requests for burial are dealt with through the municipality. She had brought us all the burial records since 1998, with ages and dates of death, as well as causes of death since 2007 – twenty years of data covering the time since the García-Moro article. A brilliant idea! Perhaps it was not 100 per cent, but it came pretty close. Several Rapanui people who had died in Chile wanted to be buried at home; therefore, we had their data too – something that the civil register might not contain.

Raúl said that he had been on the "Cappa Scotta" as one of the children sent to school on the mainland. Corroborating the letters of Tony Law, he remembered the Santa Claus, the Christmas tree, the nuns, and the strange site of Valparaiso with its snake-like train. More importantly, he recalls his inconsolable crying for feeling homesick, seasick, and frightened.

Ana Cecilia and I left David photographing the entire collection of burial requests and headed to the Secretaría Técnica del Patrimonio. Camila, Jacinta, and their colleagues wanted to know more about METEI so that they could help us to accomplish our goals and so that they could learn if the subject would be amenable to a public lecture. We assembled in a small, bright meeting room, and introductions were made. Camila and Jacinta were from Chile, but Lya Edmunds Hernández, Suvi Hereveri Tuki, and young Lucía Tepihe were Rapanui women committed to preserving their language and culture (figure 14.4). I set my laptop on the table and briefly presented the story of METEI through PowerPoint slides, as I had done several times before in Canada and the United States.

The little group was mesmerized by the photos of the island from fifty years earlier and thrilled to see youthful versions of familiar townsfolk, especially the young Alfonso Rapu. They grew sober at the images of people with leprosy and of a youthful Luis Pate (later Luis Avaka), known as Papa Kiko, who had been the undisputed impresario of traditional music and dance during METEI and beyond until his death in 2008. Everyone seemed to know of rapamycin, but no one realized that its discovery began with METEI. As for polio, the story of Armand

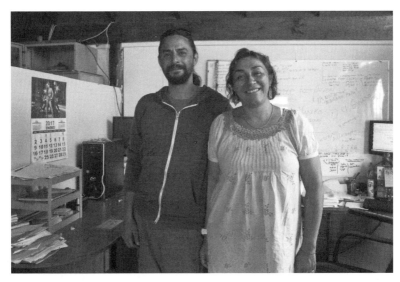

Figure 14.3 Marcos Astete Paoa and Claudia Tuki in the mayor's office at Hanga Roa. Photo author.

Boudreault's role in sending vaccine was complete news. They assured me that Peter Beighton's girlfriend, Maria Teresa Ika Pakarati, was still alive and that they would introduce us – today if we wished. We came to the picture of Stanley Skoryna and Helen Reid at the baptism of Mi Poki. Lucía said softly, "That's my mother."

"Who is your mother?" we asked.

"The baby. And that is my grandfather, my grandmother, and my aunts. They are all still here, but my mother is visiting Tahiti."

I handed Lucía the letter and photographs sent to Mi Poki from Helen Reid's children. She was astonished. We were all astonished.

The atmosphere turned giddy. Suvi had been following closely as Ana Cecilia quickly translated my words into whispered Spanish. Suvi collects the stories and memories of the elders in helping to preserve Rapanui traditions. She decided that we must appear on her regular radio broadcast that same afternoon. But first we would all convene at a restaurant nearby, and she would fetch Maria Teresa so that we could meet her. Rapanui time moves at its own pace – just as the Canadians had observed fifty-two years earlier. We waited for Suvi and Maria Teresa but eventually ordered our meals because the time for the radio show was approaching. The food was slow to come. Finally, Suvi appeared alone; Maria Teresa would meet us later. At our insistence, Suvi ordered too.

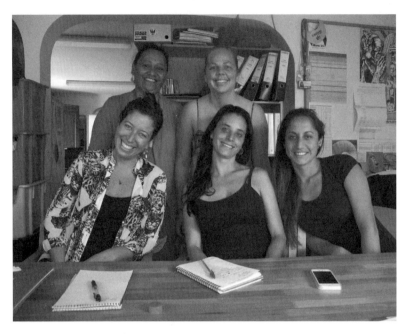

Figure 14.4 Group photo at the Secretaría Técnica del Patrimonio,
Hanga Roa. *Back row from left*, Suvi Hereveri Tuki and Lya Edmunds
Hernández. *Front row from left*, Jacinta Arthur, Camila Zurob
Dreckman, and Lucia Tepihe. Photo author.

While we sat together, Suvi explained that her opinion of METEI had
changed with our stories that morning. Born after 1965 but alert to local
legend, she had heard "bad things" about it and did not know what to
believe. Suvi had lived with a woman whose relative was in the leprosarium. The relationship of METEI to leprosy was confusing. She wondered
if memories of all the expeditions had become jumbled together. Also,
she said, METEI had induced shame. This comment was surprising and
disappointing. She explained that after METEI went home, the Rapanui
people were sad because the scientists had left many things for their use
without asking for anything in return. All along, they had been expecting
the METEI team to eventually make some kind of demand, but then, in the
end, it did not. They felt guilty that they had mistrusted the Canadians.

I could honestly assure Suvi that METEI travellers did not seem to
have experienced much skepticism from the islanders, who had been
generous in their cooperation, although some understandably hesi-
tated to participate. Suvi also told us that METEI "worked" because

the Rapanui women had decided it should work over the objections of some men who doubted its value and worried about risks in collaboration. The women perceived advantages in how it might help improve health and broaden opportunities for the islanders. They organized their children and encouraged other family members to participate. These statements confirmed the private conversations that Carlotta Hacker, Helen Reid, and Cléopâtre Montandon had documented long ago. Suvi's food came late, and she ended up taking it with her because it was now time for her broadcast.

The radio station is also located in the municipal compound. Its manager, Rafita, remembered METEI from when he was a little boy. They "gave me a needle," he said, "then a candy"; children returned the next day hoping for another candy. It was clear that in island memory, the taking of blood was not distinguished from the giving of medication. An elegant woman in her early seventies was waiting for us; she wore a brightly coloured, flowing dress, and she could speak some English. This was Maria Teresa Ika Pakarati. I could barely contain my excitement, but we were hurried into the booth and fitted with headphones. In Rapanui, Suvi introduced her program for the day, describing her guests and our objectives. She invited Maria Teresa to speak in Rapanui about her memories of METEI. Without understanding the words, we could tell that her opinion was favourable. Then, with Ana Cecilia interpreting, Suvi asked me questions in Spanish, to which I replied in English. Suvi would repeat the information in Rapanui – a cumbersome process, but Suvi seemed comfortable and in control. Back again to Maria Teresa for more Rapanui commentary. It all seemed to go well. Suvi told her listeners that we would be on the island for another week and that we were eager to hear their memories, both good and bad. She also announced that we would give a public lecture, probably at the William Mulloy Library, sometime in the coming days and that they should stay tuned for the announcement.

Suvi was now on a roll. She generated a list of people we ought to meet and assigned us appointments. Little did she know that Claudia was doing the same, and we ended up with conflicts and a tight schedule. We were to go to the library later in the afternoon to repeat the "getting-to-know-you" exercise with my PowerPoint slides and to assess whether or not a talk would be welcome.

In the little scrum outside the radio station, I gave Maria Teresa the letter from Peter Beighton. For a moment, she was speechless. Then she dissolved in tears and began a litany of questions. Was he still alive? Where? Was he married? Maria Teresa told us that she had never forgotten this wonderful man and waited seven years before she decided to

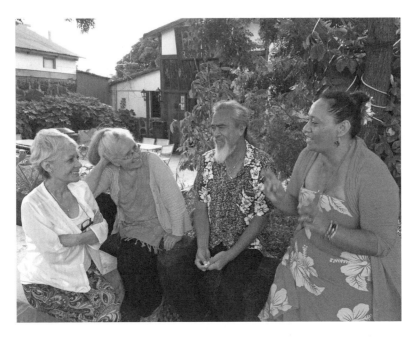

Figure 14.5 *From left*, Ana Cecilia Rodriguez de Romo, author Jacalyn Duffin, Marcos Rapu Tuki, and Suvi Hereveri Tuki at Hanga Roa, 20 January 2017. Photo Robert David Wolfe.

marry. Our knowledge of Peter Beighton, his brilliant career, and current life made Maria Teresa and Suvi our staunchest allies on Rapa Nui. She insisted that we come to her home "for coffee" on Sunday at 5:00 p.m. Suvi would bring us. Some things on Rapa Nui never change.

At the William Mulloy Library, we met librarian Katherine Marta Atán Retamales, director of communications Marlene Carolina Hernández Vasquez, and Paula Valenzuela, who is curator of the adjoining Museo Antropológico Padre Sebastián Englert. We handed over our digital and paper donations and signed documents to indicate that they were unconditional gifts and that access should be unrestricted. They decided that we would deliver a public lecture about METEI on Wednesday evening. Suvi, Katherine, and Marlene all had strong ideas about how we should handle the presentation; it seems that they disapproved of PowerPoint. But on deeper questioning, it emerged that, for them, PowerPoint meant slides with many impenetrable lines of dense prose and no pictures. We promised that our slides would be mostly pictures, just as we had been showing them; without images, our two-language talk would be slow and boring. We also agreed to the request that we close the talk with a series of pictures of people, inviting identifications and memories from the audience.

Then Suvi whisked us back to the centre of Hanga Roa to meet music-and-dancing legend Marcos Rapu Tuki (figure 14.5). We were very late (Rapanui time), but he was calmly sitting on a wall, watching the traffic rumble by. Rapanui greetings involve genuine kissing – not air kissing – on both cheeks. We all sat on the wall and chatted with the spry, elderly man with flowing white hair and beard. His eyes twinkled, and he laughed often. Of course, he remembered METEI. A teenager at the time, he worked for the team, helping to raise the ATCO trailers. No, the islanders were not paid. They pitched in because it was fun, strange, and amusing, offering many curiosities. He giggled, recalling that they had never before seen beds "with legs and mattresses." Marcos also remembered Ian Efford and Jack Mathias and how much he enjoyed helping them gather fish and animals. With the late Papa Kiko, Marcos has been the impetus behind a movement to support traditional music and dancing on the island. His troupe Kari Kari would be performing the next day. He also trained several of the other dance troupes that entertain tourists almost every evening. We acquired tickets for the next performance. Then we said goodbye to Suvi and went in search of dinner. David was in charge of logistics, food, and appointments. He found us a delicious meal at Te Moana, the fine restaurant at the southwestern end of the old METEI campsite. The sunset was beautiful, the ships stood sentinel in the bay, imitating *Cape Scott*, and the jet repeated its performance of the night before. I was feeling much happier.

MAKING CONNECTIONS

With our visit announced on the radio and at the mayor's office, we settled into a busy schedule. Some people called to make appointments, sent either by Claudia or Suvi; others found out where we were staying and dropped in unbidden. In this way, Alfredo Tuki and his nonagenarian father, master carver Manuel, showed up at the hotel on the third morning. Both had been on the mainland when METEI came, but in his work for the governor's office over many years, Alfredo had heard lots about METEI and knew its impact from a Rapanui perspective. He was the self-appointed saviour and custodian of many documents that officials had ordered destroyed and was thereby an authority on the island's legislative history.[7] They told us about carving *moai* for events in other parts of the world, and they gave us an update on current culture. Yes, Rapa Nui now had the imported problems of street drugs and sexually transmitted disease. Later we went to visit Edmundo Edwards (brother of the Chilean writer Jorge Edwards) and his daughter Alexandra, both archeologists. They are building a planetarium on Rapa Nui, and their extensive knowledge of the island and its ancient and contemporary peoples gave us more insight into the METEI legacy.[8] Edmundo knew about rapamycin and recalls the visit of one of its discoverers, whom he guided to the rim of the Rano Kao crater because the man believed that the soil containing the *Streptomyces* strain had been found there.[9] Although many islanders were aware of the wonder drug, some expressed resentment that their island did not receive a greater share of its profits.

On Sunday, we went to Mass to hear the enthusiastic singing so reminiscent of the 1960s recordings. The church is a newer, bigger building, but it occupies the same prominent site in the town. Beside it now lie the graves of four island leaders: the woman "prophetess" Angata, Nicolas Pakarati Ure Potahi, Father Eugène Eyraud, and Father Sebastian Englert. We waited for an older man who was supposed to meet us there, but he did not appear. Perhaps he saw us – we were conspicuous – and decided not to talk.

We wandered into a craft market and fell to chatting with the vendors; a woman wearing a feather headdress noticed my lousy Spanish and asked where I came from. "Canada," I replied. Wide-eyed, she indicated that I should wait, returning seconds later with the letter and photographs that we had brought for Mi Poki from Helen Reid's children. How did that letter come to her? Facebook, of course. This was Mi Poki's aunt Antonia Pate Niare, who had been photographed at the baptism with Reid and Skoryna and who had helped to raise her niece. Sixteen years old at the time, she had many memories, knew all the scientists, especially "Eskoreena" (Skoryna), and had served as a guide on their horseback explorations. She had a pass signed by the governor for guiding Ian Efford (see figures 6.13 and 6.14) and reminded us that the islanders had not been free to roam their own island. Antonia had even met her husband because of METEI: he had sailed home to Rapa Nui from school on the mainland aboard the "Cappa Scotta." He became an accountant, and they raised five biological children and fostered dozens of others. We realized everyone on the island knew about us and our project, whether they chose to speak with us or not. An introduction from Suvi or Maria Teresa helped like a passport and encouraged some of the more reticent ones to talk.

With the packed and unpredictable schedule, Ana Cecilia began to wonder if we would be going home without seeing the famous monuments. Not a chance! We took every spare moment to play tourist,

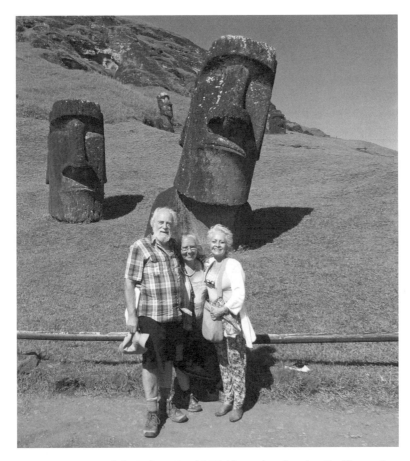

Figure 14.6 *From left*, Robert David Wolfe, author Jacalyn Duffin, and Ana Cecilia Rodriguez de Romo at Rano Raraku. No climbing allowed. Compare with figure 7.1, where Jack Mathias is atop the *moai*. Photo Robert David Wolfe.

heading out in our rickety, rented jeep to marvel at the captivating monuments and exquisite scenery (figure 14.6).

On Sunday evening we had the pleasure of dining with Maria Teresa at her new home (figure 14.7). It is painted inside and out in a familiar turquoise with orange trim – identical to the colours of METEI's ATCO trailers – the choice of which, she informed us, was no accident. Over a sumptuous meal of chicken with big glasses of juice from enormous pink guayabas, she told us her story. She had married in the early 1970s and raised four children. The family resided on the continent for some

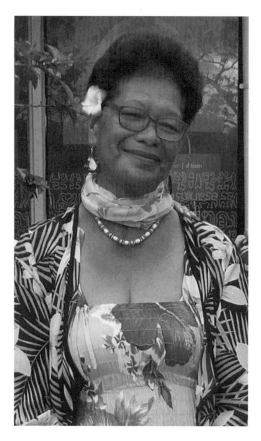

Figure 14.7 Maria Teresa Ika Pakarati,
January 2017. She is also in figure 5.21.
Photo Robert David Wolfe.

time, but she and all her progeny were now back on Rapa Nui. Divorced
many years ago and a grandmother, she had retired from working at the
hospital, where she was an administrator in maternity care. She showed
a video of her eldest son, Victor, who is a leader in traditional music and
dance; and she gave us each a compact disc recording of lovely songs
made by her daughter, Alicia, with and for her children. The news of the
letter from Peter Beighton had already made the rounds of her entire
family. They had not previously known of her first love and were eager
to establish connections. We looked at photographs taken by METEI
travellers, and Maria Teresa identified almost every islander, young and
old, and recounted their subsequent lives.

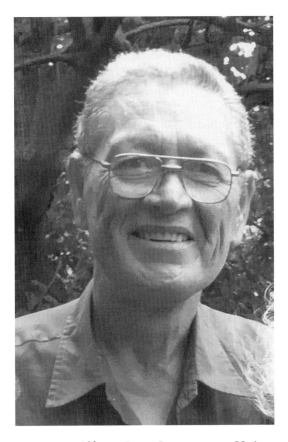

Figure 14.8 Alfonso Rapu, January 2017. He is
also in figure 4.18, the figures of chapter 6, and
figures 8.4 and 8.12. Photo Robert David Wolfe.

Young Raúl, who had helped Efford and Mathias, became a fisher-
man, but he had drowned. Her own little sister with the flaccid paralysis
was a mother, still living and walking well with support. An anonymous
woman dancing in front of a poster of President Eduardo Frei Montalva
was her cousin Selma, daughter of carver Juan Tuki. Pictures of the
"rebellion" reminded her of the cruelty of the military rulers, including Governor John Martin: two of her older brothers had been falsely
accused of theft, imprisoned, and assaulted with mutilation. The old
photographs became a method of drawing out people who were curious
to see rare images of their home and their family members, and they
became a prompt for stories.

WE MEET ALFONSO RAPU

On Monday morning, Alfonso Rapu came to meet us at the hotel (figure 14.8). Maria Teresa had told him how to find us, and she came too. Lean, quiet, and thoughtful, Rapu greeted us warmly, pleased to share memories of METEI. His younger brother, Sergio, had been at school in Chile when *Cape Scott* docked at Valparaiso. Sergio intercepted Rapu's famous letter and conveyed it to journalists. (Sergio Rapu later obtained a doctorate in archeology in the United States and served as governor of the island from 1984 to 1990.) Through both Sergio and Dr Guido Andrade, word went back to Rapa Nui about *Yelcho* bringing armed marines, who were charged with finding Rapu and killing him. Alfonso believes that his letter caused Frei to soften the orders because he saw reason in the requests. The marines were instructed to proceed with restraint and to negotiate, which is indeed what happened. "METEI saved my life," he said.

Did Alfonso have a copy of the famous letter? No, he did not. An aged uncle might have a copy, but Alfonso did not know how to find it. Where was the letter published? Both in the magazine *Ercilla*, he said, which we had already found and which had printed a summary rather than a transcript, and in the newspaper *Mercurio*. Little did we know that there were many Chilean papers called *Mercurio*, one in almost every city. Rapu said that the many copies of the letter scattered around the island had been hidden in odd places, like inside sacks of flour or under rocks, to be forgotten, lost, or accidentally thrown away. Shortly after METEI went home, the people of Rapa Nui obtained full citizenship in Chile. He corroborated the story of the special ceremony of 1966 (see chapter 11): the first citizen was the oldest woman, the second was Rapu, and the third and fourth were Alfredo Tuki and his father, Manuel, followed by everyone else.[10] Rapu gave up teaching to serve in politics, but after a second election in 1970, he gave up politics for agriculture and fishing. Nevertheless, this quiet, thoughtful man is deeply respected and continues to serve on many committees concerned with island welfare, development, and heritage. He carries what Ana Cecilia identified as "great moral weight" among his people. His granddaughter is a medical student who was working at the Rapa Nui hospital for the summer.

MORE CONNECTIONS

Edmundo and Alexandra Edwards took us to meet Ana Lola Tuki, born in 1928. Her modest home surrounded by banana trees lies off the main street in a neighbourhood known affectionately as "the far west." Pregnant at the time of METEI with the last of her fifteen children, Ana Lola ran a café and regaled us with tales of feeding hungry travellers who were seeking better fare than pumpernickel bread and cook Collin Gillingham's monotonous meals. She remembered "Eskoreena" well – "a good man," she said. Indeed, Skoryna was invoked with esteem and admiration by almost everyone who could recall the expedition, and his was the name most often volunteered. Although he had conducted none of the hands-on science, his effort to make friends and establish himself as leader had convinced the islanders, if not his team. "He did not discriminate, unlike others," we were told over and over. "He respected us and liked the children."

We soon established a routine: for lunch, it was fruit and drinks from the local grocery store and a delicious, warm empanada from the *pastelería* next door. One day, as we ate outside in the bakery shade, a bright red pickup truck loaded with people screeched to a halt in front of us. Out jumped Lucía Tepihe and her mother, Halina Irene Pont Pate ("Mi Poki"), just arrived from Tahiti; it was her fifty-second birthday, and a celebration was planned. She had already heard that we were on the island with greetings from her godparent Helen Reid's children – Mi Poki's Canadian "siblings." We exchanged hugs and took photos but did not see her again.

One day a woman called, insisting on a meeting at our hotel. She was Maruka Tepano, daughter of Margarita ("Uka") Tepano Kaituoe, who had been fundamental to the METEI laboratory. Margarita had died back in 2004. Her daughter spoke excellent English, accented with a southern American twang. She refused to use Spanish, even when searching for words, because "at school, the nuns forced us to speak Spanish and beat us when we did not." She was sixteen when METEI came and has lots of memories. Her mother used to bring home food from the Camp Hilton stores; that was how she was paid. In 1971 Maruka married an American soldier and moved to the United States, where her son and grandson still live; she did not return until 1998. She wanted to know if the METEI blood samples had been preserved, but her main purpose seemed to be to correct impressions that we may have formed. Not only were the nuns brutal, she said, but Father Sebastian too was not a saint. We must be careful not to believe all the stories written in books; a wise rule for all historians. Maruka claimed to know why METEI came. She had a hypothesis, but first she wanted to hear my version. I embarked on a synopsis, but she interrupted, eager to explain her view and because she was in a hurry.

"Honey! I know this because I figured it out when I was in the USA. They [METEI] were sent by the Americans! Think about it. Right after they left, the Americans came. The Canadians were sent to check it out for them beforehand." Her evidence included the observation that the food, brought home as modest payment by her mother, had borne labels showing that "all the cans came from the USA." I asked why she thought that the Americans would send Canadians. "You figure it out," she said. I expressed doubt: some Americans were indeed involved – graduate student Bob Meier and epidemiologists John Cutler and Elliot Alpert, who drew their public health salaries – but when asked, American institutions had declined to help with the cost overrun. She viewed all these facts as more evidence for her theory: why would the Canadians approach the American entities if they did not feel entitled to do so? Her mission accomplished, she left abruptly for sing-ing-and-dancing practice for the Tapati festival.

With the help of Marcos Astete Paoa, we made an appointment to meet the governor in order to ask for permission to see the civil register. Marcos came with us. We arrived early and found Alfredo Tuki, now our friend, in the lobby. The governor was in a meeting; in a half-hour, she would be free. Alfredo kept ducking into the governor's office, returning to assure us that we were next. Finally, after an hour, we were told that "unfortunately" the governor was too busy; our meeting was cancelled and would not be rebooked.

Disappointed, we stopped in at the registry office next door to see what would happen. I took a number and sat with people waiting to renew their driver's licences. When it was my turn, Ana Cecilia and Marcos stood by my side. The young woman behind the counter was adamant and rude: "No – no access can be given. The register is not here. No, you cannot have the address of the ministry in Chile to seek per-mission. I'm too busy. Get out." On the miserable stroll back to the *casa azul*, Marcos and I were apologizing to each other: he for having failed and for someone else's lack of manners; me for having put him in that horrible situation. He shrugged and said he had expected it. He thought that my letter of introduction with its embassy stamps, a copy of which I had sent ahead, may have hindered rather than helped the quest.

One evening, we caught up with Cristián Moreno Pakarati, a brilliant, young Rapanui historian, who had completed his graduate studies on the mainland and was back making his living as a guide for lucky tourists. Several scholars had urged us to get in touch with him. His knowledge of the island's history and prehistory was impressive, and I had already exam-ined some of his scholarly contributions about the island's political and social history.[11] Over beer at La Kaleta, he described his personal project:

a massive genealogical study conditioned by oral tradition and bolstered by his long-term access to the civil register and other official documents. He was not surprised that we had encountered difficulty with access, but he endorsed Claudia's fallback technique with the burial records. He kept track of causes of death when he found them. He pointed out the rise in identity consciousness and the tension with Chile as a colonial power. A kind of competitiveness existed between those who were more (or less) Rapanui than others, as expressed in their surnames and also in claims for genealogical "purity." There were additional pretentions to aristocracy within the "pure" group, creating stratifications within the native cohort. For different reasons, this issue was the motivator for Father Sebastian's lists, it lurked in earlier scientific publications, notably those on blood groups, and it had plagued METEI's foiled attempts to locate the anticipated but nonexistent genetic homogeneity. We agreed to swap databases: I would give Cristián my transcription of the METEI census, which contained many birth dates and household relationships, if not biological ones; he would give me his database. He kept his promise, and I kept mine.

OUR RAPA NUI TALKS ABOUT METEI: MIXED REVIEWS

We did another radio program for Suvi in advance of our public talk on Wednesday evening at the William Mulloy Library. That evening, about fifty people wandered into the large room, where the chairs were arranged lecture style facing a small screen. Katherine Atán made a generous introduction, emphasizing the METEI "gifts" that I had brought to the island. Ana Cecilia translated my words, sentence by sentence, to the backdrop of PowerPoint images containing a few words in Spanish. The room's big windows and doors stood open to the garden and the sea amid the constant movement of people as some came late and others left early. Gasps of pleasure and recognition announced the surprise and enjoyment of audience members at seeing long-gone friends; they called out identifications and comments.

As soon as the session opened for questions, however, a woman lit into us with angry invective. She claimed that all researchers take things away from the island and never give anything back. METEI had been "very bad," she said. It knew all about leprosy and did nothing – *nothing!* – for the victims. She accused me of writing a book that would make me lots of money and bring nothing to Rapa Nui. Who had said I could write a book? I needed permission, and she would refuse to give it. The image of the METEI records had set her off. Why were the records in the Chilean embassy in Ottawa? Why did Chile have them at all? She had

come to the talk a half-hour late and had not heard about our "gifts." All
the while, Ana Cecilia tried to whisper her complaints in my ear. Others
tried to ask questions, but she drowned them out, along with my feeble
attempts at reply. Eventually, Alfonso Rapu, who had been sitting quietly at the back, called out, "No more questions. It is finished," and she
stopped. Everyone stood up and milled about, chatting, and a television
crew asked for a quick on-camera interview with Ana Cecilia.

We later learned from Ana Maria Arredondo that the woman who had
confronted us was Isabel Pakarati Tepano and that she was an important
citizen: she and her mother had been generous and much appreciated
sources of history about island traditions, especially the Kai Kai string
craft.[12] Her maternal grandfather was Juan Tepano, who had advised
both Katherine Routledge and Alfred Métraux so long ago. Upset to
have provoked the outburst, I worried that her opinion represented a
widespread but suppressed sentiment that we needed to hear but probably would not.

In the aftermath, Jacinta Arthur and Francisco Torres of the museum
told me that the woman was not alone in this negative view and that
many presentations ended in this way. Alfonso Rapu explained that the
islanders were weary of scientists coming to investigate the prehistory,
ancient art, or ecology, with no interest in present-day people and their
problems. Feelings of exploitation and abuse spill over to all researchers,
whether merited or not. They fuel the repatriation movement for human
remains, one of the more romantic aspects of which is the search for the
skull of the legendary hero Hotu Matu'a, allegedly stolen by Francis
Mazière and now hiding somewhere in France. Those who had allowed
human remains to leave the island were said to have been punished with
ill health and destitution.[13] The METEI medical records must have seemed
like one more theft, although, for us, it was the opposite: a rediscovery and
a restitution. Maria Teresa, who had arrived early and sat silently in the
front row, told me not to worry; she would explain matters to Isabel.

On a happier note, following the talk, Mi Poki's daughter, Lucía,
introduced us to her grandfather and aunt, who also remembered METEI
fondly, especially Skoryna and Helen Reid, who had kept in touch over
the years. Mi Poki's sister had long been jealous of the letters and little
gifts that came from Canada. Several people that evening remembered
their own METEI encounters as children, describing the blood tests as
injections of medicine. Some also recalled being given a pill by nuns at
school ostensibly to prevent (or treat) leprosy or tuberculosis. But they
believed that it was provided by Chilean authorities and designed to
"poison" them and make them sick. "Why would the nuns do that?" we

asked. They shrugged, "to give people something to do." It was Skoryna who had told them that they could stop taking it. This pill kept recurring throughout our visit, the story shifting slightly each time. We were asked if we could identify what it had been, but we were never able to do so with certainty. Islanders mentioned various names, some similar to "conteben" (thioacetazone, an anti-tuberculosis drug also used to control leprosy).[14] Recognizing that the taking of blood had been remembered as the giving of injections, the widest possible hypotheses should be entertained for explaining its use.

At Camila Zurob's request, we gave another shorter presentation to the Comisión Asesora de Monumentos Nacionales Rapa Nui. Meeting at a pavilion in the shady grove beside the governor's office, this advisory group keeps tabs on all the research being done on the island. Chickens wandered in and out of the room as several projects were summarized and interrogated before our own. This time, Camila translated, giving Ana Cecilia a break. Word of the outburst at the library had reached the commission, and I was only seconds into my talk before someone demanded to know about the METEI physical examination records and why I would not give them back. I had not planned to make the records part of this ten-minute talk, but I quickly found and projected the picture of Georges Nógrády's boxes and explained how they had come to be with Chilean diplomats in Ottawa. Paula Valenzuela, curator of the museum, began copying the numbers on the boxes, but I assured her that I had a complete index, which I could make available. The mood then settled, and we finished amicably. A young woman who was part of the group said that she and her husband were going to move to Canada. Another woman volunteered that part of the old METEI fence was used around a house near the school.

THE MAYOR, THE LEPROSARIUM, THE HOSPITAL, AND POST-AIRPORT LIFE

Finally, we were able to meet with the *alcalde* (mayor), Pedro Edmunds Paoa, in his handsome office at the municipal compound. It was on his initiative that Marcos Astete Paoa and Claudia Tuki had been helping us with the burial records, appointments, and information. By this time, we wanted only to say, "Thank you." In his mid-fifties and the son of a mayor appointed by Pinochet, he had been *alcalde* for twenty-four years – six terms – but this would be his last. Having studied administration at the University of California, Los Angeles, he spoke flawless English. He was pleased that the burial records had helped but did not comment on our

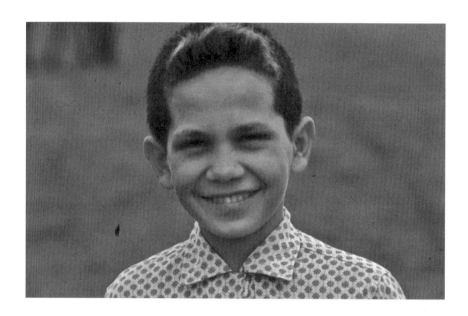

Figure 14.9 *Above*: Pedro Edmunds Paoa in 1965. Photo Archibald Wilkinson.
Below: Pedro Edmunds Paoa, long-time mayor of Rapa Nui, in 2017.
Photo Robert David Wolfe.

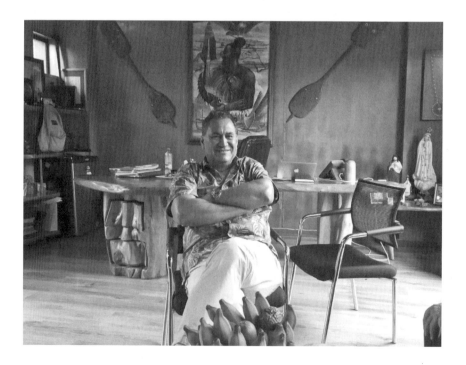

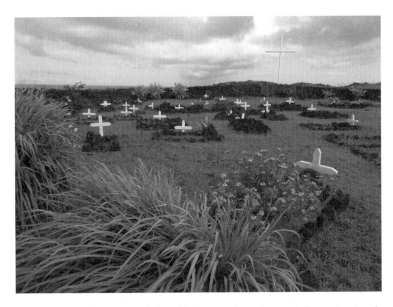

Figure 14.10 Cemetery of the old leprosarium, beautifully maintained.
The two flat stones bearing the names of the people buried there are
in the wall on either side of the giant cross. Cook Bay is visible in the
distance (*left*). Photo author.

trouble accessing the civil registry, except to remind us that Rapa Nui was
a colony, and he cautioned us about relying too much on the census. Until
the late 1980s or early 1990s, the census had been unreliable, listing random, unverifiable answers to causes of death; it would be better for recent
years. At first hesitant, perhaps fearing we wanted something that he could
not provide, the *alcalde* warmed up when we showed a few photos from
our collection, especially one of a cute little boy whom others had already
identified as the *alcalde* himself (figure 14.9). "Heh! That's him," he
exclaimed, grinning at his young self. The trailers of Camp Hilton, he told
us, had been dispersed: some to the leprosarium, some to the infirmary,
and some for dwellings. One is still a house near Liceo Aldea School, on
the grounds of the old leprosarium, and he gave directions. Delighted to
see photos of Jeep Mea Mea in action, he said, "Ha! A good truck, served
us well. We sold it for scrap only six years ago when we could no longer
get parts." METEI's truck had served the Rapanui for forty-six years!

Immediately after this meeting, we raced out to the school, looking for
the ATCO-trailer home. The gate was locked because summer holidays had
just begun. Peering carefully from a wooded hill, we made out the familiar

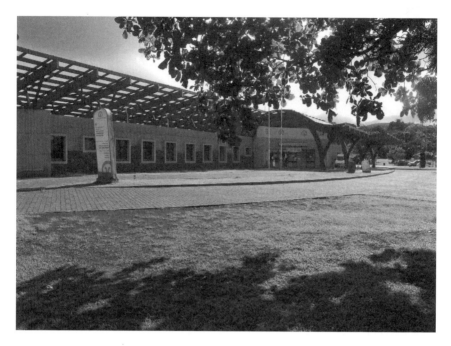

Figure 14.11 Exterior (*above*) and waiting room (*below*) of hospital at Hanga Roa, January 2017. Photos author.

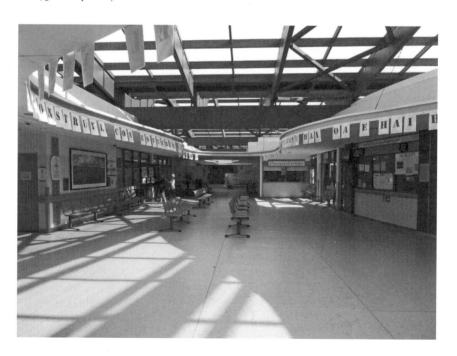

dimensions and unmistakable turquoise of what seemed to be the dwelling that the *alcalde* indicated. We also looked in town for the other house with METEI's wire fence (squares not diamonds) and thought we found it near the central school. It was clear: the remains of Camp Hilton could be everywhere around us but invisible. We were not likely to identify them in our short visit, if ever, because of the islanders' latent fear of being accused – fifty years after the fact – of stealing objects given freely.

We wanted to pay our respects at the leprosarium cemetery, which lay beyond the school, but the road was barred at the school gate. Following the coastal trails that lead northeast out of Hanga Roa toward caves and cliffs, we came on foot to a checkpoint and were asked to show our passes. We started to head inland in the general direction of where the cemetery ought to be, but the guard waved us back, trying to stop us. "Nothing important lies that way," he said. Ana Cecilia explained and asked if was forbidden to visit. He shrugged and replied that there never was leprosy on Easter Island; it all came from foreigners. We were stubborn, and he let us go but was not happy. Surrounded by a low wall in the midst of an uncultivated, rocky landscape, the grassy graveyard was well tended and filled with small white crosses, each marking a small mound of black volcanic rock (figure 14.10). Two erect, flat stones set in the wall bore the names of sixty-two people, their ages, and years of death. We found the grave of the carver Gabriel Hereveri, who had died in late 1965 soon after METEI left. The most recent burial was from 2013.

Maria Teresa also arranged for us to meet the hospital director, Juan Pacomio. We had been told such a meeting would be unlikely because he was so busy and important. But she insisted that it would be no problem: he was her nephew. The new hospital is architecturally breathtaking, with in-patient beds, operating and renal dialysis facilities, out-patient clinics, and social services (figure 14.11). On the appointed morning, she brought us to the intelligent, young director who was cordial but guarded about how much he could help. Still trying to compensate for the civil register, I had been hoping that the hospital would retain a register of deaths with causes. He admitted that such a document existed and, after an internal phone call, confirmed that his records went back to at least the year 2000; however, he cautioned that it would be a poor reflection of causes of death on Rapa Nui because so many of the seriously ill people were flown to Valparaiso or Santiago, returning only for burial – if at all. He encouraged us to use the online census statistics provided by the Instituto Nacional de Estadísticas, and he demonstrated its components for causes of death, sometimes stratified for regions. We parted friends.

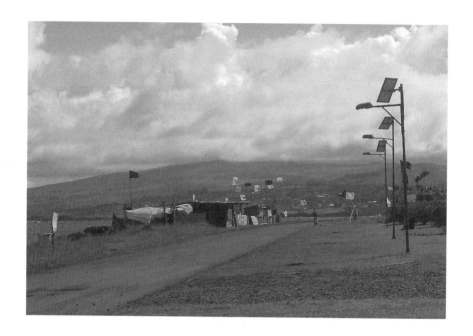

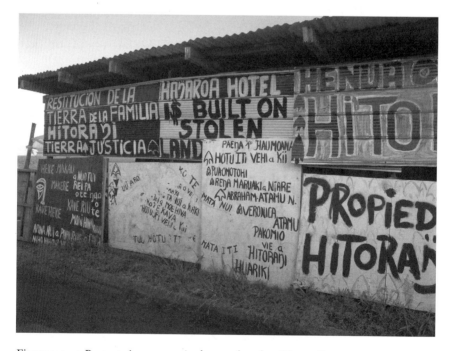

Figure 14.12 Protest signs opposite luxury hotel at Hanga Roa.
Photos Robert David Wolfe.

From our many conversations, we learned of enormous economic and ecological problems. Some Rapanui love the development projects, the prosperity, and the prospect of making ever more money from the visitors through hotels, restaurants, crafts, entertainment, and tours. Others fret over the fragility of the island's health, heritage, language, and ecosystem, threatened by the steady influx of travellers and the attendant construction, pollution, roads, garbage disposal, and indiscriminate drilling of wells.[15] The disruptions seemed to have affected all aspects of the biosphere. We were alarmed to hear that since 1984 the semi-wild horses had been dying, possibly from consuming toxins in an invasive plant that had been introduced post-METEI to control erosion; its potential to harm humans and the role of nefarious land-use practices are matters for debate.[16]

Some people opined that we were denied access to the civil register because our analysis might reveal new problems that would cost Chile even more money. Not only does friction pervade Rapa Nui's relationships with its colonial masters in Santiago and with outside researchers, but tensions also swirl among the islanders about how these challenges should be managed in the future and who should be in charge. Road blockades in 2015 and a permanent display of threatening banners and protest signs outside the most luxurious hotel reflect the anger and confusion (figure 14.12). In this subtropical place, David kept finding similarities with the public administration and cultural aspirations of Indigenous peoples in Canada's Far North.

SAYING FAREWELL AND FINDING NORMA

Exhausted from the intense visiting and talking – not to mention the heat and a couple episodes of fever and diarrhea – we began saying our goodbyes. We'd done our best and had enough information to fill weeks of analysis, even if it was not quite what we had been expecting. We'd also made friends and caught the fever of aspiration and optimism.

On our final afternoon, we made one last tour of the island. Maria Teresa's daughter, Alicia, was competing in the Tapati athletic games in the crater of the Rano Raraku volcano. Entry would be free – even for those who had already used their park passes – but the traffic and crowds were impenetrable and the heat oppressive. So, instead, we happily admired the rollers at the unreconstructed *ahu* sites along the southern shore, strolled dazzled and humbled in the shadow of Tongariki's fifteen implacable *moai*, and swam at Anakena, where Thor Heyerdahl had camped and METEI scientists had spent their rare days off. Nearby

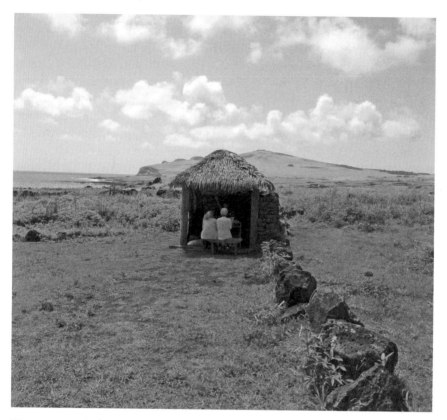

Figure 14.13 Author Jacalyn Duffin (*left*) and Ana Cecilia Rodriguez de Romo
listening like schoolgirls to Tauranga (Norma Hucke Atán) in her hut at Ahu te
Pito Kura on La Pérouse Bay. The Poike volcano is in the distance.
Photo Robert David Wolfe.

in the middle of the northeast coast, between Anakena and Poike, we
came to the deserted site of Te Pito Kura, with its giant reclining *moai*,
Paro, said to be the largest ever transported to an *ahu* and the last to be
toppled. Sated with monuments, Ana Cecilia announced that she would
stay in the jeep to rest.

David and I ambled along the hot, dusty path to one of the tiny
thatched huts. To our surprise, it contained a lonely park official in her
bright blue uniform shirt waiting to check park passes on a day when
everybody else was at the Tapati festival or the beach. Her name was
Tauranga, she said, derived from the land surrounding this *ahu*, which
belonged to her family. For her record book, she wanted to inscribe the

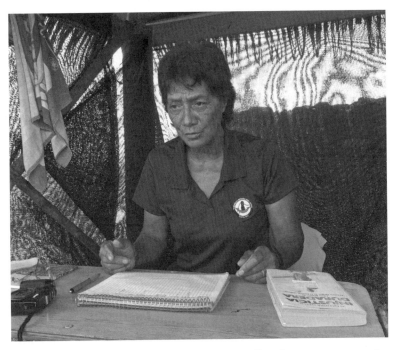

Figure 14.14 Tauranga (Norma Hucke Atán) telling her METEI memories in her hut at Ahu te Pito Kura on La Pérouse Bay. She is also in figures 5.3 and 5.5. Photo Robert David Wolfe.

name of our country, Canada. Her eyes grew wide and she began speaking rapidly in Spanish. We heard "Eskoreena," "METEI," "laboratorio," "Cappa Scotta."

"Ana Cecilia! We need you!"

Tauranga is Norma Hucke Atán, who at age sixteen had worked in the METEI lab. Seated like schoolgirls on a squat bench in front of her little table, we listened carefully while she instructed us in her views – the opposite of those expressed by Isabel Pakarati Tepano during our presentation at the library (figures 14.13 and 14.14). Before METEI, everything was utter "chaos." After METEI, Rapa Nui had democracy, citizenship, better health, and better education. We protested that the sequence of events did not imply cause and effect. She disagreed. Skoryna had invited families to send their children to help the expedition and, above all, to learn; her parents thought it would be a good idea, although others did not.

In that lab, Fred Joyce (she called him "Johnson") was her boss, and he taught her many techniques and scientific principles. These lessons made a huge difference to her future. We asked if she was paid. She bristled at the implication that METEI had taken advantage. No, she was not paid, but the education mattered far more. At his departure, Skoryna had told her that she must keep her newfound knowledge and use it to look after her people. She took it literally. Still without pay, Tauranga worked in the infirmary performing the laboratory work that METEI had taught her until new rules in 1970 created a contract with a salary.

At a moment when we had all but abandoned our Camp Hilton quest, Tauranga became our best source on its dispersal. She confirmed that the original *campamento* had been slowly dismantled: some ATCO trailers had gone to the leprosarium, some to dwellings, and some to the naval hospital, and when a newer hospital had replaced the little infirmary, one trailer had become her own home, given in belated recognition for her years of unremunerated work. There, she and her husband had raised five children. The laboratory equipment had stayed behind, but the X-ray machine had been taken to Chile shortly after METEI's departure. The truck, as we already knew, had also stayed on the island; however, the governor had tried to co-opt it too. Alcalde Alfonso Rapu had resisted, relying on the paperwork that gave it to the people, which Skoryna had insisted on signing while he kept *Cape Scott's* angry captain waiting. Two of Tauranga's daughters are physicians; she herself serves the community as the local "minister of health."

We asked about leprosy. It was Skoryna who ended it, Tauranga said. This opinion also seemed too far-fetched to be believed. She insisted that when Georges Nógrády's survey revealed little to no active leprosy, "Skoryna told President Frei" that he must send an expert to Rapa Nui to confirm that it had been controlled and to abolish the severe restrictions on freedom and travel. No such expert existed in Chile, but in 1968 the authorities engaged "a Dr Motta," who came from Brazil and confirmed METEI's findings.[17] Tauranga had worked in the laboratory for Motta's project too. The travel restrictions on islanders were lifted from that time on. The fact that Skoryna had declared the island free of leprosy was worth much more than money; it was a priceless gift. She shuddered; talking about leprosy made her sad. People who spoke ill of METEI, Tauranga said, had never worked for it, nor had they known it as she had. The Rapanui's memory of METEI was obliterated by the much bigger team and longer sojourn of the Americans.

We asked her, as we asked all women of a certain age, if any METEI babies were born after the expedition? "No, of course not," she retorted. "They were civilized people, unlike the Americans." Patricia Stambuk's recent book traces the history of the children born to American servicemen stationed on Rapa Nui in the late 1960s and early 1970s.[18]

Certainly, Canadian babies were possible; one or two were even thought to be gestating. But none of the sources – including Cristián Moreno Pakarati's genealogy, the census, and living memory – identify a single live birth in the seven to nine months after the final departure of *Cape Scott* – a curious lacuna given the otherwise high birth rate.

On the morning of our departure, while Ana Cecilia packed, David and I went for a last look around town. We were startled to see a glistening white, seven-storey cruise ship anchored off Hanga Piko. Passengers were being ferried to the jetty and into waiting vans for a daytrip on the island. Had they paid their US$80 fee? They might see monuments, but would they meet any people? In Hanga Roa at the Tapati festival stage, priests were saying Mass for an enormous crowd against the backdrop of giant portraits of Rapa Nui leaders: the woman "prophetess" Angata, Alfonso Rapu, the current *alcalde*, and his father. The parking lot and street were choked with cars. From the cemetery, we gazed over the town, the congregation at worship, the old METEI site, the massive cruise ship, and the now wooded slopes of Rano Kao. In the cemetery lay the remains of many people who had known METEI and had helped it with hope and anticipation. Had our little journey done justice to their contributions and kindness?

METEI-2

We had some answers for two of our questions about the dispersal of Camp Hilton and Rapanui memories of METEI. But what became of the islanders' health? From the Chilean census, Cristián Moreno Pakarati's data, and the burial records, it is evident that their health has changed since the opening of Mataveri International Airport and not entirely for the worse. For one thing, they live much longer. For another, fewer babies are born. Everyone still dies, of course, but the causes of death are different – "pathologies of progress."[19]

In 1964 islanders died young: five of the six deaths on Dr Guido Andrade's two-year watch had been children under the age of three. This impression was confirmed in the excellent article by García-Moro and colleagues, which traces Easter Island mortality from 1914 to 1996: until 1965 the median age at death had been only 8.28 years.[20] The majority of ailments afflicting the islanders had been infectious. Andrade had seen twenty-three new cases of tuberculosis and had watched over twenty-four cases of leprosy (six quarantined and eighteen ambulatory). Although asthma was frequent, heart disease and stroke seemed vanishingly rare – so much so that Richard Roberts gave up on his survey of electrocardiograms. The birth rate was high: Andrade had attended 107 deliveries in two years, and this same rate was mirrored in the seven births that METEI had witnessed in two months – the equivalent of approximately fifty annual births per 1,000 population, almost double what it had been at the height of Canada's baby boom. Helen Reid had also collected the statistics for the years 1955–59, which confirmed the high birth and death rates, as well as the predominance of infectious disease (see appendix C, table C.1).[21]

Although they live longer, Rapanui now die of the same diseases that kill their fellow citizens on the mainland and throughout the developed world, including circulatory diseases (i.e., heart and stroke), cancer, respiratory ailments, and accidents. They suffer slightly more respiratory disease (see appendix C, figure C.1). The annual birth rate has declined to approximately 15 per 1,000 population and the death rate to 4 per 1,000, both roughly equivalent to the rates in Valparaiso and Chile, the former being slightly higher and the latter slightly lower (see appendix C, figures C.2 and C.3). The average age at death has been increasing since 1997, although Rapanui still die younger than other Chileans (see appendix C, table C.2 and figure C.4). Over the most recent decade, the average age at death was 64.4 years; women live longer than men at 67.6 and 62.7 years respectively (see appendix C, figure C.5). Infant mortality, predominant in the 1960s, has virtually vanished; burial records of the past two decades include three such deaths. Government statistics confirm their rarity, with four Rapanui infant deaths since 2007, one in each of 2008, 2011, and 2014, and two in 2010.[22]

The burial records show that young men are more than twice as susceptible as women to trauma, drowning, and suicide. Five people have died by suicide in the past decade: four males by hanging and one fifteen-year-old female by carbon monoxide poisoning. Were these deaths provoked by stresses in the new way of life? Smoking, which seemed to be prevalent in the mid-1960s but was curtailed by limited access to cigarettes, now exacts a heavy toll, leading to many fatal illnesses of the heart and lungs, including cancer. The effect of alcohol abuse is also noticeable.

Leprosy is gone, although its ghost lingers. Some people examined by METEI are still alive with its sequelae: absent fingers and distorted features. Its decline was slow. Statistics reported by the World Health Organization (WHO) show a steady thirty cases per 1,000 population between 1963 and 1979, but by 1984 the rate had dropped to fewer than ten cases, and mainland Chile was rid of the disease.[23] In 1999 a decision was taken to destroy the leprosarium and replace it with a high school, but the segregated cemetery nearby is still maintained with reverence.[24] We saw how the very mention of leprosy still brings psychological distress, a problem that has been sensitively explored by scholars, notably Patricia Stambuk and Pablo Seward.[25]

Tuberculosis also has been controlled to a great extent. The deaths of only two Rapanui in the past decade were attributed to tuberculosis: both were women, aged fifty-three and sixty-nine, one of whom had been examined by METEI as a healthy twenty-year-old. Of the twenty-eight others who died with different infections, most often in the form of septic shock, all had an underlying severe illness, including chronic lung disease (thirteen), cancer (seven), and kidney failure (four). Poliomyelitis appeared in none of the records of the past decade.

Did Armand Boudreault's polio vaccine have a sparing effect? It is difficult to know, just as it is not clear if it was actually administered. At METEI's arrival, Dr Andrade confirmed that no vaccines were being given for typhoid or polio, and the Canadian serology results had indicated that the population was at risk of polio infection. Chile had begun a polio vaccination campaign in 1961, although Valparaiso province was slow on the uptake. The last new Chilean case was reported in 1975, making the country the third in the world to declare eradication. Nevertheless, people dying with the sequelae of old polio continued to appear in the Chilean health statistics until 2014 at least.[26] The records are not detailed enough to determine the incidence of acute polio on Rapa Nui after 1965. Knowing that no vaccine had been given, the people lacked immunity, and the airport was coming, Boudreault did the right thing in sending the vaccine with Carlotta and Isabel in 1967.

As METEI anticipated, new infections have come to the island with the increased contact, although they make up only a tiny proportion of the mortality statistics. The first may have been the severe influenza epidemic reported by the WHO in 1968.[27] But some stem from pathogens that had not even been imagined in METEI's time. Rapa Nui has seen several cases of AIDS and, at the time of writing, at least one of Zika virus.[28] Since 1970 dengue fever has been working its way around the globe with international trade and tourism. Rapa Nui faced a surprising epidemic of dengue in 2002, said to have come from Samoa or Tahiti and affecting more than 90 per cent of the population, an estimated 3,500 cases (according to serology), although only 639 symptomatic cases and no deaths were reported. Dengue recurred on Rapa Nui in 2006, 2008, 2009, 2011, and 2016, by which time public health officials were calling for vaccinations.[29]

Thanks to Cristián Moreno Pakarati's genealogy, personalizing the governmental health statistics with the outcomes for the specific 959 Rapanui examined by METEI shows that at least a third, or 311, had died by January 2017 at an overall average age of 65.7 years (males 65.6 and females 65.8). The ages at death ranged from ten to ninety-seven years. In the cohort of eleven people who had died at or under age thirty-one, all but one of whom were male, nine had succumbed to trauma (i.e., head injuries or drowning) and two had suffered from aspiration pneumonia. Four trauma deaths resulted from motor vehicle accidents between 2009 and 2014. None of the suicides occurred in the METEI cohort. Whereas hypertension, diabetes, obesity, and hyperlipidemia had not been prominent features of the physical examinations in 1965 (see appendix B), they grew increasingly present in this same population, especially into the 1980s and 1990s, when they were specifically noted as risk factors on the death records. Their ravages can also be detected in the rise in myocardial infarction and renal failure, which had been virtually nonexistent before and during METEI. Infections declined as a cause of death in this METEI cohort too, especially tuberculosis and leprosy, which had accounted for a combined high of about 10 per cent of deaths in the late 1970s but were merely incidental factors in 2 per cent of deaths from other causes by the 2010s.

Several islanders expressed concern to us over the high incidence of cancer and its greater frequency in certain families, relating it to pollution caused by vehicles or chemicals that may be sprayed on crops. Cancer deaths are indeed more frequent now than fifty years ago, but this shift likely owes something to better survival of infancy and childhood infections; therefore, people live long enough to contract malignancies. Not only was cancer unmasked by the increasing life span, but it was also aggravated by high rates of smoking. In 1965 Rapanui loved to smoke, but cigarettes were scarce. In the twenty-first century, increased wealth and abundant access have made the practice ubiquitous. It is confirmed by the anatomical profile of the fatal malignancies in the burial records: eighteen lung, three breast, three prostate, three gynecological, and thirteen digestive (i.e., esophagus, stomach, colon, liver, and pancreas). The rate of cancer on Rapa Nui now resembles that of mainland Chile and other developed countries.

❧

Our modest attempt at METEI-2 revealed that the Camp Hilton leavings were heavily used even if they had been widely dispersed. Memories of METEI were mixed: some were warm and enthusiastic; others were guarded or angry. We heard more of the former perspective than the latter but admit that our method might have skewed the responses. As for the health of the people and their island, things had changed. Skoryna, Boudreault, and Nógrády had predicted that the airport would bring travellers in enormous numbers to see the exotic monuments and that the Rapanui would go voyaging themselves. They were right; however, the harm of this greater contact with the outside world was not an influx of microbes but an invasion of lifestyle.

Conclusion

In our world of 1964, a world that sometimes threatens to become
addicted to technocracy, we need the humanities more than ever, so
that the "culture" of science will be counselled by the "culture" of
the humanities, for the peaceful benefit and betterment of mankind.

Lester B. Pearson

Contemplating the Medical Expedition to Easter Island half a century
later gives us much to celebrate and much to regret. For Canadians especially, the very fact of METEI is an amazing story: a signature accomplishment for its navy, an inspiring, fledgling project in the great sweep
of environmental science, and a nostalgic evocation of an optimistic time
when the country was ready and willing to do anything. On 15 February
1965, at sea in the South Pacific, METEI members raised the country's
new flag, convinced that their work was a manifestation of national
identity and more expeditions to come. Two years later, a Canadian
oceanographic ship would circumnavigate the Americas for the first
time.[1] Once lauded in Canada, Stanley Skoryna's prescient vision of
health and disease within their environmental conditions grew into one
that medicine newly respects and struggles to embrace through what
have since become the "social determinants." The gifts of the medical
equipment that METEI left behind, the revelation of polio vulnerability,
and the sending of vaccine were intended to contribute to the well-being
of Rapanui people. The discovery of rapamycin made a breathtaking
impact on global health and on medical knowledge. First among the
contributions of my research is a reminder of METEI – its origins, intent,
and outcomes – and the restoration of Canada's role in the history of
expeditions and of rapamycin.

For the Rapanui and Chileans, METEI witnessed and thereby fostered
the democracy movement on the island, saving the life of its first mayor,
Alfonso Rapu, or so he claims. Certainly, the presence of METEI meant

that information of the uprising flowed to the outside world, injecting caution into the military response. Perhaps also, it helped to bring about the lifting of feudal restrictions, born of the taint and fear of leprosy, by proving that the disease was controlled. Skoryna may be given credit for these benefits; however, he tried not to take sides, needing approval from both the governor and the "rebels" for his project to proceed. In any case, that independence movement is still not complete. Rapa Nui is free of leprosy and travel restrictions, but it remains a colony, and not everyone is happy about it. Uncovering METEI has added a new dimension to the history of this important moment in Rapa Nui's political destiny.

In an international context, METEI aimed to accomplish far more than any of the other Human Adaptability projects of the International Biological Programme (IBP) (see chapter 13). Even without its final report, many of its contributions, although obscure, are accessible in publications, archives, and museums. METEI sought advice from and placed its data in the hands of the founding leaders of the IBP, including Joseph S. Weiner and some of the most famous researchers and public figures of the era: Karl Lange Andersen in Norway, Alexander Bearn and Harry L. Shapiro in New York City, Edward O. Wilson in Boston, Henry Blackburn in Minnesota, Christy Turner in Arizona, William S. Laughlin in Madison, Thomas Hunt in London, Ian McTaggart-Cowan in Vancouver, and William Harding Le Riche, Roy J. Shephard, and Fraser Mustard in Toronto. Therefore, a major finding of my research has been to identify and collect the more than one hundred scientific papers and collections that came out of the expedition, although its leader was unaware. In a sense, the contents of appendices A and B comprise the data of the final report that Skoryna never wrote.

METEI's greatest accomplishment at the time, however, was not scientific; rather, it was the fact that it happened at all, that everyone came home safely, that no Canadians or islanders were harmed, and that for the first time ever, the world saw a plucky but flawed effort to document an entire biosphere. And in that, for once, Skoryna was vindicated: METEI enjoyed "100 per cent success." This too is another finding of my research, greatly amplified by the diaries, photographs, papers, and memories of the travellers themselves.

Beyond this book as a product of my work, the rediscovered records of more than nine hundred medical examinations and nearly two thousand photographs have now been returned to Rapa Nui. Inhabitants over the age of fifty had never before seen images of their younger selves or of their island as it was a half-century ago: barren and impoverished yet happy. Hopefully, the cranium will soon follow.

Our return to Rapa Nui in 2017 and the gathering of present-day health information represented a modest attempt to conduct the missing second half of METEI, contrasting the results with the findings of 1964–65 (appendix C). At the very least, it confirms the significant health impact wrought by the airport and greater contact with the outer world.

But so much of METEI must be regretted: the absence of a final report, the failure to make a return visit, the deeply disturbing personal animosities, and the shameful lack of respect and accountability to donors, taxpayers, and the Chilean government. METEI's inner conflict stemmed from the lack of advance planning and the failure to define specific roles, fostering confusion and competition. These inadequacies raise further questions of a psychological nature about rivalry between individuals and collectives, especially in academic settings or in intense but isolated confines, such as jury duty, submarines, and space stations. In that sense, METEI was not unusual, possibly banal. Its functioning corresponds well to the observations of sociologists who have explored how scientific research and its resultant communication often proceed as "bricolage," a piecing together or tinkering that is less direct, purposeful, and rational than intended and frequently marked by intersecting designs and disciplines. This book shows how the team set out to document a biosphere, its vulnerability to infection, and its future alterations; instead, they discovered a healthy population, experienced remarkable personal growth, and brought home the source of a wonder drug with unrelated applications – all worthy, although unintended, discoveries. Some Rapanui think that their island should be enjoying a greater share in the profits of rapamycin, the long gestation of which predated the formalization of the legal and ethical obligations of bioprospecting in the 1990s.[2] In investigating those problems, I have offered a few ideas to explain them.

The strife and the regrets also remind us that more work could be done in specific areas. For example, we could consider the career difficulties of brilliant scientists who were newcomers to Canada in the 1940s and 1950s, like Skoryna, Georges Nógrády, Edith Mankiewicz, and Surendra Nath Sehgal; the hurdles that they faced reveal the mid-century parochialism of this land of immigrants, even as national identity was beginning to change. Historians have only recently begun to address the source of these attitudes that continue to disturb, and more results will come.[3] Similarly, Armand Boudreault's previously unremembered gift of polio vaccine and its subsequent fortunes mean that Rapanui epidemiology through time deserves closer attention – not only for this one infection but also for all other communicable and noncommunicable diseases. It also prompts greater consideration of

Montreal's INRS–Institut Armand-Frappier and its role in the creation and dissemination of vaccines around the world.

This history of METEI is a case-study contribution to the scholarship on the history of expeditions, both colonial and postcolonial. It changes little in the analysis that is emerging from these works and confirms many previous observations. Given METEI's timing at the inception of medical anthropology and its focus on infection, the fact that Skoryna thought to include sociology and psychology is laudable and surprising; the projects of June Pimm and Cléopâtre Montandon are unique. However, neither approach had been his main interest; indeed, he appears to have made room for them as undersupported afterthoughts, simply because he thought it would help with appearances and funding. A medical anthropologist could have added insights about ethnology and social practices; one wonders if such a scholar might have analyzed the behaviour of the team itself, as Helen Reid wished to do and as young Cléopâtre tended to do in her diary.

Despite the good intentions, METEI's genetic and social studies could not avoid tilting toward the scientific racism and social chauvinism of their time. Having done some advanced reading, METEI members were prepared to find thieves and murderers rampant within an inbred population. These expectations had been conditioned by works of other writers, such as Thor Heyerdahl, and by the convictions of the respected German priest Father Sebastian Englert, who gleaned from the people a careful list of "pure natives." Father Sebastian had hoped to unravel the mystery of Rapanui origins through "heredity"; METEI had wanted to explore potential susceptibilities and health status for the future through "genetics." Situated between the early glow of genetic promise and the advent of molecular DNA techniques, METEI attempted to characterize Rapanui identity by the "classical" tests – for blood groups, enzymes, familial patterns of habitus, cholesterol, sugar, and urea nitrogen. Their work matched studies being conducted simultaneously all over the world. But the islanders were not inbred; they were diverse. Scholars have since confirmed their Polynesian origins, which had been suspected from the results of METEI and others, and they have shown the Rapanui's genetic affinities to be far richer and more complex than anyone imagined in the pre-DNA era.[4] Moreover, those genetic studies of populations – even after the more precise molecular techniques had come to the fore – failed to clarify questions of specificity, difference, and geographic or racial origins. In fact, they exposed new problems that challenged the very concepts of race and of genes and increased the relevance of the environmental and social sciences.[5]

But it would be wrong to claim that METEI scientists were unaware of these problems and their mistakes. From the moment of arrival, they were struck and embarrassed by their own lack of preparation, amateurism, erroneous assumptions, and arrogance about a people who were far more sophisticated and joyful than they had been anticipating. Some had doubted the claim of genetic homogeneity before leaving home, simply by contemplating the history. METEI travellers confronted their prejudices full on but were at a loss about how to express them in the nonexistent report. Some, like Archie Wilkinson, tried to keep track of all the detailed technical problems with the X-rays, mindful that the study was a "test balloon" funded by the World Health Organization and that future projects should learn from their many mistakes. Sadly, no one knew about Archie's meticulous, tape-recorded report.

METEI's relationship to the IBP invites more questions about that program and international science in general. This research has shown that METEI's numerous but unknown publications did correspond well to IBP goals, especially for understanding human adaptability. I hope that future studies will examine IBP history and its products in individual countries or various regions to reveal whether or not other ambitious ventures were correspondingly expunged and why.

Similarly, more historical work could be devoted to Canada's relationship to Chile prior to 1973 through trade, science, and culture. The fact that Chile tolerated, even welcomed, METEI when its own scientists were already embarked on similar studies still puzzles me. Maruka Tepano, in Hanga Roa, insists that it was the Americans who sent METEI as scouts for their future base. I have found no evidence to support her view, but it reveals our general ignorance of Canadian diplomacy in Latin America at that time and the islanders' shrewd mistrust of outsiders' accounts of their past.

Finally, although all its leaders were men, METEI is a story of women in science, in service, and in domestic life. Perhaps I have come to this conclusion because my sources were enriched by the wonderful, revelatory diaries and memories of the minority travellers Isabel Griffiths (now Cutler), Carlotta Hacker, Cléopâtre Montandon, and Helen Reid. Their keen observations placed the adventure on an intensely human scale – both feminine and feminist – and were reminiscent of the travails of the intrepid Katherine Routledge, whose Easter Island sojourn had preceded theirs by fifty years. But the assessment hit home on Rapa Nui when Suvi Hereveri Tuki explained that METEI "worked" because Rapanui women decided it should. Consequently, the unreasonable expectations and outrageous aspersions cast on the labour and dignity of these intelligent, feisty people in their homes, clinics, offices, and laboratories stands as one more reminder of the gendered world half a century ago.

Stanley Skoryna never understood how much of his dream was realized. In giving it substance, this work brings together the science, the scientists, their supporters, and the Rapanui people who helped, substituting for the report that he failed to write. But many historical questions remain, and the prescient health and environmental concerns that motivated his idealistic project are still with us.

Appendices

For complete references, use these lists with the Bibliography.

PUBLISHED AND UNPUBLISHED

Ajello, L., et al., "Easter Island Soils," 1972.
Allen, G.R., "Two New Species of Frogfishes," 1970.
Alpert, M.E., et al., "Staphylococcus Sampling Map," 1974.
Andersen, K.L., "Ethnic Group Differences," 1967.
Anderson, J.R., et al., "Ninety-Ninth Annual Meeting of the CMA," review of Richard Roberts's speech on METEI, 1966.
Angyal, T., "Serology of Rapa Nui Staphylococci," 1974.
Anon., "Eivind Myhre," interview, 1965.
– "Health Survey," 1965.
– "Medical Expedition," 1965.
– "Winners Fly to Easter Island," 1967.
– "Discussions and Recommendations," 1974.
– "Canadian Scientists Visit Easter Island," 1989.
Bain, B., et al., "Recommendations ... Blood and Serum Samples," 1974.
Beighton, P. "Easter Island People," 1966.
Berg, K., et al., "Inherited X-Linked Serum System," 1966.
– et al., "X-Linked Serum Marker," 1966.
Bergsdoll, M.S., et al., "Enterotoxin ... Rapa Nui Staphylococci," 1974.
Boudreault, A., "Huit semaines," 1965.
– "L'expédition de l'Ile de Pâques," 1965.
– et al., "Repartition des anti-corps neutralisant ... poliomyélite," 1966.
– et al., "Repartition des anti-corps inhibiteurs ... rougeole," 1966.
– et al., "Epidémiologie des infections virales," 1968.
– "Comment on the Technical Facilities of Sample Preservation," abstract, nd.
Boulanger, P., et al., "Serological Survey ... Domestic Animals on Easter Island," 1968.
Boutilier, J.A., "METEI," 1984.
– "METEI," 1992.
Brody, G.S., "Early Flight to Isla de Pascua," 2013.
Brydon, J.E., et al., "Examination of Some Soil Samples," abstract, nd.
Caldwell, D.K., et al., "Cantherhines tiki ... Easter Island Filefish," 1967.
Canadian Broadcasting Corporation, R. Williams, et al., Canadian Expedition to Easter Island, documentary, 1965.
Chagnon, A., et al., "Incidence of Rubella Antibodies," 1969.
– et al., "Epidemiological Studies on Rubella," 1970.

Clecner, B., et al., "Acquisition de la propriété hémolytique ... chez *Staphylococcus aureus*," 1966.

Clecner-Gray, B., et al., "Study of Extrachromosomic Genetic Factors ... in Staphylococci," 1974.

Comtois, R.D., "Phage Types of Rapa Nui Staphylococci," 1974.

Conway, D.J., et al., "Easter Island Families," nd.

Cutler, J.L., "Programmed Census," 1966.

– et al., "Census of the Sampled," 1974.

D.M.P. [navy], "Expedition Lands on Easter Island," 1965.

Drapkin, I., et al., "Evidence of Staphylococcal Diseases," 1974.

Ekblom, B., "Med testcykel till 'Världens Navel,'" newspaper article, 1965.

– "Oskrivna lagar," newspaper article, 1965.

– "Revolution på Påskön," newspaper article, 1965.

– et al., "Maximal Oxygen Uptake," 1968.

Embil, J.A., et al., "Prevalence of Cytomegalovirus," 1969.

Farkas-Himsley, H., et al., "Survey of Easter Island Staphylococci," 1969.

– "Survey of Penicillinase Production by Rapa Nui Staphylococci," 1974.

Fell, E.J., "Echinoids of Easter Island," 1974.

Fitzgerald, R.G., "Isolation and Characterization of Human Carciogenic [sic] Streptococci," abstract, nd.

Gibbs, H.C., "Survey on the Incidence of Enterobiasis," 1966.

– "Parasites in Rapa Nui Natives," abstract, nd.

Goodson, C.S., et al., "Easter Islander Palmar Dermatoglyphics," 1986.

– et al., "Topological Description of Easter Islander Palmar Dermatoglyphics," 1986.

Greenfield, D.W., et al., "Damselfishes (Pomacentridae)," 1970.

Hacker, C., "Aku-Aku: L'expédition canadienne," 1965.

– "Aku-Aku and Medicine Men," 1965.

– "L'expédition de l'Ile de Pâques," 1965.

– *And Christmas Day*, 1968.

– "Revolt in the Easter Islands [sic]," nd.

Haldane, E.V., et al., "Serological Study of Cytomegalovirus," 1969.

– et al., "Comparative Epidemiology of Cytomegalovirus," 1970.

H.C.W. [navy], "1964 in Review," 1965.

Hermansen, L., et al., "Physical Fitness," 1967.

Hrischenko, G., "Easter Island," 2014–15.

Ingram, D.G., "Immunoconglutinin Levels," 1974.

– "Anthropozoonosis Antibodies," abstract, nd.

Jablon, J.M., "Fluorescence-Antibody Technique," abstract, nd.

Joyce, F. "*Cape Scott* Solves Dilemma," 1964.

Kami, H.T., "New Subgenus and Species of Pristipomoides," 1973.

Kevan, D.K.McE., "Orthopteroid Insects," 1965.

Kohn, A.J., "Ecological Shift ... *Conus miliaris* at Easter Island," 1978.

Lawlor, R., et al., "Comparison of ... *Staphylococcus aureus*," 1974.

Macfarlane, D.B. Numerous articles, *Montreal Star*, 1964–68.

Magnusson, S., "Comparison of Virus Inactivating Capacity," abstract, 1969.

Mankiewicz, E., "Antibodies against Typical and Atypical Mycobacteria," abstract, 1969.

Mason, W.R.M., "Endemic Subspecies of *Echthromorpha agrestoria*," 1974.

Meerovitch, E., et al., "Intestinal Parasitic Infections," 1969.

Meier, R.J., "Medical Expedition to Easter Island," 1967.

– "Easter Islander," doctoral dissertation, 1969.

– "Review of ... Rupert I. Murrill," 1969.

– "Dermatoglyphics of Easter Islanders," 1975.

– "Penrose Analysis of Easter Island Biological Relationships," 1975.

– "Sequential Developmental Components of Digital Dermatoglyphics," 1981.

– et al., "Relationship between Dermatoglyphics and Body Measurements," 1987.

Mockford, E.L., "Psocoptera Records," 1972.

Möller-Christensen, V., "Early Signs of Leprosy," abstract, 1969.

Montandon, C., "Easter Island: A Case of Social Change," 1966.

– "Μια Ελληνιδα Στο Νησί Του Πασχά," magazine article, 1966.

– et al., "District Map of Hanga Roa" and "Map Indicating Houses," 1974.

– "Easter Island: A Case of Social Change," 1978.

– "L'Ile de Pâques: Un cas de changement social," nd.

Mydans, C., "Isle of Stone Heads," 1966.

Myhre, E., "Blood Groups of the Easter Islanders," 1969.

National Film Board and H. Lemieux, *Island Observed*, documentary, 1966.

Nógrády, G.L., "Soil Specimens," 1967.

– "Planning ... Antibiosis Project," abstract, 1969.

– et al., "Planning ... Mycobacteria Project," abstract, 1969.

– ed., *Symposium of the Medical Expedition to Easter Island*, abstracts, 1969.

– "District-House and House-District Listings," 1974.

– "Finding Lists of Rapa Nui Human Staphylococcus," 1974.

– ed., *Microbiology of Easter Island* (Rapa Nui), vol. 1, 1974 (see below).

– "Planning ... Staphylococcus Studies," 1974.

– "Easter Island Stone Basins," 1976.

– "Facial Reconstruction," poster, 1981.

Pimm, J., "Developmental Trends in an Isolated Culture," 1973.

Porteous, J.D., "METEI," 1989.

Pulverer, G., "Human and Animal Origin of Rapa Nui Staphylococci," 1974.

Randall, J.E., et al., "New Butterfly Fish," 1973.

– "Endemic Shore Fishes," 1976.

Reid, H.E., "Easter Island," 1965.

– *World Away*, 1965.

– "Physical Development," 1968.

Roberts, R.H., "Report on the Easter Island Medical Expedition," unpublished report, 1965.

– "Results of the Easter Island Expedition," unpublished conference paper, 1966.

– "Health and Hygienic Conditions," abstract, 1969.

– "Easter Island Expedition (1964–65)," unpublished conference paper, 1984.

Roberts, S.M.H., "Lecture in London," unpublished speech, nd.

Shewell, G.E., "Two Records of Agromyzidae," 1967.

Simpson, N.E., "Genetics of Esterases in Man," 1968.

Skoryna, S.C., et al., "Preliminary Report," 1965.

– "Operation METEI," 1966.

– "Objectives of the Canadian Medical Expedition to Easter Island," abstract, 1969.

– "METEI: An Epilogue," 1992.

Smyth, C.J., et al., "Easter Island Staphylococci," abstract, 1968.

– et al., "Survey of Easter Island Staphylococci," 1968.

Sonea, S., et al., "High Yield of Avirulent Staphylococcus aureus," 1966.

Tanner, F., "Sample Collection," abstract, nd.

Taylor, A.G., "Medical Expedition to Easter Island," 1965.

– "Dental Conditions," 1966.

– "Dental Health," abstract, nd.

Tector, A., "Delightful Revolution," 2014.

Toutant, R., et al., "Méthode d'étude," 1966.

Turner II, C.G., et al., "Dentition of Easter Islanders," 1977.

– "Life and Times," 2013.

Vézina, C., "Antimicrobial Activity of Streptomycetes," abstract, 1969.

Wells, J.W., "Notes ... Scleractinian Corals from Easter Island," 1972.

Williams, R.E.O., et al., "Certain Characters of Rapa Nui Staphylococci," 1974.

Wilson, E.O., "Ants of Easter Island," 1973.

Wishart, F.O., "Report of the Laboratory Section," 1966.

Zipkin, I., "Fluoride Exposure of Rapa Nui Inhabitants," abstract, nd.

GEORGES NÓGRÁDY'S VOLUME I

Listed here from the first section are the contents of volume 1 of Georges Nógrády's *Microbiology of Easter Island.*

Alpert, M.E., et al., "Staphylococcus Sampling Map," 1974.

Angyal, T., "Serology of Rapa Nui Staphylococci," 1974.

Bain, B., et al., "Recommendations ... Blood and Serum Samples," 1974.

Bergsdoll, M.S., et al., "Enterotoxin ... Rapa Nui Staphylococci," 1974.

Chile, "Map of Rapa Nui," 1974.

Clecner-Gray, B., et al., "Study of Extrachromosomic Genetic ... in Staphylococci," 1974.

Comtois, R.D., "Phage Types of Rapa Nui Staphylococci," 1974.

Cutler, J.L., et al., "Census of the Sampled," 1974.

Drapkin, I., et al., "Evidence of Staphylococcal Diseases," 1974.

Farkas-Himsley, H., "Survey of Penicillinase Production by Rapa Nui Staphylococci," 1974.

Ingram, D.G., "Immunoconglutinin Levels," 1974.

Lawlor, R., et al., "Comparison of ... *Staphylococcus aureus*," 1974.

Montandon, C., et al., "District Map of Hanga Roa" and "Map Indicating Houses," 1974.

Nógrády, G.L., "District-House and House-District Listings," 1974.

– "Finding Lists of Rapa Nui Human Staphylococcus," 1974.

– "Planning ... Staphylococcus Studies," 1974.

Pulverer, G., "Human and Animal Origin of Rapa Nui Staphylococci," 1974.

Williams, R.E.O., et al., "Certain Characters of Rapa Nui Staphylococci," 1974.

GEORGES NÓGRÁDY'S VOLUME 2

Listed here are abstracts, some included in the first section, and speeches possibly destined for the unpublished volume 2 of Georges Nógrády's *Microbiology of Easter Island*.

Boudreault, A., "Comment on the Technical Facilities of Sample Preservation," abstract, nd.

Brydon, J.E., et al., "Examination of Some Soil Samples," abstract, nd.

Clark, W.A., Microbiological Serum Sample Preservation Methods," abstract, nd.

Fitzgerald, R.G., "Isolation and Characterization of Human Carciogenic [sic] Streptococci," abstract, nd.

Gibbs, H.C., "Parasites in Rapa Nui Natives," abstract, nd.

Ingram, D.G., "Anthropozoonosis Antibodies," abstract, nd.

Jablon, J.M., "Fluorescence-Antibody Technique," abstract, nd.

Roberts, R.H., "Kokongo Epidemic," speech, nd.

– "Presentation Number 20," speech on expedition overview, nd.

– "Presentation Number 24," speech on tuberculosis and leprosy, nd.

– "Presentation Number 37," speech on kokongo, nd.

Scott, F., "Studies on an Intradermal Test," abstract, nd.

Tanner, F., "Sample Collection," abstract, nd.

Taylor, A.G., "Dental Health," abstract, nd.

Wilt, J.C. "Anthropozoonoses in the Northwest [America] ...," abstract, nd.

Zipkin, I., "Fluoride Exposure of Rapa Nui Inhabitants," abstract, nd.

Table B.1 Urinalysis on 301 Rapanui, 1965

Glucose negative	Protein negative	Protein trace	Protein +	Protein ++	Protein +++	pH range	Microscopic
304 (all)	222	52	20	1	3	5–9	2*

* 1 male, normal; 1 female, pus and blood

Note: 301 people (208 male; 91 female; 2 unknown) from 93 different families provided 304 samples (3 duplicated); 25 male family heads did not provide a sample, although their partners and children did.

Source: These results were sent by Helen Reid to Richard Roberts, 30 May 1966, LAC, Roberts Papers, vol. 1, file 22.

Table B.2 Haptoglobin type analysis of 173 Rapanui, 1965

	Tested	Haptoglobin type, 1:1 (%)	Haptoglobin type, 2:1 (%)	Haptoglobin type, 2:2 (%)
Male	87	33 (38)	46 (52.9)	8 (9.2)
Female	86	34 (39.5)	38 (44.2)	14 (16.3)
Total	173	67 (38.7)	84 (48.6)	22 (12.7)

Note: The age range is 3.5 to 75 years. For a contemporary explanation of these results, see Hirschhorn, "Recent Advances," 345–6.

Source: Starch gel electrophoresis analysis done by Dr D.J. Conway and Elena Ross, Department of Pediatrics, University of Ottawa, LAC, Roberts Papers, vol. 1, file 19.

Table B.3 Milk precipitin analysis of 176 Rapanui, 1965

	Tested	Milk precipitin, positive	Milk precipitin (%)	Average age of positive (yrs)
Male	90	9	10	18.8
Female	86	5	5.8	16.6
Total	176	14	8	18

Note: The age range is 3.5 to 75 years. These immune complexes were thought to reflect the possibility of sensitivity to milk. For a contemporary discussion of their role in detecting food allergies, see Goldstein and Heiner, "Clinical and Immunological Perspectives."

Source: Analysis done by Dr D.J. Conway and Elena Ross, Department of Pediatrics, University of Ottawa, LAC, Roberts Papers, vol. 1, file 19.

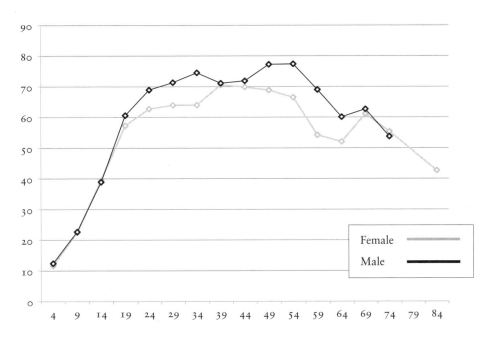

Figure B.1 Average weight (kg) of 929 Rapanui by age and sex, 1965. N = 470 males and 459 females, or 97.5% of the population. LAC, Roberts Papers, vol. 1, file 12.

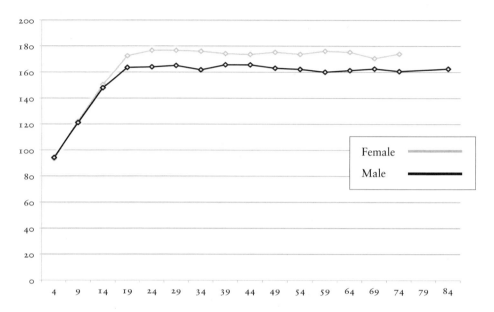

Figure B.2 Average height (cm) of 806 Rapanui by age and sex, 1965. N = 407 males and 399 females, or 84.6% of the population. LAC, Roberts Papers, vol. 1, file 12.

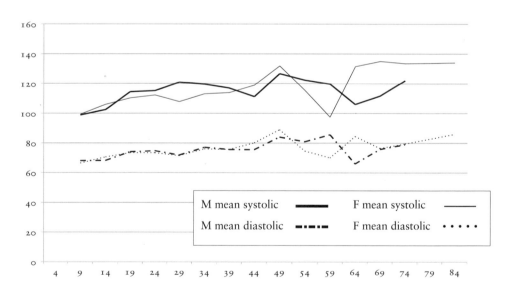

Figure B.3 Systolic and diastolic blood pressure of 638 Rapanui by age and sex, 1965. N = 322 males and 317 females, or 88 % of the population > 4 yrs. The mean pressures were calculated for each age group in quintiles. Normal systolic pressure is 120 mm; normal diastolic pressure is 80 mm. LAC, Roberts Papers, vol. 1, file 12.

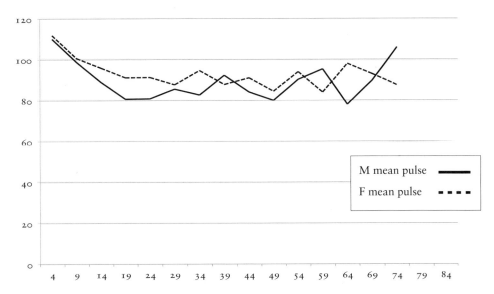

Figure B.4 Pulse of 842 Rapanui by sex and age, 1965. N = 422 males and 420 females, or 88.4% of the population. The mean pulse was calculated for each age group in quintiles. Normal pulse is about 72 beats per minute. LAC, Roberts Papers, vol. 1, file 12.

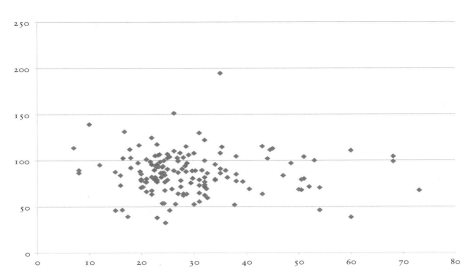

Figure B.5 Mean nonfasting glucose (mg/dl) of 419 Rapanui in 152 families by mean family age, 1965. Normal < 140 mg/dl. Each point represents the mean glucose level of a family of individuals (range 1–8 people, mean 2) by average age of each family group (average age 29.3 years). Some of these people would have taken the simplified glucose tolerance test (see chapter 5). LAC, Roberts Papers, vol. 1, file 12.

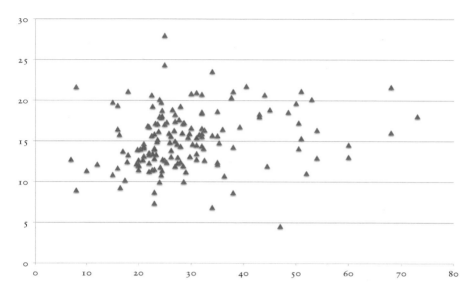

Figure B.6 Mean blood urea nitrogen (mg/dl) of 421 Rapanui in 153 families by mean family age, 1965. Normal 7–20 mg/dl. Each point represents the mean BUN level of a family of individuals (range 1–8, mean 2) by mean age of each family group (average mean age 29.3 years). BUN is a measure of kidney function; when it is elevated, problems are suspected. LAC, Roberts Papers, vol. 1, file 12.

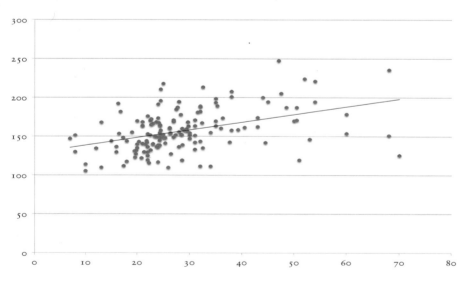

Figure B.7 Mean cholesterol (mg/dl) of 442 Rapanui in 157 families by mean family age, 1965. Normal < 200 mg/dl. Each point represents the mean cholesterol level of a family of individuals (range 1–8, mean 2) by mean age of each family group (average mean age 28.8 years). LAC, Roberts Papers, vol. 1, file 12.

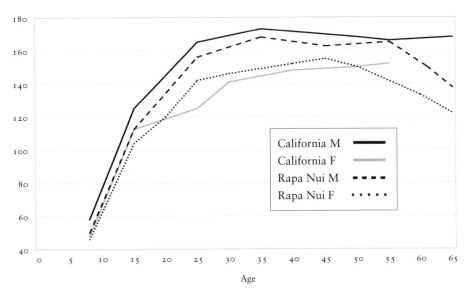

Figure B.8 Rapanui weight (lbs) compared with Californians by age and sex, 1965. The Rapanui men and women have comparable weights with the Californians until after age 50, when they weigh less. This graph did not have numerical data attached, and no source for the Californian levels was provided. Epidemiologist John Cutler was living in California when this graph was prepared. LAC, Roberts Papers, vol. 1, file 20.

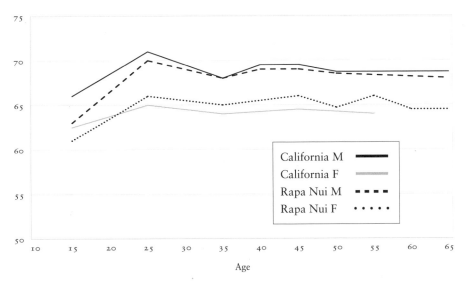

Figure B.9 Rapanui height (inches) compared with Californians by age and sex, 1965. The Rapanui men and women have comparable heights with the Californians throughout their lives. No source for the Californian levels was provided. Epidemiologist John Cutler was living in California when this graph was prepared. LAC, Roberts Papers, vol. 1, file 20.

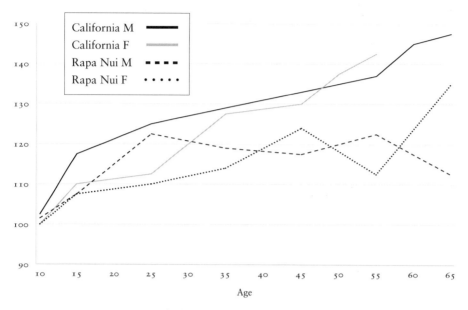

Figure B.10 Rapanui systolic blood pressure compared with Californians by age and sex, 1965. The Rapanui men and women have lower systolic blood pressure, especially after age 25. No source for the Californian levels was provided. Epidemiologist John Cutler was living in California when this graph was prepared. LAC, Roberts Papers, vol. 1, file 12.

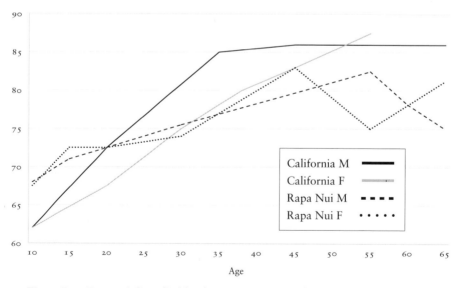

Figure B.11 Rapanui diastolic blood pressure compared with Californians by age and sex, 1965. The Rapanui men and women have lower diastolic blood pressure, especially after age 30. No source for the Californian levels was provided. Epidemiologist John Cutler was living in California when this graph was prepared. LAC, Roberts Papers, vol. 1, file 12.

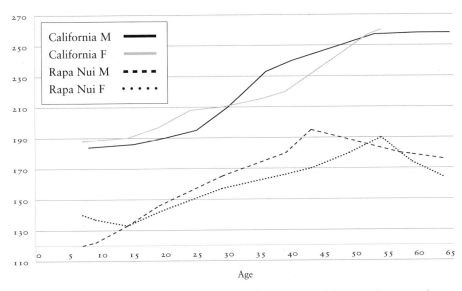

Figure B.12 Rapanui cholesterol levels compared with Californians by age and sex, 1965. Normal < 200 mg/dl. The Rapanui men and women have much lower levels. This graph did not have numerical data attached, and no source for the Californian levels was provided. Epidemiologist John Cutler was living in California when this graph

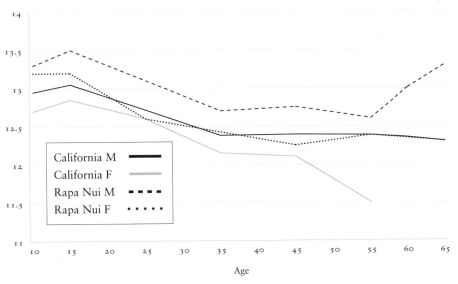

Figure B.13 Rapanui ponderal index compared with Californians by age and sex, 1965. Like the body mass index (BMI), the ponderal index is a ratio of height in inches to weight in pounds. Rapanui men and women had a higher ponderal index than Californians, especially over age 55, suggesting that they were leaner. No source for the Californian levels was provided. Epidemiologist John Cutler was living in California when this graph was prepared. LAC, Roberts Papers, vol. 1, file 20.

Table C.1 1950s health statistics gathered by Helen Reid, 1964–65

Year	Population	Births	Rate per 1,000	Deaths	Rate per 1,000
1955	862	37	42.9	13	15.1
1956	884	59	66.7	4	4.5
1957	906	53	58.5	10	11.0
1958	1053	59	56	9	8.5
1959	1088	57	52.4	13	11.9

Common diseases found	1955	1956	1957	1958	1959
Grippe	980	423	172	268	854
Meningitis	5	1	0	1	3
Tetanus	1	0	0	0	0
Parotitis (mumps)	2	0	0	0	0
Varicella (chicken pox)	0	0	2	0	59
Coqueluche (whooping cough)	0	0	0	108	0
Infectious hepatitis	0	0	0	3	0
Gonorrhea	24	4	1	0	2

Note: A 1958 survey of 234 people for *syphilis* using the Kahn test (a modification of the Wassermann test) found 32 positives and 9 people with the tertiary stage of the disease. In 1959 there were 5 new cases of *tuberculosis* (4 pulmonary and 1 peritonitis). When in operation, the leprosarium housed 7 patients with *leprosy*, and there were 19 active and convalescent cases outside.

Source: Reid Diary, nd, 31–32v, 101v–102; Murphy Diary. Reid obtained these statistics possibly from the infirmary or from a combination of the governor's office and Dr Guido Andrade's lecture on Rapanui health (see chapter 4).

Table C.2 Average age at death, Chile, Valparaiso, and Rapa Nui, 1997–2014

	1997	2002	2014
Chile	65.1	66.9	70.1
Valparaiso	67.7	69.3	72.5
Rapa Nui	43.9	55.4	63.5

Note: Figures are for males and females combined.

Source: Calculated based on Chile, Instituto Nacional de Estadísticas, *Anuario de Estadísticas Vitales*.

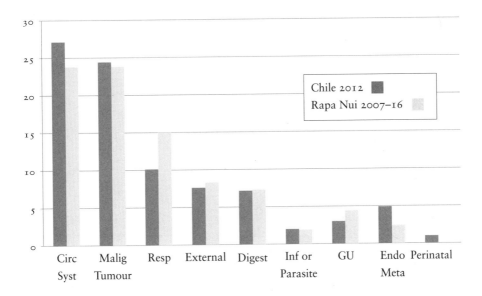

Figure C.1 Causes of death, Chile 2012 and Rapa Nui 2007–16. Percentage of total deaths. The categories are derived from the International Classification of Diseases: circ syst (heart, cardiovascular, and cerebrovascular disease), malig tumour (cancers), resp (respiratory disease), external (trauma and accidents), digest (digestive disorders affecting the gastrointestinal tract), inf or parasite (infectious and parasitc diseases), GU (genitourinary conditions, including kidney disease), endo meta (endocrine and metabolic disorders), perinatal (fetal or neonatal death). Chile, Instituto Nacional de Estadísticas, *Anuario de Estadísticas Vitales*; Municipalidad de Rapa Nui, *Autorizaciós de Sepultación*.

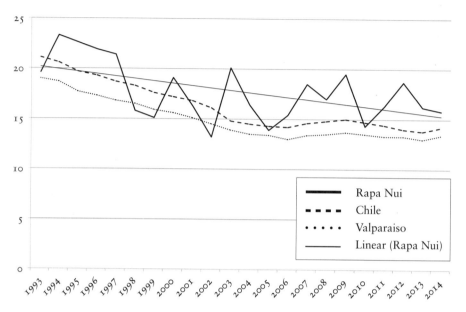

Figure C.2 Births per 1,000 population, Chile, Valparaiso, and Rapa Nui, 1993–2014. The smaller number of Easter Island births gives the apparently wider variation. Note the linear trendline. Chile, Instituto Nacional de Estadísticas, *Anuario de Estadísticas Vitales*.

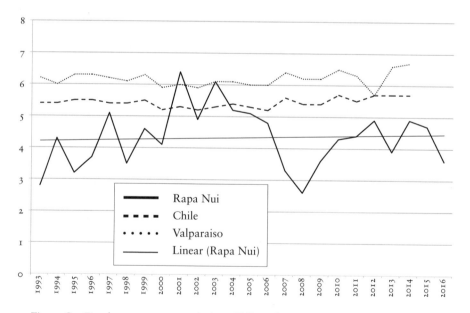

Figure C.3 Deaths per 1,000 population, Chile, Valparaiso, and Rapa Nui, 1993–2016. The smaller number of Rapa Nui deaths gives the apparently wider variation. Note the linear trendline. Chile, Instituto Nacional de Estadísticas, *Anuario de Estadísticas Vitales*.

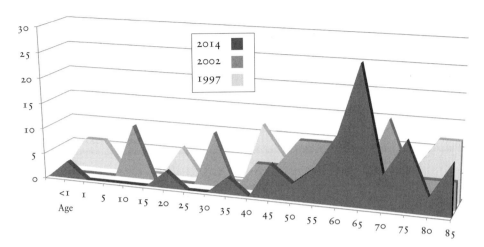

Figure C.4 Ages at death (by quintiles) on Rapa Nui in 1997 (*back*), 2002 (*middle*), and 2014 (*front*). Percentage of total deaths. Note the trend to death at increasing age across this seventeen-year period. Chile, Instituto Nacional de Estadísticas, *Anuario de Estadísticas Vitales*.

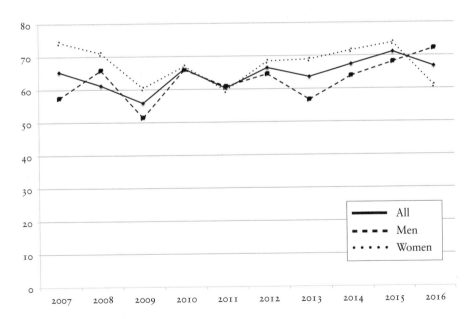

Figure C.5 Average age at death on Rapa Nui, 2007–16. N = 91 (48 males and 43 females; excludes 3 deaths < 1 yr). Although 158 burial records with death dates go back to 1998, for 42% of burials prior to 2007 the age at death could not be determined for lack of a date of birth. Municipalidad de Rapa Nui, *Requests for Burial*.

APPENDIX D: METEI CONSULTANTS, SHIP'S OFFICERS, CABINS

Table D.1 Honorary consultants to METEI

Bearn, Dr Alexander	Genetics	New York
Bauer, Herbert		
Broadbent, G. Clifford		
Burke, B.L.	Technology	Hydro-Dynamic, Montreal
Conway, Dr Dominick J.	Pediatrics	Ottawa
Christensen, A.H.		
Christensen, Fai		
Delafield, Charles	Communications	Montreal
Denton, Dr Ronald	Hematology	Montreal Children's Hospital
Dorfman, Dr O.		
Esslinger, William	Nutrition	C-A Sales Corp., St Laurent, QC
Fanzoi, Mlle Daniele		
Farquharson, Dr Ray	Medical research	Toronto
Fowler, Charles A.	Architect	Halifax
Fraser, Dr R.	Radiology	Royal Victoria Hospital, Montreal
Fredette, Dr Victorien	Microbiology	Université de Montréal
Gagliardi, Samuel	Technology	Dominion Tar Co., St Laurent, QC
Garrido Pulido, Prof. Miguel		
Gialloreto, Dr Osman	Cardiology	Institute of Cardiology, Montreal
Haidasz, Dr Stanley	Public health	Ottawa
Henderson, Mrs Carol		
Heyerdahl, Thor		Oslo, Norway
Hunt, Dr Thomas	Medical research	St Mary's Hospital, London, UK
Hurum, Mrs Gerd	Communications	Montreal
Kahn, Dr David S.	Medical research	St Mary's Hospital, Montreal

Kennedy, T.J.J.	Banking	Bank of Montreal, Montreal
Kingston, Dr Paul		
Kinnear, Dr David	Gastroenterology	Montreal General Hospital
Kuchar, Joseph	Insect control	Record Chemical Co., Montreal
Layton, Dr Basil D.B.	Public health	Dept Health and Welfare, Ottawa
Leigh, Jack H.	Land transportation	General Motors of Canada, Montreal
Le Riche, Dr William H.	Biometrics	University of Toronto
Makuch, Stanley	Lawyer	Montreal
Malley, Bryan P.	Water supply	Domtar News Prints Ltd, Montreal
Maquignaz, Edward	Land transportation	General Motors of Canada, Montreal
McCulloch, Mrs Joyce	Communications	Vancouver
Mikan, George		
Molson, Robert	Engineering	Canadian Industries Ltd, Montreal
Montandon, Dr André	Medical research	Geneva, Switzerland
Mustard, Dr J. Fraser	Medical research	University of Toronto
Noble, Dr Alan P.		
Polud, Miss Jane	Agriculture, feeds	Ralston Purina Co., Brussels, Belgium
Peirce, C.B.	Radiology	Royal Victoria Hospital, Montreal
Pfrimmer, Keith		
Powell, Ray E.	Donor	Alcan Aluminum; McGill University, Montreal
Rose, Dr Bram	Sociology	Royal Victoria Hospital, Montreal
Salisbury, Prof. Richard	Sociology	McGill University, Montreal
Shaughnessy, W.G. Lord	Communication	Montreal
Shoenauer, Prof. Norbert	Design	McGill University, Montreal
Sonea, Prof. Sorin	Microbiology	Université de Montréal
Steinman, Miss Marion		
Strub, Henry	Communication	Montreal

Takatsy, A. de	Financing	Paris, France
Tindale, William		
Turner, Dr Gilbert	Administration	Royal Victoria Hospital, Montreal
Waldron-Edward, Dr D.	Biochemistry	McGill University, Montreal
Watzka, O.C.	Optical instruments	Montreal
Webster, Dr D. Ronald	Medical research	McGill University, Montreal
Williams, Graham		
Wilson, Richard D.		
Zukel, Dr William J.	Epidemiology	National Institutes of Health, Bethesda, MD

Source: Two different lists are integrated here. McGill University Archives (MUA), RG 49, box 66, file 10436; box 64, file 01374.

Table D.2 Officers of HMCS *Cape Scott*, November 1964 to March 1965

Barlow, Cdr James R.	electrical installation
Bérubé, Sg.Lt Dr Gilbert Joseph	ship's doctor (and opera singer)
Billard, LCdr Robert Arthur	campsite installation supervisor
Gillis, LCdr Channing D.	deputy commander
Law, Cdr C. Anthony	commander
Manzer, Lt Robert B.	cargo on ship
Moore, LCdr Ernest E. ("Pony")	beachmaster
Pennie, LCdr Duff M.	engineering technical advisor generators and water
Shaw, LCdr Alfred E.	logistics and supply
Thompson, LCdr Ross E.	cargo officer
Westropp, Lt Charles L.	navigator

Note: All lived in Nova Scotia except Bérubé, whose home was in Quebec.

Table D.3 Cabin and trailer allocations

Trailer	Passengers
5A	Eivind Myhre and Björn Ekblom
5B	Bob Williams and Robert Fulton
6A	Einar Gjessing and Harry Crosman
6B	Ian Efford and Jack Mathias
7A	Richard and Maureen Roberts
7B	Garry Brody and Gonzalo Donoso
8A	Rita Dwyer and Mary King
8B	Denys and Cléopâtre Montandon
9A	Ana Maria Eccles and Isabel Griffiths
9B	Helen Reid and Carlotta Hacker
10A	Stanley Skoryna and John Easton
15A	Georges Nógrády and Carl Mydans
15B	Colin Gillingham and George Hrischenko
16A	Al Taylor and Peter Beighton
16B	Elliot Alpert and John Cutler
17A	Archie Wilkinson and Armand Boudreault
17B	Bob Meier and Jim Nielsen
18A	Hal Gibbs and David Murphy
18B	Hector ("Red") Lemieux and Fred Joyce

Note: Most pairings on the ship were the same as in the *campamento*. Gillingham was originally to share with Fulton, and Hrischenko was put with Williams. But Hrischenko preferred to stay with Gillingham and did. I have therefore shown Williams as sharing with Fulton. After Donoso left, Brody had a trailer to himself. It is possible that other variations took place.

Source: "METEI: Information Circular #3 for Landing and Setting Up Period," 2, nd, LAC, Law Scrapbook, vol. 2, "Notes, Reports, Orders."

APPENDIX E: MAPS OF RAPA NUI

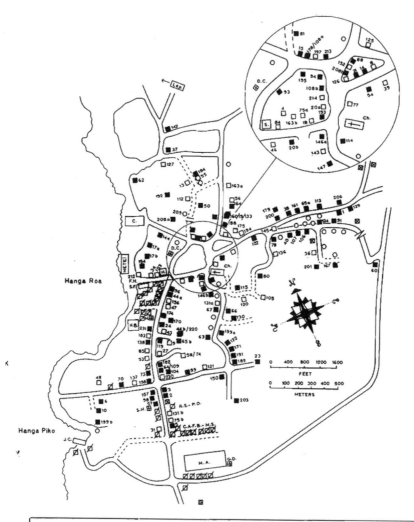

Lep.	Leprosarium	M.A.	Mataveri Airstrip
C.	Cemetery	G.D.	Gasoline Depot
H.	Hospital	△	Triangulation
S.	School	□	House of non-sampled
Ch	Church		native family
M E T E i	Expedition's Camp	■	House of sampled
F.H.	Fishermen's House		native family
S.F.	Soccer Field	⊞	House used for other than
M.	Museum		dwelling purposes
N.B.	Naval Base	/	House occupied by
D.C.	Dental Clinic		several families
R.S.- P.O.	Radio Station - Post Office	⊠	House of Chilean family
C A F B -M.S	Chilean Airforce Base-	⊠	Unidentified house
	Meteorology Station	▣	Governor's house
J C.	Jetty - 5 ton crane	○	Unoccupied house
S H.	Slaughter House		

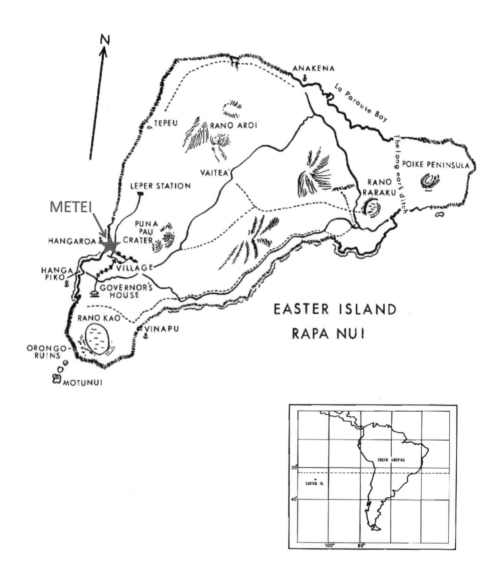

Figure E.1 *Opposite* METEI's bacterial sampling map of Hanga Roa. The location of METEI is clearly indicated. The numbers of houses correspond to those assigned to each family. See also the sketch by Cléopâtre Montandon in figure 5.10. Alpert, Nógrády, and Montandon, "Staphylococcus Sampling Map."

Figure E.2 *Above* Map of Rapa Nui in 1965. Used as endpapers for Helen Reid's book *A World Away* (1965). Reid Papers, file 5.

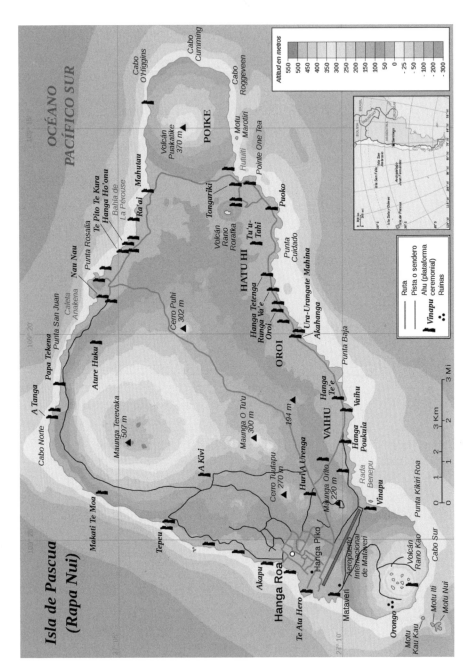

Figure E.3 Map of Rapa Nui in 2017. Note the airport, the many roads, and the reconstructed sites. Wikimedia Commons, https://commons.wikimedia.org/wiki/File:Easter_Island_map-en.svg.

Notes

INTRODUCTION

1 University of British Columbia (UBC) Archives, Efford Papers, METEI, boxes 1–3.
2 Reid, "Physical Development."
3 Reid, *World Away*.
4 Boutilier, "METEI [Part I and Part II]." See also Porteous, "METEI"; and Tector, "Delightful Revolution."
5 See, for example, Fischer, "German-Chilean Expedition"; Heyerdahl, *Aku Aku*; Mazière, *Fantastique*; Métraux, *Ethnology*; and Routledge, *Mystery*.
6 See, for example, Macleod, ed., *Nature and Empire*; Osborne, *Nature*; Pratt, *Imperial Eyes*; Stepan, *Picturing Tropical Nature*; and Van Tilburg, *Among Stone Giants*.
7 Anderson, *Colonial Pathologies*; Anderson, *Collectors of Lost Souls*; Anderson, "Hybridity, Race, and Science."
8 Appel, *Shaping Biology*; Greenaway, *Science International*; Schleper, "Conservation Compromises."
9 Osseo-Asare, *Bitter Roots*.
10 Hayden, *When Nature Goes Public*.
11 Kwa, "Representations of Nature"; Bocking, *Ecologists*; Bocking, *Nature's Experts*.
12 Lipphardt, "From 'Races' to 'Isolates'"; Lock, "From Genetics to Postgenomics"; Meier, "Critique"; Nash, *Genetic Geographies*; Rheinberger and Müller-Wille, *Gene*; Sussman, *Myth of Race*; Wade, *Troublesome Inheritance*; Widmer and Lipphardt, eds, *Health and Difference*, 1–6; Yudell, *Race Unmasked*.
13 Hagelberg, "Genetic Affinities."

14 Fischer, *Island*, 212–14; Haoa Rapahango, *Leprosario*; Joves, "Re-Imagining"; Porteous, *Modernization*, 170–3; Stambuk, *Rongo*, 265–74; Stambuk, *Iorana*; Seward, "Between 'Easter Island' and 'Rapa Nui,'" 252; Young, "Unwriting Easter Island."

CHAPTER ONE: DREAM PLAN FOR A TROUBLED WORLD

1 Cuetos and Palmer, *Medicine and Public Health*, 139–53; Greenaway, *Science International*.

2 Larson and Ebner, "Significance of Strontium-90 in Milk."

3 Boyer, *By the Bomb's Early Light*, 352–7, esp. 354. For more on the impact of the nuclear age on culture, see Weart, *Nuclear Fear*, 191–5; and Wuthnow, *Be Very Afraid*.

4 Mundey, "Civilianization."

5 Regnault, "France's Search."

6 Reiss, "Strontium-90 Absorption."

7 Geiger, Sidel, and Lown, "Medical Consequences"; Sidel, Geiger, and Lown, "Medical Consequences."

8 Webb, "History of IRPA."

9 Donaldson, *Nature against Us*, 22–6; Sharpless, "World Population Growth"; Wilmoth and Ball, "Arguments and Action."

10 Chapman, *IGY: The Year of Discovery*.

11 Canadian National Committee for the International Geophysical Year, *Report on the Canadian Program*; Canadian National Committee for the International Geophysical Year and Meek, *Report on the Canadian Program*, esp. 147–51 (list of stations and disciplines). See also Powell, "Science, Sovereignty and Nation."

12 Wilson, *I.G.Y.*, 321.

13 Prat, *Métamorphose explosive*, vol. 2, 307, 310.

14 Rudolph Peters, cited in Worthington, ed., *Evolution of IBP*, 3.

15 On the history of the IBP, see Greenaway, *Science International*, 172–6; Appel, *Shaping Biology*, 226, 230, 232, 263–7; Hagen, *Entangled Bank*, 169–81; and Bocking, *Ecologists*, 50–1, 80–1, 88, 112, 139, 142, 169–70.

16 Anon., "International Council of Scientific Unions."

17 Stebbins, "International Biological Program," 768, 770.

18 Stinson, Bogin, and O'Rourke, *Human Biology*, 31–6; Little and Collins, "Joseph S. Weiner"; Little, "Human Population Biology."

19 Osborne, *Nature*, 2.

20 Stepan, *Picturing Tropical Nature*.

21 Worboys, "Colonial World."

22 Lopes and Podgorny, "Shaping of Latin American Museums."

23 Weiner, "Human Adaptability."

24 Baker and Weiner, eds, *Biology of Human Adaptability.*

25 Lewin, "Ten Years."

26 Ibid.

27 Anon., "Surgeons College Honors Finsterer"; Anon., "Hans Finsterer"; Peale, *Power of Positive Thinking*, ch. 11, 171–2. Finsterer met Truman for five minutes on 16 November 1949, according to "The President's Day" calendar online at the Harry S. Truman Library and Museum, http://www.trumanlibrary.org/calendar/. On Skoryna's connection to Finsterer, see Dinan, *St. Mary's Hospital*, 87.

28 Skoryna, "Über die Nachbehandlung operierter Karzinome."

29 Skoryna, Ross, and Rudis, "Histogenesis of Sebaceous Gland Carcinomas."

30 Skoryna to Peyton Rous, 21 August 1951; Peyton Rous to Skoryna, 29 August 1951, Archives of the American Philosophical Society (APS), Peyton Rous Papers, Mss.B.R77, box 61. Thanks to Earl Spamer of the APS for providing these documents.

31 Skoryna, Webster, and Kahn, "New Method"; Skoryna to Peyton Rous, 22 February 1960, Archives of the APS, Peyton Rous Papers, Mss.B.R77, box 61.

32 Mumford, "War Weapons Condemned," 8E.

33 Anon., "Hot Ashes"; Baldwin, "Radioactivity-II"; Laurence, "Waste Held Peril."

34 Skoryna et al., "Incidence and Distribution."

35 Skoryna, "Systemic Factors in Carcinogenesis."

36 Skoryna, "Systemic Factors in Neoplasia."

37 Skoryna, "Medical Meetings."

38 Skoryna and Kahn, "Late Effects of Radioactive Strontium."

39 This series of articles appeared in the CMAJ from 1 August 1964 to 12 September 1970. The first 1964 article has been cited forty-four times.

40 Waldron-Edward, Paul, and Skoryna, "Suppression of Intestinal Absorption."

41 Iber, "Review of Skoryna, *Pathophysiology*."

42 Skoryna, "Stochastic Processes."

43 Hustak, *At the Heart of St. Mary's*, 92, 138. Several METEI members used the word "operator" in describing Skoryna in interviews for this book.

44 Appel, *Shaping Biology*, 267.

45 Weiner, "Human Adaptability," 15.

46 Heyerdahl, *Kon-Tiki*; Heyerdahl, *Aku-Aku.*

47 On the postcontact history of Easter Island, see Gonschor, "Facing Land Challenges"; Haun, *Inventing "Easter Island"*; Porteous, *Modernization*;

Fischer, *Island*; Ramirez Aliaga, *Rapa Nui*, 104–13; Stambuk, *Rongo*; and Stambuk, *Iorana*.

48 Sharp, ed., *Journal of Jacob Roggeveen*, 95.

49 Corney, ed. and trans., *Voyage of Captain Don Felipe Gonzalez*, 43–9.

50 Beaglehole, ed., *Journals of Captain James Cook*, vol. 2, 336–60, esp. 341, 345 (man shot), 349 (shipping), 353 (difference with Roggeveen), 357 (want of materials).

51 Gaziello, *L'expédition de Lapérouse*, 225–7.

52 Fischer, *Island*, 103.

53 Volz, "Beiträge zur Anthropologie der Südsee."

54 Fischer, *Island*, 139–42. For a translation of the treaty, see Gonschor, "Law as a Tool," appendix D, 286–8.

55 Seward, "Between 'Easter Island' and 'Rapa Nui.'"

56 Porteous, *Modernization*, 167.

57 Cañellas-Bolta et al., "Vegetation Changes"; Diamond, *Collapse*, 79–119; Jarman et al., "Diet"; Mann et al., "Drought."

58 Routledge, *Mystery*. On Routledge, see Van Tilburg, *Easter Island*, 14–18; and Van Tilburg, *Among Stone Giants*. See also Van Tilburg, "Writing Routledge."

59 Métraux, *Ethnology*.

60 Englert, *La tierra*, 54–68; Englert, *Island*, 167; Ramirez Aliaga, *Rapa Nui*, 47–50.

61 Hagelberg, "Genetic Affinities," 185; Hagelberg et al., "DNA from Ancient Easter Islanders."

62 Simmons and Graydon, "Blood Group Genetical Survey."

63 *Aku-aku* are strong spirits that may be human. Routledge had described them in her study. More recently, however, according to Seward, an islander contends that Heyerdahl invented them, hinting that he may have been as often duped as duping. Routledge, *Mystery*, 238–9; Seward, "Between 'Easter Island' and 'Rapa Nui,'" 257.

64 Heyerdahl described only two deaths. Heyerdahl, *Aku-Aku*, 114–20. But the islanders remember three: the teacher Lorenzo Baeza and two children, Elena Atán and Carlos Pakomio. Stambuk, *Rongo*, 229–34.

65 Heyerdahl, *Aku-Aku*, 63, 197 (airport), 114–20 (school outing).

66 Van Tilburg, *Among Stone Giants*, 170; Fischer, *Island*, 186–7.

67 Heyerdahl, *Aku-Aku*, 217.

68 Fischer, "German-Chilean Expedition."

69 Mazière, *Fantasique*; Mazière, *Mysteries*.

70 Fischer, *Island*, 166–72; Foerster, Ramírez, and Moreno Pakarati, *Cartografía y conflicto*; Fuentes and Moreno Pakarati, "Towards a

Characterization"; Routledge, *Mystery*, 140–9; Stambuk, *Rongo*, 29–47; Van Tilburg, *Among Stone Giants*, 150–61.

71 Boutilier, "METEI [Part II]," 50; La Fay and Abercrombie, "Easter Island."

72 Heyerdahl, *Aku-Aku*, 45; Métraux, *Ethnology*, 25–6.

73 The letters were dated 19 September and 7 December 1962. They have not been found but were referenced in Salisbury to Skoryna, 19 August 1964, McGill University Archives (MUA), RG 2, box 293, file 10669.

74 Boudreault, "Composition"; Prat, *Métamorphose explosive*. On Prat and eugenics, see McLaren, *Our Own Master Race*, 128.

75 See, for example, Cruz-Coke, "Ecología humana"; Cruz-Coke, Nagel, and Etcheverry, "Effects of Locus MN"; Etcheverry, "Blood Groups"; and Nagel, Etcheverry, and Guzman, "Haptoglobin Types."

76 Cruz-Coke, Etcheverry, and Nagel, "Influence of Migration."

77 "Annex C: Subventions à des chercheurs individuels," 2 (Skoryna's grant), in World Health Organization, *Rapport du Directeur général*; Anon., "Health Survey." I thank Reynald Erard at the Archives of the WHO for tracking the evidence and products of this grant.

CHAPTER TWO: CONVINCING CANADA, BUILDING A TEAM

1 Since 1950 the US army's William Beaumont Society had been conducting an epidemiological survey of gastrointestinal bleeding involving over 2,000 patients from across the United States. William Beaumont Society, United States Army, "Seasonal Incidence." On Roberts's 1958 paper on peptic ulcer disease in the navy, see Roberts, "Problems of Peptic Ulceration"; and Roberts to CMAJ editor A.D. Kelly, 21 June 1958, Library and Archives Canada (LAC), Roberts Papers, vol. 2, file 7.

2 Skoryna to Roberts, 4 October 1963; Roberts to Skoryna, 12 October 1963, LAC, Roberts Papers, vol. 1, file 1.

3 Skoryna to Roberts, 16 October 1963, LAC, Roberts Papers, vol. 1, file 1.

4 Roberts to Skoryna, 27 November 1963, LAC, Roberts Papers, vol. 1, file 1.

5 "Memorandum" and "Objectives and Organization," [probably January 1964], LAC, Haidasz Papers; Anon., "Scientific Aid."

6 "Memorandum" and "Objectives and Organization," [probably January 1964], LAC, Haidasz Papers.

7 On Norman, see Whitaker and Marcue, *Cold War Canada*, 402–26. On the Avro Arrow, see Campagna, *Storms of Controversy*.

8 Grant, *Lament for a Nation*. On Bomarc missile protests, see Dufresne, "'Let's Not Be Cremated Equal.'"

9 See Pearson, *Diplomacy*; Azzi, *Walter Gordon*, 111–32.

10 Peter M. Laing of Chisholm, Smith, Davis, Anglin, Laing, Weldon & Courtois, Barristers and Solicitors, to S.C. Skoryna, 14 January 1964, McGill University Archives (MUA), RG 2, box 293, file 10669.

11 Forsey, "Gerd Hurum."

12 The 310 Wilno Wing had been founded in 1953 by Polish-immigrant veterans of the Polish air force under the umbrella of the Royal Canadian Air Force. It hosted an annual Blue Ball, usually at the elegant Ritz Carleton Hotel in Montreal. Zmyślony, "Edward Hajdukiewicz."

13 Haidasz to Prime Minister Pearson, 13 January 1964; Haidasz to Hellyer, 13 January 1964, LAC, Haidasz Papers; LAC, Canada and Agencies, Lester B. Pearson Papers, 1963–1965.

14 Haidasz to Skoryna, 28 January 1964; Skoryna to Haidasz, 29 January 1964, LAC, Haidasz Papers.

15 Pearson to Hellyer, 3 February 1964 (Haidasz's copy), LAC, Haidasz Papers.

16 Haidasz to Skoryna, 19 February 1964, LAC, Haidasz Papers.

17 A.J. Pick to Mary Macdonald, Office of the Prime Minister, 28 January 1964, LAC, Haidasz Papers; Anon., "Alfred John Pick."

18 Skoryna to Haidasz, 6 March 1964, LAC, Haidasz Papers. Nógrády was a talented caricaturist. My source for his designing the logo is Judith Hermann, personal communication, 6 May 2016. Alternatively, Isabel Cutler (formerly Griffiths) says that the logo was designed by the artist wife of engineer Robert Molson.

19 Hellyer to Haidasz, 6 March 1964, LAC, Haidasz Papers.

20 Haidasz to Skoryna, 11 March 1964, LAC, Haidasz Papers.

21 Several versions of the list of honorary consultants are kept in various archives: thirty-two names and sixty names appear on two different undated lists in MUA, RG 49, box 64, file 01374, and box 66, file 10436.

22 Hellyer, *Damn the Torpedoes*; Mayne, "Years of Crisis"; Milner, *Canada's Navy*, 240–61.

23 Reid to Hellyer, 9 January 1964; Hellyer to Reid, 16 January 1964; Reid to Hellyer's secretary (Miss Bulger), 20 January and 5 February 1964. These letters are in an envelope that was returned to Helen Reid by her publisher, Ryerson Press. Reid Papers, file 1. Curiously, Reid's original letters are not in the files at LAC.

24 Cadieux to Martin, 30 April 1964, LAC, Haidasz Papers. See also Canada, "Naval Support."

25 Statement by Professor Stanley C. Skoryna, 7 April 1964, LAC, Haidasz Papers; Robert Molson to Richard Roberts, 6 April 1964, LAC, Roberts Papers, vol. 2, file 1.

26 Cadieux to Martin, 30 April 1964, LAC, Haidasz Papers.

27 Fischer, *Island*, 216; National Security Archive, with Kornbluh, "Chile 1964."
28 Anon., "Easter Island Expedition."
29 Ambassador Mario Rodriguez to Haidasz, 22 April and 21 May 1964; Haidasz to Martin, 22 May 1964, LAC, Haidasz Papers.
30 Skoryna to Farquharson, 17 August 1961, 24 January 1962, and 12 March 1962, LAC, Dorothy Wright Papers.
31 Marcel Cadieux to Haidasz, 2 and 8 October 1964, LAC, Haidasz Papers.
32 Cadieux to Martin, 30 April 1964, LAC, Haidasz Papers.
33 Haidasz to G.D.W. Cameron, 28 April 1964; Cameron to Haidasz, 5 May 1964, LAC, Haidasz Papers.
34 Haidasz to Paul Martin, 13 August 1964; Haidasz to Skoryna, 13 August 1964, LAC, Haidasz Papers. An unidentified clipping, probably from a Montreal paper, reported that the Atkinson Charitable Foundation had provided $7,500 toward equipment "for measuring clots." The report cited the "inbred nature" of the population. Anon., "Easter Isle Researchers Given Grant," clipping [possibly *Montreal Gazette*, ca. 31 December 1964], Wilkinson Papers.
35 Haidasz to H.O. Moran, 19 August 1964; Moran to Haidasz, 24 August 1964, LAC, Haidasz Papers. The External Aid Office became the Canadian International Development Agency (CIDA).
36 Designs are available at the website of the McGill School of Architecture, http://cac.mcgill.ca/schoenauer/index.htm.
37 Anon., "Shoeboxes for the Navel of the World." Special thanks to ATCO archivist Debbie Taylor.
38 MUA, RG 2, box 293, file 10669.
39 Anon., "Easter Island Expedition"; and unidentified clipping with same photos [*Montreal Gazette?*], MUA, RG 49, box 64, file 01376.
40 Brody Diary, 30 November 1964.
41 Skoryna to McTaggart-Cowan, 3 April 1964; Skoryna to Efford, 13 July 1964, University of British Columbia (UBC) Archives, Efford Papers, METEI, box 1, file 1; Hawthorn, "Ian McTaggart-Cowan."
42 Maureen Roberts to Skoryna, 31 July 1964; Skoryna to Maureen and Richard Roberts, 21 August 1964; Nancy Simpson to Maureen Roberts, 10 November 1964, LAC, Roberts Papers, vol. 2, file 1.
43 Marion Turner to Thomas Kent, 6 July 1964; F.A. Milligan to Marion Turner, 20 July 1964, LAC, Haidasz Papers.
44 A personnel list dated 5 October 1964 included Glynn, but by 7 October he had withdrawn. LAC, Law Scrapbook, vol. 2, "Members of Medical Expedition, 5 October 1964"; Reid Papers, file 5.

45 Hellyer to Reid, 24 August 1964, Reid Papers, file 1. On Glynn, see Reid to Skoryna, 10, 22, and 29 September 1964, 7 October 1964; and Griffiths to Reid, 7 October 1964, Reid Papers, files 1 and 10.

46 Skoryna to Reid, 10 and 27 August 1964; Reid to Skoryna, 5 and 15 August 1964, Reid Papers, file 1.

47 Reid to Skoryna, 24 September 1964, Reid Papers, file 10.

48 Reid to Hellyer, 28 August 1964, Reid Papers, file 1.

49 Myhre, "Effect of Corticotrophin."

50 The blood samples collected from ear lobes of fifty-one Easter Islanders by Dr Emil Gjessing, who had been with Heyerdahl, were sent to Australia for analysis. Simmons and Graydon, "Blood Group Genetical Survey."

51 Nagel, Etcheverry, and Guzman, "Haptoglobin Types"; Etcheverry, "Blood Groups."

52 Hunt, "History"; Clarke and Jones, "Thomas Cecil Hunt."

53 In his IBP collaboration, Laughlin served with Canadians J.S. Hart and Jack A. Hildes (see chapter 13). US National Committee for the International Biological Program, *Research Studies*, 2.

54 Robert Meier to Maureen Roberts at Rockefeller Institute, New York, 29 September 1964, LAC, Roberts Papers, vol. 2, file 1. The letter was forwarded to Halifax and annotated that a reply was sent 26 October.

55 Cutler, "Cerebrovascular Disease."

56 Alpert and Levison, "Epidemic of Tuberculosis."

57 On Salisbury, see Silverman, *Ethnography and Development*.

58 Salisbury referred to his earlier letters of 19 September and 7 December 1962; they have not been found. Salisbury to Skoryna, 19 August 1964, MUA, RG 2, box 293, file 10669.

59 See, for example, Hubert Soltan to Maureen Roberts, 21 January 1964, LAC, Roberts Papers, vol. 2, file 1; John R. Paul, Yale University, to C.E. Van Rooyen, Dalhousie University [forwarded to R. Roberts], 14 October 1964 ("loot"), LAC, Roberts Papers, vol. 1, file 1; and J.R. Paul to R. Roberts, 19 November 1964, LAC, Roberts Papers, vol. 1, file 1. See also Macfarlane, "Volunteers by the Boatload"; Tunis to photographer Bob Brooks of Vancouver, 4 January 1965, MUA, RG 49, box 64, file 01372.

60 Hacker, *And Christmas Day*, 144–5.

61 Ralph Graves to Stanley Skoryna, 13 October 1964 (contract); Albert A. Tunis to Carl Mydans, 19 October 1964, MUA, RG 49, box 64, file 01375.

62 Agreement between S.R. Kennedy of CBC and Skoryna, 13 November 1964, MUA, RG 49, box 64, file 01375.

63 Roberts to Skoryna, 25 August 1964; Roberts to Surgeon Commodore Walter Elliot, 27 August 1964, LAC, Roberts Papers, vol. 1, file 1.

64 Anon., "Expedition Commander"; Jessup, "C. Anthony Law"; Jessup, "C.
    Anthony Law Master and Commander"; Art Gallery of Nova Scotia, "C.
    Anthony Law."

65 C.A. Law, "CONFIDENTIAL Proposed Programme – Easter Island
    Expedition," 12 June 1964, LAC, Law Scrapbook, vol. 2, "Notes, Reports,
    Orders." On the June meeting, see also Roberts to Molson, 28 May 1964,
    LAC, Roberts Papers, vol. 1, file 1.

66 "Cargo List," LAC, Law Scrapbook, vol. 2, "Notes, Reports, Orders."

67 "Orders to C. Anthony Law Promulgated"; "Logistical Coordination,
    Medical Expedition to Easter Island"; "CONFIDENCIAL [sic] Easter Island
    Isla de Pascua"; C.A. Law, "CONFIDENTIAL Proposed Programme –
    Easter Island Expedition," 12 June 1964, LAC, Law Scrapbook, vol. 2,
    "Notes, Reports, Orders."

68 Molson to Roberts, 10 March 1964, LAC, Roberts Papers, vol. 2, file 1,
    "Correspondence."

69 Molson to Roberts, 6 April 1964; Skoryna to Roberts, 21 April 1964,
    LAC, Roberts Papers, vol. 2, file 1.

70 Maloney, "Secrets of the Bomarc."

71 Easton, cited in Campagna, *Storms of Controversy*, 152. See also Dow,
    Arrow; and Peden, *Fall of an Arrow*.

72 Roberts to Skoryna, 25 August 1964, LAC, Roberts Papers, vol. 1, file 1.
    See also T.L. Fisher of the Canadian Medical Protective Association to
    Roberts, 15 October 1964, LAC, Roberts Papers, vol. 1, file 1.

73 Roberts to Skoryna, 28 May 1964, LAC, Roberts Papers, vol. 1, file 1.

74 Skoryna to R. Roberts, 9 October 2016, LAC, Roberts Papers, vol. 2, file 1.

75 Helen Reid to Rocke Robertson, 20 November 1967, MUA, RG 2, box
    340, file 12524. On Ellis, see Dale, "Roy Gilmore Ellis."

76 Dozens of Tom Galley's black and white photographs can be found, with-
    out his name, in both LAC and MUA. A few were reproduced with credit
    in Reid, *World Away*. He appeared in a photograph published soon after
    the journey in Macfarlane, "Mysterious Moai," 20. His identity was con-
    firmed by his son Tom Galley of Nova Scotia, personal communication,
    22 August 2016. See LAC, Law Scrapbook, vol. 3, unnumbered files 2 and
    3; and MUA, RG 49, box 426, 1040D.

77 Anon., "Two Wrens Making Trip"; Lt Cmdr R[oss]. E. Thompson, "Cape
    Scott Has Numerous 'Firsts' to Her Credit," unidentified clipping,
    Wilkinson Papers; H.C.W., "1964 in Review," 17. On navy women, see
    Milner, *Canada's Navy*, 104, 216.

78 For trying (unsuccessfully) to trace Mary King, special thanks to Roy
    Bishop, physicist at Acadia University; Randall Brooks, retired curator of
    the Canadian Museum of Science and Technology; Paul Gray and Paul

Chapman of the Royal Astronomical Society; Marcin Sawicki of St Mary's University; and Debbie Reid, archivist with the *Chronicle Herald*, personal communications, July 2016 and April 2018.

79 Hacker, *And Christmas Day*, 144–5.

CHAPTER THREE: THE JOURNEY OUT

1 C.A. Law, "CONFIDENTIAL Proposed Programme – Easter Island Expedition," 12 June 1964, Library and Archives Canada (LAC), Law Scrapbook, vol. 2, "Notes, Reports, Orders."

2 García-Moro et al., "Epidemiological Transition"; Mazière, *Fantastique*; Mazière, *Mysteries*.

3 Nagel, Etcheverry, and Guzman, "Haptoglobin Types." See also Etcheverry, Nagel, and Guzman, "Encuesta"; and Etcheverry, "Blood Groups."

4 A twenty-two-page "Cargo List" with twenty categories is in LAC, Law Scrapbook, vol. 2, "Notes, Reports, Orders."

5 "Orders to C. Anthony Law promulgated"; "Logistical Coordination, Medical Expedition to Easter Island"; "CONFIDENCIAL [*sic*] Easter Island Isla de Pascua"; C.A. Law, "CONFIDENTIAL Proposed Programme – Easter Island Expedition," 12 June 1964, LAC, Law Scrapbook, vol. 2, "Notes, Reports, Orders."

6 "Logistical Coordination, Medical Expedition to Easter Island"; "CONFIDENCIAL [*sic*] Easter Island Isla de Pascua," LAC, Law Scrapbook, vol. 2, "Notes, Reports, Orders."

7 Reid, *World Away*, 8.

8 Hacker, *And Christmas Day*, 148, 155.

9 Ibid., 150.

10 Ibid..

11 Ibid., 151; Reid Diary, 16 November 1964.

12 Montandon Diary, all translations from Cléopâtre Montandon's original French are my own.

13 Hacker, *And Christmas Day*, 155.

14 Meier Diary, 16 November 1964.

15 Law to Jane, 20 November 1964, LAC, Law Scrapbook, vol. 2, "Personal Correspondence."

16 Reid Diary, 17 November 1964, 11:30 p.m.

17 Hacker, *And Christmas Day*, 154. See also Reid Diary, 17 November 1964, 10:00 p.m.; Meier Diary, 17 November 1964; and Montandon Diary, 17 November 1964.

18 Maureen Roberts to Mrs Cox, [ca. 1 December 1964], LAC, Roberts Papers, vol. 1, file 7.

19 Law to Sir, report of *Cape Scott*, 2 December 1964, LAC, Law Scrapbook, vol. 2, "Notes, Reports, Orders."

20 Law to Jane, 20 November 1964, LAC, Law Scrapbook, vol. 2, "Personal Correspondence."

21 Meier Diary, 18 November 1964.

22 Montandon Diary, 18 November 1964.

23 Tony Law, interview, 1976, cited in Boutilier, "METEI [Part II]," 50.

24 Skoryna to Tunis, [20 November 1964], "nearing Bermuda," McGill University Archives (MUA), RG 49, box 64, file 01375.

25 Hacker, *And Christmas Day*, 155.

26 Skoryna to Tunis, [20 November 1964], "nearing Bermuda," MUA, RG 49, box 64, file 01375.

27 Meier Diary, 21 November 1964.

28 Montandon Diary, 21 November 1964.

29 Hacker, *And Christmas Day*, 148.

30 Montandon Diary, 24 November 1964.

31 A blank preliminary form and the code sheet for transfer to computer cards are in LAC, Roberts Papers, vol. 1, file 11. Meier supplied a blank copy of the final form for physical examinations.

32 Law to Sir, report of *Cape Scott*, 2 December 1964, LAC, Law Scrapbook, vol. 2, "Notes, Reports, Orders."

33 Montandon Diary, 22 November 1964.

34 Meier Diary, 21 and 23 November 1964; Montandon Diary, 21 November 1964 ("un film anglais à l'ancienne mode").

35 Reid Diary, 28–29 November 1964.

36 Hacker, *And Christmas Day*, 159–60; Montandon Diary, 22 November 1964.

37 Law to Sir, report of *Cape Scott*, 2 December 1964, LAC, Law Scrapbook, vol. 2, "Notes, Reports, Orders." See also Law to Jane, 26 November 1964, LAC, Law Scrapbook, vol. 2, "Personal Correspondence."

38 Montandon Diary, 30 November 1964.

39 Mathias Diary, 4 December 1964.

40 Law to Jane, 26 and 29 November 1964, LAC, Law Scrapbook, vol. 2, "Personal Correspondence."

41 Hacker, *And Christmas Day*, 154.

42 Law to Jane, 29–30 November 1964, LAC, Law Scrapbook, vol. 2, "Personal Correspondence"; Montandon Diary, 30 November 1964.

43 Gillingham's address was 121 Charlotte Street. Anon., "Two Ottawa People"; Reid, *World Away,* 24; Françoise Gillingham, personal communication, December 2016.

44 Joyce, "Cape Scott Solves Dilemma"; Anon., "Easter Island Expedition Creates Flag," unidentified clipping, LAC, Law Scrapbook, vol. 3, "Clippings"; Montandon Diary, 23 November 1964.

45 "CONFIDENCIAL [*sic*] Easter Island Isla de Pascua," 8, LAC, Law Scrapbook, vol. 2, "Notes, Reports, Orders."

46 Montandon Diary, 28 November 1964.

47 Brody Diary, 4 and 5 December 1964.

48 Skoryna to Tunis, undated, handwritten note sent en route to Balboa, probably from San Juan, MUA, RG 49, box 64, file 01375.

49 Law to Jane, 26 November 1964, LAC, Law Scrapbook, vol. 2, "Personal Correspondence."

50 Reid Diary, 1 December 1964, 14; Reid to "Darlings," 1 December 1964, Reid Papers, file 2.

51 Montandon Diary, 26 November 1964.

52 C. Anthony Law, "Report of Her Majesty's Canadian Ship CAPE SCOTT under My Command for November 1964," LAC, Law Scrapbook, vol. 2, "Notes, Reports, Orders."

53 Law to Jane, 29 November 1964, LAC, Law Scrapbook, vol. 2, "Personal Correspondence."

54 Reid to "Darlings," 1 December 1964, Reid Papers, file 2.

55 Hrischenko, "Easter Island," 25.

56 Montandon Diary, 3 December 1964.

57 Ibid.

58 Reid Diary, 3 December 1964. She continued, "Donoso, Efford and Brody wax heated tonight in the Ward room about Jewry – it sounds as though Donoso is punishing them."

59 Brody Diary, 2 December 1964.

60 Montandon Diary, 3 December 1964.

61 Anon., "Hammie Picks Up Expedition!" See also Anon., "Dad Pacing Deck"; Harris, "All the Way to Easter Island"; and Anon., "Hams Filling Air Waves."

62 Allard, "5,000 Mile Gap."

63 Brody Diary, 3 December 1964.

64 Armand Boudreault to Armand Frappier, 1 December 1964, Archives de l'Institut national de recherche scientifique (INRS), Boudreault Papers, my translation.

65 Mathias Diary, 10 December 1964.

66 Montandon Diary, 4 and 5 December 1964.

67 Dozens of photographs were taken. A script of the ceremony is in Montandon Diary, 6 December 1964; and in LAC, Law Scrapbook, vol. 3.

68 Mathias Diary, 6 December 1964.

69 Detailed notes for off-loading with six appendices, "Easter Island Expedition, Operation Orders #1, 3 December 1964, at Sea," LAC, Law Scrapbook, vol. 2, "Notes, Reports, Orders."

70 Mathias Diary, 10 December 1964.

71 C.A. Law, "CONFIDENTIAL Proposed Programme – Easter Island Expedition," 12 June 1964, LAC, Law Scrapbook, vol. 2, "Notes, Reports, Orders."

72 Montandon Diary, 9 December 1964. For the journalists, she used the expression "se tourner les pouces."

73 Reid Diary, 28–29 November 1964, 13v; Reid, *World Away*, 12.

74 Mathias Diary, 9 December 1964.

75 Reid Diary, 28–29 November 1964, 13v; Reid, *World Away*, 12.

76 Reid Diary, 8 December 1964, 17.

77 Montandon Diary, 25 November 1964.

78 Reid, *World Away*, 62; Reid Diary, 5 December 1964, 16; Mathias Diary, 5 December 1964.

79 Mathias Diary, 7 and 10 December 1964.

80 Meier Diary, 7 and 8 December 1964; Hacker, *And Christmas Day*, 157; Montandon Diary, 10 December 1964.

81 Montandon Diary, 12 December 1964.

82 A complete copy of Cléopâtre's blank questionnaire is in Montandon Diary, 2 December 1964.

83 Reid Diary, 21 December 1964; Mathias Diary, 7 December 1964. See chapter 5.

84 Hacker, *And Christmas Day*, 157.

85 Ibid., 157–8.

86 Montandon Diary, 30 November 1964.

87 Hacker, *And Christmas Day*, 158–9.

88 On Christmas seals in Canada, see Bernier, *Médecine et idéologies*, 103–4.

89 Macfarlane, "Centre Planned for Natives."

90 Ibid.

91 Ibid.

92 Conoley, "Your Stamp Album." See also Anon., "The Realm of Stamps: Easter Island Deal," *Montreal Gazette*, [November 1964], clipping; and Anon., "Seal Marks Expedition's Unique Trip," [December 1964], unidentified clipping, Wilkinson Papers.

93 Heyerdahl, *Aku-Aku*, 120.

94 Several METEI members expressed this opinion in interviews, notably ecologist Ian Efford, anthropologist Bob Meier, and physician Peter Beighton.

95 Mathias Diary, 9 December 1964.

96 Montandon Diary, 12 December 1964.

97 Hacker, *And Christmas Day*, 160

98 Mathias Diary, 7 December 1964.

99 Brody Diary, 4 December 1964.

100 "Cargo List" 20, LAC, Law Scrapbook, vol. 2, "Notes, Reports, Orders."

101 Hacker, *And Christmas Day*, 156; Reid Diary, 10 December 1964; Mathias Diary, 10 December 1964.

102 Mathias Diary, 8 December 1964.

103 Brody Diary, 5 December 1964.

104 Reid Diary, 10 December 1964.

105 Macfarlane, "E-Day."

106 Meier Diary, 13 December 1964; Mathias Diary, 13 December 1964; Reid, *World Away*, 14–15.

107 Hacker, *And Christmas Day*, 161.

108 Macfarlane, "Easter Island Gives Ovation."

CHAPTER FOUR: RAISING CAMP HILTON

1 Hacker, *And Christmas Day*, 161; Matthias Diary, 13 December 1964.

2 Heyerdahl, *Aku-Aku*, 197, 205.

3 "CONFIDENCIAL [*sic*] Easter Island Isla de Pascua," 2; "Logistics," 3 December 1964, Library and Archives Canada (LAC), Law Scrapbook, vol. 2, "Notes, Reports, Orders."

4 Meier Diary, 13 December 1964.

5 Reid Diary, 13 December 1964.

6 Montandon Diary, 13 December 1964.

7 Ibid.

8 Ibid.

9 Ibid.

10 Hacker, *And Christmas Day*, 163–4.

11 Reid, *World Away*, 16–17.

12 Mathias Diary, 13 December 1964.

13 Law to Jane, 22 December 1964, LAC, Law Scrapbook, vol. 2, "Personal Correspondence."

14 Montandon Diary, 13 December 1964.

15 Hacker, *And Christmas Day*, 164.

16 Law provided many details of the unloading operation in Skoryna and Law, "Preliminary Report," 6–15, esp. 7.

17 C.A. Law, "Feeding Arrangements," 3 December 1964, LAC, Law Scrapbook, vol. 2, "Notes, Reports, Orders."

18 Reid Diary, 13 December 1964.

19 Meier Diary, 14 December 1964.

20 Ibid.

21 Reid, *World Away*, 16.

22 Montandon Diary, 14 December 1964.

23 Reid Diary, 16 December 1964.

24 Brody Diary, 25 December 1964.

25 Hacker, *And Christmas Day*, 166.

26 Law to Jane, 22 December 1964, LAC, Law Scrapbook, vol. 2, "Personal Correspondence"; Meier Diary, 14 December 1964.

27 Brody Diary, 25 December 1964.

28 Hacker, *And Christmas Day*, 166.

29 G. Archibald Wilkinson, Cassette 2A, at 17 mins, 50 secs, 9 February 1965, Wilkinson Audiotapes.

30 Montandon Diary, 16 December 1964.

31 Ibid.

32 Hacker, *And Christmas Day*, 166.

33 Reid Diary, 16 December 1964.

34 Montandon Diary, 16 December 1964.

35 Reid, *World Away*, 21–2; Reid Diary, 16 December 1964, 22v.

36 Law to Jane, 22 December 1964, LAC, Law Scrapbook, vol. 2, "Personal Correspondence."

37 Hacker, *And Christmas Day*, 170–1.

38 Fischer, *Island*, 210–11.

39 Law to Jane, [28?] December 1964, LAC, Law Scrapbook, vol. 2, "Personal Correspondence."

40 Stambuk, *Rongo*, 265–74, esp. 271 (Allende family).

41 Chile, *Informe . . . con Pueblos Indígenas*, vol. 1, part 1, "El Pueblo Rapa Nui," 275–342, esp. 308–9. In 2006–07 Alfonso Rapu and his mother, Reina Haoa, recounted this story to Patricia Stambuk. Stambuk, *Rongo*, 271. According to the METEI census, Alfonso and Carlos were twins (same birthdate), but the genealogy of Cristián Moreno Pakarati confirms that Carlos was two years younger.

42 Reid, *World Away*, 42; Reid Diary, 8 January 1964, 8:00 p.m., 46; Hacker, *And Christmas Day*, 214.

43 Reid Diary, 17 December 1964, 25.

44 Reid Diary, 2 February 1965, 77v. See also Hacker, *And Christmas Day*, 212. The woman was Maria Pakarati. Three years earlier, a beautiful

photo of her with long tresses had appeared in *National Geographic*. La Fay and Abercrombie, "Easter Island," 99.

45 Boutilier, "METEI [Part I]," 30; Mazière, *Mysteries*, 16, 22, 33.

46 Reid, *World Away*, 42. Several pages in Mazière's book also suggest 1964. Mazière, *Mysteries*, 22, 31, 185.

47 Law to Jane, [28?] December 1964, LAC, Law Scrapbook, vol. 2, "Personal Correspondence."

48 Mazière, *Mysteries*, 32.

49 Ibid., 182.

50 Fischer, *Island*, 210. See also McCall, "End of the World."

51 Reid, *World Away*, 42. So thoroughly did Reid subscribe to the view that the Mazière visit had caused all the political problems on Easter Island that she expressed it in a letter to *Time* magazine, which had reviewed the English translation of his book. Reid to Reviewer c/o *Time*, 17 March 1970, Reid Papers, file 11. For the review, see *Time*, 8 August 1969, 76–7.

52 Law to Jane, [28?] December 1964, LAC, Law Scrapbook, vol. 2, "Personal Correspondence."

53 Reid, *World Away*, 142.

54 Ibid., 12; Brody Diary, 2 December 1964.

55 Law to Jane, [28?] December 1964, LAC, Law Scrapbook, vol. 2, "Personal Correspondence."

56 Hacker, *And Christmas Day*, 171.

57 Skoryna and Law, "Preliminary Report," 10–11.

58 Montandon Diary, 18 December 1964.

59 Reid, *World Away*, 23–4.

60 Maureen Roberts to Mrs Cox, [ca. 12 January 1965], LAC, Roberts Papers, vol. 1, file 7.

61 Montandon Diary, 18 December 1964.

62 Law to Jane, 22 December 1964, LAC, Law Scrapbook, vol. 2, "Personal Correspondence." See also Macfarlane, "Canadian Medical Expedition Helps"; and Anon., "Cape Scott's Arrival Relieves Food Shortage," unidentified clipping, 17 December 1964, LAC, Law Scrapbook, vol. 3, "Clippings."

63 Reid, *World Away*, 65. Reid Diary, nd, 101v-102; Murphy Diary, nd.

64 Reid Diary, 16 December 1964.

65 Ibid., 19 December 1964.

66 Ibid., 17 December 1964.

67 Ibid., 28 December 1964; Reid, *World Away*, 63; Hacker, *And Christmas Day*, 200.

68 Law to Jane, 22 December 1964, LAC, Law Scrapbook, vol. 2, "Personal Correspondence."

69 Ian Efford, personal communication, 17 December 2016; Reid Diary, 17 December 1964.

70 Reid Diary, 19 December 1964.

71 Reid, *World Away*, 41.

72 Montandon Diary, 18 December 1964.

73 Law to Jane, 22 and [28?] December 1964, LAC, Law Scrapbook, vol. 2, "Personal Correspondence."

74 Jim Nielsen, personal communication, 12 August 2016.

75 Fischer, *Island*, 219–21; Porteous, *Modernization*, 172–3; Stambuk, *Iorana*, 39–50.

76 Brody, "Another Early Flight"; Maddock, "First Plane Flight"; Reid, *World Away*, 40; Reid Diary, 21 December 1964, 11 January 1965 (conversation with former governor Martin).

77 Hacker, *And Christmas Day*, 170.

78 Anon., "Historia viva."

79 Minutes of meeting, 17 December 1964, LAC, Roberts Papers, vol. 1, file 2. See also Boutilier, "METEI [Part I]," 32; and Reid, *World Away*, 26.

80 Skoryna to Tunis, [20 December 1964], McGill University Archives (MUA), RG 49, box 64, file 01372.

81 "Roster of Doctors on Call," LAC, Roberts Papers, vol. 1, file 2.

82 Skoryna to Tunis, [20 December 1964], MUA, RG 49, box 64, file 01372.

83 Gerd Hurum, "Statement," 4 January 1965, MUA, RG 49, box 64, file 01372.

84 Reid to A.L. Chute, 19–21 December 1964, Reid Papers, file 2.

85 Meier Diary, 21 December 1964.

86 Beighton, "Easter Island People," 350; Macfarlane, "Discontent in Paradise"; Meier Diary, 12 February 1965; Skoryna and Law, "Preliminary Report," 11.

87 Law to Jane, 22 December 1964, LAC, Law Scrapbook, vol. 2, "Personal Correspondence."

88 Ibid.

89 Law to Jane, [28?] December 1964, LAC, Law Scrapbook, vol. 2, "Personal Correspondence."

CHAPTER FIVE: THE STUDY BEGINS

1 Reid Diary, 23 December 1965.

2 Reid, *World Away*, 27.

3 Skoryna to Reid, December 1965, Reid Papers, file 15.

4 "Preliminary Reports," University of British Columbia (UBC) Archives, Efford Papers, METEI, box 1, file 1. These reports were written by

individual scientists and are not to be confused with Skoryna and Law, "Preliminary Report," which synthesized the individual reports.

5 G. Archibald Wilkinson, Cassette 2A and 2B, 9 February 1965, Wilkinson Audiotapes.

6 Reid, *World Away*, 93.

7 Nógrády, ed., *Microbiology*, vol. 1, "Acknowledgements." See also Boutilier, "METEI [Part I]," 33; Reid, *World Away*, 47–8, and caption opposite 55; and Hacker, *And Christmas Day*, 185–6. Norma and her siblings were recorded in the METEI census as Hucke Tepihe, but the family is known as Hucke Atán.

8 Hacker, *And Christmas Day*, 188–9.

9 Ibid., 185.

10 Meier Diary, 12 January 1965.

11 Reid Diary, 26 and 27 December 1964; Reid, "Easter Island," 23; Reid, *World Away*, 29.

12 Reid Diary, 23 and 24 December 1964. G. Archibald Wilkinson, Cassette 4, 24–25 December 1964, Wilkinson Audiotapes.

13 Montandon Diary, 25 December 1964.

14 Hacker, *And Christmas Day*, 175–6. Hacker never provided the last name of her friend Georgina; however, she mentioned that she was a mother of four. According to the METEI census, she was likely Georgina Beri Beri [Hereveri] Pakarati.

15 Montandon Diary, 25 December 1964.

16 Hacker, *And Christmas Day*, 176. Mentioned with no last name in several diaries and memoirs, "Big Carlo" may have been Carlos Teao Ika, forty-five years old and married with six children, according to METEI's "Census on the Population of Easter Island," 9 February 1965, UBC Archives, Efford Papers, METEI, box 1.

17 Reid Diary, 23 December 1964.

18 Hacker, *And Christmas Day*, 178–9. See also Reid Diary, 25 December 1964; and Montandon Diary, 25 and 26 December 1964.

19 Hacker, *And Christmas Day*, 158, 182.

20 Ibid., 178–9. For a photo of Carlotta with her "cow," see figure 5.9, and for a photograph of the resultant meal preparation, see Montandon Diary, 3 January 1965.

21 Hacker, *And Christmas Day*, 179–80.

22 Stambuk, *Rongo*, 265–310; Anon., "Historia viva."

23 Reid, *World Away*, 34; Hacker, *And Christmas Day*, 182–3; Reid Diary, 28 December 1964. This story may not be entirely accurate, although it has oft been repeated based on the books of Reid and Hacker, including by Boutilier, "METEI [Part I]," 31. In July 1965, Skoryna wrote that the

first family – that of Juan Atán – came willingly to the camp; it was on the *second* day that a family failed to appear. Helen replied that she did not plan to change the passage in her book because it was "unimportant" whether it happened on the first or second day and because the story was "more dramatic as it is." Reid to Skoryna, 6 July 1965, Reid Papers, file 10. Reid's diary does not mention Stanley's drive to town.

24 Meier Diary, 28 December 1964.

25 Reid, *World Away*, 41; G. Archibald Wilkinson, Cassette 2B, at 2 mins, 9 February 1965, Wilkinson Audiotapes.

26 Hacker, *And Christmas Day*, 183.

27 CBC, Williams, and Hrischenko, *Canadian Expedition to Easter Island*.

28 Meier Diary, 22 January 1965.

29 Hacker, *And Christmas Day*, 195–7. Located on the side of a cliff far from the camp at the Poike end of the island, the Ana o Keke cave was allegedly a place for confining young girls to keep their skin fair. It had figured in several earlier accounts; and many were said to have died there of starvation during a smallpox epidemic when no one brought food. Heyerdahl, *Aku-Aku*, 74–82.

30 Skoryna and Law, "Preliminary Report," 44–6.

31 Reid, *World Away*, 98.

32 Ibid., 97.

33 Reid to Roberts, 30 May 1966, Library and Archives Canada (LAC), Roberts Papers, vol. 1, file 22.

34 H.C. Gibbs, "Interim Report on Parasitological Survey," UBC Archives, Efford Papers, METEI, box 1.

35 Meier Diary, 31 December 1964.

36 Reid Diary, 1 January 1965; Montandon Diary, 3 January 1965. Meier attended a party with "much food and music" at the home of Maria Pakarati [Tepano?]. It may have been the same party as the Montandons attended.

37 Garry Brody, email correspondence, 17 August 2017; Brody Diary, 25 December 1964.

38 Hagelberg, "Genetic Affinities," 186; Métraux, *Ethnology*, 123–4.

39 Hacker, "Aku-Aku and Medicine Men"; Reid, *World Away*, 107–8, 121–3; Reid Diary, 2 February 1965; Brody Diary, 25 December 1964; Macfarlane, "No One She Can Marry"; Macfarlane, "Mysterious Moai," 21.

40 Meier, "Easter Islander," 79–86.

41 Hacker to Reid, 12 August [1967], Reid Papers, file 10.

42 Hacker, *And Christmas Day*, 204–5; Mydans, "Isle of Stone Heads."

43 Hacker, *And Christmas Day*, 204.

44 Reid, *World Away*, 107.

45 Reid Diary, 5 January 1964; Reid, *World Away*, 48; Hacker, *And Christmas Day*, 186.

46 Reid Diary, 25 December 1964, 1 February 1965; Montandon Diary, 24 January 1964.

47 Reid Diary, 1 and 12 February 1965.

48 Nógrády's collection has many pictures of the Ika Pakarati family on the island and several of himself with a large wooden crate addressed to them from Montreal. He wanted to adopt Jorge and bring him to school in Canada, but the boy's father refused. Maria Teresa Ika Pakarati, personal communication, 22 January 2017.

49 Reid, *World Away*, 107–9, 121–3.

50 Reid to A.L. Chute, 20 December 1964, Reid Papers, file 2.

51 Reid Diary, 9 January 1965.

52 Reid, *World Away*, 88, 90.

53 Hacker, *And Christmas Day*, 189.

54 Reid to P.M. Laing, 8 June 1965, Reid Papers, file 10.

55 Roberts, "Report on the Easter Island Medical Expedition," esp. 2–3.

56 Montandon Diary, 24 January 1965.

57 Reid, *World Away*, 88, 91.

58 Hacker, *And Christmas Day*, 189.

59 Skoryna, "Metei: An Epilogue," 70.

60 Hacker, *And Christmas Day*, 187, 189; Reid Diary, 2 and 3 January 1965; King to Reid, Sunday, 28 [November? 1965], Reid Papers, file 15.

61 Reid to A.L. Chute, 7–8 January 1965, Reid Papers, file 2.

62 Reid Diary, 3 January 1965.

63 Ibid.

64 Hacker, *And Christmas Day*, 191.

65 Reid Diary, 21 December 1964.

66 See "Continuation with [James R.] Barlow on Immorality," Reid Diary, 19 February 1965.

67 Reid to A.L. Chute, 7–8 January 1965, Reid Papers, file 2.

68 Ibid.

69 Ibid.

70 Ibid.

71 Etcheverry, Nagel, and Guzman, "Encuesta"; Barzelatto, "Endemic Goiter in Chile."

72 Hacker, *And Christmas Day*, 189.

73 Reid to Chute, 25 February 1965, Reid Papers, file 2.

CHAPTER SIX: REVOLUTION, POLITICS, AND DISEASE

1 Anon., "Historia viva"; Boutilier, "METEI [Part II]"; Delsing, "Issues of Land"; Fischer, *Island*, 210–18; Grifferos A., "Colonialism"; Grifferos A., "Entre palos e piedras"; Porteous, *Modernization*, 170–3; Stambuk, *Rongo*, 275–310; Tector, "Delightful Revolution."

2 Reid Diary, 29 December 1964; Montandon Diary, 28 December 1964; Anon., "French Barred."

3 Maureen Roberts to Mrs Cox, [ca. 12 January 1964], Library and Archives Canada (LAC), Roberts Papers, vol. 1, file 7.

4 Anon., "Chile Marines Sent"; Anon., "Chilean Marines to Easter Island."

5 Reid Diary, 1 January 1965, 3:30 p.m.

6 Reid to A.L. Chute, 8 January 1965, Reid Papers, file 2. This letter did not reach its destination until March.

7 Ralph Graves to Skoryna, 13 October 1964, McGill University Archives (MUA), RG 49, box 64, file 01375.

8 Chilean media identify the informants as Leonardo Pakarati and Mariano, possibly his son. Anon., "Medidas para incorporar"; Anon., "Situación de Isla de Pascua"; Anon., "Diversas versiones"; Anon., "Los habitantes"; Anon., "Nave de la Armada."

9 Anon., "Inquietud en Pascua."

10 George V. Cutler to Albert Tunis, 3 January 1965; Tunis to Cutler, 6 January 1965, MUA, RG 49, box 64, file 01372.

11 Anon., "Canadian Group Reports Quiet."

12 Hacker, *And Christmas Day*, 214–15.

13 Reid, *World Away*, 43–4.

14 Anon., "French Barred."

15 Montandon Diary, 3 January 1965.

16 Hacker, *And Christmas Day*, 189.

17 Reid Diary, 3 January 1965.

18 Ibid., 5 January 1965.

19 Reid, *World Away*, 44.

20 Martin is described as meting out inappropriately severe punishment, including beatings and the shaving of heads. For example, he did not believe Carlos Rapu, brother of Alfonso, and punished him when he complained of unwanted sexual attention by dentist Julio Flores. Chile, *Informe ... con Pueblos Indígenas*, vol. 1, part 1, "El Pueblo Rapa Nui," 275–342, esp. 308–9; Stambuk, *Rongo*, 267–70.

21 Reid Diary, 5 January 1965.

22 Ibid., 3–4 January 1965, midnight.

23 Chile, *Informe*, vol. 3, part 1, "Informe preparado por los senores Mario Tuki Hey y otros (Rapa Nui)," 445–82, esp. 465.

24 Pencilled annotation in Reid Diary, 19 December 1965.

25 Hacker, *And Christmas Day*, 215; Inostrosa, "Agitación." See also the report of discussion on the same day in the Chilean legislature. Chile, Labor Parlamentaria, "Creación de la comuna subdelegacion."

26 Anon., "Historia viva."

27 Reid, *World Away*, 45.

28 Hacker, *And Christmas Day*, 218

29 Ibid., 219; Reid Diary, 9 January 1965, 49. This story was confirmed by Isabel Cutler (formerly Griffiths), personal communication, July 2016.

30 Reid Diary, 8 January 1965.

31 Ibid., 8:00 p.m.

32 Meier Diary, 8 January 1965.

33 Reid Diary, 8 January 1965.

34 Meier Diary, 8 January 1965; Reid Diary, 8 January 1965, 49.

35 Reid Diary, 21 January 1965, 63v; Montandon Diary, 13 January 1965. The exact number of votes differs slightly in these two sources.

36 Reid Diary, 12 January 1965; Montandon Diary, 13 January 1965.

37 G. Archibald Wilkinson, Cassette 3A and 3B, 17 January 1965, Wilkinson Audiotapes. See also Reid Diary, 17 January 1965; and Montandon Diary, 17 January 1965.

38 These dates are established from the METEI census. University of British Columbia (UBC) Archives, Efford Papers, METEI, box 1. There are three families with four to six children headed by a "Jorge Tepano" (aged 26, 28, and 39); it is not possible to determine which family belonged to the councillor. Nevertheless, all three Jorge Tepano families were examined *after* the election.

39 Van Tilburg, *Among Stone Giants*, 170; Heyerdahl, *Aku-Aku*, 217.

40 Reid, *World Away*, 58–9, 61–2; Boutilier, "METEI [Part II]," 46; Roberts, "Results of the Easter Island Expedition," 14. See also Macfarlane, "Easter Islanders"; and Anon., "Canadians Studying Rare Disease ... Didn't Bring Cocongo," unidentified clipping, Wilkinson Papers.

41 Reid, *World Away*, 61–2.

42 Reid Diary, 10 January 1965.

43 Mydans, "Isle of Stone Heads"; Montandon Diary, 9 January 1965.

44 Reid Diary, 11 January 1965.

45 Ibid. Later, Reid summarized the five-day clinical course of *kokongo*: two cases were complicated by pneumonia, five by otitis media, and one by dizziness and a "list to the left on sudden movement." Ibid., 22 January 1965, 64 r-v.

46 Georges Nógrády, "Preliminary Report on Bacteriological Examination," 6, UBC Archives, Efford Papers, METEI, box 1, file 1.

47 Reid Diary, nd, 87 (Boudreault), 97 (Nógrády). See also notes of interviews for *Maclean's*, nd, Reid Papers, file 5. Boudreault referred to the epidemic in his own article, promising a separate publication devoted to *kokongo* in the future – one that never appeared. Boudreault and Pavilanis, "Epidémiologie."

48 Reid, "Easter Island"; Reid, *World Away*, 60–1. This hypothesis, expressed in her *Maclean's* article, garnered some criticism from readers, especially a former diplomat, but she patiently defended it with reference to the principles of transmission. Boutilier, "METEI [Part II]," 47; James Midwinter to Reid, 9 June 1965; Reid to Midwinter, 15 June 1965, Reid Papers, file 12.

49 Roberts, "Results of the Easter Island Expedition," 14.

50 Meier Diary, 9 January 1965.

51 Hacker, *And Christmas Day*, 187.

52 Reid Diary, 20 January 1965.

53 On leprosy and the leprosarium, see Haoa Rapahango, *Leprosario*; and Stambuk, *Rongo*, 173–93.

54 Reid Diary, undated insert ("Andrade's figures"), 31r-v and 32r-v. I have been unable to identify the leprologist. More than 4,000 smears implies several per individual.

55 Reid Diary, nd, 70–1 (interview with Father Ricardo Rainer).

56 Hacker, *And Christmas Day*, 192–3.

57 "Cargo List," 22, LAC, Law Scrapbook, vol. 2, "Notes, Reports, Orders."

58 Reid Diary, 99–100. Four of the names on the ambulatory list were not in the METEI census, suggesting that they were not on the island, had avoided examination, or had died. A similar file is likely with Roberts's papers, although it is sealed until 2070. LAC, Roberts Papers, vol. 1, file 18.

59 Reid, *World Away*, 69; Reid Diary, 4 February 1965, 78; Hacker, *And Christmas Day*, 207–9.

60 McCall, "End of the World."

61 Seward, "Between 'Easter Island' and 'Rapa Nui,'" 257.

62 Reid Diary, 22 December 1964.

63 Greve Hernández, "Planificación"; Montes, "Aspectos clínicos."

64 Reid, *World Away*, 100–1.

65 Armand Boudreault, personal communication, 13 January 2017. Given her date of birth and name, the child was likely Cecilia Rita Riroroko Pakarati, born 21 January 1965.

66 Reid, *World Away*, 109; Meier Diary, 31 January 1965.

67 On Aurelio's journey, see Stambuk, *Rongo*, 205–12. Esteban Pakarati described his own 1943 journey to the Montandons. Montandon Diary, 3 January 1965.

68 Reid, *World Away*, 100–11, 126–7.

69 Isabel Cutler (formerly Griffiths), email correspondence, 12 January 2016.

70 Reid, *World Away*, 67.

71 Ibid.

72 Heyerdahl, *Aku-Aku*, 120.

73 Meier Diary, 21 January 1965. See also the report on a talk given by Helen Reid in Anon., "No Feeling for Animals."

74 Hacker, *And Christmas Day*, 207.

75 Ibid., 190.

CHAPTER SEVEN: PLANTS, ANIMALS, MORES, AND MICROBES

1 Compare the original plan in the first four pages of Efford's diary with his summary in Skoryna and Law, "Preliminary Report," March 1965. Ian Efford, "Easter Island – Data," 156 unnumbered pages, University of British Columbia (UBC) Archives, Efford Papers, METEI, box 2 (hereinafter Efford Diary). See also Ian Efford, "Preliminary Report," UBC Archives, Efford Papers, METEI, box 1, file 5.

2 Efford Diary, 16 December 1964, unnumbered pp. 39–43 (marked "1–5").

3 In 2017 islanders identified these boys from photographs as Gerardo Manutomatoma Pate (aged fifteen) and Raúl Pakarati (aged fourteen).

4 Hacker, *And Christmas Day*, 202.

5 Efford Diary, 22, 23, and 27 December 1964, unnumbered pp. 12 (marked "6"), 25, 28, and 32.

6 Ibid., nd, unnumbered p. 70.

7 Ibid., 26 December 1964 (turtle), unnumbered pp. 16 (marked "10) and 31; 6, 13, and 19 January and 4 February 1965 (sharks), unnumbered pp. 21 (marked "24"), 72, 73, and 77.

8 Ibid., 21 January 1965, unnumbered p. 76; another octopus was caught at Apina Iti. Ibid., 18 January 1965, unnumbered p. 73. See also Meier Diary, 22 January 1965.

9 Efford Diary, 28 December 1964, unnumbered pp. 18 (marked "15") and 57.

10 Ibid., nd, unnumbered p. 87.

11 Ibid., nd, unnumbered p. 95.

12 Ibid., 5 January 1965, unnumbered p. 107.

13 Maunder et al., "Conservation of the Toromiro Tree."

14 Compare Efford Diary, nd, unnumbered pp. 2–5 (marked "1–4"), with Efford's statements in CBC, Williams, and Hrischenko, *Canadian Expedition to Easter Island*, part 2, at 21 mins; and in Skoryna and Law, "Preliminary Report," 50–8.

15 Efford Diary, 31 December 1964, unnumbered p. 49 (marked "18").

16 Ibid., 29 December 1964, unnumbered p. 36.

17 Ibid., 5 January 1965, unnumbered p. 37.

18 Ibid., nd, unnumbered p. 95.

19 Ibid., nd, unnumbered p. 82.

20 Gibbs, "Survey"; Skoryna and Law, "Preliminary Report," 40–1.

21 Efford Diary, 6, 7, and 8 January 1965, unnumbered pp. 84, 87, and 95.

22 Ibid., 28 January 1965, unnumbered p. 74.

23 Ibid., nd, unnumbered p. 95.

24 Ibid., 30 December 1964, unnumbered pp. 3, 19 (marked "22"), and 67.

25 Ibid., 26 December 1964, unnumbered p. 46 (marked "16").

26 Ibid., 4 February 1965 and nd, unnumbered pp. 91, 93, 100, and 101.

27 Reid Diary, nd, 117–18. For more on Rapanui traditional healing, see Holdsworth, "Preliminary Study"; and Joves, "Re-Imagining."

28 Efford Diary, unnumbered pp. 15 (marked "9") (Brody), 69 (Easton), 77 (Nielsen), and 112 (Roberts).

29 Ibid., 1 January 1965, unnumbered p. 68.

30 Skoryna and Law, "Preliminary Report," 50–8.

31 Ibid., 54.

32 Ibid., 57–8.

33 Ibid., 49.

34 Meier Diary, 15 January 1965.

35 Montandon Diary, 28 December 1964. A typewritten "Dictionary" with 1,500 Rapanui words was provided to METEI, a copy of which resides in Wilkinson Papers.

36 Montandon Diary, 27 December 1964.

37 Ibid., 3 January 1965.

38 Ibid., 27 December 1964, 8 February 1965.

39 Ibid., 8 February 1965.

40 Ibid., 28 January 1965.

41 Cléopâtre Montandon, "Sociological Study on Easter Island," UBC Archives, Efford Papers, METEI, box 1, file 5; Skoryna and Law, "Preliminary Report."

42 Reid Diary, nd, 91v-92. Compared to Montandon's report, cited above in note 41, Reid's notes for the *Maclean's* article show differences in the figures and contain a few additional items, suggesting that the notes were

indeed based on a conversation between the two women, not on an analysis of Montandon's report.

43 Montandon Diary, 6 February 1965.

44 Denys Montandon, "Medical Examination of the Continental Population of Easter Island" and "METEI Work Summary," UBC Archives, Efford Papers, METEI, box 1, file 5. Denys Montandon's reports were excluded from the synthetic Skoryna and Law, "Preliminary Report." I have not located any other data from his study. The individual examination records may have been left on the island.

45 Montandon Diary, 8 February 1965. She had lost another week when she developed an infected wound on her ankle.

46 Montandon Diary, 8 February 1965.

47 Reid Diary, nd, 70–1. She called Father Ricardo "the modern [saint] Peter."

48 Ibid., 30 December 1964. Her source was Cléopâtre.

49 Ibid., 7 January 1965. For her other nutritional queries, see also 16 December 1964 (at school), 21 January 1965 (Juan Atán), and 25 January 1965.

50 Ibid., 26 January 1965.

51 "Mercaderías destinadas a ECA Pascua," list of goods, quantities "requested," and "supplied," five typewritten loose pages folded into the back of Reid Diary.

52 Reid, *World Away*, 95; Reid Diary, 21 January 1965 (Juan Atán), 25 January 1965, and esp. nd, 79–84, including 79v-80 (toothpaste). The position of these diary pages suggests that the work was done in February. Possibly, she made the calculations on the return journey.

53 Roberts, "Results of the Easter Island Expedition," 19.

54 Richard and Maureen Roberts, "Medical Examinations," UBC Archives, Efford Papers, METEI, box 1, file 5.

55 Reid Diary, 3 January 1965.

56 Georges Nógrády, "Preliminary Report on Bacteriological Examinations," 8–9, UBC Archives, Efford Papers, METEI, box 1, file 5. See also LAC, Roberts Papers, vol. 2, file 5.

57 Hacker, *And Christmas Day*, 191.

58 Montandon Diary, 17 January 1965; Reid Diary, 3 January 1965.

59 Montandon Diary, 30 November 1964.

60 Hacker, *And Christmas Day*, 157. See also chapter 3.

61 Nógrády and Lawlor, *Manuel et cahier*; Nógrády and Fredette, *Catalogue des films microbiologiques*; Nógrády, *L'effet de la toxine staphylococcique*; Nógrády, *Effects of Streptomycin*. The latter two items are films in the library of the Université de Montréal.

62 Hacker, *And Christmas Day*, 191–2.

63 Reid, *World Away*, 75

64 Ibid., 77. See also Hacker, *And Christmas Day*, 192.

65 Reid Diary, 1 February 1965, 76.

66 Ibid., 75.

67 Montandon Diary, 24 January 1965; Hacker, *And Christmas Day*, 190.

68 Montandon Diary, 31 January 1965.

69 Reid Diary, 23 January 1965; Meier Diary, 23 January 1965.

70 Meier Diary, 30 January 1965.

71 Reid Diary, 23 January 1965; Meier Diary, 23 January 1965.

72 Hacker, *And Christmas Day*, 199.

73 Montandon Diary, 31 January 1965.

74 Meier Diary, 26 January 1965.

75 Reid Diary, 1 February 1965.

76 Meier Diary, 2 January 1965, 2 February 1965.

77 Reid, *World Away*, 128. Shortly after Noe was hired to work in the kitchen, Ana Maria Eccles was warned that he was the only person on the island with a criminal record, having been jailed for abusing little girls. Reid Diary, 23 December 1964.

78 Montandon Diary, 11 [12] February 1965. Two entries are dated 11 February – one Thursday and one Friday – so the correct date is likely 12 February.

79 Hacker, *And Christmas Day*, 206.

80 Meier Diary, 2 February 1965 (and more recent annotation).

81 Reid, *World Away*, 89.

82 Meier Diary, 3 February 1965.

83 Hacker, *And Christmas Day*, 183.

84 Children's paintings, Reid Papers, file 3.

85 Reid Diary, 12 February 1964.

CHAPTER EIGHT: RETURN OF HMCS *CAPE SCOTT*

1 "CONFIDENCIAL [*sic*] Easter Island Isla de Pascua," 7–8 (Skoryna's suggestion with destinations), Library and Archives Canada (LAC), Law Scrapbook, vol. 2, "Notes, Reports, Orders."

2 Zahniser and Wies, "Diplomatic Pearl Harbor?"; Shannon, "'One of Our Greatest'"; Lerner, "'Big Tree of Peace and Justice.'"

3 Haidasz to Cadieux, 2 October 1965; Cadieux to Haidasz, 8 October 1965, LAC, Haidasz Papers. The proposed countries were Peru, Colombia, and Venezuela.

4 "CONFIDENCIAL [*sic*] Easter Island Isla de Pascua," 7–8; C.A. Law, "CONFIDENTIAL Proposed Programme – Easter Island Expedition," 12 June 1964, LAC, Law Scrapbook, vol. 2, "Notes, Reports, Orders."

5 Law to Jane, 17 January 1965, parts 1 and 2, LAC, Law Scrapbook, vol. 2, "Personal Correspondence."

6 Ibid.

7 Ibid.

8 Inostrosa, "Agitación." On Sister Esperanza and the letter, see Stambuk, *Rongo*, 288–98.

9 Law to Jane, 17 January 1965, parts 1 and 2, LAC, Law Scrapbook, vol. 2, "Personal Correspondence."

10 Ibid.

11 Law to Jane, 19 January 1965, part 1, LAC, Law Scrapbook, vol. 2, "Personal Correspondence."

12 "Confidential," Santiago to External Affairs, Ottawa, 5 January 1965, LAC, Canada and Agencies, Lester B. Pearson Papers, 1963–1965.

13 Law to Jane, 19 January 1965, part 1, LAC, Law Scrapbook, vol. 2, "Personal Correspondence."

14 They were likely Jorge Thornton Strahan and Jorge Paredes Wetzer. See a newspaper report from *La Prensa Austral*, 12 March 1957, cited by Jara Fernández et al., eds, *El Año Geofísico Internacional*, 294. Jorge Paredes Wetzer was later implicated in the 1973 torture of prisoners at Isla Quiriquina, a crime that he denied. See Magasich-Airola, *Los que dijeron "no."*

15 Law to Jane, 19 January 1965, part 1, LAC, Law Scrapbook, vol. 2, "Personal Correspondence."

16 Ibid.

17 Ibid., 25 January 1965.

18 The C.A.E. Fowler architectural firm would design the "brutalist" Dalhousie University Arts Centre, which opened in 1971. Charles and Dot Fowler had attended Law's farewell party in November 1964.

19 With his patrician background, history degree, and naval past, Tovell had met Law during the war. As ambassador, in 1963, he had helped negotiate the release of hostages in a Bolivian miners' strike. Rosita Tovell, active in the Canadian art scene, served the National Gallery, promoted Native art, and left more than a million dollars to the Victoria Gallery at her death in 2014. For his obituary, see Hawthorn, "Ambassador Negotiated Release"; and for her memorial and announcement of the bequest, see Chamberlain, "Art Gallery Receives."

20 Law to Jane, 2 February 1965, LAC, Law Scrapbook, vol. 2, "Personal Correspondence." Images of the erotic pre-Colombian pottery abound on

the Internet. Rafael Larco Herrera founded the private museum, which was carried on by his son, Rafael Larco Hoyle, who was collecting and publishing on erotic art at the time of Law's visit. See Larco Hoyle, *Checan*.

21 Law to Jane, 2 February 1965, LAC, Law Scrapbook, vol. 2, "Personal Correspondence."

22 Ibid., 10 February 1965. The fire is confirmed by the ship's log, 6 February 1965 at 08:50. It resulted in reduced speed for two hours. LAC, Ships Logs, February 1965.

23 Reid, *World Away*, 157.

24 Ibid., 161.

25 Meier Diary, 30 January 1965 (Taylor packing), 5 and 6 February 1965 (museum), 8 February 1965 (boat).

26 Montandon Diary, 11 February 1965.

27 Ibid., 9 February 1965.

28 Ibid., 13 February 1965.

29 Reid, *World Away*, 163.

30 Montandon Diary, 10 February 1965; Meier Diary, 7 February 1965.

31 G. Archibald Wilkinson, Cassette 2A and 2B, 9 February 1965, Wilkinson Audiotapes.

32 Meier Diary, 11 February 1965.

33 Law to Jane, 23 February 1965, LAC, Law Scrapbook, vol. 2, "Personal Correspondence."

34 Hacker, *And Christmas Day*, 229.

35 Ibid., 230.

36 Law to Jane, 10 and 22 February 1965, LAC, Law Scrapbook, vol. 2, "Personal Correspondence."

37 Hacker, *And Christmas Day*, 229.

38 Montandon Diary, 11 February 1965.

39 Meier Diary, 11 February 1965.

40 Skoryna to Law, 12 February 1965, LAC, Law Scrapbook, vol. 2, "Correspondence."

41 Reid Diary, 30 January 1965.

42 Reid Diary, 12 February 1965.

43 Meier Diary, 12 February 1965.

44 Hacker, *And Christmas Day*, 232–3.

45 Montandon Diary, 11 [12] February 1965.

46 Law to Jane, 10 and 22 February 1965, LAC, Law Scrapbook, vol. 2, "Personal Correspondence."

47 Ibid., 23 February 1965.

48 Montandon Diary, 13 February 1965.

49 Ibid.

50 Citing Reid, Wilkinson, and Dr Robert G. Fraser, Skoryna announced Reid's idea of a comparison study in his McGill lecture at the Leacock Building. Macfarlane, "500 Montreal, Toronto Children."

51 Reid Diary, nd, 116v.

52 Ibid., nd, 87–98. The "questionnaire" and original notes are with the Reid Papers, file 5.

53 Meier Diary, entries of 13 to 24 February 1965.

54 Skoryna to Pearson, 25 June 1964, 1 and 17 December 1964; Jules Pelletier for P.M. Pearson to Skoryna, 10 December 1964, LAC, Canada and Agencies, Lester B. Pearson Papers, 1963–1965.

55 "Order of Service," LAC, Law Scrapbook, vol. 2. "Memorabilia."

56 Milner, *Canada's Navy*, 249; Anon., "New Flag." Featured on page 3 of the issue of *Crowsnest* that published the latter article is a photograph of a nuclear test explosion off Hawaii witnessed by HMCS *Fraser*.

57 "HMCS *Cape Scott*, Order of Service on the Proclamation of the Canadian Flag," LAC, Law Scrapbook, vol. 2., "Memorabilia."

58 Reid Diary, 15 February 1965.

59 Montandon Diary, 15 February 1965.

60 Rapa Nui Science Club certificates are dated 20 February 1965. Most travellers still have the newsletters. A copy and all the "rules" are in Montandon Diary, 10 March 1965, and LAC, Law Scrapbook, vol. 2, "Rapa Nui Science Club."

61 Montandon Diary, 15 February 1965.

62 Reid Diary, 19 February 1965.

63 Ibid.

64 Law to Jane, 23 February 1965, LAC, Law Scrapbook, vol. 2, "Personal Correspondence."

65 Meier Diary, 21 February 1965.

66 Montandon Diary, 21 February 1965.

67 Reid Diary, 24 February 1965.

68 Reid to Bob Williams, 8 September 1965, Reid Papers, file 10.

69 Beighton to Nielsen, 3 April 1965, Nielsen Papers.

70 Reid, *World Away*, 91, 157; Hacker, *And Christmas Day*, 230–1.

71 Reid Diary, 12 February 1965.

72 Songs in LAC, Law Scrapbook, vol. 2. "Memorabilia." The travellers kept these certificates; some framed them. Cléopâtre and Denys Montandon put theirs in Montandon Diary, 5 December 1965.

73 Regulations "do not permit women to take passage in naval vessels except with the express permission of the government." Rear Admiral

Robert Willard to Albert A. Tunis, 23 February 1965, McGill University Archives (MUA), RG 49, box 66, file 10436.

74 Montandon Diary, 25 February 1965.

75 Ibid.

76 Reid to Chute, 28 February and 2 March 1965, Reid Papers, file 2; Reid Diary, entries of 25 to 28 February 1965.

77 Reid Diary, 28 February 1965, 111. See also Reid, "Easter Island," 23.

78 Chute to Reid, 7 and 14 February 1965; Reid to Chute, 25 February 1965, Reid Papers, file 2.

79 Boudreault to Frappier, 25 February 1965, Archives de l'Institut national de recherche scientifique (INRS), Boudreault Papers.

80 Reid to Chute, "3 or 4" March 1965, Reid Papers, file 2.

81 Following Colombia, Dier would be posted to South Vietnam and was instrumental in peace talks early in the conflict. Anon., "South Viet Makes Peace Deal." During the October Crisis of 1970, Dier would be one of two diplomats held at gunpoint by the Federation de Libération de Québec kidnappers of James Cross on their escape flight to Cuba aboard a Royal Canadian Air Force plane. See Hilliker, Halloran, and Donaghy, *Canada's Department of External Affairs,* vol. 3, 97.

82 Montandon Diary, 7 March 1965. For a report on a METEI interview conducted in Cartagena, see Lee, "State of the Most Isolated Humans."

83 Reid to Chute, 25 February, 2, 4, and 6 March 1965, Reid Papers, file 2.

84 On Parque el Canada, see Robinson, *Diplomat in Environmentalist's Clothing,* 79–85. The flag donation was more appropriate than Reid knew. When diplomat Raymond M. Robinson first saw the pathetic site in the early 1960s, the Canadian ensign was flying upside down (79). See also "History of the Parque el Canada," 5 August 1964, typescript, 2 pages; and explanation of the donation of the *Cape Scott* flag, 1 page, Reid Papers, file 5.

85 Ambassador Dier used the flag made by Charles Fowler for the opening of the school but thought that it belonged in Canada. He sent it to Prime Minister Pearson, who thanked him. Dier copied the correspondence to Helen Reid with a letter explaining what happened. Dier to Reid, 14 May 1965; Dier to Pearson, 25 March 1965; Pearson to Dier, 7 April 1965, Reid Papers, file 22. Tony Law's flag went to the navy museum. Fowler's has not been located.

86 Mathias and Nielsen have vivid memories of their escapade. Isabel and Carlotta printed a description in Rapa Nui Science Club, *Newsletter,* 21 May 1965, University of British Columbia (UBC) Archives, Efford Papers, METEI, box 1, file 2.

87 They held typewritten letters from Commandante Daniel Alfonso Gomez Tellez, Departamento Policio Bolivar, Cartagena, 4 March 1965, and from Roberto Galán Ponce de León, Department of Biology, and Gerardo Reichel-Dolmatoff, Head of the Department of Anthropology, both at Universidad de Los Andes, Bogotá, 7 March 1965. The anthropologist attended the METEI symposium in Bogotá, possibly with the biologist. After Nielsen and Mathias encountered difficulties, they had another letter of introduction from Rezack Mohammed in Guajira, Venezuela, addressed to his brother Hatim Mohammed in Trinidad, 13 March 1965. Nielsen Papers.

88 Reid confided, "We shed about half the expedition here, a great refreshing change." Reid to Chute, 28 February 1965, Reid Papers, file 2. Cléopâtre wrote, "Several expedition members left us at Balboa. As we left the quay, we felt the difference right away and I dare say with no regret." Montandon Diary, 25 February 1965.

89 Reid to Chute, 25 February 1965, Reid Papers, file 2.

90 Reid to Chute, 3 or 4 March 1965, Reid Papers, file 2.

91 Chute to Reid, 24 November 1964, Reid Papers, file 2.

92 Haidasz's speech on behalf of the government is in LAC, Haidasz Papers.

93 "Procedures for Arrival of Cape Scott, 17 March 1965," handwritten notes, 2 pages, MUA, RG 49, box 66, file 10436.

94 McKeen to Robertson, 19 March 1965, MUA, RG 2, box 293, file 10670.

95 "CDR COCKS LOSS IS DR REIDS GAIN / WE HAD WONDERFUL WEATHER AS HOMEWARD WE CAME / HERES THANKS TO YOU FROM ALL CAPE SCOTTS / WE NEVER HAD WIND OVER TWENTY-FOUR KNOTS / SO HAVE THE POSTMAN TAKE HIS LOAD / TO DR REID 77 GOLFDALE ROAD / AND SO IT WONT BE OVERDUE / APPEND TO THE BOTTOM TORONTO ONE TWO." *Cape Scott* to *Yukon*, 16 March 1965, Reid Papers, file 22. Reid must have thanked the navy, for she received a second telex: "DELIGHTED TO HAVE PAID FOR A FAIR PASSAGE FOR A FAIR LADY." *Yukon* to *Cape Scott*, 18 March 1965, Reid Papers, file 22.

96 [Macfarlane?], "Mission Over; Research Starts." See also Anon., "Mission Accomplished."

97 Templeton, "Expedition Leader," 3. The island remains Motu Nui.

98 Macfarlane, "500 Montreal, Toronto Children."

99 Macfarlane, "Most Islanders Free." See also *Sun Life Review*, July 1965, 14–15.

CHAPTER NINE: PERSONAL AND POPULAR RESULTS

1 Copies of Skoryna and Law, "Preliminary Report," abound. Several are in Library and Archives Canada (LAC) with the papers of Commander Tony Law, Richard Roberts, Stanley Haidsaz, and Lester B. Pearson (under Canada and Agencies). The report was sent to all METEI members whose private records have been available to me. Copies may also have been sent to every seaman on *Cape Scott*, as the report was once available on the Internet at the personal website of sailor George Goodwin – a site about his Canadian navy career that, sadly, has been taken down.

2 A complete set of the Rapa Nui Science Club's *Newsletter* is in University of British Columbia (UBC) Archives, Efford Papers, METEI, box 1, file 2. Incomplete sets are scatted in LAC, Roberts Papers; LAC, Law Papers; and Reid Papers.

3 Rapa Nui Science Club, *Newsletter*, 28 April (leaves Rapa Nui), 21 May (asking for news of him), and 19 August 1965 (Beighton found), UBC Archives, Efford Papers, METEI, box 1, file 2.

4 Rapa Nui Science Club, *Newsletter*, 19 August, 1 November, and 20 December 1965, UBC Archives, Efford Papers, METEI, box 1, file 2.

5 Hacker to Reid, "Tuesday," [October 1965], Reid Papers, file 5.

6 Macfarlane, "Mysterious Moai."

7 Reid, "Easter Island."

8 Hacker to Reid, 20 April 1965, Reid Papers, file 10.

9 Corrected galleys of Reid's *Maclean's* article, Reid Papers, file 11.

10 Reid to Bob Williams, 8 September 1965, Reid Papers, file 10.

11 Boudreault, "Huit semaines."

12 Memo for the Prime Minister, 18 May 1965, and various handwritten notes; Jules Pelletier to Skoryna, 6 April 1965, LAC, Canada and Agencies, Lester B. Pearson Papers, 1963–1965.

13 Anon., "PM, Wife Receive Gifts"; Anon., "PM Decrees." Negatives for official photos of the occasion are in LAC, Photograph Room, file 28, box 03764.1, negative sleeve 10385. The statue lived in the basement of the official residence at 22 Sussex Drive until Pierre Elliott Trudeau was defeated by Joe Clark in 1979. It now resides in storage at the Museum of History, accession no. 1979-026-001; its acquisition file contains photographs of it with the elder Trudeau. Thanks to Alan Elder, Elise Rowsome, and Sarah Smith for their help in locating it.

14 Anon., "Gift of Appreciation." See also photos with letter from L.A. Bourgeois to Dr Chute [Reid], Reid Papers, file 1.

15 Canada, Office of the Auditor General, *Report of the Auditor General*, 47.

16 Canada, *House of Commons Debates*, 26th Parliament, 2nd Session, 16 December 1964; Canada, *House of Commons Debates*, 27th Parliament, 1st Session, 4 April 1966.

17 Hacker, "Aku-Aku and Medicine Men"; Hacker, "Aku-Aku: L'expédition." The newspaper article likely appeared in January or February 1965, as the story was filed "from Easter Island." Only one clipping testifies to its existence, Hacker, "Revolt in the Easter Islands [*sic*]."

18 Montandon, "Μια Ελληνιδα Στο Νησί Του Πασχά."

19 Ekblom's article "Med testcykel till 'Världens Navel'" appeared in three parts in the leading Swedish newspaper, *Dagens Nyheter*, 9 May 1965.

20 Rapa Nui Science Club, *Newsletter*, 28 April and 21 May 1965, UBC Archives, Efford Papers, METEI, box 1, file 2.

21 Roger Belcourt to Reid, 13 December 1965, Reid Papers, file 15.

22 Reid to Skoryna, 19 May and 2 June 1965, Reid Papers, file 14, "Legal Hassles."

23 Hacker to Reid, 31 May 1965; Reid to Skoryna, 2 June 1965; Skoryna to Reid, 2 and 4 June 1965; Laing to Reid, 7 June 1965, Reid Papers, file 14.

24 Using the coded records of 312 adults and excluding child examinations, Cutler discovered that Helen Reid had examined 27.24 per cent, Maureen Roberts 24.03 per cent, Peter Beighton 22.75 per cent, Richard Roberts, 21.79 per cent, and David Murphy 2.56 per cent, the remainder being blank or marked "other." Cutler to Roberts, 20 April 1966, LAC, Roberts Papers, vol. 1, file 17, "Leprosy."

25 Reid to R.F. Laing, 8 June 1965, Reid Papers, file 14.

26 One-page sequence of events, Reid Papers, file 14. See also Reid Papers, "tape running," cover of file 9, "Manuscript."

27 R.F. Laing to Helen Reid, 7 June 1965, Reid Papers, file 14; "Considerations," McGill University Archives (MUA), RG 49, box 64, file 01372.

28 Reid to Skoryna, 19 May and 2 June 1965, Reid Papers, file 14; Reid, *All Silent*, 125.

29 Reid Papers, cover of file 9, "Manuscript."

30 Mary King to Reid, 27 October 1965, Reid Papers, file 5.

31 Boudreault to Reid, 2 February 1967, Reid Papers, file 8, "Easter Island Children."

32 Anon., "She Wrote a Book."

33 Hacker to Reid, nd, Reid Papers, file 8, "Easter Island Children."

34 Mydans to Law, 21 September 1965, LAC, Law Scrapbook, vol. 2, file 5.

35 On the contract with *Life* magazine, see Managing Editor Ralph Graves to Stanley Skoryna, 13 October 1964, MUA, RG 49, box 64, file 01375. In exchange for exclusivity, *Life* covered Mydans's expenses and donated $5,000 to METEI.

36 Mydans to Tunis, 18 July 1966, MUA, RG 49, box 64, file 01372.

37 For Carl Mydans's images of Easter Island and METEI, see http://images. google.com/hosted/life/d94762dd4951e679.html.

38 Reid, *World Away*, 91.

39 Hacker to Reid, nd, Reid Papers, file 8, "Easter Island Children."

40 Hacker to Reid, "Tuesday," [1966?], Reid Papers, file 5.

41 Hacker to Reid, nd, Reid Papers, file 8, "Easter Island Children."

42 Pratt, *Imperial Eyes*, 3.

43 Skoryna to Pearson, 7 October; R.H. Bélanger to Skoryna, 13 October 1965, LAC, Canada and Agencies, Lester B. Pearson Papers, 1963–1965.

44 Some are now collectors' curiosities. See item uploaded 15 November 2014 at the stamp collectors' website the Stamp Forum under "Canada: Cinderellas," http://thestampforum.boards.net/thread/1325/ canada-cinderellas?page=9.

45 Correspondence relating to these talks is in MUA, RG 2, box 293, file 10671.

46 "List of Invoices Not to Be Paid, According to Dr. Skoryna," MUA, RG 49, box 66, file 10436.

47 Skoryna to Law, 7 March 1966, LAC, Law Scrapbook, vol. 2, "Correspondence."

48 Skoryna, "Operation METEI."

49 Reid Papers, file 11.

50 Anon., "Free Trip to Easter Island," advertisement, 640, published with Hacker, "Aku-Aku and Medicine Men."

51 Rapa Nui Science Club, *Newsletter*, 12 January 1967, UBC Archives, Efford Papers, METEI, box 1, file 2; Anon., "Winners Fly."

52 "List of Invoices Not to Be Paid, According to Dr. Skoryna," MUA, RG 49, box 66, file 10436.

53 Bob Williams to Helen Reid, 25 August 1965, Reid Papers, file 10.

54 Beighton to Nielsen, 18 September 1965, Nielsen Papers.

55 Easter Island Expedition Foundation, "Statement of Cash Receipts and Disbursements," 1966, MUA, RG 2, box 293, file 10671.

56 CBC, Williams, and Hrischenko, *Canadian Expedition to Easter Island*. I thank Darren Yearsley of the CBC Archives and Barry B. Smith of the Nova Scotia Archives for making this film available.

57 Williams to Reid, 31 August 1965, Reid Papers, file 10.

58 NFB and Lemieux, *Island Observed*. In 2015 this film was uploaded from
    Rapa Nui to YouTube at https://www.youtube.com/watch?v=4Xox
    PDkJAzc.

59 Hacker to Reid, "Tuesday," [1966?], Reid Papers, file 5.

60 Griffiths to Reid, 6 December 1965, Reid Papers, file 15; Rapa Nui
    Science Club, *Newsletter*, 27 October 1966, UBC Archives, Efford Papers,
    METEI, box 1, file 2.

CHAPTER TEN: THE SCIENTIFIC PAPERS BEGIN

1   Beighton, "Easter Island People."

2   Weiner, "Report of the Convener," 28. Karl Lange Andersen was men-
    tioned in this report.

3   Holdsworth, "Preliminary Study."

4   The collections of Efford and Mathias are acknowledged in the following
    works published between 1965 and 1978: Allen, "Two New Species";
    Caldwell and Randall, "*Cantherhines tiki*"; Fell, "Echinoids of Easter
    Island"; Greenfield and Hensley, "Damselfishes"; Kami, "New Subgenus";
    Kevan, "Orthopteroid Insects"; Kohn, "Ecological Shift"; Mason,
    "Endemic Subspecies"; Mockford, "Psocoptera Records"; Randall,
    "Endemic Shore Fishes"; Randall and Caldwell, "New Butterfly Fish";
    Shewell, "Two Records of Agromyzidae"; Wells, "Notes on Indo-Pacific";
    and Wilson, "Ants of Easter Island."

5   The catalogue numbers of the Rapa Nui fish at the Beaty Museum are
    UBC 650400, 650461, 650820-21, and 650823. Special thanks to Don
    McPhail and Eric Taylor of the University of British Columbia for helping
    to locate them.

6   Gibbs, "Survey."

7   Boulanger, Gibbs, and Murphy, "Serological Survey."

8   Meerovitch and Gibbs, "Intestinal Parasitic Infections."

9   On Kevan, see Vickery, "D. Keith McE. Kevan." Special thanks to
    Stéphanie Boucher of the Lyman Museum for tracking down these insects
    of Rapa Nui.

10 Kevan, "Orthopteroid Insects."

11 Mason, "Endemic Subspecies"; Shewell, "Two Records of Agromyzidae."

12 Mockford, "Psocoptera Records"; Wilson, "Ants of Easter Island."

13 Ajello and Alpert, "Survey of Easter Island Soils."

14 Taylor, "Medical Expedition"; Taylor, "Dental Health."

15 Reid to Robertson, 20 November 1967, McGill University Archives
    (MUA), RG 2, box 340, file 12524; Bob Meier, personal communication,
    19 November 2015. I thank Arleyn Simon, Christopher Stojanovksi, and

Gary Schwartz of Arizona State University, who, in late November 2015, confirmed the presence of these casts in their collection.

16 Turner, "Life and Times," 23.

17 Hermansen and Ekblom, "Physical Fitness."

18 Andersen, "Ethnic Group Differences."

19 Shephard, "Proceedings."

20 Ekblom and Gjessing, "Maximal Oxygen Uptake."

21 Weiner, "Foreword," ix-x. In Shephard, *Human Physiological Work Capacity*, the work of Ekblom and Gjessing is cited and compared to other groups: maximal heart rate (45), aerobic power (66–7), height-weight ratios in children (196–7), and maximum O_2 uptake in children (214).

22 Hacker to Reid, 12 August 1967, Reid Papers, file 10.

23 Alice E. Johannson to G.A. Wilkinson, 13 October 1965, Wilkinson Papers.

24 Fraser to Dr J. Gilbert Turner, Executive Director, 12 April 1965, Wilkinson Papers, "Lectures."

25 Fraser to Wilkinson, 24 February 1966, Wilkinson Papers, "Lectures."

26 CBC, Williams, and Hrischenko, *Canadian Expedition to Easter Island*, part 1, narrator at 14 mins, 14 secs (Reid); part 2, Roberts at 10 mins, 17 secs (Fraser).

27 Reid to Wilkinson, 13 April, 12 July, 20 September, and 4 December 1965; Reid to Fraser, 29 October and 6 November 1965; Fraser to Reid, 4 November and 4 December 1965; Wilkinson to Reid, 1 December 1965, Wilkinson Papers.

28 G. Archibald Wilkinson, "Easter Island Radiological Survey," Wilkinson Papers.

29 G. Archibald Wilkinson, "Easter Island Radiological Survey," Library and Archives Canada (LAC), Roberts Papers, vol. 2, file 18.

30 Reid to Cutler, 8 September 1966, 22 January, 13 February, and 10 April 1967; Cutler to Reid, 23 June and 14 September 1966, 22 February and 18 April 1967; Reid to Roberts, 4 March 1967, Reid Papers, file 13.

31 Reid to William Gruelich, 1 April 1967; Gruelich to Reid, 20 June 1967, Reid Papers, file 16; Greulich and Pyle, *Radiographic Atlas*.

32 Reid Papers, file 13.

33 Reid, "Physical Development."

34 Reid Diary, 17 December 1964 (weaning), undated loose paper with names and ages (onset of menstruation). See also Reid to Cutler, 13 February and 10 April 1967, Reid Papers, file 13.

35 Roberts to John [Cutler], 22 April 1968, LAC, Roberts Papers, vol. 1, file 5.

36 Roberts to John [Cutler], 23 January 1968; Roberts to John [Cutler], 22 April 1968, LAC, Roberts Papers, vol. 1, files 4 and 5.

37 LAC, Roberts Papers, vol. 1, file 7.

38 Libby McKean, "Women We Meet Show Appreciation with Shell Necklaces," unidentified clipping [Halifax *Mail Star?*], LAC, Roberts Papers, vol. 2, file 22.

39 Gray, "Profiles: Maureen Roberts."

40 Cutler to Roberts, 22 April 1966, LAC, Roberts Papers, vol. 1, file 17, "Leprosy"; Wilkinson to Roberts, 9 May 1966, and short "Radiological Observations," Wilkinson Papers. The report was sent to Roberts, Nógrády, and Skoyrna but was never published. See also Wilkinson's full "Radiological Survey," LAC, Roberts Papers, vol. 2, file 18, and Wilkinson Papers.

41 Roberts, "Results of the Easter Island Expedition," 16. This speech was repeated almost verbatim in Toronto for a symposium in April 1969 (see chapter 12).

42 H.E. Lewis to Roberts, 7 June 1966, LAC, Roberts Papers, vol. 1, file 4. See also Zamel et al., "Asthma on Tristan da Cunha."

43 Roberts, "Results of the Easter Island Expedition," 8.

44 Correspondence with CMAJ editors, 1958, LAC, Roberts Papers, vol. 2, file 7.

45 Anderson and Godden, "Ninety-Ninth Annual Meeting of the CMA," 236.

46 Reid, "Physical Development."

47 Roberts, "Report on the Easter Island Medical Expedition."

48 Cutler to Roberts, 20 April 1966, LAC, Roberts Papers, vol. 1, file 17, "Leprosy."

49 See Cruz-Coke, "Ecología humana"; Cruz-Coke, "Estudios biomédicos"; Nagel, Etcheverry, and Guzman, "Haptoglobin Types"; and Valdés et al., "Factores."

50 Blackburn to Cutler, 29 June 1966, LAC, Roberts Papers, vol. 1, file 14. See also Blackburn to Cutler, 11 February 1966; and Cutler to Blackburn, 14 February 1966, LAC, Roberts Papers, vol. 1, file 4.

51 Reid to Roberts, 30 May 1966, LAC, Roberts Papers, vol. 1, file 22.

52 On these methods, see Hagelberg, "Genetic Affinities"; Hagelberg et al., "DNA from Ancient Easter Islanders"; and Hirschhorn, "Recent Advances."

53 See, for example, Nagel, Etcheverry, and Guzman, "Haptoglobin Types"; and Simmons and Graydon, "Blood Group Genetical Survey." See also Hagelberg, "Genetic Affinities."

54 Métraux, *Ethnology*, 25–6.

55 Shapiro, "Distribution of Blood Groups." On Father Sebastian's likely encounter with anthropologist Harry L. Shapiro in New York City in late 1968, see Dos Passos, *Easter Island*, 3–5. On Shapiro, the yacht *Zaca*,

and its owner, Templeton Crocker, see Anderson, "Hybridity, Race, and Science."

56 Simmons and Graydon, "Blood Group Genetical Survey."

57 Ibid.

58 In this expedition, samples came from "36 'pure natives,' and 126 'admixed.'" Nagel, Etcheverry, and Guzman, "Haptoglobin Types"; Cruz-Coke, "Ecología humana."

59 Cruz-Coke, "Ecología humana"; Etcheverry, "Blood Groups."

60 Heyerdahl, *Aku-Aku*, 296, 358–9.

61 Myhre, "Blood Groups."

62 Skoryna to Roberts, 4 October 1963, LAC, Roberts Papers, vol. 1, file 1.

63 Nancy E. Simpson to Maureen Roberts, 21 January 1965, LAC, Roberts Papers, vol. 1, file 15.

64 "Genealogy," LAC, Roberts Papers, vol. 1, files 15 and 16.

65 Simpson to Maureen Roberts, 12 December 1966, LAC, Roberts Papers, vol. 1, file 4.

66 Simpson, "Genetics of Esterases."

67 Berg and Bearn, "Inherited X-Linked Serum System"; Berg and Bearn, "Common X-Linked Serum Marker."

68 Maureen Roberts to Alexander G. Bearn, [1965]; Kari Berg to Maureen Roberts, 4 April 1966, LAC, Roberts Papers, vol. 1, files 3 and 4.

69 Hacker to Reid, 12 August 1967, Reid Papers, file 10.

70 Conway and Ross, "Easter Island Families."

71 Maureen Roberts to Denton, 30 May 1966, LAC, Roberts Papers, vol. 1, file 4.

72 Denton to Bearn, 6 June 1966, LAC, Roberts Papers, vol. 1, file 4.

73 Skoryna to Roberts, 27 February 1967, LAC, Roberts Papers, vol. 1, file 4.

74 Hacker to Reid, 12 August [1967?], Reid Papers, file 10.

75 Meier to Roberts, 20 October 1968, LAC, Roberts Papers, vol. 1, file 5.

76 Denton to Maureen Roberts, 7 November 1968, LAC, Roberts Papers, vol. 1, file 5.

77 Roberts to Joyce, 12 November 1968, LAC, Roberts Papers, vol. 1, file 5.

78 Joyce to Roberts, 8 December 1968, LAC, Roberts Papers, vol. 1, file 5.

79 Mustard to Roberts, 5 June 1967; Roberts to Mustard, 9 June 1967, LAC, Roberts Papers, vol. 1, file 5.

80 Roberts to Cutler, 9 June 1967, LAC, Roberts Papers, vol. 1, file 5.

81 Mustard to Roberts, 14 June 1967, LAC, Roberts Papers, vol. 1, file 5.

82 Cutler annotation on Roberts's copy of Cutler to Mustard, 7 July 1967, LAC, Roberts Papers, vol. 1, file 5.

83 Reid to Robertson, 20 November 1967, MUA, RG 2, box 340, file 12524.

84 Skoryna to Robertson, 8 December 1967, MUA, RG 2, box 340, file 12524.

85 Skoryna to Robertson, 8 December 1967; Robertson to Reid, 1 February 1968, MUA, RG 2, box 340, file 12524.

86 Roberts, "Results of the Easter Island Expedition," 10–11.

87 Tabulation of results, LAC, Roberts Papers, vol. 1, file 12, "Tabulations: Haptoglobins; Urines; ECGs."

88 Cutler to Roberts, [ca. 12 January 1968], LAC, Roberts Papers, vol. 1, file 17.

89 Roberts, "Easter Island Expedition."

90 Meier, "Medical Expedition"; Meier, "Easter Islander"; Meier "Review."

91 Meier, "Dermatoglyphics of Easter Islanders"; Meier, "Penrose Analysis"; Meier, "Sequential Developmental Components"; Goodson and Meier, "Topological Description"; Goodson and Meier, "Easter Islander"; Meier and Jamison, "Relationship."

92 Cléopâtre Montandon, "Ile de Pâques: Un cas de changement social," [1967?], LAC, Roberts Papers, vol. 2, file 20.

93 Montandon, "Development of Science."

94 Montandon, "Easter Island."

95 Montandon and Nógrády, "Map Indicating Houses"; Alpert, Nógrády, and Montandon, "Staphylococcus Sampling Map."

CHAPTER ELEVEN:
VIROLOGY, PSYCHOLOGY, AND RETURN VISITS

1 Peter Beighton to R. Roberts, [between May and July 1965], Library and Archives Canada (LAC), Roberts Papers, vol. 1, file 3.

2 Rosenberg, "Pathologies of Progress."

3 Mona Wilson to Dr Roberts, 6 January 1965 [1966]; Mona Wilson to Dr Roberts and Mr Mydans, 4 March 1966 ("on the high seas en route to Valparaiso"), LAC, Roberts Papers, vol. 1, file 4. On Mona Wilson (1884–1981), see Baldwin, "Interconnecting the Personal."

4 Efford to Reid, 5 January 1966, 22 January 1967, Reid Papers, file 15.

5 Ian Efford, email correspondence, 28 January 2016.

6 "Easter Island Manuscript," nd, University of British Columbia (UBC) Archives, Efford Papers, METEI, box 1, file 4.

7 Skoryna to Efford, 14 November 1966; Efford to John E. Randall, 8 April 1968; Randall to Efford, 13 April 1968, UBC Archives, Efford Papers, METEI, box 1, file 1.

8 Boudreault, Pavilanis, and Chagnon, "Répartition des anticorps neutralisant"; Boudreault, Pavilanis, and Podoski, "Répartition des anticorps inhibiteurs."

9   Chagnon and Pavilanis, "Incidence of Rubella"; Chagnon and Pavilanis, "Epidemiological Studies."

10 Boudreault and Pavilanis, "Epidémiologie."

11 Embil et al., "Prevalence of Cytomegalovirus Infection"; Haldane, Embil, and Wall, "Serological Study"; Haldane and Embil, "Comparative Epidemiology."

12 Riley, "History of the Cytomegalovirus"; Ho, "History of Cytomegalovirus."

13 Armand Boudreault, personal communication, 13 January 2017. On his techniques, see Armand Boudreault, "Comments on the Technical Facilities of Sample Preservation during the Expedition," LAC, Roberts Papers, vol. 2, file 16.

14 Anon., "Informations épidémiologiques," 241.

15 Reid, "Physical Development," 196.

16 Boudreault and Pavilanis, "Epidémiologie," 404, my translation.

17 Skoryna to Frappier, 23 February 1967 (annotation), Archives de l'Institut national de recherche scientifique (INRS), Vézina Papers. On the INRS-Institut Armand-Frappier, see Malissard, "Les 'Start-Ups.'"

18 Katz, "Measles Elimination."

19 Macey et al., "Rubella Elimination."

20 Skoryna to Roberts, 27 February 1967, LAC, Roberts Papers, vol. 1, file 4.

21 Gerd Hurum to J.E. Murhee, Mechanical Equipment Company New Orleans, 8 March 1967, McGill University Archives (MUA), RG 49, box 64, file 01375.

22 Tuki, "Historia de la 'Ley Pascua.'"

23 Fischer, Island, 217.

24 Grifferos A., "Entre palos e piedras."

25 Stambuk, Iorana.

26 Rapa Nui Science Club, Newsletter, 18 August 1967, UBC Archives, Efford Papers, METEI, box 1, file 2.

27 Flint, "Expedition Fulfills Women's Dream."

28 Boudreault and Pavilanis, "Epidémiologie," 404.

29 Borgoño and Corey, "Chilean Experience"; De Quadros et al., "Eradication of Wild Poliovirus"; Laval R., "Anotaciones."

30 Georges Nógrády, "General Informations and Medical Problems on Easter Island," LAC, Roberts Papers, vol. 2, file 19.

31 Fischer, Island, 221; Stambuk, Iorana, 96.

32 David, "And Christmas Day."

33 Rapa Nui Science Club, Newsletter, 12 January 1967, UBC Archives, Efford Papers, METEI, box 1, file 2.

34 Press release, nd, LAC, Roberts Papers, vol. 1, file 6.

35 June Pimm, "Developmental Trends in an Isolated Culture," unpublished article, Pimm Papers.

36 Macfarlane, "Prosperity in Easter Island."

37 Herzog and Saulnier, "Les mystères"; Fischer, *Island*, 207.

38 Mulloy, "Foreword," 12; Rapa Nui Science Club, *Newsletter*, 28 August 1967, UBC Archives, Efford Papers, METEI, box 1, file 2; Dos Passos, *Easter Island*, 194.

39 Garry Brody, email correspondence with author and eight METEI alumni, 18 January 2016.

CHAPTER TWELVE:
NÓGRÁDY'S LEGACY AND A WONDER DRUG

1 Reid Diary, 29 December 1964.

2 Nógrády, "Easter Island Stone Basins."

3 Reid Diary, nd, 98.

4 Georges Nógrády, "Reports or Papers Delivered or Published by the Contributors of the Medical Expedition to Easter Island," [ca. 1969], Library and Archives Canada (LAC), Roberts Papers, vol. 1, file 6; Reid Papers, file 5. See also note 18 below.

5 Nógrády to Reid, 1 and 18 December 1965, Reid Papers, file 15.

6 Nógrády to Law, [ca. May 1972], LAC, Law Scrapbook, vol. 2, file 4.

7 Nógrády to Richard and Maureen [Roberts], 3 December 1966, with typewritten list titled "Comparison of Polynesian-Maori Words with Similar Hungarian Words, Based on Uxbond, 1928," LAC, Roberts Papers, vol. 2, file 2. Eighty-four pages of symbols from *rongorongo* script blown up to a size of 8 by 10 inches that Nógrády sent to the Robertses are in LAC, Roberts Papers, vol. 1, file 26.

8 Nógrády to Richard and Maureen Roberts, 20 June 1978, LAC, Roberts Papers, vol. 2, file 4. The unnamed Macfarlane Burnet book was likely his gloomy *Endurance of Life: The Implications of Genetics for Human Life* (1979). Based on studies of genetics and aging, Burnet endorsed euthanasia and abortion, but public opinion likened these "eugenicist" views to Adolf Hitler. Even more controversial had been Burnet's *Genes, Dreams, and Realities* (1971), in which he claimed that major discoveries in biological sciences had peaked and that the modest gains in coping with "intrinsic disease" were offset by the rise of the diseases of civilization: lung cancer, coronary artery disease, road accidents, alcoholism, and drug addiction.

9 Georges Nógrády, "General Informations and Medical Problems on Easter Island," LAC, Roberts Papers, vol. 2, file 19.

10 The Nógrády-Toutant paper appears on Nógrády's list but not in the abstracts of the papers read at the annual meeting of the ACFAS for 1966 or any other year. Either the paper was rejected, or it was a last-minute add-on to the program. Georges Nógrády, "Reports or Papers Delivered or Published by the Contributors of the Medical Expedition to Easter Island," [ca. 1969], LAC, Roberts Papers, vol. 1, file 6.

11 Nógrády and Fredette, *Catalogue des films microbiologiques*; Nógrády, *L'effet de la toxine staphylococcique*; Nógrády, *Effects of Streptomycin*. The latter two items are films in the library of the Université de Montréal.

12 Georges Nógrády, "Soil Specimens," abstract, LAC, Roberts Papers, vol. 1, file 21. The Culture Collection in Lausanne closed in the 1990s; the lyophilized strains were preserved, but the archive holds no record of Nógrády's gift. I thank Silvano Landert, Dr Guy Prod'hom, and Professor Gilbert Greub for conducting this search.

13 On Paul Hauduroy, see the biographical sketch that accompanies the description of his papers, which entered the Archives Cantonales Vaudoises by happy accident in 2011, following their discovery in the hands of a *brocanteur*. See http://www.davel.vd.ch/qfpdavel/o/D4403.pdf.

14 Lapage, "World Federation"; Uruburu, "History and Services."

15 List of delegates, in Martin, ed., *Culture Collections*.

16 "Camille Guérin," Nobel Prize Nomination Database, http://www.nobelprize.org/nomination/archive/show.php?id=12517.

17 Canetti et al. "Mycobacteria." On Canada's experience, see Bernier, *Médecine et idéologies*, 89–93; Feldberg, *Disease and Class*, 158–65; and Malissard, "La controverse."

18 Nógrády to Recteur R. Gaudry, 22 January 1968, with "Progress Report of the Ulterior Work on Mycology, Bacteriology, Immunology, Dental Caries, and Sample Preservation," 20 December 1967, 5 pages, Archives de l'Université de Montréal. A copy of this same report was sent to Tony Law, LAC, Law Scrapbook, vol. 2, file 7. For other "editions," see note 4 above. I thank Professor Hugo Soudeyns for his interest and help in tracing this document.

19 The text of this speech might be Nógrády's undated, ten-page paper "General Informations and Medical Problems on Easter Island," LAC, Roberts Papers, vol. 2, file 19.

20 Upjohn Company, "1973 Price List," http://www.upjohn.net/catalog/1973/1973price.htm; Upjohn Company, "Timeline," http://www.upjohn.net/corporate/timeline/timeline.htm.

21 Griffith, "Introduction to Vancomycin"; Griffith, "Vancomycin Use"; Levine, "Vancomycin"; Moellering, "Vancomycin."

22 Hilliard, "Keith John Roy Wightman."

23 Nógrády, ed., *Symposium of the Medical Expedition*. See also UBC Archives, Efford Papers, METEI, box 1, file 1.

24 Nógrády to Roberts, 20 January 1969, LAC, Roberts Papers, vol. 2, file 11.

25 Skoryna, "Objectives."

26 Roberts, "Health and Hygienic Conditions"; Richard Roberts, "The Health and Hygienic Conditions of the Easter Islanders, 1964–65," typescript, 12 pages, LAC, Roberts Papers, vol. 2, file 10, "Speeches."

27 Reid to Boudreault, 7 April 1969, Reid Papers, file 5.

28 Drapkin, "Reminiscences of Medical Experience." On Drapkin, see Fischer, *Island*, 187–9; and Landau and Sebba, eds, *Criminology in Perspective*.

29 Möller-Christensen, "Osteological and Pathological Survey."

30 Nógrády, "Planning and Execution of the Antibiosis Project."

31 Nógrády, Dionne, and Morin, "Planning and Execution of Mycobacteria Project."

32 Anon., "Edith Marion Mankiewicz"; Anon., "Edith Mankiewicz"; McArthur, "Edith Marion Mankiewicz."

33 Mankiewicz, "Antibodies."

34 Magnusson, "Comparison of Virus."

35 Toranzo, Barja, and Hetrick, "Antiviral Activity."

36 Claude Vézina, "Curriculum Vitae," ca. 1982, Archives de l'Institut national de recherche scientifique (INRS), Vézina Papers.

37 Vézina, "Antimicrobial Activity."

38 Lehmann to Roberts, LAC, Roberts Papers, vol. 2, file 11.

39 Nógrády had written in advance to Kenneth F. Girard, acting director of diagnostic laboratories in the Massachusetts Department of Public Health, advising him about the display and hoping that they might meet. Girard replied politely with apologies for not meeting, but he let Georges know that he and his wife had visited his "fascinating exhibit." Girard had studied at McGill in the 1950s. Girard to Nógrády, 7 May 1970, LAC, Roberts Papers, vol. 1, file 6.

40 Minneapolis "is the most attractive American city [I] ever saw. Completely a different world. Charming individuals, polished people everywhere, all official, in brand new, uniform, simple, energetic management." Nógrády to Cléo and Denys [Montandon], 2 July 1971, Montandon Papers; Nógrády to Roberts, 10 March 1981, LAC, Roberts Papers, vol. 1, file 6. I thank Jeff Kerr of the American Society for Microbiology for confirming Nógrády's paper at the 1981 conference.

41 Nógrády to Cléo and Denys [Montandon], 2 July 1971, Montandon Papers.

42 Ibid.

43 Ibid.

44 Ibid.

45 For the authors and contents of the 1974 volume, as listed in the Bibliography, see appendix A, section 2.

46 Feinstein, "Pablo Neruda Poisoning"; Semeniuk, "Researchers Hope"; Bonnefoy, "Cancer Didn't Kill."

47 Kevan, "Orthopteroid Insects."

48 Routledge, *Mystery*, 210; Heyerdahl, *Aku-Aku*, 129–30.

49 Nógrády to Law, 8 December 1975 and 12 January 1976; Georges Nógrády, "Entomomicrobiology: Discussions and Recommendations," LAC, Law Scrapbook, vol. 2, file 3.

50 Routledge, *Mystery*, 218, 240–1; Owsley et al., "Demographic Analysis."

51 Knowledge of this unpublished presentation came from one of Nógrády's bibliographical lists (see notes 4 and 18 above); however, Bob Meier had a copy of the poster and kindly provided it. I thank him and Jerome Cybulski, who remembers supervising the making of the plastic cast. I also thank Annamária Bárány, zoologist at the Hungarian National Museum in Budapest, for confirming the presence and provenance of the sculptures, and Ontario coroner Dr Dirk Huyer.

52 Gill and Stefan, "Descriptive Skeletal Biology." Reconstructed faces from paleopathological material, amplified by genetics, are featured in the Canadian History Hall of the Museum of History, which opened in July 2017, and in a documentary featuring this technique, *The First Brit: Secrets of the 10,000 Year Old Man*, aired on Britain's Channel 4 in February 2018.

53 Nógrády to Roberts, 10 March and 19 May 1981, LAC, Roberts Papers, vol. 1, file 6. See also LAC, Roberts Papers, vol. 2, file 15, "Correspondence re Vol. 2 Microbiology Proceedings."

54 Nógrády to Roberts, 10 March 1981, LAC, Roberts Papers, vol. 1, file 6.

55 Nógrády to Roberts, 27 August 1981, LAC, Roberts Papers, vol. 2, file 15.

56 Roberts to Nógrády, 3 September 1981; Nógrády to Roberts, 19 September 1981, LAC, Roberts Papers, vol. 2, file 15.

57 For the titles of these bilingual abstracts in Roberts's papers, see appendix A, section 3. As listed in the Bibliography, they are authored by A. Boudreault (U Montréal), W.A. Clark (Rockville, Maryland), R.G. Fitzgerald (VA Hospital, Miami), H.C. Gibbs (Macdonald College, McGill), D.G. Ingram (Ontario Veterinary College, Guelph), J.M. Jablon (U Miami), F. Scott (Loon Lake, Saskatchewan), F. Tanner (Lausanne, Switzerland), J.C. Wilt (U Manitoba); A. Taylor (CFB Chilliwack, British Columbia); and I. Zipkin (U California).

58 Roberts, "Presentation Number 20," "Presentation Number 24," "Presentation Number 37," and "Kokongo Epidemic."

59 Zipkin, "Fluoride Exposure."

60 Brydon and MacLean, "Examination of Some Soil Samples."

61 Nógrády to Roberts, 10 March 1981, LAC, Roberts Papers, vol. 1, file 6.

62 On Sehgal, see Canadian Society of Transplantation, "In Memoriam"; and Sehgal, "Surendra Nath Sehgal." I am grateful to his widow, Uma Sehgal, and son, Ajai, for their memories.

63 On Gibbons, see Murray, "Contributor to Systemic Bacteriology."

64 Examples are US Patent No. 3,929,992, 1975; Canada Patent No. 1,000,631, 1976; and British Patent No. 1,436,447, 1976. Claude Vézina, "Curriculum Vitae," Archives de INRS, Vézina Papers.

65 Vézina, Kudelski, and Sehgal, "Rapamycin"; Sehgal, Baker, and Vézina, "Rapamycin."

66 Garber, "Rapamycin's Resurrection"; Sehgal, "Story of Rapamune."

67 Baker et al., "Rapamycin"; Eng, Sehgal, and Vézina, "Activity of Rapamycin"; Singh, Sun, and Vézina, "Rapamycin."

68 Swindells, White, and Findlay, "X-Ray Crystal Structure."

69 Findlay and Radics, "On the Chemistry."

70 Martel, Klicius, and Galet, "Inhibition of the Immune Response."

71 Sehgal, quoted in Garber, "Rapamycin's Resurrection."

72 Houchens et al., "Human Brain Tumor"; Broome et al., "Biochemical and Biological Effects."

73 Eng, Sehgal, and Vézina, "Activity of Rapamycin."

74 Letters of application, offer, and acceptance, Archives de INRS, Vézina Papers.

75 Gifford, "Does a Real Anti-Aging Pill?" The exclusivity of *Streptomyces hygroscopicus* to Rapa Nui may have been overblown; Sehgal once told transplant surgeon Vivian McAlister that he had found "an even more potent source of rapamycin in soil taken from the woods behind his house in Princeton." Vivian McAlister, personal communication, 18 August 2018.

76 Garry Brody, email correspondence, 29 August 2017.

77 Sehgal, "Sirolimus."

78 Brown et al., "Mammalian Protein"; Heitman, Movva, and Hall, "Targets for Cell-Cycle Arrest."

79 Bjornsti and Houghton. "TOR Pathway."

80 Gifford, "Does a Real Anti-Aging Pill?"; Herald, *Beyond Human*, 172–3; Tector, "Delightful Revolution." See also Das, "Pharma Companies Switch Gears."

81 US Department of Justice, Office of Public Affairs, "Wyeth Pharmaceuticals Agrees to Pay."

82 Sorkin and Wilson, "Pfizer Agrees to Pay."

83 Hoy, "Living with Lymphangioleiomyomatosis."

84 Jeff Kerr of the ASM Center for the History of Microbiology explains that a record is kept only of those delegates reading papers: Sehgal spoke in 1978 and Nógrády in 1981.

85 Sehgal, "Surendra Nath Sehgal."

CHAPTER THIRTEEN: FORGETTING METEI AND THE IBP

1 Ambassador Glen Buick to Allan E. Gottlieb, Undersecretary of State for External Affairs, 20 January 1981, Library and Archives Canada (LAC), Department of External Affairs, Health Research Canada with Other Countries, RG 25-A-3-C, vol. 16954, file 46-11-1-Easter Island.

2 Stebbins, "International Biological Program," 768, 770; Appel, *Shaping Biology*, 226; Aronova, Baker, and Oreskes, "Big Science and Big Data."

3 Hildes, "Circumpolar People."

4 Collins and Weiner, *Human Adaptability*, 7–9.

5 Weiner, "Report of the Convener."

6 Beighton, "Easter Island People."

7 A search through the CCIBP papers in Library and Archives Canada did not permit identification of the missing HA projects, although it revealed other projects and personnel. LAC, National Research Council – International Biological Program, 1967–68, MG 28-I-79, vol. 143, file 2.

8 Hayes, *Chaining of Prometheus*.

9 CCIBP, *Canadian Participation*.

10 Shephard, *Human Physiological Work Capacity*, 8–10, 36–47, 66–77, 196–7, 214.

11 Roy J. Shephard, email correspondence, 13 March 2016.

12 Simpson, "Genetics of Esterases."

13 CCIBP, *Summary*; Simpson, "Polyacrylamide Electrophoresis," which is article no. 155 in CCIBP, *Collected Reprints of Scientific Papers*, vol. 5.

14 Collins and Weiner, *Human Adaptability*, 69–77.

15 Worthington, ed., *Evolution of IBP*, 166–7.

16 Cook, "IBP – Internationally and Nationally."

17 Appel, *Shaping Biology*, 263. On CCIBP funding for each section, see Cook, "IBP – Internationally and Nationally."

18 CCIBP, *Organization and Activities*. See also Cook, "Overview," 1.

19 Roberts to John [Cutler], 23 January 1968, LAC, Roberts Papers, vol. 1, file 5.

20 Cameron and Billingsley, eds, *Energy Flow*.

21 Efford and Hall, "Marion Lake"; Hughes, "International Study of Eskimos"; Demirjian et al., "Somatic Growth of Canadian Children." Registered but unreported projects appeared in an appendix to Cameron and Billingsley, eds, *Energy Flow*. Could the latter two have been the missing HA-2 and HA-4 projects?

22 CCIBP, *Collected Reprints of Scientific Papers*, vol. 5.

23 Cook, "IBP – Internationally and Nationally." This information also comes from the acknowledgments in the various publications.

24 Nelson G. Hairston, quoted in Appel, *Shaping Biology*, 265. See also Hagen, *Entangled Bank*, 169–72.

25 Collins and Weiner, *Human Adaptability*.

26 On the IBP's role in formation of the Man and the Biosphere Programme, see Schleper, "Conservation Compromises." See also Greenaway, *Science International*, 134, 182, 186, 195; and UNESCO, "Man and the Biosphere Programme."

27 Bridgewater, "Man and the Biosphere Programme"; Cuetos and Palmer, *Medicine and Public Health*, 153–6; Dayala, "Islands at a Glance"; Ishwaran, "Diversity, Protected Areas"; Kwa, "Representations of Nature."

28 Macnamara, Mitchell, and Miles, "Study of Immunity to Rubella."

29 Physician-historian Erwin H. Ackerknecht captured this sentiment well. Around 1950, an awestruck clinician told him that he was a lucky man: all diseases would soon be wiped out, and the only professor left in the medical school would be the historian. Ackerknecht, *Therapeutics*, 2.

30 On Gajdusek, see Anderson, *Collectors of Lost Souls*.

31 Dorolle, "Old Plagues in the Jet Age."

32 The twenty-four volumes of the IBP synthesis series were republished in 2009 by Cambridge University Press; the list of titles can be found at http://www.cambridge.org/de/academic/subjects/life-sciences/series/international-biological-programme-synthesis-series?page=1.

33 The news item was Anon., "Health Survey." The two other articles, published in the *Bulletin of the World Health Organization* in 1968 and 1969 respectively, were Boudreault and Pavilanis, "Epidémiologie"; and Haldane, Embil, and Wall, "Serological Study." Thanks to Reynald Erard at the Archives of the WHO for helping with this search.

34 Elliot Alpert went on to conduct research in Uganda and to work at Massachusetts General Hospital in Boston before returning to Montreal as chief of medicine at the Jewish General Hospital. He retired as professor emeritus in 2009 and moved to California. Special thanks to Fern D. Charles and Dean David Eidelman of McGill's Faculty of Medicine for their help in trying to locate Dr Alpert.

35 Duffin, "Peter Beighton."

36 McArdle, Katch, and Katch, *Exercise Physiology*, lv-lvi.
37 I am grateful to Ambassador Alejandro Marisio Cugat, Rodrigo Meza Goto, and the late Elena Bornand of the Chilean embassy in Ottawa, as well as to Gail Paech of Associated Medical Services and to Brechin Group Incorporated. One digitized copy is in the Queen's University Archives. None of these entities whose contributions were essential to the project were recognized when the repatriation was described as the culmination of "two years' effort." See Chile, Servicio Nacional de Patrimonio Cultural, "Rapa Nui celebra," my translation. In fact, the return of the medical records came thirteen months after we informed Rapa Nui of their existence and of Georges Nógrády's hope to repatriate them (see chapter 14).
38 Salinas, "How the Chilean Coup"; Duran, "Chile"; Aguirre, *Something Fierce*; Westhead, "How Canada Helped."
39 Robertson to Frei, 17 February 1965, McGill University Archives (MUA), RG 49, box 66, file 10436.
40 Skoryna to Robertson, 29 October 1966; Stanley Skoryna, "Proposal Concerning the Transfer of the US Pavilion for International Biological Center for Data Transfer," 6 pages, MUA, RG 2, box 293, file 10671.
41 Skoryna and Waldron-Edward, eds, *Guidelines to Radiological Health*.
42 Marion Turner to Haidasz, 15 September 1969; Haidasz to Minister of National Revenue J.-P. Côté, 17 September 1969; Haidasz to Minister of Finance E. Benson, 18 September 1969; Benson to Haidasz, 22 September 1969; Haidasz to Skoryna, nd, with congratulations on charitable status approved on 3 October 1969; Penfield to Haidasz, 16 October 1969, LAC, Haidasz Papers.
43 Anon., "Scientists Seek"; Ham and Skoryna, "Generation of Amyloid A Protein"; Ham and Skoryna, "Cellular Defense."
44 Death notice of Halina Irene Skoryna, unidentified clipping, LAC, Law Scrapbook, vol. 3, "Clippings"; Maciej Matthew Syzmański, *Pamięta Remembers*, vol. 2, 152, online book originally at http://szymanski.biulpol. net/ja-jo/JA-JO_vol__2.pdf (accessed 23 July 2017) but now missing.
45 Skoryna to P.E. Trudeau, 3 March 1969, LAC, Haidasz Papers.
46 Roberts to John [Cutler], 23 January 1968, LAC, Roberts Papers, vol. 1, file 5.
47 On body-voyaging, see Ehrenberger, "Autopsy, Authority.".

CHAPTER FOURTEEN: METEI 2017

1 Fischer, *Island*, 236–54; Haun, *Inventing "Easter Island,"* xiii-xv; Seward, "Between 'Easter Island' and 'Rapa Nui.'"
2 Arthur, "Reclaiming Mana."

3 See, for example, Loret and Tanacredi, eds, *Easter Island*; Stefan and Gill, eds, *Skeletal Biology*.

4 Easter Island Statue Project, http://www.eisp.org.

5 García-Moro et al., "Epidemiological Transition."

6 Nógrády to Law, 5 May 1972, Library and Archives Canada (LAC), Law Scrapbook, vol. 2, "Notes Reports, Orders.

7 Tuki, "Historia de la 'Ley Pascua.'"

8 Edwards and Edwards, *When the Universe Was an Island*.

9 George Nógrády did not return to Easter Island and Surendra Nath Sehgal never went. Judith Hermann, personal communication, 25 January 2017; Uma and Ajai Sehgal (wife and son of Suren), personal communication, 12 July 2017. I have been unable to locate Bernard Le Duc, said by the Sehgals to have led Wyeth Pharmaceuticals' journey to Rapa Nui in 2001.

10 Tuki, "Historia de la 'Ley Pascua'"; Delsing, "Issues of Land."

11 Fuentes and Moreno Pakarati, "Towards a Characterization"; Foerster, Ramírez, and Moreno Pakarati, *Cartografía y Conflicto*.

12 Ramírez Aliaga, *Rapa Nui*, 4; UNESCO, Santiago Office, "Chile's Living Human Treasures."

13 On the skull of Hotu Matu'a, see Arthur, "Reclaiming Mana" 209–13; McCall, "End of the World"; Seward, "Between 'Easter Island' and 'Rapa Nui,'" 219; and Thomas and Mariani, "Le crâne de Hotu Matu'a."

14 Conteben, called tibione in the United States, was developed by the German Nobel laureate Gerhard Domagk. By 1970 a survey of more than 3,000 patients from eight countries on three continents had revealed the full extent of its gastric, cutaneous, and neurological side effects. Notwithstanding its toxicity, the drug is still available and is being reconsidered for treatment of resistant tuberculosis. Ahmad et al., "History of Drug Discovery," 2–3; Miller et al., "Second International Co-operative Investigation"; Anon., "Antileprosy Drugs"; Belardinelli and Morbidoni, "Recycling and Refurbishing"; Caminero et al., "Best Drug Treatment."

15 Nakadaira et al., "Concentration of Metals"; Errol L. Montgomery & Associates, Water Resource Consultants, *Condiciones hidrogeológicas*; Long, "Trouble in Paradise."

16 Alvarez, "Restoration on Rapa Nui"; Arzt and Mount, "Hepatotoxicity"; Fisher, "Trouble Festering in Paradise"; Gonschor, "Facing Land Challenges"; Gonschor, "Law as a Tool."

17 I have been unable to identify Motta or locate his report. He may have been Dr Célio Paula Motta, who was involved with the eradication of leprosy in Brazil and still living in 1990 but said to be deceased by 1998. Motta and Zuniga, "Time Trends"; Andrade et al., "Monitoring the

Elimination." See also Rodriguez Grunert, Castellazzi, and Ortlieb, "Estudio inmunológico."

18 Stambuk, *Iorana*.

19 Rosenberg, "Pathologies of Progress."

20 García-Moro et al., "Epidemiological Transition."

21 Reid Diary, nd., 101v-102.

22 Chile, Ministerio de Salud, "Estadísticas de Natalidad y Mortalidad."

23 World Health Organization, WHO *Weekly Epidemiological Record* 48, no. 4 (26 January 1973): 50; and 59, no. 22 (1 June 1984): 166, http://www.who.int/wer/archives/en/.

24 Fischer, *Island*, 248; Haoa Rapahango, *Leprosario*.

25 Stambuk, *Rongo*, 173–93; Seward, "Between 'Easter Island' and 'Rapa Nui.'"

26 Borgoño and Corey, "Chilean Experience"; De Quadros et al., "Eradication of Wild Poliovirus"; Laval R., "Anotaciones."

27 Anon., "Informations épidémiologiques," 241.

28 Chile, Comisión Nacional de SIDA-CONASIDA, "Caracterización epidemiológica"; Lugones Botell and Ramírez Bermúdez, "Infección por virus Zika"; Garcia et al., "Zika Virus."

29 Fernandez et al., "Detection of Dengue"; Canals et al., "Dinamica epidemiológica"; Fica et al., "Razones para recomendar la vacunación."

CONCLUSION

1 Wadhams, "Hudson-70."

2 Hayden, *When Nature Goes Public*.

3 Chicha, *Le mirage d'égalité*; Igartua, *Other Quiet Revolution*; Monnais and Wright, eds, *Doctors beyond Borders*; Sangster, "Polish 'Dionnes.'"

4 Hagelberg, "Genetic Affinities"; Fehren-Schmidt et al., "Genetic Ancestry."

5 Lock, "From Genetics to Postgenomics," 129–30. See also Lipphardt, "From 'Races' to 'Isolates'"; Meier, "Critique"; Nash, *Genetic Geographies*; Rheinberger and Müller-Wille, *The Gene*; Sussman, *Myth of Race*; Wade, *Troublesome Inheritance*; Widmer and Lipphardt, eds, *Health and Difference*, 1–6; and Yudell, *Race Unmasked*.

Bibliography

INTERVIEWS

I communicated with the people named below by letter, phone, Skype, email, and in person, sometimes many times, from May 2015 to April 2019. The unattributed quotations in this book are from those conversations.

METEI *Members and* HMCS Cape Scott

Beighton, Peter
Boudreault, Armand
Brody, Garry
Cutler (formerly Griffiths), Isabel
Efford, Ian
Ekblom, Björn
Fowler, Charles
Gibbs, Harold
Gjessing, Einar
Hall, Reid
Hellyer, Paul
Hrischenko, George
Mathias, John ("Jack")
Meier, Robert
Montandon, Cléopâtre and Denys
Murphy, David
Nielsen, James ("Jim")
Pimm, June
Westropp, Charles

Family Members, Friends, and Colleagues of the Deceased

Crosman, Harry: sons George and Bill Crosman; grandson Chris Crosman
Cutler, John: widow Isabel Cutler
Galley, Tom: son Tom Galley
Gillingham, Colin: widow Françoise Gillingham
Gillis, Channing: widow Mary Gillis; grandson Channing Guenther
Joyce, Fred: children Jim and Linda Joyce; son-in-law Ian Whitehouse
Manzer, Robert: son Robert Manzer; daughters Yvonne, Jackie, and Jennifer
Myhre, Eivind: son Professor Jan Eivind Myhre
Nógrády, Georges: Judith Hermann, Nógrády's friend and executrix;
    Dr Hugo Soudeyns, current head of Nógrády's department at the Université
    de Montréal
Reid, Helen: son Douglas Chute; daughter Judith Redfield
Roberts, Maureen and Richard: daughter Susan Roberts; sister Dr Vanora
    Haldane
Shephard, Roy J.: physiologist, University of Toronto
Simpson, Nancy E.: geneticist, Queen's University
Skoryna, Stanley C.: widow Jane Skoryna; son Christopher Skoryna;
    daughter-in-law Jean Skoryna; grandchildren Ana Maria Warren, Michael
    Burnley, Halina Skoryna, Mary Skoryna; friend Darlene Lake; nephew
    Wojtek Skoryna
Taylor, Al: widow May Taylor; friend Dr John Baumbrough
Tunis, Al: son Andrew Tunis
Wilkinson, G. Archibald: widow Sally Wilkinson; brother-in-law Tony Archer

HMCS Cape Scott *Crew*

The minister of veterans affairs refused to forward a request for information to
the Royal Canadian Navy members of METEI and their families, claiming that
informing them of my project would be an intrusion of their privacy. A complaint to the Office of the Privacy Commissioner of Canada did not help. Navy
veterans Reid Hall and Chez Walters, who sailed on HMCS *Cape Scott* to Rapa
Nui as teenagers, expressed their disappointment over that decision when they
learned of my project owing to publicity surrounding my lecture about METEI
in Halifax on 16 January 2019. I regret that the crew members' stories could
not be included here.

ARCHIVES

Public and Institutional Archives

American Philosophical Society (APS)
Peyton Rous Papers, Mss.B.R77, box 61.
Archives de l'Institut national de recherche scientifique (INRS), Montreal
Boudreault Papers.
Vézina Papers.
Archives de l'Université de Montréal
Boudreault Papers.
Library and Archives Canada (LAC)
Canada and Agencies, Lester B. Pearson Papers, 1963–1965, MG 26-N-3,
vol. 272, file 828, "WHO Easter Island."
Department of External Affairs, Health Research Canada with Other
Countries, RG 25-A-3-C, vol. 16954, file 46-11-1-Easter Island.
Haidasz, Stanley, Papers, R1273, vol. 1, file 8, "Easter Island Expedition."
Health Research Canada, Medical Expedition to Easter Island, RG 128, vol.
493.
Law, Charles Anthony Francis, Papers and Scrapbook, MG 30-E-260, vols 1,
2, and 3.
National Research Council, International Biological Programme, 1967–68,
MG 28-I-79, vols 143 and 211.
Photograph Room, file 28, box 03764.1, negative sleeve 10385, July 1965.
Roberts, Richard H., Papers, MG 31-G-26, vols 1 and 2.
Ships Logs, HMCS *Cape Scott* log books, RG 24, vol. 5532.
Wright, Dorothy, Papers (exec. assist. to president of MRC), RG 128, vol.
290, "Records."
McGill University Archives (MUA), Easter Island Expedition, 1963–68, 1979
Office of the Principal, RG 2, box 293, files 10669, 10670, 10671; RG 2, box
340, file 12524; RG 2, box 414, file 14413.
Board of Governors, RG 4, box 191, file 120; RG 4, box 538, file 12873.
Public Relations, RG 49, box 64, files 01372, 01374, 01375, 01376; RG 49,
box 66, file 10436.
Photographs, RG 49, box 426.
Municipalidad de Rapa Nui
Autorizacións de Sepultación en Cementerio Municipal de Isla de Pascua,
1998–2016.

Queen's University Archives
  Jacalyn Duffin Papers, file "METEI Records."
University of British Columbia (UBC) Archives
  Efford Papers, METEI, boxes 1, 2 (contains diary), and 3.
World Health Organization Archives

Private Archives, Papers, and Photographs

ATCO Company Archives, loaned by Debbie Taylor
Beighton Photographs, loaned by Peter Beighton, Cape Town, South Africa
Boudreault Photographs, loaned by Armand Boudreault
Brody Diary and Photographs, loaned by Garry Brody, Los Angeles, CA
Efford Photographs, loaned by Ian Efford (papers are in UBC Archives)
Joyce Photographs, loaned by Jim Joyce of Halifax, NS
Mathias Diary, loaned by Jack Mathias of Vancouver Island, BC
Meier Diary and Papers, loaned by Robert J. Meier of Bloomington, IN
Montandon Diary and Papers, loaned by Cléopâtre and Denys Montandon of
  Geneva, Switzerland
Moreno Pakarati, Cristián, "Las familias de Rapa Nui," genealogical database,
  Rapa Nui
Murphy Diary, Papers, and Photographs, loaned by David Murphy of Halifax, NS
Mydans Photographs at *Life* magazine historical websites, Time Inc., hosted by
  Google (e.g., http://images.google.com/hosted/life/a6a29aeea7699410.html;
  http://images.google.com/hosted/life/f79767c9c8f4f540.html)
Nielsen Papers and Photographs, loaned by James Neilsen of Clearwater, FL
Nógrády Photographs and Papers (medical records), loaned by Judith
  Hermann of Montreal, QC, George Demmer of Ottawa, ON, and Chilean
  Embassy, Ottawa, ON
Pimm Papers and Photographs, loaned by June Pimm of Ottawa, ON
Reid Diary, Papers, and Photographs, loaned by son Douglas Chute of
  Philadelphia, PA; daughter Judith Redfield of Columbia, MO; and grand-
  daughter Deborah Chute at family farm in Adjala-Tosorontio, ON
Wilkinson Papers, Photographs, and Audiotapes, loaned by widow Sally
  Wilkinson of Prescott, ON

SECONDARY SOURCES

Ackerknecht, Erwin H. *Therapeutics from the Primitives to the Twentieth
  Century*. New York: Hafner, 1973.
Aguirre, Carmen. *Something Fierce: Memoirs of a Revolutionary Daughter*.
  Toronto: Vintage, 2013.

Ahmad, Z., N.H. Makaya, and J. Grosset. "History of Drug Discovery: Early Evaluation Studies and the Lessons Learnt from Them." In Peter R. Donald and Paul D. Van Helden, eds, *Antituberculosis Chemotherapy*, 2–9. Basel: Karger Medical and Scientific Publishers, 2011.

Ajello, Libero, and Morton Elliot Alpert. "Survey of Easter Island Soils for Keratinophilic Fungi." *Mycologia* 64, no. 1 (1972): 161–6.

Allard, Desmond. "5,000 Mile Gap Is Bridged by Telephone Hookup." *Montreal Star*, 28 December 1964.

Allen, Gerald R. "Two New Species of Frogfishes (Antennariidae) from Easter Island." *Pacific Science* 24, no. 4 (1970): 517–22.

Alpert, Morton Elliot, and Matthew E. Levison. "An Epidemic of Tuberculosis in a Medical School." *New England Journal of Medicine* 272, no. 14 (1965): 718–21.

Alpert, Morton Elliot, G.L. Nógrády, and C. Montandon. "Staphylococcus Sampling Map of Hanga Roa Village (1964–65)." In G.L. Nógrády, ed., *Microbiology of Easter Island (Rapa Nui): Proceedings of an International Symposium, April 26–28, 1971*, vol. 1, 233. Montreal: G.L. Nógrády, 1974.

Alvarez, Regina. "Restoration on Rapa Nui." *Ecological Restoration* 28, no. 4 (2010): 422–4.

Andersen, K.L. "Ethnic Group Differences in Fitness for Sustained and Strenuous Muscular Exercise." *Canadian Medical Association Journal* 96, no. 12 (1967): 832–3.

Anderson, J.R., and J.O. Godden. "The Ninety-Ninth Annual Meeting of the CMA: Scientific Program." *Canadian Medical Association Journal* 95, no. 5 (1966): 231–9.

Anderson, Warwick. *The Collectors of Lost Souls: Turning Kuru Scientists into Whitemen*. Baltimore, MD: Johns Hopkins University Press, 2008.

– *Colonial Pathologies: American Tropical Medicine, Race, and Hygiene in the Philippines*. Manila: Ateneo de Manila University Press, 2007.

– "Hybridity, Race, and Science: The Voyage of the Zaca, 1934–1935." *Isis* 103, no. 2 (2012): 229–53.

Andrade, Vera, Paulo Chagastelles Sabroza, Maria de Fatima Militao de Albuquerque, and Celio da Paula Motta. "Monitoring the Elimination of Leprosy in Brazil." *International Journal of Leprosy* 66, no. 4 (1998): 457–63.

Angyal, Tibor. "Serology of Rapa Nui Staphylococci." In G.L. Nógrády, ed., *Microbiology of Easter Island (Rapa Nui): Proceedings of an International Symposium, April 26–28, 1971*, vol. 1, 97–101. Montreal: G.L. Nógrády, 1974.

Anon. "Alfred John Pick (1916–2010)." Obit. *Globe and Mail*, 5 March 2010.

– "Antileprosy Drugs." *British Medical Journal* 3, no. 5767 (1971): 174–6.

- "Canadian Group Reports Quiet on Easter Isle." *Globe and Mail*, 2 January 1965, 9.
- "Canadian Scientists Visit Easter Island." *Rapa Nui Journal* 3, no. 2 (1989): 8.
- "Chile Marines Sent to Quell Easter Island Revolt." *Globe and Mail*, 31 December 1964, 1.
- "Chilean Marines to Easter Island." *New York Times*, 31 December 1964, 3.
- "Dad Pacing Deck While Stork on Way." *Montreal Star*, 30 November 1964.
- "Discussions and Recommendations." In G.L. Nógrády, ed., *Microbiology of Easter Island (Rapa Nui): Proceedings of an International Symposium, April 26–28, 1971*, vol. 1, 104–16. Montreal: G.L. Nógrády, 1974.
- "Diversas versiones sobre la situación en Isla de Pascua." *El Mercurio* (Santiago), 2 January 1965.
- "Easter Island Expedition Adds Three More Experts [Roberts, Murphy, Molson]." *Montreal Star*, 24 March 1964, 23.
- "Edith Mankiewicz." Obit. *Montreal Gazette*, 21 October 2006.
- "Edith Marion Mankiewicz." Obit. *Globe and Mail*, 21 October 2006, S9.
- "Eivind Myhre, Dosent, Dr. Med." Interview. *Tidsskrift for Den Norske Laegeforening* 85, no. 11 (1965): 939–41.
- "Expedition Commander an Accomplished Artist." *Montreal Star*, 14 August 1964.
- "Free Trip to Easter Island." Advertisement. *Canadian Nurse* 61 (August 1965): 640.
- "French Barred at Easter Island." *Washington Post*, 29 December 1964, A1.
- "Gift of Appreciation." Halifax *Mail Star*, 22 July 1965, 18.
- "Hammie Picks Up Expedition ... and Lo!" *Montreal Star*, 28 November 1964.
- "Hams Filling Air Waves to 'Easter.'" Halifax *Mail Star*, 21 December 1964.
- "Hans Finsterer." Obit. *Lancet* 269, no. 6900 (1955): 1144.
- "Health Survey of an Isolated Population." WHO *Chronicle* 19 (1965): 159–60.
- "Historia viva: Un grito de libertad / Living History: A Cry for Freedom." *Moe Varua Rapa Nui*, 26 April 2010, 3–7. https://issuu.com/moevarua/docs/26 --abril-2010.
- "Hot Ashes." *New York Times*, 27 June 1954, 6.
- "Informations épidémiologiques." WHO *Weekly Epidemiological Record*, 43, no. 19 (10 May 1968): 241.
- "Inquietud en Pascua." *El Mercurio* (Santiago), 3 January 1964.
- "International Council of Scientific Unions." *Nature* 191 (19 August 1961): 752.
- "Los habitantes de la Isla de Pascua realizan asamblea con el fin de elegir autoridades." *El Mercurio* (Santiago), 3 January 1965.

– "A Medical Expedition to the Navel of the World." *Canadian Medical Association Journal* 92, no. 5 (1965): 240–1.
– "Medidas para incorporar la Isla de Pascua al proceso económico." *El Mercurio* (Santiago), 29 December 1964.
– "Mission Accomplished: Easter Island Trip Success." *Montreal Gazette*, 18 March 1965, 15.
– "Nave de la Armada zarpó anoche a Isla de Pascua." *El Mercurio* (Valparaiso), 30 December 1964.
– "The New Flag." *Crowsnest: The Royal Canadian Navy's Magazine* 17, no. 2 (1965): 6–9.
– "No Feeling for Animals." *Globe and Mail*, 29 April 1965.
– "PM Decrees Grass Skirts Are Out." Halifax *Mail Star*, 22 July 1965, W3.
– "PM, Wife Receive Gifts." *Montreal Star*, 17 July 1965.
– "Scientific Aid for the Easter Islanders." CIL *Oval* 33, no. 4 (1964): 21–2.
– "Scientists Seek to Curb Phosphate Pollution [Skoryna]." *Ottawa Citizen*, 30 July 1970.
– "She Wrote a Book in Six Weeks." *The Age* (Melbourne), 18 March 1966, 14.
– "Shoeboxes for the Navel of the World." ATCO *Newsletter*, Summer 1965, 3, 8.
– "Situación de Isla de Pascua preocupa poderes públicos." *El Mercurio* (Santiago), 30 December 1964.
– "South Viet Makes Peace Deal." *Chicago Tribune*, 18 April 1967, 6, col. 4.
– "Surgeons College Honors Finsterer." *New York Times*, 12 November 1949, 13.
– "Two Ottawa People on Expedition." *Ottawa Journal*, 10 November 1964, 13.
– "Two Wrens Making Trip to Easter Island." Halifax *Mail Star*, 14 November 1964, 22.
– "Winners Fly to Easter Island." *Canadian Nurse* 63 (February 1967): 16.
Appel, Toby A. *Shaping Biology: The National Science Foundation and American Biological Research, 1945–1975*. Baltimore, MD: Johns Hopkins University Press, 2003.
Aronova, Elena, Karen S. Baker, and Naomi Oreskes. "Big Science and Big Data in Biology: From the International Geophysical Year through the International Biological Program to the Long Term Ecological Research (LTER) Network, 1957 –Present." *Historical Studies in the Natural Sciences* 40, no. 2 (2010): 183–224.
Art Gallery of Nova Scotia. "C. Anthony Law, 1916–1996." http://www.artgalleryofnovascotia.ca/c-anthony-law.
Arthur, Jacinta. "Reclaiming Mana: Repatriation in Rapa Nui." PhD diss., University of California, Los Angeles, 2015.

Arzt, J., and M.E. Mount. "Hepatotoxicity Associated with Pyrrolizidine Alkaloid (Crotalaria Spp) Ingestion in a Horse on Easter Island." *Veterinary and Human Toxicology* 41, no. 2 (1999): 96–9.

Azzi, Stephen. *Walter Gordon and the Rise of Canadian Nationalism.* Montreal and Kingston: McGill-Queen's University Press, 1999.

Bain, Barbara, Edouard F. Potworowski, and John C. Wilt. "Recommendations for Further Studies with Rapa Nui Blood and Serum Samples." In G.L. Nógrády, ed., *Microbiology of Easter Island (Rapa Nui): Proceedings of an International Symposium, April 26–28, 1971,* vol. 1, 223–8. Montreal: G.L. Nógrády, 1974.

Baker, H., A. Sidoriwicz, S.N. Sehgal, and C. Vézina. "Rapamycin (Ay-22,989): A New Antifungal Antibiotic III: *In vitro* and *in vivo* Evaluation." *Journal of Antibiotics* 31, no. 6 (1978): 539–45.

Baker, Paul T., and Joseph S. Weiner, eds. *The Biology of Human Adaptability.* Oxford: Clarendon, 1966.

Baldwin, Douglas. "Interconnecting the Personal and Public: The Support Networks of Public Health Nurse Mona Wilson." *Canadian Journal of Nursing Research* 27, no. 3 (1995): 19–38.

Baldwin, Hanson W. "Radioactivity-II." *New York Times,* 8 November 1954.

Barzelatto, José. "Endemic Goiter in Chile." In John B. Stanbury, ed., *Endemic Goiter: Report of the Meeting of the PAHO Scientific Group on Research in Endemic Goiter, Puebla, Mexico, 27 to 29 June 1968,* 229–32. Washington, DC: Pan American Health Organization, 1969.

Beaglehole, J.C., ed. *The Journals of Captain James Cook on his Voyages of Discovery.* Vol. 2, *The Voyage of the Resolution and the Adventure, 1772– 1775.* Cambridge, UK: Cambridge University Press and Hakluyt Society, 1961.

Beighton, Peter. "Easter Island People." *Geographical Journal* 132, no. 3 (1966): 347–57.

Belardinelli, Juan M., and Héctor R. Morbidoni. "Recycling and Refurbishing Old Antitubercular Drugs: The Encouraging Case of Inhibitors of Mycolic Acid Biosynthesis." *Expert Review of Anti-Infective Therapy* 11, no. 4 (2013): 429–40.

Berg, K., and A.G. Bearn. "A Common X-Linked Serum Marker and Its Relation to Other Loci on the X Chromosome." *Transactions of the Association of American Physicians* 79 (1966): 165–76.

– "An Inherited X-Linked Serum System in Man: The Xm System." *Journal of Experimental Medicine* 123, no. 2 (1966): 379–97.

Bergsdoll, M.S., K.F. Weiss, and R.N. Robbins. "Enterotoxin Production by Certain Rapa Nui Staphylococci." In G.L. Nógrády, ed., *Microbiology of Easter Island (Rapa Nui): Proceedings of an International Symposium, April 26–28, 1971,* vol. 1, 66–70. Montreal: G.L. Nógrády, 1974.

Bernier, Jacques. *Médecine et idéologies: La tuberculose au Québec, XVIIIe-XXe siècles*. Quebec City: Presses de l'Université Laval, 2018.

Bjornsti, Mary-Ann, and Peter J. Houghton. "The Tor Pathway: A Target for Cancer Therapy." *Nature Reviews Cancer* 4, no. 5 (2004): 335–48.

Bocking, Stephen. *Ecologists and Environmental Politics: A History of Contemporary Ecology*. New Haven, CT: Yale University Press, 1997.

– *Nature's Experts: Science, Politics, and the Environment*. New Brunswick, NJ: Rutgers University Press, 2004.

Bonnefoy, Pascale. "Cancer Didn't Kill Pablo Neruda, Panel Finds. Was It Murder?" *New York Times*, 21 October 2017.

Borgoño, J.M., and G. Corey. "The Chilean Experience with Antipoliomyelitis Vaccination." *Developments in Biological Standardization* 41 (1978): 141–8.

Boudreault, Armand. "Comment on the Technical Facilities of Sample Preservation during the Expedition." Bilingual abstract. Library and Archives Canada, Roberts Papers, vol. 2, file 16, "Dental Conditions," nd [Nógrády's volume 2, 1971?].

– "Composition en acides aminés et activité biologique de diverses fractions d'une antitoxine diphtérique purifiée." PhD diss., Université de Montréal, 1954.

– "Huit semaines à l'Ile de Pâques." *Le Magazine Maclean*, 5 July 1965, 14–15, 33–6.

– "L'expédition de l'Ile de Pâques." *Bleu d'Or* 2, no. 3 (1965): np.

Boudreault, Armand, and V. Pavilanis. "Epidémiologie des infections virales dans la population de l'Ile de Pâques: Étude sérologique." *Bulletin of the World Health Organization* 39, no. 3 (1968): 389–406.

Boudreault, Armand, V. Pavilanis, and A. Chagnon. "Répartition des anti-corps neutralisant le virus de la poliomyélite chez les habitants de l'Ile de Pâques." *Canadian Journal of Public Health* 57, no. 12 (1966): 555–60.

Boudreault, Armand, V. Pavilanis, and M.O. Podoski. "Répartition des anti-corps inhibiteurs de l'hemagglutination contre la rougeole dans la population de l'Ile de Pâques." *Canadian Journal of Public Health* 57, no. 7 (1966): 313–16.

Boulanger, P., D.P. Gray, H.C. Gibbs, and D.A. Murphy. "A Serological Survey of Sera from Domestic Animals on Easter Island." *Canadian Journal of Comparative Medicine* 32, no. 2 (1968): 425–9.

Boutilier, James A. "METEI: A Canadian Medical Expedition to Easter Island, 1964–1965." Paper presented at the First International Congress on Easter Island and East Polynesia, Centro de Estudios Isla de Pasqua, Universidad de Chile, Hangaroa, Easter Island, 1984.

– "METEI: A Canadian Medical Expedition to Easter Island, 1964–1965 [Part I and Part II]." *Rapa Nui Journal* 6, no. 2 (1992): 21–3, 26–33; and no. 3 (1992): 45–53.

Boyer, Paul. *By the Bomb's Early Light: American Thought and Culture at the Dawn of the Atomic Age.* New York: Pantheon, 1985.

Bridgewater, Peter. "The Man and Biosphere Programme of UNESCO: Rambunctious Child of the Sixties, but Was the Promise Fulfilled?" *Current Opinion in Environmental Sustainability* 19 (2016): 1–6.

Brody, Garry S. "Another Early Flight to Isla de Pascua." *Rapa Nui Journal* 27, no. 1 (2013): 4.

Broome, M.G., R.K. Johnson, D.M. Silveira, and I. Wodinksy. "Biochemical and Biological Effects of Two Unique Antitumor Antibiotics: Rapamycin (NSC 226080) and Macbecin II (NSC 330500)." Abstract. *Proceedings of the American Association for Cancer Research* 24 (1983): 321.

Brown, Eric J., Mark W. Albers, Tae Bum Shin, Kazuo Ichikawa, Curtis T. Keith, William S. Lane, and Stuart L. Schreiber. "A Mammalian Protein Targeted by G1-Arresting Rapamycin-Receptor Complex." *Nature* 369 (30 June 1994): 756–8.

Brydon, J.E., and A.J MacLean. "An Examination of Some Soil Samples from Easter Island." Bilingual abstract. Library and Archives Canada, Roberts Papers, vol. 1, file 21, "Soil Analysis," nd [Nógrády's volume 2, 1971?].

Caldwell, David K., and John E. Randall. "*Cantherhines tiki*, a Junior Synonym of the Easter Island Filefish, *Cantherhines rapanui*." *Copeia*, no. 4 (1967): 857–8.

Cameron, Thomas W.M., and L.W. Billingsley, eds. *Energy Flow: Its Biological Dimensions: A Summary of the IBP in Canada, 1964–74.* Ottawa: Royal Society of Canada for the Canadian Committee for the International Biological Programme, 1975.

Caminero, J.A., G. Sotgiu, A. Zumla, and G. Battista Migliori. "Best Drug Treatment for Multidrug-Resistant and Extensively Drug-Resistant Tuberculosis." *Lancet Infectious Diseases* 10, no. 9 (2010): 621–9.

Campagna, Palmiro. *Storms of Controversy: The Secret Avro Arrow Files Revealed.* Toronto: Dundurn, 2010.

Canada. *House of Commons Debates.* 26th Parliament, 2nd Session, 16 December 1964.

– *House of Commons Debates.* 27th Parliament, 1st Session, 4 April 1966.

– "Naval Support for Scientific Expedition to Easter Island." *Cabinet Conclusions.* Library and Archives Canada, RG 2, Privy Council Office, series A-5-a, vol. 6264, access code 90, item 24960. http://www.bac-lac.gc.ca/eng/discover/politics-government/cabinet-conclusions/Pages/list.aspx?MeetingDate=1964-03-12&.

Canada, Office of the Auditor General. *Report of the Auditor General to the House of Commons for the Fiscal Year Ended March 1965.* Ottawa: Queen's Printer, 1966. https://ia802706.us.archive.org/19/items/reportofauditorg6465cana/reportofauditorg6465cana.pdf.

Canadian Broadcasting Corporation (CBC), Robert Williams (director), and George Hrischenko (sound). *Canadian Expedition to Easter Island.* Documentary. 1965.

Canadian Committee for the International Biological Programme (CCIBP). *Canadian Participation in the International Biological Programme: Report No. 1.* Ottawa: National Research Council of Canada, 1967.

– *Collected Reprints of Scientific Papers.* Vol. 5, *Human Adaptability.* 1975. Canadian National Science Library, call number QH9.5 v. 5.

– *Organization and Activities, 1964–1970.* Ottawa: National Research Council of Canada, 1971.

– *Summary: Annual Reports from Projects.* Ottawa: National Research Council of Canada, 1968–72.

Canadian National Committee for the International Geophysical Year. *Report on the Canadian Program for the International Geophysical Year, 1957–1958.* Ottawa, 1957.

Canadian National Committee for the International Geophysical Year and J.H. Meek. *Report on the Canadian Program for the International Geophysical Year [1958–59].* Ottawa, 1959.

Canadian Society of Transplantation. "In Memoriam: Suren Sehgal (1932–2003)." 2003. http://www.cst-transplant.ca/in-memoriam.html#Sehgal.

Canals, Mauricio, Christian González, Andrea Canals, and Daniela Figueroa. "Dinamica epidemiológica del dengue en Isla de Pascua." *Revista Chilena de Infectología* 29, no. 4 (2012): 388–94.

Cañellas-Bolta, Núria, Valenti Rull, Alberto Saez, Olga Margalef, Roberto Bao, Sergi Pla-Rabes, Maarten Blaauw, Blas Valero-Garcés, and Santiago Giralt. "Vegetation Changes and Human Settlement of Easter Island during the Last Millennia: A Multiproxy Study of the Lake Raraku Sediments." *Quaternary Science Reviews* 72 (2013): 36–48.

Canetti, G., S. Froman, J. Grosset, P. Hauduroy, M. Langerová, H.T. Mahler, G. Meissner, D.A. Mitchison, and L. Šula. "Mycobacteria: Laboratory Methods for Testing Drug Sensitivity and Resistance." *Bulletin of the World Health Organization* 29, no. 5 (1963): 565–78.

Chagnon, A. and V. Pavilanis. "Epidemiological Studies on Rubella." *Canadian Medical Association Journal* 102, no. 9 (1970): 933–8.

– "Incidence of Rubella Antibodies in Two Insular Populations." *Canadian Journal of Public Health* 60, no. 7 (1969): 284–6.

Chamberlain, Adrian. "Art Gallery Receives $1.1 Million from Art Collector, Philanthropist." *Victoria Times Colonist,* 17 February 2016.

Chapman, Sidney. *IGY: The Year of Discovery.* Ann Arbor: University of Michigan Press, 1959.

Chicha, Marie-Thérèse. *Le mirage de l'égalité: Les immigrées hautement qualifiées à Montréal*. Montreal: La Fondation canadienne de relations raciales, 2009.

Chile. *Informe de la Comisión Verdad Histórica y Nuevo Trato*, vol. 3, bk 1. Santiago, Chile, 2001–03. http://biblioteca.serindigena.org/libros_digitales/ cvhynt/v_iii/t_i/pueblos/v3_t1_informe_pueblo_mario_tuki_y_otros.html.

– *Informe de la Comisión Nacional de Verdad Histórica y Nuevo Trato y Reconciliación con los Pueblos Indígenas*. Santiago, Chile, 2008–10. Chile.

– "Map of Rapa Nui." In G.L. Nógrády, ed., *Microbiology of Easter Island: Proceedings of an International Symposium on the Microbiology of Easter Island (Rapa Nui), April 26–28, 1971*, vol. 1, 229. Montreal: G.L. Nógrády, 1974.

Chile, Comisión Nacional de SIDA-CONASIDA. "Caracterización epidemiológica de la infección por VIH/SIDA en Chile, diciembre de 2003." *Revista Chilena de Infectología* 22, no. 2 (2005): 169–202.

Chile, Departamento de Estadísticas e Información de Salud. *Estadísticas de Natalidad y Mortalidad*. Santiago, 2007–16.

Chile, Instituto Nacional de Estadísticas. *Anuario de Estadísticas Vitales*. Santiago, 1993–2016.

Chile, Labor Parlamentaria. "Creación de la comuna subdelegación Isla de Pascua." 6 January 1965. http://www.bcn.cl/laborparlamentaria/wsgi/ consulta/verParticipacion.py?idParticipacion=942445&idPersona=1689 &idDocumento=609065&idAkn=akn609065-ds18-p01-ds31-ds49.

Chile, Ministerio de Salud. "Estadísticas de Natalidad y Mortalidad." http:// www.deis.cl/estadisticas-de-natalidad-y-mortalidad/.

Chile, Servicio Nacional de Patrimonio Cultural. "Rapa Nui celebra el regreso de valiosa documentación médica desde Canadá." http://www.museo rapanui.cl/sitio/Contenido/Noticias/83800:Rapa-Nui-celebra-el-regreso- de-valiosa-documentacion-medica-desde-Canada.

Clark, W.A. "Microbiological Serum Sample Preservation Methods." Bilingual abstract. Library and Archives Canada, Roberts Papers, vol. 2, file 16, "Dental Conditions," nd [Nógrády's volume 2, 1971?].

Clarke, Cyril, and Francis Avery Jones. "Thomas Cecil Hunt (1901–1980)." In Royal College of Physicians, *Lives of the Fellows: Munk's Roll*, vol. 7, *1976–1983*, 286. http://munksroll.rcplondon.ac.uk/Biography/Details/2332.

Clecner, B., and S. Sonea. "Acquisition de la proprieté hémolytique de la type delta par conversion lysogénique chez *Staphylococcus aureus*." *Revue Canadienne de Biologie* 25 (1966): 145–8.

Clecner-Gray, B., and S. Sonea. "Study of Extrachromosomic Genetic Factors Responsible for Virulence and Antibiotic Resistance in Staphylococci Obtained from an Isolated Population (Rapa Nui)." In G.L. Nógrády, ed., *Microbiology of Easter Island (Rapa Nui): Proceedings of an International Symposium, April 26–28, 1971*, vol. 1, 71–9. Montreal: G.L. Nógrády, 1974.

Collins, Kenneth J., and Joseph S. Weiner. *Human Adaptability: A History and Compendium of Research in the International Biological Programme.* London: Taylor Francis, 1977.

Comtois, R.D. "Phage Types of Rapa Nui Staphylococci." In G.L. Nógrády, ed., *Microbiology of Easter Island (Rapa Nui): Proceedings of an International Symposium, April 26–28, 1971,* vol. 1, 89–96. Montreal: G.L. Nógrády, 1974.

Conoley, Ken. "Your Stamp Album: Easter Island to Mark Historic Event." *Montreal Star,* 28 November 1964.

Conway, D.J., and Elena Ross. "Easter Island Families: Haptoglobin Types and Milk Precipitins." Library and Archives Canada, Roberts Papers, vol. 1, file 19, "Haptoglobin."

Cook, W.H. "The IBP – Internationally and Nationally." In Thomas W.M. Cameron and L.W. Billingsley, eds, *Energy Flow: Its Biological Dimensions: A Summary of the IBP in Canada, 1964–74,* vii–viii. Ottawa: Royal Society of Canada for the Canadian Committee for the International Biological Programme, 1975.

– "An Overview." In Thomas W.M. Cameron and L.W. Billingsley, eds, *Energy Flow: Its Biological Dimensions: A Summary of the IBP in Canada, 1964–74,* 1–16. Ottawa: Royal Society of Canada for the Canadian Committee for the International Biological Programme, 1975.

Corney, Bolton Glanvill, ed. and trans. *The Voyage of Captain Don Felipe Gonzalez to Easter Island, 1770–1771.* Cambridge, UK: Cambridge University Press and Hakluyt Society, 1908.

Cruz-Coke, Ricardo. "Ecología humana de la Isla de Pascua." *Revista Médica de Chile* 91 (October 1963): 773–9.

– "Estudios biomédicos chilenos en Isla de Pascua (1932–1985)." *Revista Médica de Chile* 116, no. 8 (1988): 818–21.

Cruz-Coke, Ricardo, Raúl Etcheverry, and Ronald Nagel. "Influence of Migration on Blood-Pressure of Easter Islanders." *Lancet* 283, no. 7335 (1964): 697–9.

Cruz-Coke, Ricardo, Ronald Nagel, and Raúl Etcheverry. "Effects of Locus MN on Diastolic Blood Pressure in a Human Population." *Annals of Human Genetics* 28 (1964): 39–48.

Cuetos, Marcos, and Steven Palmer. *Medicine and Public Health in Latin America: A History.* Cambridge, UK: Cambridge University Press, 2014.

Cutler, J.L. "Cerebrovascular Disease in an Elderly Population." *Circulation* 36, no. 3 (1967): 394–9.

– "Programmed Census on the Easter Island Population." Unpublished, 1966. University of British Columbia Archives, Efford Papers, METEI, box 1, file 6.

Cutler, J.L., and G.L. Nógrády. "Census of the Sampled Rapa Nui Native Population in 1964–65 as Regards Staphylococci and Sera." In G.L. Nógrády, ed., *Microbiology of Easter Island (Rapa Nui): Proceedings of an International Symposium, April 26–28, 1971*, vol. 1, 181–222. Montreal: G.L. Nógrády, 1974.

Dale, Jack. "Roy Gilmore Ellis, 1906–1989." Obit. *Word of Mouth*, January 1990. https://dentistry.library.utoronto.ca/sites/dentistry.library.utoronto.ca/files/Ellis.pdf.

Das, Reenita. "Pharma Companies Switch Gears: A New Market Emerges Called 'The Fountain of Youth.'" *Forbes*, 12 February 2015.

David, John M. "And Christmas Day on Easter Island." Letter. *Geographical Journal* 135, no. 2 (1969): 324.

Dayala, P.G. "Islands at a Glance." *Environmental Management* 15, no. 5 (1992): 565–8.

De Quadros, Ciro A., Bradley S. Hersh, Jean-Marc Olivé, Jon K. Andrus, Claudio M. da Silveira, and Peter A. Carrasco. "Eradication of Wild Poliovirus from the Americas: Acute Flaccid Paralysis Surveillance, 1988–1995." *Journal of Infectious Diseases* 175, suppl. 1 (1997): S37–42.

Delsing, Riet. "Issues of Land and Sovereignty: The Uneasy Relationship between Chile and Rapa Nui." In Florencia E. Mallon, ed., *Decolonizing Native Histories: Collaboration, Knowledge, and Language in the Americas*, 54–78. Durham, NC: Duke University Press, 2012.

Demirjian, A., D.A. Bailey, J. de Pena, F. Auger, and M. Jenicek. "Somatic Growth of Canadian Children of Various Ethnic Origins." In Thomas W.M. Cameron and L.W. Billingsley, eds, *Energy Flow: Its Biological Dimensions: A Summary of the IBP in Canada, 1964–74*, 299–312. Ottawa: Royal Society of Canada for the Canadian Committee for the International Biological Programme, 1975.

Diamond, Jared. *Collapse: How Societies Choose to Fail or Succeed*. New York: Viking Penguin, 2005.

Dinan, J.J. *St. Mary's Hospital: The Early Years*. Montreal and Toronto: Optimum, 1987.

D.M.P. "Expedition Lands on Easter Island." *Crowsnest: The Royal Canadian Navy's Magazine* 17, no. 1 (1965): 2–3, 17.

Donaldson, Peter J. *Nature against Us: The United States and the World Population Crisis, 1965–1980*. Chapel Hill: University of North Carolina Press, 1990.

Dorolle, Pierre. "Old Plagues in the Jet Age: International Aspects of Present and Future Control of Communicable Disease." *British Medical Journal* 4, no. 5634 (1968): 789–92.

Dos Passos, John. *Easter Island: Island of Enigmas*. Garden City, NY: Doubleday, 1971.

Dow, James. *The Arrow*. 2nd ed. Toronto: James Lorimer, 1997.

Drapkin, Israel. "Reminiscences of Medical Experience in Rapa Nui (1934–1935)." Abstract. In G.L. Nógrády, ed., *Symposium of the Medical Expedition to Easter Island: Antibiosis and Mycobacteria Studies*, 5–6. Abstracts. Canadian Society for Chemotherapy, Park Plaza Hotel, Toronto, 1969. Library and Archives Canada, Roberts Papers, vol. 2, file 11, "Chemotherapy Symposium."

Drapkin, Israel, and Richard H. Roberts. "Evidence of Staphylococcal Diseases." In G.L. Nógrády, ed., *Microbiology of Easter Island (Rapa Nui): Proceedings of an International Symposium, April 26–28, 1971*, vol. 1, 102–3. Montreal: G.L. Nógrády, 1974.

Duffin, Jacalyn. "Peter Beighton on Rapa Nui (Easter Island), 1964–65." *South African Medical Journal* 106, no. 6 (2016): S21–2.

Dufresne, Michael Maurice. "'Let's Not Be Cremated Equal': The Combined Universities Campaign for Nuclear Disarmament, 1959–1967." In M. Athena Palaeologu, ed., *The Sixties in Canada: A Turbulent and Creative Decade*, 9–64. Montreal: Black Rose Books, 2009.

Duran, Claudio. "Chile: Revolution and Counter Revolution." *Social Praxis* 1, no. 4 (1974): 337–58.

Edwards, Edmundo, and Alexandra Edwards. *When the Universe Was an Island: Exploring the Cultural and Spiritual Cosmos of Ancient Rapa Nui*. Easter Island: Hangaroa Press, 2013.

Efford, Ian, and K.J. Hall. "Marion Lake: An Analysis of a Lake Ecosytem." In Thomas W.M. Cameron and L.W. Billingsley, eds, *Energy Flow: Its Biological Dimensions: A Summary of the IBP in Canada, 1964–74*, 199–220. Ottawa: Royal Society of Canada for the Canadian Committee for the International Biological Programme, 1975.

Ehrenberger, Kristin Ann. "Autopsy, Authority, and Affect: Body Voyaging in Anatomical Fairy Tales from 1920s to 1940s Germany." In Thomas O. Haakenson, Tirza True Latimer, Carol Hager, and Deborah Barton, eds, *Becoming Transgerman: Cultural Identity beyond Geography*, 39–67. Oxford: Peter Lang, 2019.

Ekblom, Björn. "Med testcykel till 'Världens Navel'" [With the test cycle to the "The World's Navel"]. *Dagens Nyheter*, 9 May 1965, 1, 29.

– "Oskrivna lagar mot inavel: Besökaren erbjuds bli far" [Unwritten laws against inbreeding ...]. *Dagens Nyheter*, 13 May 1965, 29.

– "Revolution på Påskön" [Revolution on Easter Island]. *Dagens Nyheter*, 18 July 1965, 31.

Ekblom, Björn, and Einar Gjessing. "Maximal Oxygen Uptake of the Easter Island Population." *Journal of Applied Physiology* 25, no. 2 (1968): 124–9.

Embil, J.A., E.V. Haldane, R.A. MacKenzie, and C.E. van Rooyen. "Prevalence of Cytomegalovirus Infection in a Normal Urban Population in Nova Scotia." *Canadian Medical Association Journal* 101, no. 12 (1969): 78–81.

Eng, C.P., S.N. Sehgal, and C. Vézina. "Activity of Rapamycin (Ay-22,898) against Transplanted Tumors." *Journal of Antibiotics* 37, no. 10 (1984): 1231–7.

Englert, Father Sebastian. *Island at the Center of the World: New Light on Easter Island*. Trans. William Mulloy. New York: Charles Scribner's Sons, 1970.

– *La tierra de Hotu Matu'a: Historia, etnología y lengua de la Isla de Pascua*. San Francisco: Padre Las Casas, 1948.

Errol L. Montgomery & Associates, Water Resource Consultants. *Condiciones hidrogeológicas Isla de Pascua, Chile*. Santiago, Chile: Gobierno de Chile, Ministerio de Obras Públicas, Direccion General de Aguas, Division de Estudios y Planificacion, 2011.

Etcheverry, Raúl. "Blood Groups in Natives of Easter Island." *Nature* 216 (18 November 1967): 690–1.

Etcheverry, Raúl, Ronald Nagel, and Carlos Guzman. "Encuesta de bocio en los nativos de la Isla de Pascua." *Revista Médica de Chile* 91 (September 1963): 683–4.

Farkas-Himsley, Hannah. "A Survey of Penicillinase Production by Rapa Nui Staphylococci." In G.L. Nógrády, ed., *Microbiology of Easter Island (Rapa Nui): Proceedings of an International Symposium, April 26–28, 1971*, vol. 1, 52–65. Montreal: G.L. Nógrády, 1974.

Farkas-Himsley, Hannah, Ruth Farkas-Himsley, and Hanna Gemeinet. "A Survey of Easter Island Staphylococci: Second Report." Abstract for Canadian Public Health Association, 36th Annual Meeting of the Laboratory Section, Seigneury Club, Montebello, 1968. *Canadian Journal of Public Health* 60, no. 1 (1969): 37.

Fehren-Schmidt, L., C.L. Jarman, K.M. Harkins, M. Kayser, B.N. Popp, and P. Skoglund. "Genetic Ancestry of Rapanui before and after European Contact." *Current Biology* 27, no. 20 (2017): 1–7, e1-e6.

Feinstein, Adam. "Pablo Neruda Poisoning Doubts Fuelled by New Forensic Tests." *Guardian* (London), 5 June 2015.

Feldberg, Georgina D. *Disease and Class: Tuberculosis and the Shaping of Modern North American Society*. New Brunswick, NJ: Rutgers University Press, 1995.

Fell, E. Julian. "Echinoids of Easter Island (Rapa Nui)." *Pacific Science* 28, no. 2 (1974): 147–58.

Fernández, J., L. Vera, J. Tognarelli, R. Fasce, P. Araya, E. Villagra, O. Roos, and J. Mora. "Detection of Dengue Virus Type 4 in Easter Island, Chile." *Archives of Virology* 156, no. 10 (2011): 1865–8.

Fica, Alberto, Marcela Potin, Gabriela Moreno, Liliana Véliz, Jaime Cerda, Carola Escobar, and Jan Wilhelm. "Razones para recomendar la vacunación contra el dengue en Isla de Pascua: Opinión del Comité de Inmunizaciones de la Sociedad Chilena de Infectología." *Revista Chilena de Infectología* 33, no. 4 (2016): 452–54.

Findlay, John A., and L. Radics. "On the Chemistry and High-Field Nuclear Magnetic Resonance Spectroscopy of Rapamycin." *Canadian Journal of Chemistry* 58, no. 6 (1980): 579–90.

Fischer, Steven Roger. "The German-Chilean Expedition to Easter Island (1957–58) (Part I and Part II)." *Rapa Nui Journal* 24, no. 1 (2010): 11–19; no. 2 (2010): 47–57.

– *Island at the End of the World: The Turbulent History of Easter Island.* London: Reaktion Books, 2005.

Fisher, Matthew. "Trouble Festering in Paradise as Easter Island Natives Push for Independence from Chile." *National Post*, 26 March 2015. http://nationalpost.com/news/world/easter-island-chile-tensions.

Fitzgerald, R.G. "Isolation and Characterization of Human Carciogenic [*sic*] Streptococci." Bilingual abstract. Library and Archives Canada, Roberts Papers, vol. 2, file 16, "Dental Conditions," nd [Nógrády's volume 2, 1971?].

Flint, Donna. "Expedition Fulfills Women's Dream." *Montreal Gazette*, 27 April 1967.

Foerster, Rolf, Jimena Ramírez, and Cristián Moreno Pakarati. *Cartografía y conflicto en Rapa Nui, 1888–2014.* Rapa Nui: Rapanui Press, 2014.

Forsey, Joan. "Gerd Hurum Has 'Easter Island' Role: Kon Tiki Godmother Still Exploring, but in Canada." *Montreal Gazette*, 19 May 1965.

Fuentes, Miguel, and Cristián Moreno Pakarati. "Towards a Characterization of Colonial Power on Rapa Nui (1917–1936)." *Rapa Nui Journal* 27, no. 1 (2013): 5–19.

Garber, Ken. "Rapamycin's Resurrection: A New Way to Target the Cancer Cell Cycle." *Journal of the National Cancer Institute* 93, no. 20 (2001): 1517–19.

Garcia, E., S. Yactayo, V. Millot, K. Nishino, and S. Briand. "Zika Virus: An Epidemiological Update." WHO *Weekly Epidemiological Record* 92, no. 15 (14 April 2017): 188–92.

García-Moro, Clara, Miguel Hernández, Pedro Moral, and Antonio González-Martín. "Epidemiological Transition in Easter Island (1914–1996)." *American Journal of Human Biology* 12, no. 3 (2000): 371–81.

Gausemeier, Bernd, Staffan Müller-Wille, and Edmund Ramsden, eds. *Human Heredity in the Twentieth Century*. London: Pickering and Chatto, 2013.

Gaziello, Catherine. *L'expédition de Lapérouse, 1785–1788: Réplique française aux voyages de Cook*. Paris: Comité des travaux historiques et scientifiques, 1984.

Geiger, H. Jack, Victor W. Sidel, and Bernard Lown. "The Medical Consequences of Thermonuclear War: Still Relevant a Half-Century Later?" *Medicine, Conflict and Survival* 28, no. 4 (2012): 278–81.

Gibbs, H.C. "Parasites in Rapa Nui Natives." Bilingual abstract. Library and Archives Canada, Roberts Papers, vol. 2, file 16, "Dental Conditions," nd [Nógrády's volume 2, 1971?].

– "A Survey on the Incidence of Enterobiasis in Easter Island Children." *Canadian Journal of Public Health* 57, no. 5 (1966): 206–8.

Gifford, Bill. "Does a Real Anti-Aging Pill Already Exist?" *Bloomberg Business*, 12 February 2015.

Gill, George W., and Vincent H. Stefan. "A Descriptive Skeletal Biology Analysis of the Ancient Easter Island Population." In Vincent H. Stefan and George W. Gill, eds, *The Skeletal Biology of the Ancient Rapanui*, 66–88. Cambridge, UK: Cambridge University Press, 2016.

Goldstein, Gerald B., and Douglas C. Heiner. "Clinical and Immunological Perspectives in Food Allergy." *Journal of Allergy* 46, no. 5 (1970): 270–87.

Gonschor, Lorenz. "Facing Land Challenges in Rapa Nui (Easter Island)." *Pacific Studies* 34, nos 2–3 (2011): 175–94.

– "Law as a Tool of Oppression: Institutional Histories and Perspectives on Political Independence in Hawai'i, Tahiti Nui, French Polynesia, and Rapa Nui." MA thesis, University of Hawaii, 2008.

Goodson, C. Sorenson, and R.J. Meier. "Easter Islander Palmar Dermatoglyphics: Sexual Dimorphism, Bilateral Asymmetry, and Family Polymorphism." *American Journal of Physical Anthropology* 70, no. 1 (1986): 125–32.

– "Topological Description of Easter Islander Palmar Dermatoglyphics." *American Journal of Physical Anthropology* 71, no. 2 (1986): 225–32.

Grant, George. *Lament for a Nation: The Defeat of Canadian Nationalism*. 1965. Reprint, Ottawa: Carleton University Press, 1989.

Gray, Charlotte. "Profiles: Maureen Roberts." *Canadian Medical Association Journal* 131, no. 10 (1984): 1285.

Greenaway, Frank. *Science International: A History of the International Council of Scientific Unions*. Cambridge, UK: Cambridge University Press, 2006.

Greenfield, D.W., and D.A. Hensley. "Damselfishes (Pomacentridae) of Easter Island, with Descriptions of Two New Species." *Copeia*, no. 4 (1970): 689–95.

Greulich, W.W., and S.I. Pyle. *Radiographic Atlas of Skeletal Development of the Hand and Wrist*. 2nd ed. Stanford, CA: Stanford University Press, 1959.

Greve Hernández, Guillermo. "Planificaión del programa de lucha contra la tuberculosis." *Revista Chilena de Pediatría* 34 (1963): 450.

Grifferos A., Alejandra M. "Colonialism and Rapanui Identity." In Christopher M. Stevenson, Georgia Lee, and F.J. Morin, eds, *Easter Island in Pacific Context: Proceedings of the Fourth International Conference on Easter Island and East Polynesia, Albuquerque, 5–10 August 1997*, 365–7. Santa Barbara, CA: Easter Island Foundation, 1998.

– "Entre palos e piedras: La reformulación de la etnicidad en Rapanui (Isla de Pascua)." *Estudios Atacameños*, no. 19 (2000): 121–34.

Griffith, Richard S. "Introduction to Vancomycin." *Reviews of Infectious Diseases* 3, suppl. (1981): S200–4.

– "Vancomycin Use: An Historical Review." *Journal of Antimicrobial Chemotherapy* 14, suppl. D (1984): 1–5.

Hacker, Carlotta. "Aku-Aku: L'expédition canadienne à l'Ile de Paques." *Infirmière Canadienne* 61, no. 9 (1965): 582–6.

– "Aku-Aku and Medicine Men." *Canadian Nurse* 61 (August 1965): 636–40.

– *And Christmas Day on Easter Island*. London: Michael Joseph, 1968.

– "L'expédition de l'Ile de Pâques." *Blue Gold* 2, no. 3 (1965): 3–4.

– "Revolt in the Easter Islands [*sic*]." 1965. Unidentified clipping. University of British Columbia Archives, Efford Papers, METEI, box 1, file 1.

Hagelberg, Erika. "Genetic Affinities of the Rapanui." In Vincent H. Stefan and George W. Gill, eds, *The Skeletal Biology of the Ancient Rapanui*, 182–201. Cambridge, UK: Cambridge University Press, 2016.

Hagelberg, Erika, Silvia Quevedo, Daniel Turbon, and J. B. Clegg. "DNA from Ancient Easter Islanders." *Nature* 369 (5 May 1994): 25–6.

Hagen, Joel Bartholemew. *An Entangled Bank: The Origins of Ecosystem Ecology*. New Brunswick, NJ: Rutgers University Press, 1992.

Haldane, E.V., and J.A. Embil. "Comparative Epidemiology of Cytomegalovirus Infection in Two Contrasting Population Groups." *Nova Scotia Medical Bulletin* 49, no. 6 (1970): 157–60.

Haldane, E.V., J.A. Embil, and A.D. Wall. "A Serological Study of Cytomegalovirus Infection in the Population of Easter Island." *Bulletin of the World Health Organization* 40, no. 6 (1969): 969–73.

Ham, Daniela, and S.C. Skoryna. "Cellular Defense against Oxidized Low-Density Lipoproteins and Fibrillar Amyloid Beta in Murine Cells of Monocyte Origin with Possible Susceptibility to the Oxidative Stress Induction." *Experimental Gerontology* 39, no. 2 (2004): 225–31.

– "Generation of Amyloid A Protein by the Cell Lines from Amyloid-Susceptible and -Resistant Mice." *Scandinavian Journal of Immunology* 59, no. 2 (2004): 117–22.

Haoa Rapahango, Betty. *Leprosario de Isla de Pascua: Memoria técnica patri-monial*. Valparaiso, Chile: Museo Fonck, 2016.

Harris, Leon. "All the Way to Easter Island: Father to Hear Daughter's Cry." *Montreal Star*, 3 December 1964, 4.

Haun, Beverley. *Inventing "Easter Island."* Toronto: University of Toronto Press, 2008.

Hawthorn, Tom. "Ambassador Negotiated Release of Hostages." Obit. of Freeman Tovell. *Globe and Mail*, 2 April 2011.

– "Ian McTaggart-Cowan Was Dedicated to Preserving B.C.'s Natural Bounty." Obit. *Globe and Mail*, 20 April 2010.

Hayden, Cori. *When Nature Goes Public: The Making and Unmaking of Bioprospecting in Mexico*. Princeton, NJ: Princeton University Press, 2003.

Hayes, F. Ronald. *The Chaining of Prometheus: Evolution of a Power Structure for Canadian Science*. Toronto. University of Toronto Press, 1973.

H.C.W. "1964 in Review." *Crowsnest: The Royal Canadian Navy's Magazine* 17, no. 1 (1965): 14–17.

Heitman, J., N.R. Movva, and M.N. Hall. "Targets for Cell-Cycle Arrest by the Immunosuppressant Rapamycin in Yeast." *Science* 253 (23 August 1991): 905–9.

Hellyer, Paul T. *Damn the Torpedoes: My Fight to Unify Canada's Armed Forces*. Toronto: McClelland and Stewart, 1990.

Herald, Eve. *Beyond Human: How Cutting-Edge Science Is Extending Our Lives*. New York: St Martin's Press, 2016.

Hermansen, L., and Björn Ekblom. "Physical Fitness of an Arctic and a Tropical Population." In Karl Evang and Karl Lange Andersen, eds, *Physical Activity in Health and Disease*, 231–4. Philadelphia, PA: Lippincott Williams and Wilkins, 1967.

Herzog, Hubert, and Tony Saulnier. "Les mystères de l'Île de Pâques." *Paris Match*, 30 March 1968, 73–88.

Heyerdahl, Thor. *Aku-Aku: The Secret of Easter Island*. London: George Allen and Unwin, 1958.

– *Kon-Tiki: Across the Pacific by Raft*. Trans. F.H. Lyon. Chicago: Rand McNally, 1950.

Hildes, Jack A. "The Circumpolar People: Health and Physiological Adaptations." In Paul T. Baker and Joseph S. Weiner, eds, *The Biology of Human Adaptability*, 497–508. Oxford: Clarendon, 1966.

Hilliard, I.M. "Keith John Roy Wightman (1914–1978)." In Royal College of Physicians, *Lives of the Fellows: Munk's Roll*, vol. 7, 1976–1983, 601. http://munksroll.rcplondon.ac.uk/Biography/Details/4751.

Hilliker, John, Mary Halloran, and Greg Donaghy. *Canada's Department of External Affairs*. Vol. 3, *Innovation and Adaptation, 1968–1984*. Toronto: University of Toronto Press, 2017.

Hirschhorn, Kurt K. "Recent Advances in Methodology of Human Genetics." *Bulletin of the New York Academy of Medicine* 40, no. 5 (1964): 343–55.

Ho, M. "The History of Cytomegalovirus and Its Diseases." *Medical Microbiology and Immunology* 197, no. 2 (2008): 65–73.

Houchens, David P., Artemio A. Ovejera, Sylvia M. Riblet, and Donald E. Slagel. "Human Brain Tumor Xenografts in Nude Mice as a Chemotherapy Model." *European Journal of Cancer and Clinical Oncology* 19, no. 6 (1983): 799–805.

Holdsworth, David K. "A Preliminary Study of Medicinal Plants of Easter Island, South Pacific." *Pharmaceutical Biology* [formerly *International Journal of Pharmacognosy*] 30, no. 1 (1992): 27–32.

Hoy, Lyndsay M. "Living with Lymphangioleiomyomatosis: An Anesthesiologist's Experience." *Anesthesiology* 124, no. 1 (2016): 235–8.

Hrischenko, George. "Easter Island: My One and Only Dxpedition [*sic*], Pt. 1 and 2." *TCA: The Canadian Amateur* 42, no. 2 (March 2014): 24–36; and 43, no. 6 (November-December 2015): 39.

Hughes, D.R. "International Study of Eskimos: Human Adaptability Section of CCIBP (Igloolik and Hall Lake)." In Thomas W.M. Cameron and L.W. Billingsley, eds, *Energy Flow: Its Biological Dimensions: A Summary of the IBP in Canada, 1964–74*, 277–98. Ottawa: Royal Society of Canada for the Canadian Committee for the International Biological Programme, 1975.

Hunt, Thomas. "History of the British Society of Gastroenterology." *Gut* 1, no. 1 (1960): 2–5.

Hustak, Alan. *At the Heart of St. Mary's: A History of Montreal's St. Mary's Hospital Center*. Montreal: Véhicule, 2014.

Iber, Frank L. "Review of Skoryna, *Pathophysiology of Peptic Ulcer*." *Archives of Internal Medicine* 113, no. 1 (1964): 905–6.

Igartua, José E. *The Other Quiet Revolution: National Identities in English Canada, 1945–71*. Vancouver: UBC Press, 2006.

Ingram, D.G. "Anthropozoonosis Antibodies in Rapa Nui Humans." Bilingual abstract. Library and Archives Canada, Roberts Papers, vol. 2, file 16, "Dental Conditions," nd [Nógrády's volume 2, 1971?].

– "Immunoconglutinin Levels in the Serum of Rapa Nui Natives (1964–65)." In G.L. Nógrády, ed., *Microbiology of Easter Island (Rapa Nui): Proceedings of an International Symposium, April 26–28, 1971*, vol. 1, 121–5. Montreal: G.L. Nógrády, 1974.

Inhorn, Marcia C., and Emily A. Wentzell, eds. *Medical Anthropology at the Intersections: Histories, Activism, and Futures*. Durham, NC: Duke University Press, 2012.

Inostrosa, Jorge. "Agitación en la Isla de Pascua: Las dos caras de la Isla de Pascua." *Ercilla* (Santiago), 6 January 1965.

Ishwaran, N. "Diversity, Protected Areas and Sustainable Development." *Nature and Resources* 28, no. 1 (1992): 18–25.

Jablon, J.M. "Fluorescence-Antibody Technique for the Detection of Cariogenic Streptococci." Bilingual abstract. Library and Archives Canada, Roberts Papers, vol. 2, file 16, "Dental Conditions," nd [Nógrády's volume 2, 1971?].

Jara Fernández, Mauricio, Pablo Mancilla González, Consuelo León Wöppke, Anelio Aguayo Lobo, Nelson Llanos Sierra, Guido Olivares Salinas, eds. *El Año Geofísico Internacional en la perspectiva histórica chilena, 1954–1958.* Valparaiso, Chile: Puntángeles Editorial, Universidad de Playa Ancha, 2012. http://antarticarepositorio.umag.cl/bitstream/handle/20.500.11894/177/01-LIBRO-AGI.pdf?sequence=3&isAllowed=y.

Jarman, Catrine L., Thomas Larsen, Terry Hunt, Carl Lipo, Reidar Solsvik, Natalie Wallsgrove, Cassie Ka'apu-Lyons, Hilary G. Close, and Brian N. Popp. "Diet of the Prehistoric Population of Rapa Nui (Easter Island, Chile) Shows Environmental Adaptation and Resilience." *American Journal of Physical Anthropology* 164, no. 2 (2017): 1–19.

Jessup, Pat. "C. Anthony Law." MA thesis, St Mary's University, 2009.

– "C. Anthony Law Master and Commander." *Canadian Forces Journal* 6, no. 3 (2005): 69–74. http://www.journal.forces.gc.ca/vo6/no3/doc/history-histoire-02-eng.pdf.

Joves, James. "The Re-Imagining of Rapu Nui Traditional Healing Arts: Explorations of Narrative Identity, Mimesis, and the Public Sphere." PhD diss., University of San Francisco, 2013.

Joyce, Fred. "Cape Scott Solves Dilemma of Ensign." Unidentified clipping. Wilkinson Papers.

Kami, Harry T. "A New Subgenus and Species of Pristipomoides (Family Lutjanidae) from Easter Island and Rapa." *Copeia*, no. 3 (1973): 557–9.

Katz, Samuel L. "Measles Elimination in Canada." *Journal of Infectious Diseases* 189, suppl. 1 (2004): S236–42.

Kevan, D. Keith McE. "The Orthopteroid Insects of Easter Island." *Entomologist's Record and Journal of Variation* 77 (1965): 283–6.

Kohn, Alan J. "Ecological Shift and Release in an Isolated Population: *Conus miliaris* at Easter Island." *Ecological Monographs* 48, no. 3 (1978): 323–36.

Kwa, Chunglin. "Representations of Nature Mediating between Ecology and Science Policy: The Case of the International Biological Programme." *Social Studies of Science* 17, no. 3 (1987): 413–42.

La Fay, Howard, and Thomas Abercrombie. "Easter Island and Its Mysterious Monuments." *National Geographic*, January 1962, 90–117.

Landau, Simha F., and Leslie Sebba, eds. *Criminology in Perspective: Essays in Honor of Israel Drapkin.* Lexington, MA: Heath, 1977.

Lapage, S.P. "World Federation for Culture Collections: Xth International

Congress for Microbiology: Minutes." *International Journal of Systematic Bacteriology* 22, no. 4 (1972): 401–2.

Larco Hoyle, Rafael. *Checan: Essay on Erotic Elements in Peruvian Art.* Geneva: Nagel, 1965.

Larson, B.L. and K.E. Ebner. "Significance of Strontium-90 in Milk. A Review." *Journal of Dairy Science* 41, no. 12 (1958): 1647–62.

Laurence, William L. "Waste Held Peril." *New York Times*, 17 December 1955, 12.

Laval R., Enrique. "Anotaciones para la historia de la poliomielitis en Chile." *Revista Chilena de Infectología* 24, no. 3 (2007): 247–50.

Lawlor, R., and J. de Repentigny. "Comparison of Canadian and Rapa Nui *Staphylococcus aureus* Strains for High Yield Avirulent Mutation Rates Obtained with Acridine Orange." In G.L. Nógrády, ed., *Microbiology of Easter Island (Rapa Nui): Proceedings of an International Symposium, April 26–28, 1971*, vol. 1, 80–8. Montreal: G.L. Nógrády, 1974.

Lee, Betty. "The State of the Most Isolated Humans on Earth." *Globe and Mail*, 15 March 1965, 7.

Lerner, Mitchell. "'A Big Tree of Peace and Justice': The Vice-Presidential Travels of Lyndon Johnson." *Diplomatic History* 34, no. 2 (2010): 357–93.

Levine, Donald P. "Vancomycin: A History." *Clinical Infectious Diseases* 42, suppl. (2006): S5–12.

Lewin, Roger. "Ten Years of International Biology." *New Scientist*, 5 June 1975, 558–9.

Lipphardt, Veronika. "From 'Races' to 'Isolates' and 'Endogamous Communities': Human Genetics and the Notion of Human Diversity in the 1950s." In Bernd Gausemeier, Staffan Müller-Wille, and Edmund Ramsden, eds, *Human Heredity in the Twentieth Century*, 55–68. London: Pickering and Chatto, 2013.

Little, Michael A. "Human Population Biology in the Second Half of the Twentieth Century." *Current Anthropology* 53, no. S5 (2012): 126–38.

Little, Michael A., and Kenneth J. Collins. "Joseph S. Weiner and the Foundation of Post–WWII Human Biology in the United Kingdom." *American Journal of Physical Anthropology* 149, suppl. 55 (2012): 114–31.

Lock, Margaret. "From Genetics to Postgenomics and the Discovery of the New Social Body." In Marcia C. Inhorn and Emily A. Wentzell, eds, *Medical Anthropology at the Intersections: Histories, Activism, and Futures*, 29–60. Durham, NC: Duke University Press, 2012.

Long, Gideon. "Trouble in Paradise for Chile's Easter Island." BBC *News*, 18 April 2014. http://www.bbc.com/news/world-latin-america-26951566.

Lopes, Maria Margaret, and Irina Podgorny. "The Shaping of Latin American Museums of Natural History, 1850–1990." In Roy Macleod, ed., *Nature and Empire: Science and the Colonial Enterprise*, 108–18. Ithaca, NY: Cornell University Press, 2000.

Loret, John, and John T. Tanacredi, eds. *Easter Island: Scientific Exploration into the World's Environmental Problems in Microcosm*. New York: Kluwer Academic, 2003.

Lugones Botell, Miguel, and Marieta Ramírez Bermúdez. "Infección por virus Zika en el embarazo y microcefalia." *Revista Cubana de Obstetricia y Ginecología* 42, no. 1 (2016): 398–411.

Macey, J.F., T. Tam, T. Lipskie, G. Tipples, and T. Eisbrenner. "Rubella Elimination, the Canadian Experience." *Journal of Infectious Diseases* 204, suppl. 2 (2011): S585–92.

Macfarlane, D.B. "Canadian Medical Expedition Helps Out Hungry Islanders." *Montreal Star*, 21 December 1964.

– "Centre Planned for Natives: McGill to Issue Special Seal to Promote Health on the Island." *Montreal Star*, 9 December 1964.

– "Discontent in Paradise: Many Flee Carefree Island." *Montreal Star*, 29 January 1965.

– "Easter Islanders Take to Expedition." *Montreal Star*, 16 January 1965.

– "Easter Island Gives Ovation to Canadian Ship." *Montreal Star*, 14 December 1964.

– "E-Day: Expedition Hits the Beach Tomorrow." *Montreal Star*, 12 December 1964.

– "500 Montreal, Toronto Children to Be Studied." *Montreal Star*, 8 April 1965.

– "Most Islanders Free from Inherited Diseases." *Montreal Star*, 27 March 1965, sec. 4, 1.

– "Mysterious Moai of Easter Island: A Canadian Medical Team Visits an Ancient People." *Weekend Magazine*, suppl. in *Montreal Star*, *Vancouver Sun*, et al., 1 May 1965, 18–22.

– "No One She Can Marry." *Montreal Star*, 7 April 1965, 42.

– "Prosperity in Easter Island Growing." *Montreal Star*, 24 January 1968.

[–?] "Mission Over; Research Starts." *Montreal Star*, 20 March 1965.

– "Volunteers by the Boatload." *Montreal Star*, 22 October 1964, 21.

MacLeod, Roy, ed. *Nature and Empire: Science and the Colonial Enterprise*. Ithaca, NY: Cornell University Press, 2000.

Macnamara, F.N., R. Mitchell, and J.A.R. Miles. "A Study of Immunity to Rubella in Villages in the Fiji Islands Using the Haemagglutination Inhibition Test." *Journal of Hygiene* 71, no. 4 (1973): 825–31.

Maddock, David. "The First Plane Flight to Easter Island: The Robert Parragué Singer Story." *Rapa Nui Journal* 27, no. 1 (2011): 25–30.

Magasich-Airola, Jorge. *Los que dijeron "no": Historia del movimiento de los marinos ...* Vol. 2. Santiago, Chile: LOM Ediciones, 2008.

Magnusson, S. "Comparison of Virus Inactivating Capacity of Rapa Nui Sea Water with North and Baltic Sea Waters." Abstract. In G.L. Nógrády, ed., *Symposium of the Medical Expedition to Easter Island: Antibiosis and Mycobacteria Studies*, 4–5. Abstracts. Canadian Society for Chemotherapy, Park Plaza Hotel, Toronto, 1969. Library and Archives Canada, Roberts Papers, vol. 2, file 11, "Chemotherapy Symposium."

Malissard, Pierrick. "La controverse de la vaccination antituberculeuse au Canada." *Canadian Bulletin of Medical History* 15 (1998): 87–128.

– "Les 'Start-Ups' de jadis: La production des vaccins au Canada." *Sociologie et Sociologies* 30, no. 1 (2000): 93–106.

Maloney, Sean. "Secrets of the Bomarc: Re-Examining Canada's Misunderstood Missile Part I." *Royal Canadian Air Force Journal* 3, no. 3 (2014): 32–43.

Mankiewicz, E. "Antibodies against Typical and Atypical Mycobacteria from Rapa Nui Inhabitants." Abstract. In G.L. Nógrády, ed., *Symposium of the Medical Expedition to Easter Island: Antibiosis and Mycobacteria Studies*, 8–9. Abstracts. Canadian Society for Chemotherapy, Park Plaza Hotel, Toronto, 1969. Library and Archives Canada, Roberts Papers, vol. 2, file 11, "Chemotherapy Symposium."

Mann, Daniel, James Edwards, Julie Chase, Warren Beck, Richard Reanier, Michele Mass, Bruce Finney, and John Loret. "Drought, Vegetation Change, and Human History on Rapa Nui (Isla De Pascua, Easter Island)." *Quaternary Research* 69, no. 1 (2008): 16–28.

Martel R., J. Klicius, and S. Galet. "Inhibition of the Immune Response by Rapamycin, a New Antibiotic." *Canadian Journal of Physiology and Pharmacology* 55, no. 1 (1977): 48–51.

Martin, S.M., ed. *Culture Collections: Perspectives and Problems: Proceedings of the Specialists' Conference on Culture Collections, Ottawa, 1962*. Toronto: University of Toronto Press, 1963.

Mason, W.R.M. "An Endemic Subspecies of *Echthromorpha agrestoria* on Easter Island (Hymenoptera: Ichneumonidae)." *Canadian Entomologist* 106, no. 9 (1974): 935–6.

Maunder, Mike, Alastair Culham, Bjorn Alden, Georg Zizka, Cathérine Orliac, Wolfram Lobin, Alberto Bordeu, Jose M. Ramirez, and Sabine Glissmann-Gough. "Conservation of the Toromiro Tree: A Case Study in Management of a Plant Extinct in the Wild." *Conservation Biology* 14, no. 5 (2000): 1341–50.

Mayne, Richard Oliver. "Years of Crisis: The Canadian Navy in the 1960s." In Richard H. Gimblett, ed., *The Naval Service of Canada, 1910–2010: The Centennial Story*, 141–59. Toronto: Dundurn, 2009.

Mazière, Francis. *Fantastique Ile de Pâques*. Paris: Laffont, 1965.

– *Mysteries of Easter Island*. New York: Tower, 1968.

McArdle, William D., Frank I. Katch, and Victor L. Katch. *Exercise Physiology: Nutrition, Energy, and Human Performance*. Philadelphia, PA: Lippincott Williams and Wilkins, 2010.

McArthur, Douglas. "Edith Marion Mankiewicz: Doctor and Researcher." Obit. 24 November 2006, *Globe and Mail*, S9.

McCall, Grant. "The End of the World at the End of the Earth: Retrospective Eschatology on Rapanui (Easter Island)." In Sebastian Job and Linda Connor, eds, *Anthropology and the Ends of Worlds*, 45–53. Sydney: Department of Anthropology, University of Sydney, 2010.

McLaren, Angus. *Our Own Master Race: Eugenics in Canada, 1885–1945*. Toronto: McClelland and Stewart, 1990.

Meerovitch, E., and H.C. Gibbs. "Intestinal Parasitic Infections in the Inhabitants of Easter Island." *Transactions of the Royal Society of Tropical Medicine and Hygiene* 63, no. 3 (1969): 370–3.

Meier, R.J. "A Critique of Race-Based and Genomic Medicine." *Collegium Antropologicum* 36, no. 1 (2012): 1–5.

– "Dermatoglyphics of Easter Islanders Analyzed by Pattern Type, Admixture Effect and Ridge Count Variation." *American Journal of Physical Anthropology* 42, no. 2 (1975): 269–75.

– "The Easter Islander: A Study in Human Biology." PhD diss., University of Wisconsin, 1969.

– "Medical Expedition to Easter Island: A Progress Report on Physical Anthropology of Islanders." *American Journal of Physical Anthropology* 27, no. 2 (1967): 244.

– "A Penrose Analysis of Easter Island Biological Relationships." *Archaeology and Physical Anthropology in Oceania* 10, no. 1 (1975): 40–54.

– "Review of Cranial and Postcranial Remains from Easter Island, by Rupert I. Murrill." *American Anthropologist* 71, no. 2 (1969): 360–1.

– "Sequential Developmental Components of Digital Dermatoglyphics." *Human Biology* 53, no. 4 (1981): 557–73.

Meier, R.J., and C. Sorenson Jamison. "The Relationship between Dermatoglyphics and Body Measurements of Adult Easter Islanders." *Collegium Antropologicum* 11, no. 2 (1987): 333–8.

Métraux, Alfred. *Ethnology of Easter Island*. Honolulu: Bernice Bishop Museum, 1940.

Miller, A.B., A.J. Nunn, D.K. Robinson, G.C. Ferguson, W. Fox, and R. Tall. "A Second International Co-operative Investigation into Thioacetazone Side-Effects." *Bulletin of the World Health Organization* 43, no. 1 (1970): 107–25.

Milner, Marc. *Canada's Navy: The First Century*. Toronto: University of Toronto Press, 1999.

Mockford, Edward L. "Psocoptera Records from Easter Island." *Proceedings of the Entomological Society of Washington* 74, no. 3 (1972): 327–9.

Moellering, Robert C., Jr. "Vancomycin: A 50-Year Reassessment." *Clinical Infectious Diseases* 42, suppl. 1 (2006): S3–4.

Möller-Christensen, V. "Osteological and Pathological Survey on the Early Signs of Leprosy: The Importance of Missing Incisors." Abstract. In G.L. Nógrády, ed., *Symposium of the Medical Expedition to Easter Island: Antibiosis and Mycobacteria Studies*, 7–8. Abstracts. Canadian Society for Chemotherapy, Park Plaza Hotel, Toronto, 1969. Library and Archives Canada, Roberts Papers, vol. 2, file 11, "Chemotherapy Symposium."

Monnais, Laurence, and David Wright, eds. *Doctors beyond Borders: The Transnational Migration of Physicians in the Twentieth Century*. Toronto: University of Toronto Press, 2016.

Montandon, Cléopâtre. "The Development of Science in Geneva in the XVIIIth and XIXth Centuries: The Case of a Scientific Community." PhD diss. Columbia University, 1973.

– "Easter Island: A Case of Social Change." Unpublished, 1966.

– "Easter Island: A Case of Social Change." *Ethnologische Zeitschrift Zürich* 1 (1978): 5–44.

– "L'Ile de Pâques: Un cas de changement social." Unpublished, nd. Library and Archives Canada, Roberts Papers, vol. 2, file 20.

– "Μια Ελληνιδα Στο Νησί Του Πασχά" [A Greek on Easter Island]. *ΕΛΛΗΝΙΚΑ ΘΕΜΑΤΑ*, 1966, 227–31.

Montandon, Cléopâtre, and G.L. Nógrády. "District Map of Hanga Roa" and "Map Indicating Houses with Identical Numbers." In G.L. Nógrády, ed., *Microbiology of Easter Island (Rapa Nui): Proceedings of an International Symposium, April 26–28, 1971*, vol. 1, 231 and 235. Montreal: G.L. Nógrády, 1974.

Montes, Osvaldo. "Aspectos clínicos de la T.B.C. infantil." *Revista Chilena de Pediatría* 35 (1964): 265–6.

Motta, Célio Paula, and Manuel Zuniga G. "Time Trends of Hansen's Disease in Brazil." *International Journal of Leprosy* 58, no. 3 (1990): 453–61.

Mulloy, William. "Foreword." In Father Sebastian Englert, *Island at the Center of the World: New Light on Easter Island*, trans. William Mulloy, 9–15. New York: Charles Scribner's Sons, 1970.

Mumford, Lewis. "War Weapons Condemned." *New York Times*, 27 November 1955, 8E.

Mundey, Lisa M. "The Civilization of a Nuclear Weapon Effects Test: Operation Argus." *Historical Studies in the Natural Sciences* 42, no. 4 (2012): 283–321.

Murray, R.G.E. "Contributor to Systemic Bacteriology: Norman Edwin

Gibbons, 1906–1977." *International Journal of Systematic Bacteriology* 28,
no. 2 (1978): 338–9.

Mydans, Carl. "The Isle of Stone Heads." *Life*, 4 February 1966, 48–68.

Myhre, Eivind. "Blood Groups of the Easter Islanders: A Genetical Study."
Zeitschrift für Morphologie und Anthropologie 60, no. 3 (1969): 315–22.

– "Effect of Corticotrophin and Cortisone on the Healing of Gastric Ulcer." In
Stanley C. Skoryna, ed., *Pathophysiology of Peptic Ulcer*, 233–43. Montreal:
McGill University Press, 1963.

Nagel, Ronald, Raúl Etcheverry, and Carlos Guzman. "Haptoglobin Types in
Inhabitants of Easter Island." *Nature* 201 (11 January 1964): 216–17.

Nakadaira, Hiroto, Ivan Serra, Yamamotu Masamaru, and Ruth Rogers.
"Concentration of Metals and Other Elements in the Hair of Easter
Islanders." *Archives of Environmental Health* 51, no. 1 (2002): 85–6.

Nash, Catherine. *Genetic Geographies: The Trouble with Ancestry.*
Minneapolis: University of Minnesota Press, 2015.

National Film Board (NFB) and Hector Lemieux (cinematography, writer, and
director). *Island Observed.* Documentary, colour, 30 mins. 1966.

National Security Archive, with Peter Kornbluh. "Chile 1964: CIA Covert
Support in Frei Election Detailed: Operational and Policy Records Detailed
for the First Time." Press release, 25 September 2004. http://nsarchive.gwu.
edu/news/20040925/index.htm.

Nógrády, G.L. "District-House and House-District Listings in Hanga Roa
Village." In G.L. Nógrády, ed., *Microbiology of Easter Island (Rapa Nui):
Proceedings of an International Symposium, April 26–28, 1971*, vol. 1, 237–
46. Montreal: G.L. Nógrády, 1974.

– "Easter Island Stone Basins." *Journal of the Polynesian Society* 85, no. 3
(1976): 381–2.

– *The Effects of Streptomycin.* Film. nd.

– "Facial Reconstruction of an Easter Island Skull." Poster presented at a
meeting of the Hungarian Medical Association of America, Toronto, May
1981, and at a speleology conference, Kentucky, July 1981.

– "Finding Lists of Rapa Nui Human Staphylococcus Isolates and Human
Serum Samples." In G.L. Nógrády, ed., *Microbiology of Easter Island (Rapa
Nui): Proceedings of an International Symposium, April 26–28, 1971*, vol. 1,
126–80. Montreal: G.L. Nógrády, 1974.

– *L'effet de la toxine staphylococcique.* Film. nd.

– "Planning and Execution of the Antibiosis Project." Abstract. In G.L.
Nógrády, ed., *Symposium of the Medical Expedition to Easter Island:
Antibiosis and Mycobacteria Studies*, 3. Abstracts. Canadian Society for
Chemotherapy, Park Plaza Hotel, Toronto, 1969. Library and Archives
Canada, Roberts Papers, vol. 2, file 11, "Chemotherapy Symposium."

– "Planning and Execution of Staphylococcus Studies." In G.L. Nógrády, ed., *Microbiology of Easter Island (Rapa Nui): Proceedings of an International Symposium, April 26–28, 1971*, vol. 1, 2–16. Montreal: G.L. Nógrády, 1974.

– "Soil Specimens Taken in the Easter Island for Bacteriological Studies." Abstract. *Bulletin d'Information: International Centre for Information on and Distribution of Type-Cultures* (Lausanne) 2, no. 1 (1967): 32.

– ed. *Microbiology of Easter Island (Rapa Nui): Proceedings of an International Symposium, April 26–28, 1971*. Vol. 1. Montreal: G.L. Nógrády, 1974.

– ed. *Symposium of the Medical Expedition to Easter Island: Antibiosis and Mycobacteria Studies*. Abstracts. Canadian Society for Chemotherapy, Park Plaza Hotel, Toronto, 1969. Library and Archives Canada, Roberts Papers, vol. 2, file 11, "Chemotherapy Symposium."

Nógrády, G.L., P. Dionne, and G. Morin. "Planning and Execution of Mycobacteria Project: Bacterioscopic Examination of Nasal Smears for Mycobacterium Leprae." Abstract. In G.L. Nógrády, ed., *Symposium of the Medical Expedition to Easter Island: Antibiosis and Mycobacteria Studies*, 6–7. Abstracts. Canadian Society for Chemotherapy, Park Plaza Hotel, Toronto, 1969. Library and Archives Canada, Roberts Papers, vol. 2, file 11, "Chemotherapy Symposium."

Nógrády, G.L., and V. Fredette. *Catalogue des films microbiologiques avec resumés français et anglais*. Montreal: Departement de Bacteriologie de la Faculté de Médecine, Université de Montréal, 1964.

Nógrády, G.L., and R. Lawlor. *Manuel et cahier de travaux pratiques en microbiologie et immunologie*. Montreal: La Librarie de l'Université de Montréal, 1972.

Osborne, Michael A. *Nature, the Exotic and the Science of French Colonialism*. Bloomington and Indianapolis: Indiana University Press, 1994.

Osseo-Asare, Abena Dove. *Bitter Roots: The Search for Healing Plants in Africa*. Chicago: University of Chicago Press, 2014.

Owsley, Douglas W., Vicki E. Simon, Kathryn G. Barca, Jo Anne Van Tilburg, and Deidre Whitmore. "Demographic Analysis of Modified Crania from Rapa Nui." In Vincent H. Stefan and George W. Gill, eds, *The Skeletal Biology of the Ancient Rapanui*, 253–68. Cambridge, UK: Cambridge University Press, 2016.

Pakarati, Leo (writer and director). *Te Kuhane O Te Tupuna: El espíritu de los ancestros*. Documentary. Hanga Roa, Rapa Nui: Mahatua Productions, 2015.

Peale, Norman Vincent. *The Power of Positive Thinking*. New York: Prentice Hall, 1954.

Pearson, Lester B. *Diplomacy in the Nuclear Age*. Toronto: S.J. Reginald Saunders and Company, 1959.

Peden, Murray. *Fall of an Arrow*. Toronto: Dundurn, 2003.

Pimm, June. "Developmental Trends in an Isolated Culture." Paper presented at the 15th Inter-American Congress of Psychology, Sao Paulo, Brazil, 1973.

Porteous, J. Douglas. "METEI: The Canadian Medical Expedition to Easter Island." *Rapa Nui Journal* 3, no. 3 (1989): 11.

– *The Modernization of Easter Island*. Victoria, BC: University of Victoria Press, 1981.

Powell, R.C. "Science, Sovereignty and Nation: Canada and the Legacy of the International Geophysical Year 1957–58." *Journal of Historical Geography* 34, no. 4 (2008): 618–38.

Prat, Henri. *Métamorphose explosive de l'humanité*. 2 vols. Paris: Société d'édition d'enseignement supérieur, 1960.

Pratt, Mary Louise. *Imperial Eyes: Studies in Travel Writing*. London and New York: Routledge, 1992.

Pulverer, Gerhard. "Human and Animal Origin of Rapa Nui Staphylococci." In G.L. Nógrády, ed., *Microbiology of Easter Island (Rapa Nui): Proceedings of an International Symposium, April 26–28, 1971*, vol. 1, 17–29. Montreal: G.L. Nógrády, 1974.

Ramírez Aliaga, José Miguel. *Rapa Nui: El Ombligo del Mundo*. Santiago, Chile: Banco Santander and Museo Chileno del Arte Precolombino, 2008.

Randall, J.E. "The Endemic Shore Fishes of the Hawaiian Islands, Lord Howes Island, and Easter Island: Colloque Commorson, 1973." *Travaux et Documents* ORSTOM [*Office de la recherche scientifique et technique d'outre-mer*] 47 (1976): 49–73.

Randall, J.E., and D.K. Caldwell. "A New Butterfly Fish of the Genus *Chaetodon* and a New Angelfish of the Genus *Centropyge* from Easter Island." *Contributions in Science* (Natural History Museum, Los Angeles), no. 237 (1973): 1–11.

Regnault, Jean-Marc. "France's Search for Nuclear Test Sites, 1957–1963." *Journal of Military History* 67, no. 4 (2003): 1223–48.

Reid, Helen Evans. *All Silent, All Damned: The Search for Isaac Barr*. Toronto: Ryerson, 1968.

– "Easter Island: A Forgotten Race Is Taken over by the Jet Age." *Maclean's*, 19 June 1965, 20–3, 45–7.

– "Physical Development and Health of Easter Island Children." *Canadian Medical Association Journal* 98, no. 12 (1968): 584–9.

– *A World Away: A Canadian Adventure on Easter Island*. Toronto: Ryerson Press, 1965.

Reiss, Louise Z. "Strontium-90 Absorption by Deciduous Teeth." *Science* 134 (24 November 1961): 1669–73.

Rheinberger, Hans Jörg, and Staffan Müller-Wille. *The Gene: From Genetics to*

Post-Genomics. Trans. Adam Bostanci. Chicago: University of Chicago Press, 2018.

Riley, H.D., Jr. "History of the Cytomegalovirus." *Southern Medical Journal* 90, no. 2 (1997): 184–90.

Roberts, Richard H. "The Easter Island Expedition (1964–65): An Exercise in Specialized Medical Logistics." Paper presented at the Canadian Federation of Medical Students Clinical Conference, 1984. Library and Archives Canada, Roberts Papers, vol. 2, file 23.

– "The Health and Hygienic Conditions of the Easter Islanders." Abstract. In G.L. Nógrády, ed., *Symposium of the Medical Expedition to Easter Island: Antibiosis and Mycobacteria Studies*, 2. Abstracts. Canadian Society for Chemotherapy, Park Plaza Hotel, Toronto, 1969. Library and Archives Canada, Roberts Papers, vol. 2, file 11, "Chemotherapy Symposium."

– "Kokongo Epidemic." 4 pp. Library and Archives Canada, Roberts Papers, vol. 2, file 10, "Miscellaneous Speeches," nd [Nógrády's volume 2, 1971?].

– "Presentation Number 20." Expedition overview. Abstract. Library and Archives Canada, Roberts Papers, vol. 2, file 10, "Miscellaneous Speeches," nd [Nógrády's volume 2, 1971?].

– "Presentation Number 24." On tuberculosis and leprosy. Abstract. Library and Archives Canada, Roberts Papers, vol. 2, file 10, "Miscellaneous Speeches," nd [Nógrády's volume 2, 1971?].

– "Presentation Number 27." On *kokongo*. Abstract. Library and Archives Canada, Roberts Papers, vol. 2, file 10, "Miscellaneous Speeches," nd [Nógrády's volume 2, 1971?].

– "Problems of Peptic Ulceration in a Naval Environment." *Canadian Medical Association Journal* 79, no. 11 (1958): 902–5.

– "Report on the Easter Island Medical Expedition, 1964–65." Report prepared for Surgeon Rear Admiral Walter Elliot, Canadian Forces, 24 February 1965. Library and Archives Canada, Roberts Papers, vol. 1, file 9.

– "The Results of the Easter Island Expedition." Paper presented at the Annual Meeting of the Canadian Medical Association, Edmonton, Alberta, 15 June 1966. Library and Archives Canada, Roberts Papers, vol. 2, file 9.

Roberts, Sheila Maureen Howell. "Lecture in London." nd. Library and Archives Canada, Roberts Papers, vol 1., file 7, sd.

Robinson, Raymond M. *A Diplomat in Environmentalist's Clothing: A Memoir*. Toronto and New York: BPS Books, 2014.

Rodriguez Grunert, Leonardo, Zino Castellazzi, and Patricia Ortlieb. "Estudio inmunológico de la población de Isla de Pascua para detectar infección Hanseniasica." *Revista Médica de Chile* 113, no. 3 (1985): 183–5.

Rosenberg, Charles E. "Pathologies of Progress: The Idea of Civilization as Risk." *Bulletin of the History of Medicine* 72, no. 4 (1998): 714–30.

Routledge, Katherine. *The Mystery of Easter Island.* 1919. Reprint, New York: Cosimo Classics, 2005.

Salinas, Eve. "How the Chilean Coup Forever Changed Canada's Refugee Policies." *Globe and Mail*, 6 September 2013.

Sangster, Joan. "The Polish 'Dionnes': Gender, Ethnicity, and Immigrant Workers in Post –Second World War Canada." *Canadian Historical Review* 88, no. 3 (2007): 469–500.

Schleper, Simone. "Conservation Compromises: The MABs and the Legacy of the International Biological Program, 1964–1974." *Journal of the History of Biology* 50, no. 1 (2017): 133–67.

Scott, F. "Studies on an Intradermal Test to Detect Human Amebiasis." Bilingual abstract. Library and Archives Canada, Roberts Papers, vol. 2, file 16, "Dental Conditions," nd [Nógrády's volume 2, 1971?].

Sehgal, Ajai, "The Story of Rapamune." 2001. http://www.sehgal.net/story_of_rapamune.htm.

– "Surendra Nath Sehgal." 2003. http://www.sehgal.net/surenshistory.htm.

Sehgal, S.N. "Sirolimus: Its Discovery, Biological Properties and Mechanism of Action." *Transplantation Proceedings* 35, no. 3, suppl. (2003): 7S–14S.

Sehgal, S.N., H. Baker, and C. Vézina. "Rapamycin (Ay-22,989), a New Antifungal Antibiotic. II. Fermentation, Isolation and Characterization." *Journal of Antibiotics* 28, no. 10 (1975): 727–32.

Semeniuk, Ivan. "Researchers Hope Dead Chilean Poet Has One More Story to Tell." *Globe and Mail*, 24 February 2016, A1, A10, A11.

Seward, Pablo. "Between 'Easter Island' and 'Rapa Nui': The Making and Unmaking of an Uncanny Lifeworld." *Berkeley Undergraduate Journal* 27, no. 2 (2014): 217–77.

Shannon, Matthew K. "'One of Our Greatest Psychological Assets': The New Frontier, Cold-War Public Diplomacy, and Robert Kennedy's 1962 Goodwill Tour." *International History Review* 36, no. 4 (2014): 767–90.

Shapiro, H.L. "The Distribution of Blood Groups in Polynesia." *American Journal of Physical Anthropology* 26, no. 1 (1940): 409–16.

Sharp, Andrew, ed. *The Journal of Jacob Roggeveen.* Oxford: Clarendon, 1970.

Sharpless, John. "World Population Growth, Family Planning, and American Foreign Policy." *Journal of Policy History* 7, no. 1 (1995): 72–102.

Shephard, Roy J. *Human Physiological Work Capacity.* Cambridge, UK: Cambridge University Press, 1978.

– "Proceedings of the International Symposium on Physical Activity and Cardiovascular Health Held in Toronto, Ontario, October 11–13, 1966 and Sponsored by the Ontario Heart Foundation, the Ontario Medical

Association, and the Canadian Medical Association." *Canadian Medical Association Journal* 96, no. 12 (1967): 695–6.

Shewell, G.E. "Two Records of Agromyzidae from Chile and Easter Island (Diptera)." *Canadian Entomologist* 99, no. 3 (1967): 332–3.

Sidel, Victor W., H. Jack Geiger, and Bernard Lown. "The Medical Consequences of Thermonuclear War. II. The Physician's Role in the Post-Attack Period." *New England Journal of Medicine* 266 (1962): 1137–45.

Silverman, Marilyn, ed. *Ethnography and Development: The Work of Richard F. Salisbury.* Montreal: McGill University Libraries, 2004.

Simmons, R.T., and J.J. Graydon. "A Blood Group Genetical Survey in Eastern and Central Polynesians." *American Journal of Physical Anthropology* 15, no. 3 (1957): 357–66.

Simpson, Nancy E. "Genetics of Esterases in Man." *Annals of the New York Academy of Sciences* 151, no. 2 (1968): 699–707.

– "Polyacrylamide Electrophoresis Used for the Detection of C5+ Cholinesterase in Canadian Caucasians, Indians, and Eskimos." *American Journal of Human Genetics* 24, no. 3 (1972): 317–20.

Singh, Karta, Sheila Sun, and Claude Vézina. "Rapamycin (Ay-22,989), a New Antifungal Antibiotic. IV. Mechanism of Action." *Journal of Antibiotics* 32, no. 6 (1979): 630–45.

Skoryna, S.C. "Medical Meetings: Seventh International Cancer Congress: Canadian Contributions." *Canadian Medical Association Journal* 79, no. 4 (1958): 288–9.

– "METEI: An Epilogue." *Rapa Nui Journal* 6, no. 4 (1992): 69–73.

– "Objectives of the Canadian Medical Expedition to Easter Island." Abstract. In G.L. Nógrády, ed., *Symposium of the Medical Expedition to Easter Island: Antibiosis and Mycobacteria Studies,* 1. Abstracts. Canadian Society for Chemotherapy, Park Plaza Hotel, Toronto, 1969. Library and Archives Canada, Roberts Papers, vol. 2, file 11, "Chemotherapy Symposium."

– "Operation METEI." *Abbottempo* 3 (1966): 2–7.

– "Stochastic Processes in the Causation of Peptic Ulcer." In Stanley C. Skoryna, ed., *Pathophysiology of Peptic Ulcer,* 481–97. Montreal: McGill University Press, 1963.

– "Systemic Factors in Carcinogenesis." *Canadian Medical Association Journal* 80, no. 9 (1959): 689–97.

– "Systemic Factors in Neoplasia." *Lancet* 1, no. 7082 (1959): 1101–2.

– "Über die Nachbehandlung operierter Karzinome des Verdauungstraktes mit Blastolysine" [About the follow-up treatment of operated cancer of the digestive tract with blastolysine]. *Der Krebsarzt* 1 (1946): 214–25.

– ed. *Pathophysiology of Peptic Ulcer.* Montreal: McGill University Press, 1963.

Skoryna, S.C., D.P. Goel, A. Szekerese, D.S. Kahn, and D.R. Webster. "Incidence and Distribution of Bone Tumors Produced by Radioactive Strontium in Rats." Abstract. *Revue Canadienne de Biologie* 16 (1957): 517.

Skoryna, S.C., and David S. Kahn, "The Late Effects of Radioactive Strontium on Bone: Histogenesis of Bone Tumors Produced in Rats by High Sr89 Dosage." *Cancer* 12, no. 2 (1959): 306–22.

Skoryna, S.C., and C.A. Law. "Preliminary Report: Medical Expedition to Easter Island and H.M.C.S. Cape Scott (November 16, 1964 – March 17, 1965)." 1965. Many copies of this type-written document exist in public and private archives.

Skoryna, S.C., Roderick C. Ross, and L.A. Rudis. "Histogenesis of Sebaceous Gland Carcinomas Produced in Rats by 2-Acetylaminofluorine." *Journal of Experimental Medicine* 94, no. 1 (1951): 1–8 with 5 plates.

Skoryna, S.C., and Deirdre Waldron-Edward, eds. *Guidelines to Radiological Health: Summaries of Lectures Presented at the International Conference at McGill University, Montreal ...* Montreal: McGill University, 1967.

Skoryna, S.C., D.R. Webster, and D.S. Kahn. "New Method of Production of Experimental Gastric Ulcer: Effects of Hormonal Factors on Healing." *Gastroenterology* 34, no. 1 (1958): 1–10.

Smyth, C.J., and H. Farkas-Himsley. "A Survey of Easter Island Staphylococci." Abstract. *Canadian Journal of Public Health* 59, no. 1 (1968): 36–7.

– "A Survey of Easter Island Staphylococci." *Canadian Journal of Public Health* 59, no. 8 (1968): 313–17.

Sonea, S., R. Lawlor, and J. de Repentigny. "High Yield of Avirulent *Staphylococcus aureus* Obtained with Acridine Orange." *Bacteriological Proceedings (66th Annual Meeting of the American Society for Microbiology)* (1966): 36.

Sorkin, Andrew Ross, and Duff Wilson. "Pfizer Agrees to Pay $68 Billion for Rival Drugmaker Wyeth." *New York Times*, 25 January 2009.

Stambuk, Patricia. *Iorana & Goodbye: Una base yanqui en Rapa Nui.* Santiago, Chile: Pehuén, 2016.

– *Rongo: La historia oculta de Isla de Pascua.* Santiago, Chile: Pehuén, 2010.

Stebbins, G. Ledyard. "International Biological Program." *Science* 137 (7 September 1962): 768–70.

Stefan, Vincent H., and George W. Gill, eds. *The Skeletal Biology of the Ancient Rapanui.* Cambridge, UK: Cambridge University Press, 2016.

Stepan, Nancy Leys. *Picturing Tropical Nature.* London: Reaktion Books, 2001.

Stinson, Sara, Barry Bogin, and Dennis O'Rourke. *Human Biology: An Evolutionary and Biocultural Perspective.* Hoboken, NJ: John Wiley and Sons, 2012.

Sussman, Robert Wald. *The Myth of Race: The Troubling Persistence of an Unscientific Idea*. Cambridge, MA: Harvard University Press, 2014.

Swindells, D.C.N., P.S. White, and J.A. Findlay. "X-Ray Crystal Structure of Rapamycin C51H79NO13." *Canadian Journal of Chemistry* 56, no. 18 (1978): 2491–2.

Tanner, F. "Sample Collection of the Canadian Medical Expedition to Easter Island Microbiology Project." Bilingual abstract. Library and Archives Canada, Roberts Papers, vol. 2, file 16, "Dental Conditions," nd [Nógrády's volume 2, 1971?].

Taylor, A.G. "Dental Conditions among the Inhabitants of Easter Island." *Journal of the Canadian Dental Association* 32, no. 5 (1966): 286–90.

– "Dental Health of Easter Islanders in 1964–65." Bilingual abstract. Library and Archives Canada, Roberts Papers, vol. 2, file 16, "Dental Conditions," nd [Nógrády's volume 2, 1971?].

– "Medical Expedition to Easter Island." *Royal Canadian Dental Corps Quarterly* 6, no. 2 (1965): 15–25.

Tector, Amy. "The Delightful Revolution: The Canadian Medical Expedition to Easter Island, 1964–65." *British Journal of Canadian Studies* 27 no. 2 (2014): 181–93.

Templeton, Owen. "Expedition Leader Says Island May Be Named McGill." *Montreal Gazette*, 30 March 1965, 3.

Thomas, Stéphanie, and Dyphy Mariani. "Le crâne de Hotu Matu'a en France." Podcast. *France Culture*, 30 September 2014. http://www.france culture.fr/emissions/sur-les-docks-14-15/le-crane-de-hotu-matua-en-france.

Toranzo, Alicia E., Juan L. Barja, and Frank M. Hetrick. "Antiviral Activity of Antibiotic-Producing Marine Bacteria." *Canadian Journal of Microbiology* 28, no. 2 (1982): 231–8.

Toutant, R., and G.L. Nógrády. "Méthode d'étude de symbiose et de l'antibi-ose bactérienne: Croissance parabiotique d'un staphylococcus oral avec les streptococques originaires de l'Ile de Pâques." Association canadienne-française pour l'avancement des sciences (ACFAS), Quebec, 1966.

Tuki, Alfredo. "Historia de la 'Ley Pascua': Ley No. 16,441 / History of the 'Easter Island Law': Law No. 16,441." *Moe Varua Rapa Nui* 9, no. 102 (2016).

Turner II, Christy G. "Life and Times of a Dental Anthropologist." In G. Richard Scott and Joel D. Irish, eds, *Anthropological Perspectives on Tooth Morphology: Genetics, Evolution, Variation*, 16–30. Cambridge, UK: Cambridge University Press, 2013.

Turner II, Christy G., and G.R. Scott. "Dentition of Easter Islanders." In Albert A. Dahlberg and Thomas M. Graber, eds, *Orofacial Growth and Development*, 229–49. The Hague: Mouton de Gruyter, 1977.

United Nations Educational, Scientific and Cultural Organization (UNESCO). "Man and the Biosphere Programme." http://www.unesco.org/new/en/ natural-sciences/environment/ecological-sciences/man-and-biosphere -programme/.

United Nations Educational, Scientific and Cultural Organization (UNESCO), Santiago Office. "Chile's Living Human Treasures Honored by President Bachelet." 19 December 2017. http://www.unesco.org/new/en/santiago/ press-room/single-new/news/tesoros_humanos_vivos_de_chile_son_ galardonados_por_la_presi/.

Uruburu, Federico. "History and Services of Culture Collections." *International Microbiology* 6, no. 2 (2003): 101–3.

US Department of Justice, Office of Public Affairs. "Wyeth Pharmaceuticals Agrees to Pay $490.9 Million for Marketing the Prescription Drug Rapamune for Unapproved Uses." 30 July 2013. https://www.justice.gov/ usao-wdok/pr/wyeth-pharmaceuticals-agrees-pay-4909-million-marketing- prescription-drug-rapamune-unapproved.

US National Committee for the International Biological Program. *Research Studies Constituting the U.S. Contribution to the International Biological Program: Report #3.* Washington, DC: National Research Council, National Academy of Sciences, and National Academy of Engineering, 1967.

Valdés, Gloria, Ricardo Cruz-Coke, Javier Lagos, José Lorenzoni, Rodrigo Concha, and Berríos Ximena. "Factores de riesgo de hipertensión arterial en nativos de Isla de Pascua" [Risk factors for arterial hypertension in the natives of Easter Island]. *Revista Médica de Chile* 118, no. 10 (1990): 1077–84.

Van Tilburg, Jo Anne. *Among Stone Giants: The Life of Katherine Routledge and Her Remarkable Voyage to Easter Island.* New York: Scribner, 2003.

– *Easter Island: Archaeology, Ecology, and Culture.* London: British Museum Press, 1994.

– "Writing Routledge: Her Field Notes and Their Value to Science." Easter Island Statue Project, 2009. http://www.eisp.org/818/.

Vézina, C. "Antimicrobial Activity of *Streptomycetes* and Fungi Isolated from Rapa Nui Soil Samples." Abstract. In G.L. Nógrády, ed., *Symposium of the Medical Expedition to Easter Island: Antibiosis and Mycobacteria Studies,* 4. Abstracts. Canadian Society for Chemotherapy, Park Plaza Hotel, Toronto, 1969. Library and Archives Canada, Roberts Papers, vol. 2, file 11, "Chemotherapy Symposium."

Vézina, C., A. Kudelski, and S.N. Sehgal. "Rapamycin (Ay-22,989), a New Antifungal Antibiotic. I. Taxonomy of the Producing Streptomycete and Isolation of the Active Principle." *Journal of Antibiotics* 28, no. 10 (1975): 721–6.

Vickery, Vernon R. "D. Keith McE. Kevan." *Cultural Entomology Digest*, no. 3 (1994): np. https://www.insects.orkin.com/ced/issue-3/keith-kevan/.

Volz, Wilhelm. "Beiträge zur Anthropologie der Südsee." *Archiv für Anthropologie* 23 (1895): 96–170.

Wade, Nicholas. *A Troublesome Inheritance: Genes, Race, and Human History*. New York: Penguin, 2014.

Wadhams, Peter. "Hudson-70: The First Circumnavigation of the Americas." *Oceanography* 22, no. 3 (2009): 226–35.

Waldron-Edward, D., T.M. Paul, and S.C. Skoryna. "Suppression of Intestinal Absorption of Radioactive Strontium by Naturally Occurring Non-Absorbable Polyelectrolytes." *Nature* 205 (13 March 1965): 1117–18.

Webb, Geoffrey. "The History of IRPA up to the Millennium." *Journal of Radiological Protection* 31, no. 2 (2011): 177–204.

Weart, Spencer R. *Nuclear Fear: A History of Images*. Cambridge, MA: Harvard University Press, 1988.

Weiner, Joseph S. "Human Adaptability." In E.B. Worthington, ed., *The Evolution of IBP*, 14–16. Cambridge, UK: Cambridge University Press, 1975.

– "Foreword." In Roy J. Shephard, *Human Physiological Work Capacity*, ix–x. Cambridge, UK: Cambridge University Press, 1978.

– "Report of the Convener of the HA Sectional Committee." *IBP News*, no. 3 (1965): 26–31.

Wells, John W. "Notes on Indo-Pacific Scleractinian Corals Part 8: Scleractinian Corals from Easter Island." *Pacific Science* 26 (1972): 183–90.

Westhead, Rick. "How Canada Helped Keep the Junta at Bay." *Toronto Star*, 11 February 2007.

Whitaker, Reg, and Gary Marcue. *Cold War Canada: The Making of a National Insecurity State, 1945–1957*. Toronto: University of Toronto Press, 1994.

Widmer, Alexandra, and Veronika Lipphardt, eds. *Health and Difference: Rendering Human Variation in Colonial Engagements*. Oxford and New York: Berghahn Books, 2016.

William Beaumont Society, United States Army. "Seasonal Incidence of Upper Gastrointestinal Tract Bleeding: Report of the Standing Committee on Upper Gastrointestinal Bleeding." *Journal of the American Medical Association* 198, no. 2 (1966): 184–5.

Williams, R.E.O., and M.T. Parker. "Certain Characters of Rapa Nui Staphylococci." In G.L. Nógrády, ed., *Microbiology of Easter Island (Rapa Nui): Proceedings of an International Symposium, April 26–28, 1971*, vol. 1, 30–51. Montreal: G.L. Nógrády, 1974.

Wilmoth, J.R., and P. Ball. "Arguments and Action in the Life of a Social Problem: A Case Study of Overpopulation, 1946–1990." *Social Problems* 42, no. 3 (1995): 318–43.

Wilson, Edward O. "Ants of Easter Island and Juan Fernandez." *Pacific Insects* 15, no. 2 (1973): 285–87.

Wilson, J. Tuzo. *I.G.Y.: The Year of the New Moons*. Toronto: Longmans, 1961.

Wilt, J.C. "Anthropozoonoses in the Northwest [America] ..." Bilingual abstract. Library and Archives Canada, Roberts Papers, vol. 2, file 16, "Dental Conditions," nd [Nógrády's volume 2, 1971?].

Wishart, F.O. "Report of the Laboratory Section: 33rd Annual Meeting, Sheraton Toronto, December 1–2, 1965." *Canadian Journal of Public Health* 57, 10 (1966): 488.

Worboys, Michael. "The Colonial World as Mission and Mandate: Leprosy and Empire, 1900–1940." In Roy Macleod, ed., *Nature and Empire: Science and the Colonial Enterprise*, 207–18. Ithaca, NY: Cornell University Press, 2000.

World Health Organization (WHO). *Rapport du Directeur général: Examen du projet de programme et de budget pour 1966: Programme de recherches médicales*. 15 January 1965.

Worthington, E.B., ed. *The Evolution of IBP*. Cambridge, UK: Cambridge University Press, 1975.

Wuthnow, Robert. *Be Very Afraid: The Cultural Response to Terror, Pandemics, Environmental Devastation, Nuclear Annihilation, and Other Threats*. New York: Oxford University Press, 2010.

Young, Forrest Wade. "Unwriting Easter Island; Listening to Rapa Nui." PhD diss., University of Hawaii, 2011.

Yudell, Michael. *Race Unmasked: Biology and Race in the 20th Century*. New York: Columbia University Press, 2014.

Zahniser, Marvin R., and W. Michael Wies. "A Diplomatic Pearl Harbor? Richard Nixon's Goodwill Mission to Latin America in 1958." *Diplomatic History* 13, no. 2 (1989): 163–90.

Zamel N., P.A. McClean, P.R. Sandell, K.A. Siminovitch, and A.S. Slutsky. "Asthma on Tristan da Cunha: Looking for the Genetic Link." *American Journal of Respiratory and Critical Care Medicine* 153, no. 6, pt 1 (1996): 1902–6.

Zipkin, I. "Fluoride Exposure of Rapa Nui Inhabitants and Its Implication in Dental Caries." Abstract. Library and Archives Canada, Roberts Papers, vol. 2, file 16, "Dental Conditions," nd [Nógrády's volume 2, 1971?].

Zmyślony, Wojciech. "Edward Hajdukiewicz." Trans. Diana Dale. http://www.polishairforce.pl/hajdukiewiczeng.html.

Index